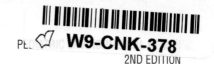

# Pediatric Environmental Health

*2nd Edition*

Author: Committee on Environmental Health
American Academy of Pediatrics

Ruth A. Etzel, MD, PhD, Editor
Sophie J. Balk, MD, Associate Editor

The American Academy of Pediatrics gratefully acknowledges the generous support provided by the following organizations:

Agency for Toxic Substances and Disease Registry
National Institute for Child Health and Human Development
US Environmental Protection Agency

Suggested Citation: American Academy of Pediatrics Committee on Environmental Health. [chapter title]. In: Etzel RA, ed. *Pediatric Environmental Health*. 2nd ed. Elk Grove Village, IL: American Academy of Pediatrics; 2003:[page number]

2nd Edition
1st Edition — 1999

Library of Congress Control Number: 2002114969
ISBN: 1-58110-111-2
MA0234

The recommendations in this publication do not indicate an exclusive course of treatment or serve as a standard of medical care. Variations, taking into account individual circumstances, may be appropriate.

Please note: Inclusion in this publication does not imply an endorsement by the American Academy of Pediatrics (AAP). The AAP is not responsible for the content of the resources mentioned. Addresses, phone numbers, and Web site addresses are as current as possible, but may change at any time.

# Table of Contents

## VI. Appendices

# Committee on Environmental Health
## 2003–2004

Michael W. Shannon, MD, MPH, Chair
Dana Best, MD, MPH
Helen J. Binns, MD, MPH
Christine L. Johnson, MD
Janice J. Kim, MD, MPH, PhD
Lynnette J. Mazur, MD, MPH
David W. Reynolds, MD
James R. Roberts, MD, MPH
William B. Weil, Jr, MD

**Former Chair**
Sophie J. Balk, MD

**Former Committee Members**
Katherine M. Shea, MD, MPH
Benjamin A. Gitterman, MD
Mark D. Miller, MD, MPH

**Liaison Representatives**
Robert W. Amler, MD
*Agency for Toxic Substances and Disease Registry/Centers for Disease Control and Prevention*
Elizabeth Blackburn, RN
*US Environmental Protection Agency*
Martha Linet, MD
*National Cancer Institute*
Robert W. Miller, MD, DrPH
*National Cancer Institute*
Walter J. Rogan, MD
*National Institute of Environmental Health Sciences*

**AAP Staff**
Paul Spire

**Former Staff**
Lauri A. Sweetman

# Preface

The publication of *Pediatric Environmental Health*, 2nd Edition, reflects continued advances in our understanding of the etiology, identification, and management of diseases linked to the environment. First published in 1999, the handbook is intended for pediatricians and others who are interested in preventing children's exposures to environmental hazards during infancy, childhood, and adolescence.

In this handbook, we present updated summaries of the evidence that has been published in the scientific literature about environmental hazards to children, and provide guidance to pediatricians about how to diagnose, treat, and prevent childhood diseases linked to environmental exposures. Ten new chapters have been introduced in this edition, including topics such as preconceptional and prenatal exposures, irradiation of food, chemical-biological terrorism, and environmental health advocacy. Major modifications have been made to all 33 chapters from the first edition. Knowledge, research, and information relevant to pediatric practice have been growing at an exponential rate since the children's environmental health and disease prevention research programs were established by the US Environmental Protection Agency and the National Institute for Environmental Health Sciences. New associations are being discovered and our knowledge of existing ones is constantly being refined and expanded. As the field of pediatric environmental health evolves, appropriate guidance may change with the publication of additional research findings.

Although all of the 59 contributors to this handbook are from North America, most of the information presented here should be useful to those in other parts of the world. Exposures to many contaminants may be higher in the developing world than in North America; nonetheless, the book can be expected to provide reliable background information for clinicians in other countries who are faced with providing practical advice to parents and communities. A new chapter on environmental threats to children's health in developing countries gives pediatricians in North America a glimpse of the array of problems facing children growing up in a variety of international settings.

The book is meant to be practical, containing information that is useful in office practice, but that could also be helpful to a clinician preparing a grand rounds presentation for colleagues or testimony before a group of state legislators. Throughout the book, I have taken the liberty of combining the contributions of multiple authors in each chapter. I hope that the information presented in the handbook will foster an informed understanding of environmental health among those who care for children.

Parents of young children are intensely interested in the impact of the environment on their children's health. They may look to their pediatrician for guidance about how to evaluate news reports about potential hazards in the air, water, and food. Yet the history of such well-established hazards as the exposure of children to environmental tobacco smoke shows many years of epidemiologic and laboratory research before the weight of the evidence compels a consensus. While the evidence is accumulating, what should a worried parent do? Prudently avoid exposure after the first study suggesting problems is published? At what point should the pediatrician advocate a specific action? Obviously, there are no easy answers to these questions. Issues of value, scientific understanding, and cost are involved. Each hazardous exposure must be considered in the context of other problems facing the child and financial, emotional, and intellectual resources available to surmount them. After fully understanding the facts and uncertainties, reasonable pediatricians may choose different ways to respond to the accumulating evidence.

I have many people to thank for their contributions to this book. First, I am grateful to those who contributed the 33 chapters to the first edition because their outstanding work provided an excellent foundation for this revision. Fifteen committees and sections of the American Academy of Pediatrics (AAP) reviewed and provided comments on new and revised chapters of the handbook. I owe special thanks to Paul Spire for his commitment to excellence and his superb work in keeping this book on track, and to Kate Larson, copyeditor, Linda Diamond, graphic designer, Darlene Mattefs, department assistant, and Barbara Drelicharz, division assistant, for their help in its preparation. I am immensely thankful to the committee chair and associate editor, Sophie Balk, MD, for ensuring the most up-to-date information was included in the handbook and for her meticulous attention to detail. Thanks also to the hardworking members of the Committee on Environmental Health, whose dedication to an evidence-based approach to environmental health has had a major impact on the handbook. I owe special thanks to Gary Q. Peck, MD, of the AAP Board of Directors for his comprehensive review of the book for consistency with AAP policy.

Though the second edition is 75% longer than the first, there are still many aspects of environmental health that could not be covered. The committee gave priority to those topics that appeared to have the greatest effect on child health, or to be of concern to parents. I hope that this handbook will help you in your practice and in counseling parents about preventing their children's exposure to environmental hazards.

Ruth A. Etzel, MD, PhD
Editor

# Contributors

The American Academy of Pediatrics (AAP) gratefully acknowledges the invaluable assistance provided by the following individuals who served as reviewers and contributors to the second edition of *Pediatric Environmental Health* and/or who were primary contributors to the first edition. Their expertise, critical review, and cooperation were essential to the committee's development of recommendations for the recognition, treatment, and prevention of diseases linked to environmental exposures.

Every attempt has been made to recognize all those who contributed to this effort; the AAP regrets any omissions that may have occurred.

Organizational affiliations are provided for identification purposes only.

Robert W. Amler, MD; *Agency for Toxic Substances and Disease Registry; Atlanta, GA*

Susan Aronson, MD; *The Children's Hospital; Philadelphia, PA*

Sophie J. Balk, MD; *Children's Hospital of Montefiore, Albert Einstein College of Medicine; Bronx, NY*

Lauren B. Ball, DO, MPH; *Tampa, FL*

Cynthia F. Bearer, MD, PhD; *Rainbow Babies and Children's Hospital; Cleveland, OH*

Nancy B. Beck, PhD; *AAAS Fellow at US Environmental Protection Agency; Washington, DC*

Dana Best, MD, MPH; *Children's National Medical Center; Washington, DC*

Elizabeth Blackburn, RN; *US Environmental Protection Agency; Washington, DC*

Jerome M. Blondell, PhD, MPH; *US Environmental Protection Agency; Washington, DC*

Irena Buka, MB, ChB; *University of Alberta; Edmonton, AB, Canada*

John Carl, MD; *Rainbow Babies and Children's Hospital; Cleveland, OH*

J. Milton Clark, PhD; *US Environmental Protection Agency; Chicago, IL*

Deon Corkins, MPH; *County Health Department; Salt Lake City, UT*

Adolfo Correa, MD, PhD; *Centers for Disease Control and Prevention; Atlanta, GA*

Karen M. Emmons, PhD; *Dana-Farber Cancer Institute; Boston, MA*

Ruth A. Etzel, MD, PhD; *George Washington University School of Public Health & Health Services; Washington, DC*

Henry Falk, MD, MPH; *Centers for Disease Control and Prevention; Atlanta, GA*

Laurence J. Fuortes, MD, MS; *University of Iowa; Iowa City, IA*

Steven K. Galson, MD, MPH; *Food and Drug Administration; Rockville, MD*

Benjamin A. Gitterman, MD; *Children's National Medical Center; Washington, DC*

Lynn R. Goldman, MD, MPH; *Johns Hopkins Bloomberg School of Public Health; Baltimore, MD*

Birt Harvey, MD; *Palo Alto, CA*

Molly Hicks, MPA; *American Academy of Pediatrics; Washington, DC*

Christine L. Johnson, MD; *Uniformed Services University of the Health Sciences; Bethesda, MD*

Janice J. Kim, MD, MPH, PhD; *California Environmental Protection Agency; Oakland, CA*

Richard Kreutzer, MD; *California Department of Health Services; Emeryville, CA*

Philip J. Landrigan, MD, MSc; *Mount Sinai School of Medicine; New York, NY*

Martha Linet, MD; *National Cancer Institute; Rockville, MD*

Lynnette J. Mazur, MD, MPH; *University of Texas Health Science Center; Houston, TX*

Susan W. Metcalf, MD; *Agency for Toxic Substances and Disease Registry; Atlanta, GA*

Mark D. Miller, MD, MPH; *California Environmental Protection Agency; Oakland, CA*

Robert W. Miller, MD, DrPH; *National Cancer Institute; Bethesda, MD*

Howard Mofenson, MD; *Winthrop University Hospital; Mineola, NY*

Mary Ellen Mortensen, MD; *McNeil Consumer & Specialty Pharmaceuticals; Fort Washington, PA*

Lawrie Mott, MS; *Natural Resources Defense Council; San Francisco, CA*

Herbert Needleman, MD; *University of Pittsburgh School of Medicine; Pittsburgh, PA*

Raymond Neutra, MD, PhD; *California Department of Health Services; Emeryville, CA*

Philip Ozuah, MD, MSEd, PhD; *Children's Hospital at Montefiore; Bronx, NY*

Kathleen Eaton Paterson, MPH; *Community Health Connections; Montpelier, VT*

Jerome A. Paulson, MD; *George Washington University Medical Center; Washington, DC*

Gary Q. Peck, MD; *AAP Board of Directors; New Orleans, LA*

Rossanne M. Philen, MD; *Centers for Disease Control and Prevention; Atlanta, GA*

Susan H. Pollack, MD; *Kentucky Injury Prevention & Research Center; Lexington, KY*

J. Routt Reigart, MD; *Medical University of South Carolina; Charleston, SC*

David W. Reynolds, MD; *Community Pediatrician; Birmingham, AL*

James R. Roberts, MD, MPH; *Medical University of South Carolina; Charleston, SC*

Walter J. Rogan, MD; *National Institute of Environmental Health Sciences; Research Triangle Park, NC*

Christine L. Rosheim, DDS, MPH; *Agency for Toxic Substances and Disease Registry; Atlanta, GA*

Lawrence M. Schell, PhD; *School of Public Health, State University of New York; Albany, NY*

Michael W. Shannon, MD, MPH; *Children's Hospital; Boston, MA*

Katherine M. Shea, MD, MPH; *Duke University Medical Center; Durham, NC*

Peter R. Simon, MD, MPH; *Rhode Island Department of Health; Providence, RI*

Gina Solomon, MD, MPH; *Natural Resources Defense Council; San Francisco, CA*

Babasaheb Sonawane, PhD; *US Environmental Protection Agency; Washington, DC*

Catherine J. Staes, BSN, MPH; *Salt Lake City, UT*

Robert C. Thompson; *US Environmental Protection Agency; Washington, DC*

Michael A. Wall, MD; *Oregon Health Sciences University School of Medicine; Portland, OR*

William B. Weil, Jr, MD; *Michigan State University; East Lansing, MI*

Peter Weyer, PhD; *University of Iowa; Iowa City, IA*

Mary C. White, ScD; *Centers for Disease Control and Prevention; Atlanta, GA*

Alan D. Woolf, MD, MPH; *Children's Hospital; Boston, MA*

# 1
# Introduction

Environmental hazards are among the top health concerns many parents have for their children.[1,2] Little time is spent during medical school and residency training on environmental hazards and their relationship to illness.[3,4] General medical and pediatric textbooks devote scant attention to illness as a result of environmental factors. Information pertinent to pediatric environmental health is widely scattered in scientific, epidemiological, and specialty journals not regularly read by clinicians.[5]

Forty-six years have passed since the formation of the American Academy of Pediatrics' (AAP) first committee on environmental health. In that time rapid progress has been made in understanding the role of the environment in the illnesses of childhood and adolescence. Consideration of illnesses traditionally associated with the environment, such as waterborne and food-borne diseases, has expanded to include study of toxic chemicals and other environmental hazards that derive from the rapid expansion of industry and technology in the developed world.[6]

This book, written to be useful to practicing pediatricians, is organized into 5 sections. The first section gives background information. The second and third sections focus on chemical and physical hazards and on specific environments. The fourth section addresses a variety of complex environmental situations. The fifth section provides information on communicating about environmental hazards.

Most chapters on chemical and physical hazards are organized in sections that describe the pollutant, routes of exposure, systems affected, clinical effects, diagnostic methods, treatment, and prevention of exposure and include suggested responses to questions that pediatricians may have or that parents may ask. Most chapters contain a list of pertinent resources. Appendix B refers readers to additional resources when further help is needed.

The AAP Committee on Environmental Health recognizes that pediatric environmental health is a field in the early stages of development. Knowledge in some areas has evolved rapidly, whereas in other areas there are more questions than answers. The authors have attempted to make readers aware of the controversial areas and gaps in scientific data. Given the state of knowledge for any pollutant or situation, this handbook tries to provide the pediatrician with the most accurate and prudent information needed to advise parents and children.

**History of Pediatric Environmental Health**
In 1954 errant fallout from a nuclear weapons test on Bikini Island, an atoll of the Marshall Islands, caused acute burns from beta radiation to develop in neighboring islanders. Subsequently, severe hypothyroidism developed in 2 children exposed to fallout prior to 1 year of age. Of 18 children exposed before 10 years of age, 14 developed thyroid neoplasia (13 benign and 1 malignant), and 1 developed leukemia.[7] At about the same time, fallout in southwestern Utah from tests in Nevada apparently caused sickness in sheep, and people who were exposed worried about later effects. In 1956 expert committees of the National Academy of Sciences (NAS) and the British Medical Research Council reported on the biological effects of ionizing radiation in humans. These reports led to a marked reduction in unnecessary exposures from the use of radiotherapy for benign disorders and fluoroscopy. Therefore, in 1957, because of concerns about fallout from weapons testing and fears of nuclear war, the AAP, in keeping with its tradition of promoting research and advocacy for child health, established the Committee on Radiation Hazards and Congenital Malformations to develop policy on exposure of children to ionizing radiation. This was the forerunner of the present Committee on Environmental Health.

In 1961, as the interests of the committee broadened, its name was changed to the Committee on Environmental Hazards. In 1966 an expert overview of the effects of radiation on children was organized by the Committee on Environmental Hazards—the Conference on the Pediatric Significance of Peacetime Radioactive Fallout.[8] The participants included pediatricians, radiobiologists, scientists from relevant government health agencies, and Dr Benjamin Spock, who spoke about the psychological effects of radioactive fallout in children.

The committee, recognizing that man-made chemicals were increasingly permeating the environment, organized the Conference on the Susceptibility of the Fetus and Child to Chemical Pollutants, held in 1973 in Brown's Lake, WI.[9] Fresh thinking was sought by bringing together scientists knowledgeable about the effects of chemicals on the environment but not about child health and pediatricians who knew about child health but had not given much thought to environmental effects. This meeting led to more interaction between pediatric experts and federal agencies concerned with the environment to discuss the possible effects of the environment on the health of children.

The Conference on Chemical and Radiation Hazards to Children, held in 1981 to enhance knowledge by expert consultation, enabled the exchange of concerns and information with the pediatric community[10] and led to further interactions between the committee and federal environmental health agencies. The Council on Pediatric Research called for including pediatricians in meetings of government agencies and on other committees that make policy or deliberate on environmental matters of national importance. To foster relations with other groups, the committee, which met twice a year, held every other meeting at an organization concerned with environmental research, such as the US Environmental Protection Agency (EPA), the National Institute of Environmental Health Sciences (NIEHS), the Kettering Laboratories, and the National Institute of Child Health and Development.

In 1991 the name of the Committee on Environmental Hazards
was changed to the Committee on Environmental Health to emphasize prevention.

Increasingly, academic and health organizations were studying
the impact of the environment on infant and child health. In 1993
the publication of a report by the NAS, titled *Pesticides in the Diets of
Infants and Children,*[11] was instrumental in highlighting environmental hazards unique to children and the relative paucity of information
relating environmental exposures and child health. In October 1995
EPA Administrator Carol Browner directed the agency to formulate a
new national policy requiring, for the first time, that the health risks to
children and infants from environmental hazards be considered when
conducting environmental risk assessments.[12]

In 1996 the Food Quality Protection Act became law. One requirement of this new act was that the EPA use an additional safety factor
in risk assessments when risks for children are uncertain.

On April 21, 1997, President Clinton issued Executive Order 13045,
Protection of Children from Environmental Health Risks and Safety
Risks, which directed agencies to ensure that policies, programs, activities, and standards address disproportionate risks to children that
result from environmental health risks or safety risks. A task force,
cochaired by the secretary of the US Department of Health and
Human Services and the administrator of the EPA, was established
to recommend federal environmental health and safety policies,
priorities, and activities to protect children.

A number of new initiatives, among them the 12 children's environmental health and disease prevention research programs funded
by the EPA and NIEHS, have stimulated more research into the impact
of the environment on the health of children.

The Pediatric Environmental Health Specialty Units (PEHSUs),
established in 1998 by the Association of Occupational and Environmental Clinics, with funding from the Agency for Toxic Substances

and Disease Registry (ATSDR), have increased awareness and knowledge of health care providers and health agency officials about pediatric environmental health.

The first edition of the AAP *Handbook of Pediatric Environmental
Health* was published in October 1999.[13] It was distributed to more
than 20,000 pediatricians and pediatric residents and was widely used,
in the United States and other countries, to teach about the health
hazards of contaminants in the environment. It prompted the World
Health Organization to begin developing materials on children's
health and the environment for an international audience.[14,15]

In 2000 the Committee on Environmental Health initiated the first
in a series of 4 annual workshops on pediatric environmental health
for incoming pediatric chief residents held at the annual meeting of
the Pediatric Academic Societies. This effort was funded by the Office
of Children's Health Protection at the EPA.

In March 2001 the Committee on Environmental Health held a
workshop, with funding from the ATSDR, to bring together pediatricians from each chapter of the AAP with experts in pediatric environmental health from the regional offices of federal agencies (including
the ATSDR and EPA). The proceedings of this conference were
published in a special supplement to *Pediatrics*.[16]

In 2002 the Ambulatory Pediatric Association launched the first
formal fellowship training programs in pediatric environmental
health. These 3-year training programs are designed to provide pediatricians with specific competencies[17] to enable them to undertake
environmental health research, teaching, and advocacy. The first
textbook to focus on environmental threats to child health was published in 2003.[18] These and other activities should further enhance
our understanding of the effects of environmental hazards on
children's health.

## References

1. Stickler GB, Simmons PS. Pediatricians' preferences for anticipatory guidance topics compared with parental anxieties. *Clin Pediatr.* 1995;34:384–387

2. US Environmental Protection Agency. *Public Knowledge and Perceptions of Chemical Risks in Six Communities: Analysis of a Baseline Survey.* Washington, DC: US Environmental Protection Agency; 1990. EPA 230-01-90-074

3. Pope AM, Rall DP, eds. *Environmental Medicine: Integrating a Missing Element into Medical Education.* Washington, DC: National Academies Press; 1995

4. Roberts JR, Gitterman BA. Pediatric environmental health education: a survey of US pediatric residency programs. *Ambul Pediatr.* 2003;3:57–59

5. Etzel RA. Introduction. In: *Environmental Health: Report of the 27th Ross Roundtable on Critical Approaches to Common Pediatric Problems.* Columbus, OH: Ross Products Division, Abbott Laboratories; 1996:1

6. Chance GW, Harmsen E. Children are different: environmental contaminants and children's health. *Can J Public Health.* 1998;89(suppl 1):S9–S13

7. Merke DP, Miller RW. Age differences in the effects of ionizing radiation. In: Guzelian PS, Henry CJ, Olin SS, eds. *Similarities and Differences Between Children and Adults: Implications for Risk Assessment.* Washington, DC: International Life Sciences Institute; 1992:139–149

8. American Academy of Pediatrics Committee on Environmental Hazards. Conference on the Pediatric Significance of Peacetime Radioactive Fallout. *Pediatrics.* 1968;41:165–378

9. American Academy of Pediatrics Committee on Environmental Hazards. The susceptibility of the fetus and child to chemical pollutants. *Pediatrics.* 1974;53:777–862

10. Finberg L. *Chemical and Radiation Hazards to Children: Report of the Eighty-fourth Ross Conference on Pediatric Research.* Columbus, OH: Ross Laboratories; 1982

11. National Research Council. *Pesticides in the Diets of Infants and Children.* Washington, DC: National Academies Press; 1993

12. US Environmental Protection Agency. *Environmental Health Threats to Children.* Washington, DC: US Environmental Protection Agency; 1996. EPA 175-F-96-001

13. American Academy of Pediatrics Committee on Environmental Health. Etzel RA, ed. *Handbook of Pediatric Environmental Health.* Elk Grove Village, IL: American Academy of Pediatrics; 1999

14. European Environment Agency. *Children's Health and Environment: A Review of Evidence. A Joint Report From the European Environment Agency and the WHO Regional Office for Europe.* Luxembourg: Luxembourg Office for Official Publications of the European Communities; 2002. Environmental issue report No. 29

15. United Nations Environment Programme, United Nations Children's Fund, World Health Organization. *Children in the New Millenium: Environmental Impact on Health.* 2002

16. Balk SJ, ed. A partnership to establish an environmental safety net for children. *Pediatrics.* 2003;112:209–264

17. Etzel RA, Crain EF, Gitterman BA, et al. Pediatric environmental health competencies for specialists. *Ambul Pediatr.* 2003;3:60–63

18. Wigle DT. *Child Health and the Environment.* New York, NY: Oxford; 2003

# 2
# Developmental Toxicity: Special Considerations Based on Age and Developmental Stage

This chapter discusses the scientific basis for the unique vulnerability of children to environmental hazards. It describes differences between adults and children and among children in different developmental stages, in physical, biological, and social environments. It explains why children should not be treated as "little adults." Six developmental stages are considered: fetus (although there are multiple stages of development for the fetus), newborn (birth–2 months of age), infant/toddler (2 months–2 years of age), preschool child (2–6 years of age), school-aged child (6–12 years), and adolescent (12–18 years).

## Critical Windows of Vulnerability
The developing fetus and child are susceptible to certain drugs and environmental toxicants. Well-known adverse outcomes for the developing fetus due to transplacental exposure include the effects of thalidomide on limb development, ethanol on brain development, and diethylstilbestrol on the reproductive system. Postnatal effects include lead's effects on the developing brain of the infant and toddler. Fetal and childhood development occur rapidly and may be easily deranged. The importance of the timing of exposures with regard to developmental outcome is a concept that has recently received scientific attention. In embryonic or fetal stages, some narrow "critical windows of exposure"[1]—highly susceptible periods of organogenesis—have been defined. In contrast, there are very few actual "critical windows" known in childhood. Because data are lacking, there is significant uncertainty about many of the effects of environmental toxicants on children. This area is the subject of intense investigation. Some of the work on "critical windows" has been

published in a supplement to *Environmental Health Perspectives* (http://ehpnet1.niehs.nih.gov/docs/2000/suppl-3/toc.html).

## Human Environments

A child's environment can be thought of as having 3 components: physical, biological, and social. The physical environment is anything that comes in contact with the body. Air, for example, which is in constant contact with our lungs and skin, is a large part of the physical environment. To define the physical environment more precisely, it may be necessary to divide a large environment (a macro environment) into smaller units, called micro environments. (The macro environment may be Detroit, a micro environment may be the floor of the kitchen of a house in Detroit.) Micro environments can differ enormously between adults and children. For example, in a room in which the air is contaminated with mercury, the mercury vapor may not be evenly dispersed—air near the floor may have a higher concentration of mercury than air near the ceiling.[2] The environment of an infant lying on the floor therefore would be different from that of a standing adult. The biological environment consists of the internal physiological interactions of the body with the chemicals it contacts. The absorption, distribution, metabolism, and toxic action of chemicals may vary with the developmental stage of the child. The social environment includes the day-to-day circumstances of living as well as regulations that may affect day-to-day living.

## Exposure: The Physical Environment

A child's exposure is the sum of the exposures in several environments during the course of a day, including the home, school, child care setting, and play areas. Estimates of exposure often are retrospective because it is difficult to monitor children. Even if the total duration of exposure to a toxicant is the same for 2 children, different patterns of exposure may have different health effects. For example, ingestion of nitrates in well water may cause the hemoglobin to become reduced to methemoglobin.[3] However, if the nitrates are ingested at a slow enough rate for enzymes to oxidize the methemoglobin back to hemo-globin, no deleterious health effects occur. This is an example of a threshold effect; the health problem will not occur until the toxicant reaches a particular level in the body.

## Exposure From Conception to Adolescence

In most instances, exposures to the fetus are from the pregnant woman. However, premature infants who spend months in the neonatal intensive care unit have very different exposures from healthy full-term infants (eg, exposure to noise, light, compressed gases, intravenous solutions, benzyl alcohol, etc).[4]

Exposures to newborns, infants, toddlers, preschool children, school-aged children, and adolescents occur with changes in physical location, breathing zones, oxygen consumption, types of foods consumed, amount of food consumed, and normal behavioral development.[5]

## Physical Location

Physical location changes with development. Newborn exposures usually are similar to those experienced by the mother. Moreover, the newborn frequently spends prolonged periods in a single environment, such as a crib. Because infants and toddlers frequently are placed on the floor, carpet, or grass, they have more exposure to chemicals associated with these surfaces, such as pesticide residues. Infants who are unable to walk or crawl may experience sustained exposure to some agents because they cannot remove themselves from their environment (eg, prolonged exposure to the sun).

Preschool children may spend part of their day in child care settings with varied environments, including some time outdoors.

School-aged children may be exposed to toxicants when schools are built near highways (resulting in exposure to motor vehicle emissions). Adolescents not only have a school environment, but also are beginning to select other physical environments, often misjudging or ignoring the risks to themselves. For example, listening to loud music may result in permanent hearing loss. Many adolescents work part-time in hazardous physical environments.[6]

## Breathing Zones

The breathing zone for an adult is typically 4 to 6 ft above the floor. For a child, it is closer to the floor, depending on the height and mobility of the child. Within lower breathing zones, chemicals heavier than air, such as mercury, may concentrate.[7,8]

## Oxygen Consumption

Children are smaller than adults, and their metabolic rates are higher relative to their size. Thus they consume more oxygen than adults and produce more carbon dioxide ($CO_2$) per pound of body weight. This increased $CO_2$ production requires higher minute ventilation. Minute ventilation for a newborn and adult are approximately 400 mL/min per kilogram and 150 mL/min per kilogram, respectively.[9] Thus children's exposure to air pollutants may be greater than that of adults.

## Quantity and Quality of Food Consumed

The amount of food that children consume per pound of body weight is higher than that of the adult because children not only need to maintain homeostasis as adults do, but they also are growing. Figure 2.1 shows grams of food (dry weight) per kilogram of body weight per day consumed. The difference is 3-fold between a child younger than 1 year and an adult. Unfortunately, data do not exist for further subdivisions of children (eg, a newborn vs a 6-month-old infant).

In addition, children consume different types of food, and the diversity of the foods they eat is much smaller than adults. The diet of many newborns is limited to breast milk. The diet of children contains more milk products and certain fruits and vegetables than the typical adult diet.[4,5] Figure 2.2 shows the differences for apples, beef, and potatoes for different age groups.

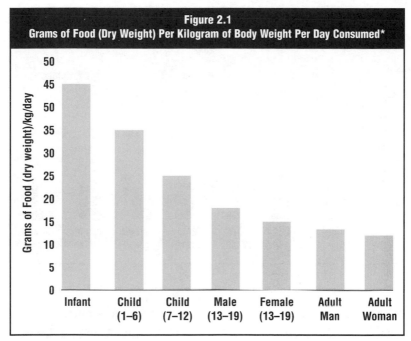

**Figure 2.1**
**Grams of Food (Dry Weight) Per Kilogram of Body Weight Per Day Consumed***

*From Plunkett LM, Turnbull D, Rodricks JV.[10]

## Water

The average newborn consumes 5 oz of breast milk or formula per kilogram of body weight (for the average male adult, this is equivalent to drinking 30 12-oz cans of soda a day). If the newborn drinks reconstituted formula, the water will all be from a single tap water source; such newborns are a subpopulation heavily exposed to any contaminants in water. Differences in water consumption for different age groups are shown in Figure 2.3. If the water or liquid contains a contaminant, children may receive more of it relative to their size than adults.[3,11]

## Normal Behavioral Development

Children pass through a developmental stage of intense oral exploratory behavior. Therefore, normal oral exploration may place children

13

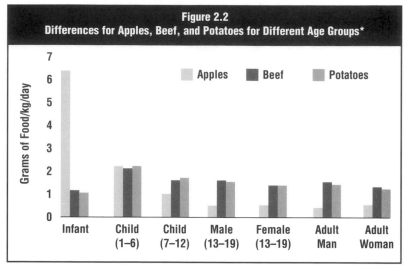

Figure 2.2
Differences for Apples, Beef, and Potatoes for Different Age Groups*

*From Plunkett LM, Turnbull D, Rodricks JV.[10]

at risk, such as in environments with high levels of lead dust. Wood used in some playground equipment is treated with arsenic and creosote, thus exposing children when they place their mouths directly on these materials, or when they place their hands in their mouths after playing on these materials. Additionally, children lack the cognitive ability to recognize hazardous situations.

Ambulatory children may be exposed to used drums containing potentially harmful chemicals while playing in abandoned areas. Adolescents, as they gain freedom from parental authority, may be less protected from some exposures. While at a stage of development where physical strength and stamina are at a peak, they are still acquiring abstract reasoning skills and often fail to consider cause and effect, particularly delayed effects. Thus adolescents may place themselves in situations with greater risk than would an adult.

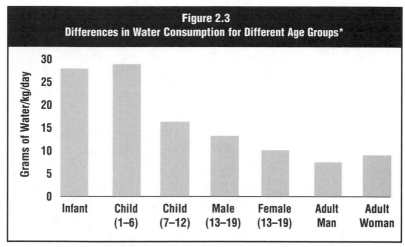

**Figure 2.3**
**Differences in Water Consumption for Different Age Groups***

*From Plunkett LM, Turnbull D, Rodricks JV.[10]

Note: The citation of grams of water consumed per kilogram per day in this table is considerably underestimated because water consumed as breast milk was not included in the analysis. Thus for total water consumption per kilogram per day, the values in the text are accurate.

## Absorption, Distribution, Metabolism, and Target Organ Susceptibility: The Biological Environment

### Absorption

Absorption generally occurs by 1 of 4 pathways: transplacental, percutaneous, respiratory, and gastrointestinal. The type of toxicant and the developmental stage of the child determine the pathway of absorption.

### Transplacental

Several toxicants readily cross the placenta, including compounds with low molecular weight such as carbon monoxide, those that are fat soluble, and specific elements such as calcium and lead. Because carbon monoxide has a higher affinity for fetal hemoglobin than adult hemoglobin, the concentration of carboxyhemoglobin is higher in the fetus than in the pregnant woman.[12,13] Therefore, the infant may have a reduced level of oxygen delivered to tissues. Lipophilic compounds, such as polycyclic aromatic hydrocarbons (found in cigarette smoke), methylmercury, and ethanol, also readily gain access to the fetal circulation.

## Percutaneous

The skin undergoes enormous change with developmental stage, which changes the properties of absorption. Pathways of absorption through the skin are particularly important for fat-soluble compounds. Although chemicals such as nicotine and cotinine have been described in amniotic fluid,[14] their absorption through the fetal skin has not been studied. The dermis of a fetus lacks the exterior dead keratin layer, one of the major barriers of fully developed skin. The acquisition of keratin occurs over 3 to 5 days following birth. Therefore, the skin of a newborn remains particularly absorptive up to about 2 to 3 weeks of life.[15] Epidemics involving absorption of chemicals through the skin in newborns include hypothyroidism from iodine in Betadine scrub solutions,[16] neurotoxicity from hexachlorophene,[17] and hyperbilirubinemia from a phenolic disinfectant used to clean hospital equipment.[18]

An additional factor in percutaneous absorption is the larger surface-to-body mass ratio of newborns compared with older children and adults. The newborn has a surface-to-body mass ratio 3 times larger than an adult, and the child has a surface-to-body mass ratio 2 times larger than an adult. Thus children will absorb more pound for pound than the amount absorbed by an adult.[10]

## Respiratory

The fetus makes breathing motions. Some chemicals in the amniotic fluid may come into contact with the lining of the respiratory tract. Studies on this pathway of exposure to foreign chemicals are limited.

Lung development proceeds through proliferation of pulmonary alveoli and capillaries until the ages of 5 to 8 years.[19] Thereafter, the lungs grow through alveolar expansion.[20] The surface absorptive properties of the lung do not change during development.

## Gastrointestinal

The gastrointestinal tract undergoes numerous changes during development. Certain pesticides as well as chemicals from tobacco smoke are present in amniotic fluid,[14] but it is not known if the fetus, which actively swallows amniotic fluid, absorbs them. Following birth, stomach acid secretion is relatively low, but achieves adult levels by several months of age, markedly affecting absorption of chemicals from the stomach. If acidity levels are too low, bacterial overgrowth in the small bowel and stomach may result in the information of chemicals that can be absorbed. For example, several cases of methemoglobinemia in infants in Iowa were traced to well water contaminated with nitrate that was converted to nitrite by intestinal bacteria.[3]

The small intestine transports certain chemicals to the blood and may respond to increased nutritional needs by increasing absorption of that particular nutrient. For example, the bones of infants and children absorb more calcium from food sources than do adults. Lead, which may be absorbed in place of calcium, also may be absorbed to a greater extent: an adult absorbs 10% of ingested lead, whereas a 1- to 2-year-old absorbs 50%.[21]

### Distribution

The distribution of chemicals within the body varies with body composition such as fat and water content, which are known to vary with developmental stage. For example, animal models have shown that lead is retained to a larger degree in the infant animal brain than in the adult animal brain.[22] Lead also may accumulate more rapidly in children's bones.[23]

### Metabolism

Metabolism of a chemical may result in its activation or deactivation.[24] The activity in each step of these metabolic pathways is determined by the child's developmental stage and genetic susceptibility. Therefore, some children are genetically more susceptible to adverse effects from certain exposures. For example, children (and adults) with glucose-6-phosphate dehydrogenase (G6PD) deficiency are at risk of hemolytic anemia if exposed to certain chemicals such as naphthalene. Large differences also exist in the activity of enzymes in various developmental stages. The same enzyme may be more or less active depending on the age of the child. Two examples are the enzymes involved in the P450 cytochrome family, which metabolizes such xenobiotics as theophylline and caffeine,[25] and alcohol dehydrogenase, which converts ethanol to acetaldehyde.[26]

The differences between metabolism in children and adults may harm or protect children from environmental hazards or drugs. Such is the case for acetaminophen. In the adult, high levels of acetaminophen are metabolized to products that may cause hepatic failure. Infants born to women with high blood acetaminophen levels have similar acetaminophen levels, but do not sustain liver damage because their metabolic pathways have not yet developed enough to break down acetaminophen into harmful metabolites.[27–30]

### *Target Organ Susceptibility*

During growth and maturation the organs of children may be affected by exposure to harmful chemicals.[31] Following cellular proliferation, individual cells undergo 2 further processes to become the adult organism: differentiation and migration. Differentiation occurs when cells take on specific tasks within the body and lose the ability to divide. The trigger for differentiation may be hormonal, so chemicals that mimic hormones could alter the differentiation of some tissues. Because organ systems in children, including the reproductive system, continue to differentiate, chemicals that mimic hormones may have effects on the development of those organ systems.

Cell migration is necessary for certain cells to reach their destination. Neurons, for example, originate in a structure near the center of the brain, then migrate to a predestined location in one of the many layers of the brain. Chemicals may have a profound effect on this process (eg, ethanol and fetal alcohol syndrome).

Synaptogenesis occurs rapidly during the first 2 years.[32] Waves of synapses are formed as learning occurs throughout life. Dendritic trimming is the active removal of synapses. A 2-year-old's brain contains more synapses than at any other age. These synapses are trimmed back to allow more specificity of the resulting neural network. There are some data to suggest that low-dose lead may interfere with this synapse trimming.[33]

Some organs continue developing for several years, and development is not complete until adolescence, increasing the vulnerability of these organs. For example, brain tumors frequently are treated by radiation therapy in adults with uncomfortable but reversible side effects. However, in infants, radiation therapy generally is avoided because of the profound and permanent effects on the developing central nervous system. Similarly, lead and mercury affect the brain and nervous system of children. The brain attains four fifths of its adult size by the end of the second year of life.[20] By adolescence there are no gross changes in brain morphology[20]; electroencephalographic studies demonstrate continued neurodevelopmental maturation.[20]

Exposure to environmental tobacco smoke (ETS) compromises lung development. The rate of growth of lung function in children exposed to ETS is slower than that of nonexposed children. The forced expiratory volumes in 1 second of children exposed to ETS are measurably lower than those of children without exposure.[34]

Tissues undergoing growth and differentiation are particularly susceptible to cancer due to the shortened period for deoxyribonucleic acid (DNA) repair and the changes occurring within the DNA during cell growth. The epidemic of scrotal cancer among adolescent chimney sweeps of Victorian England illustrates the likelihood that the scrotum at this stage of development has increased susceptibility to the chemicals in soot.[35] Although occupational exposure at that time to cancer-causing chemicals such as soot was common in many occupations, scrotal tumors were uncommon except in young male chimney sweeps.

## Regulations and Laws: The Social Environment

Regulatory policies usually do not take into account the unique combinations of developmental characteristics, physical environment, and biological environment that place children at risk. Most laws and regulations are based on studies using adult men weighing an average of 70 kg and, hence, are intended to protect adult men. However, recent advances have been made to change regulations to protect children. For example, the Food Quality Protection Act of 1996 states that pesticide tolerances must be set to protect the health of infants and children. New rules on cigarette vending machines make cigarettes less available to children. The US Environmental Protection Agency enacted more stringent regulations on outdoor air quality to protect children.

How can a clinician integrate information about children's developmental susceptibility into practice? The roles of educator, investigator, and advocate are extremely important. The most important intervention is the education of parents and children about exposures. Prevention efforts have the most impact when developmentally appropriate. Parents, children, teachers, community leaders, and policy makers need to be educated about the unique vulnerability of children to environmental pollution. The role of the clinician as investigator also is very important. Most diseases caused by environmental factors have been diagnosed by an alert clinician, and publication of case studies has enabled further description of these illnesses. Finally, clinicians must advocate for children, working to ensure that regulatory policies take into account their unique vulnerability.

## References

1. Selevan SG, Kimmel CA, Mendola P. Identifying critical windows of exposure for children's health. *Environ Health Perspect.* 2000;108(suppl 3): 451–455

2. Agocs MM, Etzel RA, Parrish RG, et al. Mercury exposure from interior latex paint. *N Engl J Med.* 1990;323:1096–1101

3. Lukens JN. Landmark perspective: the legacy of well-water methemoglobinemia. *JAMA.* 1987;257:2793–2795

4. Bearer CF. Occupational and environmental risks to the fetus. In: Fanaroff AA, Martin RM, eds. *Neonatal-Perinatal Medicine: Diseases of the Fetus and Infant.* 6th ed. St Louis, MO: Mosby-Year Book; 1997:188–199

5. Guzelian PS, Henry CJ, Olin SS, eds. *Similarities and Differences Between Children and Adults: Implications for Risk Assessment.* Washington, DC: ILSI Press; 1992

6. Pollack SH, Landrigan PJ, Mallino DL. Child labor in 1990: prevalence and health hazards. *Annu Rev Public Health.* 1990;11:359–375

7. Leaderer BP. Assessing exposures to environmental tobacco smoke. *Risk Anal.* 1990;10:19–26

8. Foote RS. Mercury vapor concentrations inside buildings. *Science.* 1972;177:513–514

9. Snodgrasss WR. Physiological and biochemical differences between children and adults as determinants of toxic response to environmental pollutants. In: Guzelian PS, Henry CJ, Olin SS, eds. *Similarities and Differences Between Children and Adults: Implications for Risk Assessment.* Washington, DC: ILSI Press; 1992:35–42

10. Plunkett LM, Turnbull D, Rodricks JV. Differences between adults and children affecting exposure assessment. In: Guzclian PS, Henry CJ, Olin SS, eds. *Similarities and Differences Between Children and Adults: Implications for Risk Assessment.* Washington, DC: ILSI Press; 1992:79–94

11. Shannon MW, Graef JW. Lead intoxication in infancy. *Pediatrics.* 1992;89:87–90

12. Longo LD, Hill EP. Carbon monoxide uptake and elimination in fetal and maternal sheep. *Am J Physiol.* 1977;232:H324–H330

13. Longo LD. Carbon monoxide in the pregnant mother and fetus and its exchange across the placenta. *Ann N Y Acad Sci.* 1970;174:312–341

14. VanVunakis H, Langone JJ, Milunsky A. Nicotine and cotinine in the amniotic fluid of smokers in the second trimester of pregnancy. *Am J Obstet Gynecol.* 1974;120:64–66

15. Holbrook KA. Structure and biochemical organogenesis of skin and cutaneous appendages in the fetus and newborn. In: Polin RA, Fox WW, eds. *Fetal and Neonatal Physiology.* Philadelphia, PA: WB Saunders; 1998:729–752

16. Clemens PC, Neumann RS. The Wolff-Chaikoff effect: hypothyroidism due to iodine application. *Arch Dermatol.* 1989;125:705

17. Shuman RM, Leech RW, Alvord EC Jr. Neurotoxicity of hexachlorophene in the human: I. A clinicopathologic study of 248 children. *Pediatrics.* 1974;54:689–695

18. Wysowski DK, Flynt JW Jr, Goldfield M, Altman R, Davis AT. Epidemic neonatal hyperbilirubinemia and use of a phenolic disinfectant detergent. *Pediatrics.* 1978;61:165–170

19. Dietert RR, Etzel RA, Chen D, et al. Workshop to identify critical windows of exposure for children's health: immune and respiratory systems work group summary. *Environ Health Perspect.* 2000;108(suppl 3):483–490

20. Behrman RE, Kleigman RM, Jenson HB. *Nelson Textbook of Pediatrics.* 16th ed. Philadelphia, PA: WB Saunders; 2000

21. US Environmental Protection Agency. *Review of the National Ambient Air Quality Standards for Lead: Exposure Analysis Methodology and Validation.* Washington, DC: Air Quality Management Division, Office of Air Quality Planning and Standards, US Environmental Protection Agency; 1989

22. Momicilovic B, Kostial K. Kinetics of lead retention and distribution in suckling and adult rats. *Environ Res.* 1974;8:214–220

23. Barry PS. A comparison of concentrations of lead in human tissues. *Br J Ind Med.* 1975;32:119–139

24. Faustman EM, Silbernagel SM, Fenske RA, Burbacher TM, Ponce RA. Mechanisms underlying children's susceptibility to environmental toxicants. *Environ Health Perspect.* 2000;108(suppl 1):13–21

25. Nebert DW, Gonzalez FJ. P450 genes: structure, evolution, and regulation. *Annu Rev Biochem.* 1987;56:945–993

26. Card SE, Tompkins SF, Brien JF. Ontogeny of the activity of alcohol dehydrogenase and aldehyde dehydrogenases in the liver and placenta of the guinea pig. *Biochem Pharmacol.* 1989;38:2535–2541

27. Byer AJ, Traylor TR, Semmer JR. Acetaminophen overdose in the third trimester of pregnancy. *JAMA.* 1982;247:3114–3115

28. Kurzel RB. Can acetaminophen excess result in maternal and fetal toxicity? *South Med J.* 1990;83:953–955

29. Rosevear SK, Hope PL. Favourable neonatal outcome following maternal paracetamol overdose and severe fetal distress. Case report. *Br J Obstet Gynaecol.* 1989;96:491–493

30. Stokes IM. Paracetamol overdose in the second trimester of pregnancy. Case report. *Br J Obstet Gynaecol.* 1984;91:286–288

31. World Health Organization. *Environmental Health Criteria 59. Principles for Evaluating Health Risks From Chemicals During Infancy and Early Childhood: The Need for a Special Approach.* Geneva, Switzerland: World Health Organization; 1986

32. Adams J, Barone S Jr, LaMantia A, et al. Workshop to identify critical windows of exposure for children's health: neurobehavioral work group summary. *Environ Health Perspect.* 2000;108(suppl 3):535–544

33. Goldstein GW. Developmental neurobiology of lead toxicity. In: Needleman HL, ed. *Human Lead Exposure.* Boca Raton, FL: CRC Press; 1992:125–135

34. Tager IB, Weiss ST, Munoz A, Rosner B, Speizer FE. Longitudinal study of the effects of maternal smoking on pulmonary function in children. *N Engl J Med.* 1983;309:699–703

35. Nethercott JR. Occupational skin disorders. In: LaDou J, ed. *Occupational Medicine.* Norwalk, CT: Appleton & Lange; 1990

# 3
# Breastfeeding

Breastfeeding is good for infants. The American Academy of Pediatrics (AAP),[1] World Health Organization,[2] and US Surgeon General[3] have considered the problem of environmental contaminants in human milk and continue to recommend breastfeeding. So far, despite literature that is now almost 50 years old, there are very few instances in which morbidity has been described in a nursling from a pollutant chemical in milk. There is good evidence that little if any morbidity is occurring from the more common and well-studied chemical agents.

In 1951 Laug and colleagues[4] reported the presence of the persistent pesticide dichlorodiphenyltrichloroethane (DDT) in human milk. Dichlorodiphenyltrichloroethane or one of its derivatives, usually the very stable metabolite dichlorodiphenyldichloroethene (DDE), has since been found in the lipid of essentially all human milk tested worldwide. Hexachlorobenzene; the cyclodiene pesticides, such as dieldrin, heptachlor, and chlordane; and industrial chemicals, such as polychlorinated biphenyls (PCBs) and similar compounds, have been, and in some cases continue to be, common contaminants. These residues are present in the breast milk of women without occupational or other special exposure (see Table 3.1).[5,6] Infant formula is free of these residues because the lipid comes from coconuts or other sources low on the food chain. Dairy cows do not have much exposure; in addition, a cow makes tons of milk during her lifetime production, keeping the concentrations of pollutants low in any given volume of milk.

Human milk is the major dietary source of these stable pollutants for young children. The quantities transferred, 20% or more of maternal body burden in 6 months of lactation, are much larger than children would receive otherwise and leave breastfed children with a

**Table 3.1**
**Pollutants That May Be Found in Human Milk**

| Chemical Agent |
| --- |
| DDT, DDE |
| PCB/PCDF |
| TCDD (Dioxin) |
| Chlordane |
| Heptachlor |
| Hexachlorobenzene |
| Volatile organic compounds<br>   Tetrachloroethylene, trichloroethylene<br>   Halothane<br>   Carbon disulfide |
| Nicotine |
| Metals<br>   Lead<br>   Methylmercury |

detectable higher body burden of pollutants for years.[7] The relatively high concentration of fat in breast milk means that fat-soluble substances will, in effect, concentrate there. The persistent fat-soluble agents that are discussed here are the best-studied human milk contaminants, but volatile organic hydrocarbons, metals, and organometals can contaminate milk, although almost always at levels that are of much less toxicological concern than the persistent fat-soluble agents. Asbestos fibers or fine particulate air pollution are not found in human milk. Drugs, of course, may appear but this topic is discussed elsewhere.[8] For a table of the prevalent concentrations of the persistent fat-soluble chemicals found in human milk, estimates of daily intakes for breastfed infants, comparisons with the concentrations permitted in infant foods, and comparisons with the recommended maximum daily intakes, see Rogan.[5] Many of the chlorinated aromatic compounds are carcinogenic in the laboratory, which has led to questions of delayed, irreversible toxicity from early life exposure, however low.

For a discussion of this topic, and for a table with the carcinogenic potencies, estimated life-time cancer risk from consumption of contaminated human milk, and a comparison with mortality attributable to not breastfeeding, see Rogan and colleagues.[9] For a comprehensive review of the older literature, see Jensen.[6]

## Specific Agents

### *Dichlorodiphenyltrichloroethane and Dichlorodiphenyldichloroethene*

Dichlorodiphenyltrichloroethane, an organochlorine pesticide once used widely in the United States, was banned from manufacture in 1972 after 4 decades of extensive global use. This decision was based on, among other things, its widespread appearance in human tissue and its effects on wildlife, especially reproduction in pelagic birds. The metabolites $o,p'$-DDT and DDE are weak estrogens, and $p,p'$-DDE is a potent anti-androgen.[10] In a prospective study of more than 700 children, there was a large difference in lactation performance between women at the extremes of the DDE distribution. The 75 women with DDE levels above 5 ppm in fat had median durations of lactation of 10 weeks, whereas 259 women whose levels were below 2 ppm breast-fed for 26 weeks.[11] In a similar study of approximately 230 nursing women in Mexico, where levels of DDE in breast milk were higher, women showed a similar decrease in the length of lactation, at least among second and later children.[12] This is plausibly related to the estrogenicity of DDE because prolactin is inhibited peripherally by the high estrogen levels during pregnancy, and lactation is initiated at very low levels of estrogen postpartum. The possibility that DDE might interfere with lactation performance or have other toxicity (an association with preterm birth has been reported)[13] was of primarily academic interest until the recent resurgence of interest in DDT for malaria control.[14] Control of malaria vectors with affordable, effective methods in developing countries will present public health dilemmas if DDT is deemed the most suitable agent and yet has the potential to increase mortality by producing preterm birth and early weaning.[15] Results from a Catalonian birth cohort showed that prenatal exposure to $p,p'$-DDE was associated with a delay in mental and psychomotor development at 13 months. Long-term breastfeeding was found to be beneficial to neurodevelopment, potentially counterbalancing the impact of exposure to these chemicals through breast milk.[16]

**Polychlorinated Biphenyls and Polychlorinated Dibenzofurans**
Exposure to commonly encountered levels of PCBs is associated with lower developmental/IQ test scores, including lower psychomotor scores from the newborn period through 2 years of age,[17] defects in short-term memory in 7-month-olds[18] and 4-year-olds,[19] and lowered IQs in 42-month-olds[20,21] and 11-year-olds.[22] Prenatal exposure to PCBs from the mother's body burden, rather than exposure through human milk, seems to account for most, but not all,[21] of the findings.

Polychlorinated dibenzofurans (PCDFs) are partially oxidized PCBs that appear in PCB mixtures subjected to high heat or explosions. They are responsible for some of the toxicity seen in workers cleaning up office building transformer fires[23] and also in 2 Asian outbreaks of PCB poisoning from contaminated cooking oil[24] (see Chapter 25). In the Asian poisonings, infants do seem to have been affected by exposure through breast milk.[25,26] Background exposure to PCDFs probably comes mostly from diet, especially contaminated fish.[27]

**Chlordane**
In 1970 inadvertent injection of chlordane, an organochlorine insecticide, into the heating ducts of a military home resulted in air contamination when the heat was turned on. The US Air Force performed studies in almost 500 dwellings and found that while most homes had very little chlordane in the air, occasionally values were as high as 260 $\mu g/m^3$. The symptoms abated and the air cleared when appropriate repairs were made.[28] Among women who lived in homes treated with

chlordane, breast milk levels of chlordane increased during the following 5 years.[29] There are no reports of morbidity due to this exposure.

### Heptachlor

The agricultural use of heptachlor, an organochlorine cyclodiene pesticide, resulted in 2 major mishaps: one in Hawaii, the other in Arkansas. In January 1982 routine analysis of cow milk by the Hawaii State Health Department turned up an unexpected amount of heptachlor epoxide, the stable metabolite. The contamination was traced to the practice of feeding dairy cows "green chop," which is the leafy portion of the pineapple plant. In this case, the pineapple plants had been treated with heptachlor to control aphids and were harvested too soon. Retrospective testing of green chop samples showed that heptachlor was present as far back as June 1981. Human milk in Hawaii had previously been quite low in heptachlor epoxide; during this episode the levels increased 3-fold, but into the range of values of those reported from the US mainland.[30] In 1986 cow milk in Arkansas was found to be contaminated. This time, the cows had been fed mash left over from the fermentation of grain to produce ethanol for addition to gasoline. Nine hundred forty-two samples collected contemporaneously with the exposure have been analyzed, and breast milk concentrations of heptachlor epoxide do not seem to be higher in Arkansas than in the adjoining southeastern states.[31] There has thus far been no morbidity attributable to these exposures, but research continues in Hawaii. (See http://www.lava.net/~hhref/ for a description of current activities.)

### Hexachlorobenzene

The fungicide hexachlorobenzene in human milk has caused disease in nurslings. After an epidemic of hexachlorobenzene poisoning in Turkey (1957–1959), breastfed children did not get porphyria as seen in adults, but rather *pembe yara* (pink sore), characterized by weakness, convulsions, and an annular papular rash. The case fatality rate was approximately 95%, and cohorts of children died in some of the villages. The chemical was present in human milk but not quantitated at the time; 20 years later, 20 samples had an average of 0.23 ppm of hexachlorobenzene.[32] If it is assumed that analysis was per gram of milk fat, then levels were still at about 15 times background levels.

### *Volatile Organic Compounds*

There is a single case report of a child who developed cholestatic jaundice while being breastfed.[33] His mother lunched daily with her husband, who was a dry cleaner, and perchloroethylene was found in her milk. The child's jaundice resolved with cessation of breastfeeding. Whether the perchloroethylene in the milk actually caused the child's jaundice has never been determined. In the many years since this case was reported, there have been no other reported occurrences, so it may have been coincidence or the levels of perchloroethylene may now be low enough so that it does not occur.

Because halothane has been detected in the milk of a lactating anesthesiologist,[34] it may be presumed to be present in lactating women who undergo anesthesia using halothane. Volatile agents similar to anesthetic gases may be excreted through expired air, and their concentration in human milk should decline rapidly once exposure ceases. Many other commonly encountered volatile organic compounds, such as benzene, freon, and methylene chloride, have been found in breast milk but are of no known clinical significance.

### *Nicotine*

Nicotine, its metabolites, and probably other components of cigarette smoke appear in the milk of smokers.[35] Smokers tend to wean early, but whether this is caused by smoking is not known.[36] There is no evidence of a smoking effect on the child from components of smoke in breast milk—indeed, there is some evidence that the increase in lower respiratory infections seen in the offspring of smoking mothers is prevented by 6 months of breastfeeding. Although no one should smoke cigarettes, the AAP encourages women who cannot quit to breastfeed nonetheless.

## *Metals*

Lead levels in human milk are low, and there are no modern reports of lead toxicity in a nursed child from an asymptomatic mother. Lead was known historically to be toxic to the nurslings of women who worked with it. Earlier this century, there was much more lead in canned formula and evaporated milk than in breast milk because of the soldered seams in the cans. The levels are lower now, but probably still higher than in human milk.[37]

Levels of cadmium, arsenic, and metallic mercury are low in human milk. Methylmercury, although relatively nonpolar, associates with protein and appears in milk at levels lower than those in serum. In Iraq in 1972, methylmercury-treated seed wheat inadvertently used to make bread produced levels in human milk of about 200 ppb, which is 50 to 100 times background exposure. There were thousands of cases of illness (see Chapter 20), including some that may have resulted from exposure to human milk alone.[38] The upper end of background exposure to methylmercury has been studied among children in the Seychelles Islands[39] and Faroe Islands[40] who have relatively high dietary exposure from ocean fish or mammals; these studies are inconsistent, with some effects seen from transplacental exposure in the Faroes but not in the Seychelles. In neither case were effects seen that could be attributed to breast milk exposure.

## Diagnostic Methods

Many laboratories have equipment to measure some or all of the contaminant residues in human milk. However, any such analysis must be regarded as research because there are no standard quality assurance methods, no established normal values, and some evidence that, at least for PCBs, the variability of test results between laboratories is too great to allow a single sample to be interpretable. Analysis of human milk for these chemicals is not clinically useful.

Professional organizations, including the World Health Organization and AAP,[1] that have considered the issue of pollutants in human milk continue to recommend breastfeeding and do not recommend testing of breast milk.

## Regulations

There are no regulations for chemical contaminants in human milk. Although it is tempting to apply the numbers used for infant formula, the risk-benefit situation is not comparable. The alternative to contaminated formula is uncontaminated formula. There likely is no such thing as uncontaminated human milk. The most difficult situation is encountered with the persistent fat-soluble agents, such as PCBs, because their levels in human milk have been at or near the upper regulatory allowances for formula or infant foods. For the other environmental contaminants, amounts in human milk are relatively low.

The most important action is to eliminate exposure to persistent bioaccumulating toxic chemicals. The manufacture and use of DDT, all the cyclodienes (ie, dieldrin), and most PCBs have been stopped in the United States, but not in many other parts of the world. Because 25% of the US food supply is imported, global action is necessary.

## Frequently Asked Questions

Q  *Should I get my breast milk tested for chemical pollutants?*

A  No. Residue levels of many chemicals can be found in milk; quantitating them is difficult, and there are no programs to promote quality assurance. Even if a very good laboratory generates results, there are no accepted normal or safe values against which to evaluate them.

Q  *Might an illness occurring in a breastfed child be due to a contaminant in milk?*

A  Nursing infants have been poisoned by contaminant chemicals in breast milk, although in most cases the mother herself also was ill. Investigating such a case would be research, and the phenomenon is extraordinarily rare.

Q  *Would dieting during lactation increase the levels of contaminants because the same amount of contaminants would be dissolved in a smaller amount of fat? Or would weight loss mobilize the contaminants out of fat and allow them to be excreted?*

A  No one has measured the levels of these chemicals in breast milk during weight loss. The greatest reported average weight loss among long-term breastfeeding women is 4.4 kg[41] at 1 year, compared with a 2.4-kg loss in non-breastfeeding women. Other studies find little or no weight loss among breastfeeding women.[42] Overweight breastfeeding women who exercise and restrict calories can achieve that weight loss faster and lose it mostly as fat.[43] Theoretically, because the same amount of chemical would be stored in 4.4 kg less tissue, mostly fat, weight loss might increase the concentration of the fat-soluble contaminants by up to 25%.

Breastfeeding does decrease the amount of these contaminants in the mother's body. The concentration per unit of milk would be higher if the mother had lost body fat, but there should be no "mobilization" beyond that. Because there is little evidence that background exposure to contaminated breast milk produces any morbidity in children, and because there is reasonable evidence that obesity in the mother does have consequences, a woman probably should not avoid a sensible diet and exercise on the basis that she might increase the concentration of contaminants in her milk and thus harm her child.

## References

1. American Academy of Pediatrics Committee on Environmental Health. PCBs in breast milk. *Pediatrics.* 1994;94:122–123

2. Consultation on assessment of the health risk of dioxins; re-evaluation of the tolerable daily intake (TDI): executive summary. *Food Addit Contam.* 2000;17:223–240

3. Office of Women's Health. *HHS Blueprint for Action on Breastfeeding.* Washington, DC: US Department of Health and Human Services; 2000

4. Laug EP, Kunze FM, Prickett CS. Occurrence of DDT in human fat and milk. *Arch Indust Hyg Occup Med.* 1951;3:245–246
5. Rogan WJ. Pollutants in breast milk. *Arch Pediatr Adolesc Med.* 1996;150:981–990
6. Jensen AA. Chemical contaminants in human milk. *Residue Rev.* 1983;89:1–128
7. Niessen KH, Ramolla J, Binder M, Brugmann G, Hofmann U. Chlorinated hydrocarbons in adipose tissue of infants and toddlers: inventory and studies on their association with intake of mothers' milk. *Eur J Pediatr.* 1984;142:238–244
8. American Academy of Pediatrics Committee on Drugs. Transfer of drugs and other chemicals into human milk. *Pediatrics.* 2001;108:776–789
9. Rogan WJ, Blanton PJ, Portier CJ, Stallard E. Should the presence of carcinogens in breast milk discourage breastfeeding? *Regul Toxicol Pharmacol.* 1991;13:228–240
10. Kelce WR, Stone CR, Laws SC, Gray LE, Kemppainen JA, Wilson EM. Persistent DDT metabolite p,p'-DDE is a potent androgen receptor antagonist. *Nature.* 1995;375:581–585
11. Rogan WJ, Gladen BC, McKinney JD, et al. Polychlorinated biphenyls (PCBs) and dichlorodiphenyl dichloroethene (DDE) in human milk: effects on growth, morbidity, and duration of lactation. *Am J Public Health.* 1987;77:1294–1297
12. Gladen BC, Rogan WJ. DDE and shortened duration of lactation in a northern Mexican town. *Am J Public Health.* 1995;85:504–508
13. Longnecker MP, Klebanoff MA, Zhou H, Brock JW. Association between maternal serum concentration of the DDT metabolite DDE and preterm and small-for-gestational-age babies at birth. *Lancet.* 2001;358:110–114
14. Roberts DR, Manguin S, Mouchet J. DDT house spraying and re-emerging malaria. *Lancet.* 2000;356:330–332
15. Rogan WJ. The DDT question. Lancet. 2000;356:1189
16. Ribas-Fito N, Cardo E, Sala M, et al. Breastfeeding exposure to organo-chlorine compounds, and neurodevelopment in infants. *Pediatrics.* 2003;111:e580–e585
17. Rogan WJ, Gladen BC. PCBs, DDE, and child development at 18 and 24 months. *Ann Epidemiol.* 1991;1:407–413
18. Jacobson SW, Fein GG, Jacobson JL, Schwartz PM, Dowler JK. The effect of intrauterine PCB exposure on visual recognition memory. *Child Dev.* 1985;56:853–860

19. Jacobson JL, Jacobson SW, Humphrey HE. Effects of in utero exposure to polychlorinated biphenyls and related contaminants on cognitive functioning in young children. *J Pediatr.* 1990;116:38–45

20. Patandin S, Lanting CI, Mulder PG, Boersma ER, Sauer PJ, Weisglas-Kuperus N. Effects of environmental exposure to polychlorinated biphenyls and dioxins on cognitive abilities in Dutch children at 42 months of age. *J Pediatr.* 1999;134:33–41

21. Walkowiak SJ, Wiener JA, Fastabend A, et al. Environmental exposure to polychlorinated biphenyls and quality of the home environment: effects on psychodevelopment in early childhood. *Lancet.* 2001;358:1602–1607

22. Jacobson JL, Jacobson SW. Intellectual impairment in children exposed to polychlorinated biphenyls in utero. *N Engl J Med.* 1996;335:783–789

23. Schecter A, Tiernan T. Occupational exposure to polychlorinated dioxins, polychlorinated furans, polychlorinated biphenyls, and biphenylenes after an electrical panel and transformer accident in an office building in Binghamton, NY. *Environ Health Perspect.* 1985;60:305–313

24. Rogan WJ, Gladen BC, Hung KL, et al. Congenital poisoning by polychlorinated biphenyls and their contaminants in Taiwan. *Science.* 1988;241:334–336

25. Harada M. Intrauterine poisoning: clinical and epidemiological studies and significance of the problem. *Bull Inst Const Med, Kumamoto Univ.* 1976;25(suppl):1–66

26. Yu ML, Hsu CC, Gladen BC, Rogan WJ. In utero PCB/PCDF exposure: relation of developmental delay to dysmorphology and dose. *Neurotoxicol Teratol.* 1991;13:195–202

27. Svensson BG, Nilsson A, Hansson M, Rappe C, Akesson B, Skerfving S. Exposure to dioxins and dibenzofurans through the consumption of fish. *N Engl J Med.* 1991;324:8–12

28. Lillie TH. Chlordane in Air Force family housing: a study of houses treated after construction. San Antonio, TX: USAF Occupational and Environmental Health Laboratory, Brooks Air Force Base; 1981. OEHL Report no. 81-45

29. Taguchi S, Yakushiji T. Influence of termite treatment in the home on the chlordane concentration in human milk. *Arch Environ Contam Toxicol.* 1988;17:65–71

30. Heptachlor epoxide in mother's milk. Oahu, August 1981–November 1982. Manoa, HI: University Hawaii at Manoa; 1983

31. Mattison DR, Wohlleb J, To T, et al. Pesticide concentrations in Arkansas breast milk. *J Ark Med Soc.* 1992;88:553–557

32. Cripps DJ, Gocmen A, Peters HA. Porphyria turcica. Twenty years after hexachlorobenzene intoxication. *Arch Dermatol.* 1980;116:46–50

33. Bagnell PC, Ellenberger HA. Obstructive jaundice due to a chlorinated hydrocarbon in breast milk. *Can Med Assoc J.* 1977;117:1047–1048

34. Cote CJ, Kenepp NB, Reed SB, Strobel GE. Trace concentrations of halothane in human breast milk. *Br J Anaesth.* 1976;48:541–543

35. Ferguson BB, Wilson DJ, Schaffner W. Determination of nicotine concentrations in human milk. *Am J Dis Child.* 1976;130:837–839

36. Counsilman JJ, MacKay EV. Cigarette smoking by pregnant women with particular reference to their past and subsequent breast feeding behaviour. *Aust N Z J Obstet Gynaecol.* 1985;25:101–107

37. Sinks T, Jackson RJ. International study finds breast milk free of significant lead contamination. *Environ Health Perspect.* 1999;107:A58–A59

38. Bakir F, Damluji SF, Amin-Zaki L, et al. Methylmercury poisoning in Iraq. *Science.* 1973;181:230–241

39. Myers GJ, Marsh DO, Davidson PW, et al. Main neurodevelopmental study of Seychellois children following in utero exposure to methylmercury from a maternal fish diet: outcome at six months. *Neurotoxicology.* 1995;16:653–664

40. Grandjean P, Weihe P, White RF, et al. Cognitive deficit in 7-year-old children with prenatal exposure to methylmercury. *Neurotoxicol Teratol.* 1997;19:417–428

41. Dewey KG, Heinig MJ, Nommsen LA. Maternal weight-loss patterns during prolonged lactation. *Am J Clin Nutr.* 1993;58:162–166

42. Schauberger CW, Rooney BL, Brimer LM. Factors that influence weight loss in the puerperium. *Obstet Gynecol.* 1992;79:424–429

43. Lovelady CA, Garner KE, Moreno KL, Williams JP. The effects of weight loss in overweight, lactating women on the growth of their infants. *N Engl J Med.* 2000;342:449–453

# 4
# How to Take an Environmental History

Questions about a child's environment are basic to a comprehensive pediatric health history. The answers can help the pediatrician understand the child's physical surroundings and offer appropriate suggestions to promote a healthy environment. Questions can be incorporated during visits for health supervision, illness, or symptoms that may be linked to an environmental cause. Further information about toxicants and abatement measures can be found elsewhere in the text.

## Health Supervision Visits

The following questions can be integrated into health supervision visits. Parents' answers can guide pediatricians in providing anticipatory guidance about preventing or abating exposures.

1. Where does the child live or spend time?
2. Does anyone in the home smoke?
3. Do you use well water? Tap water?
4. Are there exposures from items in the diet?
5. Is the child protected from excessive sun exposure?
6. What do parents/teenagers do for a living?

Additional questions can be added to determine whether particular environmental health risks in the community may be affecting the child. The patient's developmental stage is an important consideration during evaluation; Table 4.1 suggests when to introduce environmental questions.

### Where Does the Child Live or Spend Time?

**At Home.** Infants and toddlers spend most of their time indoors in their own homes, in a relative's home, or in a child care setting.

**Table 4.1**
**When to Introduce Environmental Questions***

| Topic | Suggested Time |
|-------|----------------|
| Home environment, smoking, environmental tobacco smoke (ETS), mold, occupational exposures, breastfeeding and bottle-feeding issues | Prenatal period |
| ETS, sun exposure, mold | When the child is 2 months old |
| Poison exposures, including household pesticides; lead poisoning | When the child is 6 months old |
| Arts and crafts exposures | Preschool period |
| Occupational exposures, exposures from hobbies | When the patient is a teenager |
| Lawn and garden products, lawn services, scheduled chemical applications | Spring and summer |
| Woodstoves and fireplaces, gas stoves | Fall and winter |

*Adapted from Balk SJ.[1]

Important features of these settings are

- *Type of Dwelling.* Private homes or apartments may have high levels of radon in basements or lower floors, or friable asbestos. Parents may need advice about testing for either or both toxicants. Building materials commonly used in mobile homes (eg, particleboard and pressed wood products) may contain formaldehyde, a respiratory and dermal irritant.
- *Age and Condition.* Buildings constructed before 1950 are likely to have leaded paint, which may peel, chip, or chalk. Lead dust can be released from poorly maintained surfaces that encounter friction, such as windows. Homes that have flooded or that have plumbing or roof leaks may have problems with mold growth. A "tight" home, built to conserve energy, may have inadequate ventilation, which may result in the trapping of pollutants indoors. When asked about whether hazards exist for the child, parents may be able to provide some information (eg, the

condition of the window wells) but not other information (the year the home was built).

- *Ongoing or Planned Renovation.* Renovation of a bedroom is common to prepare for the birth of a baby or to update the room decor as the child grows. Improper renovation procedures may expose a pregnant woman, her fetus, an infant, or a toddler to lead or other dusts, asbestos, and molds. Newly installed carpets may release irritating or toxic vapors.
- *Heating Sources.* Woodstoves and fireplaces emit respiratory irritants (nitrogen dioxide [$NO_2$], respirable particulates, and polycyclic aromatic hydrocarbons), especially when they are not properly vented and maintained. Gas stoves, which may produce $NO_2$, are used in more than half of US homes. Respiratory symptoms may occur when gas stoves are used as supplemental heat. Woodstoves, fireplaces, and other fuel-burning appliances may be sources of carbon monoxide (CO); exposure to this "silent killer" may be deadly.
- *Indoor and Outdoor Pesticides.* Children may inhale and absorb pesticide residues as they crawl or play on freshly sprayed outdoor surfaces, such as lawns and gardens, or on indoor surfaces, such as upholstery or rugs. Pesticide residues may adhere to plush toys. The hazards of spraying or "bombing" with pesticides while children are young should be explained to parents.
- *Proximity to Sites of Potential Hazardous Exposure in the Neighborhood or Community.* Exposures include polluted lakes and streams, industrial plants, highways, and dump sites. Children can be exposed to lead if they live downwind from a lead smelter, or have agricultural exposures to pesticides or other chemicals if they live on farms or at the urban-rural interface. Low-income families are more likely to live in contaminated areas.

**At School.** Many hazards found in school environments are similar to those in homes.[2] In addition, children engaging in arts and crafts activities may encounter potential hazards such as felt-tip markers (containing aromatic hydrocarbons) and oil-based paints.

Children with certain disabilities may be at more risk for toxic exposures. Children with asthma or visually impaired children working close to a project may be affected by fumes. Children who are unable to follow safety precautions may contaminate their skin or place art materials in their mouths. Emotionally disturbed children may abuse art materials, endangering themselves and others.

**Hobbies.** Hobby activity may pose a risk to school-aged children and adolescents. Shooting at an indoor firing range may result in lead exposure.[3] Toluene and other solvents may be encountered in glues used in model building.

### Does Anyone in the Home Smoke?

Exposure to environmental tobacco smoke (ETS) places children at risk for significant morbidity and mortality. If parents smoke, the pediatrician should advise them to quit and offer help in doing so. Educating parents about the associations between ETS and their child's illness may help them quit. Parents also can be informed that their children are more likely to begin smoking if the parents smoke. The US Public Health Service recommends that clinicians ask about smoking at every clinical encounter and offer smokers at least a brief (1–3 minute) intervention at each visit.[4] Pamphlets, posters, and information about programs to help parents quit may assist educational efforts. Parents should avoid exposing their children to environments that contain tobacco smoke.

Pediatricians should discuss the hazards of cigarette smoking with school-aged children and teenagers.

### Do You Use Well Water? Tap Water? Are There Exposures From Items in the Diet?

Tap water used to reconstitute infant formula may be contaminated with lead.[5] To decrease the possibility of contamination from leaded pipes and solder, water that has been standing in pipes overnight should be run for 2 minutes, or until cold, before it is used. Parents also can choose to test their water for lead.

Well water used to reconstitute infant formula may be contaminated. Infants exposed to high levels of nitrates in well water may develop methemoglobinemia, which may result in death. Well water also may contain coliform bacteria. Well water should be tested for nitrates and coliforms before being offered to an infant. High levels of nitrates or coliforms in the water may indicate the presence of pesticides.

Boiling water for infant formula is rarely necessary. Overboiling water for infant formula preparation concentrates lead and nitrates. Water brought to a rolling boil for 1 minute kills microorganisms such as *Cryptosporidium* without concentrating lead or nitrates.[6]

Dietary items include certain fish that may be contaminated with excessive amounts of mercury or polychlorinated biphenyls. Parents whose children eat these fish should be instructed to follow fish advisories issued by state and local health departments.

### Is the Child Protected From Excessive Sun Exposure?

Advice about sun protection includes covering up with clothing and hats, timing children's activities to avoid peak sun exposure, consulting the ultraviolet (UV) index, using sunscreen and reapplying frequently as needed, and wearing sunglasses.

### What Do Parents/Teenagers Do for a Living?

**Parental Occupations.** Parental occupations may produce hazards for a child. Workplace contaminants may be transported to the home on clothes, shoes, and skin surfaces.[7] Lead poisoning has been described in children of lead storage battery workers and construction workers,[8,9] asbestos-related lung diseases have been found in families of shipyard workers,[10] and elevated mercury levels have been reported in children whose parents worked in a mercury thermometer plant.[11] Parents who work with art materials at home may expose children to toxicants such as lead used in solder, pottery glazes, or stained glass.

An occupational history can be obtained when information about family composition and the family history is obtained. Workers exposed to toxic substances are legally entitled to be notified of this exposure under federal "right-to-know" and "hazard communication" laws. Parents who work with toxic substances should shower, if possible, and change clothes and shoes before leaving work. At home, children should not be allowed in rooms where parents work with toxic substances.

**Adolescent Employment.** Although employment may help teenagers become more responsible, develop skills, and earn money, work activities may carry the risk of toxic exposure or injury. Environmental exposures include UV radiation with outdoor work, ETS encountered in restaurants and bars, pesticides from lawn care and farm work, and noise from operating equipment.

Work also may interfere with an adolescent's education, sleep, and social behavior. Federal and state child labor laws regulate employment of children younger than 18 years. These laws address the minimum ages for general and specific types of employment, maximum daily and weekly number of hours of work permitted, prohibition of work during night hours, prohibition of certain types of employment, and the registration of minors for employment.[12,13]

## Visits for Illness: Considering Environmental Etiologies in the Differential Diagnosis

Environmental tobacco smoke is the most common toxicant associated with respiratory diseases such as asthma, recurrent lower and upper airway disease, and persistent middle ear effusion. Lead poisoning may present with symptoms of recurrent abdominal pain, constipation, irritability, developmental delay, seizures, or unexplained coma. Headaches may be caused by acute and chronic exposure to CO from improperly vented heating sources, formaldehyde, and chemicals used on the job. Pediatricians should ask about mold and water damage in the home when they treat infants with acute pulmonary hemorrhage.[14]

Environmental causes of illness may not always be apparent.[15] Because most environmental or occupational illnesses present as common medical problems or have nonspecific symptoms, the diagnosis may be missed unless a history of exposure is obtained, which is especially important if the illness is atypical or unresponsive to treatment.[16] The following questions may provide information about whether an illness is related to the environment:

1. Do symptoms subside or worsen in a particular location (eg, home, child care, school, or room)?
2. Do symptoms subside or worsen during a particular time? At a particular time of day? On weekdays or weekends? During a particular week or season?
3. Do symptoms worsen during a particular activity? While the child is playing outside or engaging in hobby activities, such as working with arts and crafts?
4. Are siblings or other children experiencing similar symptoms to your child's?

## Case Examples

The following are 2 case examples illustrating integrating environmental health etiologies into the differential diagnosis:

### Case 1—Asthma

*A 5-year-old boy comes to your office for follow-up. He has had mild intermittent asthma for most of his life. His known triggers for wheezing episodes are cold weather and upper respiratory infections. What else do you need to know?*

Environmental triggers that may precipitate asthma include
- Environmental tobacco smoke
- Molds
- Dust mites
- Cockroaches
- Animal allergens

- Nitrogen oxides
- Odors
- Volatile organic compounds such as formaldehyde

Most of these triggers are amenable to abatement measures. Inquiring about the details of environmental health exposures and suggesting ways to decrease exposures may result in improvement of symptoms.

### Case 2—Fever and Rash

*A 3-year-old boy comes in with a 1-week history of fever, rash, and difficulty when walking. His medical history is unremarkable. Physical examination reveals an irritable child with a temperature of 40°C; there is conjunctival injection, pharyngeal erythema, swelling of hands and feet, and a macular rash. What is in your differential diagnosis?*

The differential diagnosis includes
- Kawasaki disease
- Measles
- Scarlet fever
- Juvenile rheumatoid arthritis
- Acrodynia

Although the child described in this case turns out to have Kawasaki disease, the differential diagnosis of these symptoms includes acrodynia. Acrodynia ("pink disease"), a rare hypersensitivity reaction to mercury, mainly occurs in children. Prominent symptoms are anorexia, generalized pain, paresthesias, and apathy. Physical examination reveals hypotonia and an acral rash that is predominantly pink, papular, and pruritic and may progress to desquamation. Other features include irritability, tremors, diaphoresis, hypertension, and tachycardia.[17]

## Resources

Agency for Toxic Substances and Disease Registry (ATSDR),[16] Internet: http://www.atsdr.cdc.gov. The ATSDR offers a detailed environmental history questionnaire geared toward adults in the workplace, with examples used and principles illustrated that can be helpful to pediatricians.

Association of Occupational and Environmental Health Clinics (AOEC), Internet: http://www.aoec.org. In conjunction with the US Department of Health and Human Services and the ATSDR, the AOEC has produced *Approach to the Environmental Health History* (CD-ROM). Case examples are used to illustrate important elements of an environmental history when the child presents with a symptom that may have an environmental cause. The CD-ROM contents are available at http://www.aoec.org/PedEnvHx_files/frame.htm.

Canadian Association of Physicians for the Environment (CAPE), Internet: http://children.cape.ca. This association is dedicated to the protection and promotion of human health by addressing issues of local and global environmental degradation. Information on environmental history-taking is available on their Web site at http://children.cape.ca/history.html.

## References

1. Balk SJ. The environmental history: asking the right questions. *Contemp Pediatr.* 1996;13:19–36
2. Common teaching, hobby materials could pose significant health risks. *Environ Health Lett.* 1996;35:153
3. Goldberg RL, Hicks AM, O'Leary LM, London S. Lead exposure at uncovered outdoor firing ranges. *J Occup Med.* 1991;33:718–719
4. Fiore MC, Bailey WC, Cohen SJ, et al. *Treating Tobacco Use and Dependence: A Clinical Practice Guideline.* Rockville, MD: US Department of Health and Human Services; 2000. AHRQ Publication 00-0032
5. Baum CR, Shannon MW. The lead concentration of reconstituted infant formula. *J Toxicol Clin Toxicol.* 1997;35:371–375

6.  US Environmental Protection Agency, Office of Ground Water and Drinking Water. *Safe Drinking Water—Guidance for People With Severely Weakened Immune Systems.* Washington, DC: US Environmental Protection Agency; 1999. EPA Publication 816-F-99-005. Available at: http://www.epa.gov/safewater/crypto.html

7.  Chisolm JJ Jr. Fouling one's own nest. *Pediatrics.* 1978;62:614–617

8.  Watson WN, Witherell LE, Giguere GC. Increased lead absorption in children of workers in a lead storage battery plant. *J Occup Med.* 1978;20:759–761

9.  Whelan EA, Piacitelli GM, Gerwel B, et al. Elevated blood lead levels in children of construction workers. *Am J Public Health.* 1997;87:1352–1355

10. Kilburn KH, Lilis R, Anderson HA, et al. Asbestos disease in family contacts of shipyard workers. *Am J Public Health.* 1985;75:615–617

11. Hudson PJ, Vogt RL, Brondum J, Witherell L, Myers G, Paschal DC. Elemental mercury exposure among children of thermometer plant workers. *Pediatrics.* 1987;79:935–938

12. Rose KL, Fraser BS, Chavner I. *Minor Laws of Major Importance.* Dubuque, IA: Kendall/Hunt Publishing Co; 1994

13. Pollack SH. Adolescent occupational exposures and pediatric-adolescent take-home exposures. *Pediatr Clin North Am.* 2001;48:1267–1289

14. American Academy of Pediatrics Committee on Environmental Health. Toxic effects of indoor molds. *Pediatrics.* 1998;101:712–714

15. Goldman LR. The clinical presentation of environmental health problems and the role of the pediatric provider. What do I do when I see children who might have an environmentally related illness? *Pediatr Clin North Am.* 2001;48:1085–1098

16. Agency for Toxic Substances and Disease Registry. *Case Studies in Environmental Medicine: Taking an Exposure History.* Atlanta, GA: US Department of Health and Human Services, Agency for Toxic Substances and Disease Registry; 2000. ATSDR Publication ATSDR-HE-CS-2001-0002. Available at: http://www.atsdr.cdc.gov/HEC/CSEM/exphistory/index.html

17. Behrman RE, Kleigman RM, Jenson HB. *Nelson Textbook of Pediatrics.* 16th ed. Philadelphia, PA: WB Saunders; 2000:2155

# 5
# How to Do a Home Inventory of Environmental Hazards

Although the utility of home audit questionnaires has not been scientifically tested, some pediatricians find them helpful in obtaining an environmental history. Parents can fill out a questionnaire in the waiting room or at home after the visit. Answers that indicate possible exposure to environmental hazards can be followed up with appropriate actions such as (1) testing the child for lead poisoning, (2) testing the home for radon, (3) advising family members about prevention, or (4) advising parents about eliminating the hazard.

The following questionnaire* can be used or adapted to include environmental issues specific to a community. Basic questions are included. Information for parents can be found in the brochure *Your Child and the Environment,* by the American Academy of Pediatrics. In addition, pediatricians can seek out whether there are community-based programs to address some of the areas inquired about on the home inventory form. A more extensive environmental history questionnaire, which includes a detailed workplace exposure history form, is available.[1]

---

*This questionnaire is adapted from Sophie J. Balk, MD. The original material appeared in the manual *Kids and the Environment—Toxic Hazards,* edited by the Children's Environmental Health Network, California Public Health Foundation. The sponsors for this project were the Agency for Toxic Substances and Disease Registry and the California Department of Health Services.

The material was presented in Needleman HL, Landrigan PJ. *Raising Children Toxic Free.* New York, NY: Farrar, Strauss, Giroux; 1994.

| Where the Child Lives or Spends Time | Chapter(s) for Further Information |
|---|---|
| 1. What is the age and condition of the home? | Lead |
| 2. Are the windowsills peeling? Do the window wells contain solid material? | Lead |
| 3. Are you renovating a room or planning to? | Lead; Asbestos; Air Pollutants, Indoor |
| 4. Do you have a basement? | Asbestos; Ionizing Radiation (Including Radon) |
| 5. Are there sleeping or playing areas in the basement? | Asbestos; Ionizing Radiation (Including Radon) |
| 6. Do you have water damage or visible mold in any part of your home? Is there standing water or condensation? Is your home damp? Does it smell musty? | Asthma; Air Pollutants, Indoor |
| 7. Do you live in a mobile home? | Air Pollutants, Indoor |
| 8. Do you have a wood-burning stove or fireplace? Does smoke enter the room when you use it? | Air Pollutants, Indoor; Carbon Monoxide |
| 9. Do you have a gas stove? Does it have a pilot light? Do you use a kerosene- or propane-fueled space heater? | Air Pollutants, Indoor; Carbon Monoxide |

| Where the Child Lives or Spends Time | Chapter(s) for Further Information |
|---|---|
| 10. Do you use pesticides on your lawn or use a proprietary lawn service? Do you use pesticides in your home? | Pesticides |
| 11. What kind of thermometer does your family use? | Mercury; Air Pollutants, Indoor |
| 12. Is your home located near a polluted lake or stream, industrial area, highway, dump site, farm, etc? | Water Pollutants; Air Pollutants, Outdoor; Waste Sites; Pesticides |
| 13. Does your child play outside in the sun? | Ultraviolet Light |
| **Smoking** | |
| 14. Does anyone in the home smoke? How many people? Is smoking allowed by visitors to your home, or in the car? Does your child's caregiver smoke? | Environmental Tobacco Smoke and Smoking Cessation; Asthma; Air Pollutants, Indoor |
| **Diet—Water and Food** | |
| 15. Do you use well water? | Nitrates and Nitrites in Water; Pesticides; Water Pollutants; Arsenic |
| 16. Do you use tap water? | Lead; Water Pollutants |
| 17. Do you wash fresh fruits and vegetables? | Food Contaminants |

| Where the Child Lives or Spends Time | Chapter(s) for Further Information |
|---|---|
| 18. Do you use dietary supplements or ethnic remedies? | Herbs, Dietary Supplements, and Other Remedies |
| 19. Do you or your child eat a lot of fish? | Water Pollutants; Mercury; Polychlorinated Biphenyls, Dibenzofurans, and Dibenzodioxins |
| **Job-Related Hazards** | |
| 20. What do you and your spouse do for a living? Does your job or your spouse's job involve contact with heavy metals, dust, chemicals, pesticides, or fibers? | Workplaces |
| 21. Are teenagers employed? What kinds of work do they do? | Workplaces; Noise |
| **Hobbies** | |
| 22. Do you work at home with substances that may be hazardous? Are you or your child involved in a hobby at home? | Workplaces; Arts and Crafts; Schools; Lead; Air Pollutants, Indoor |

## Reference

1. Agency for Toxic Substances and Disease Registry. *Case Studies in Environmental Medicine: Taking an Exposure History.* Atlanta, GA: US Department of Health and Human Services, Agency for Toxic Substances and Disease Registry; 2000. ATSDR Publication ATSDR-HE-CS-2001-0002. Available at: http://www.atsdr.cdc.gov/HEC/CSEM/exphistory/index.html

# 6
# Air Pollutants, Indoor

Indoor air quality has become a health concern in recent years because energy costs have led to building designs that reduce air exchanges and new synthetic materials have become more widely used in furnishings. Furthermore, children spend an estimated 80% to 90% of their time indoors at home or at school. Exposure to indoor air contaminants may have adverse effects on health. Indoor environments have a range of airborne pollutants, including particulate matter, gases, vapors, biological materials, and fibers.[1,2] In the home, common sources of air pollutants include tobacco smoke, gas stoves and woodstoves, and furnishings and construction materials that release organic gases and vapors. Allergens and biological agents include animal dander, fecal material from house-dust mites and other insects, mold spores, and bacteria (see Chapter 34). Pollutants such as particulate matter may be brought into the indoor environment from the outdoor air by natural and mechanical ventilation. Pesticides may be sprayed in the home to reduce insect infestations. This chapter focuses on indoor air pollutants other than tobacco smoke (ie, combustion products, volatile organic compounds [VOCs], and molds). Unlike the common outdoor air pollutants, for which the US Environmental Protection Agency (EPA) has standards, there are no federal standards for indoor air pollutants in homes and schools. Clinical symptoms due to exposure to indoor air pollutants are usually acute, short-lived, and generally cease with elimination of exposure. Treatment of most indoor air pollution–related illnesses includes relief of symptoms and elimination of the pollution source. Children with persistent respiratory symptoms may require evaluation for possible infection, allergy, and asthma.

## Combustion Pollutants

### Route and Sources of Exposure

The route of exposure to combustion products is through inhalation. Combustion pollutants in the home arise primarily from gas ranges, particularly when they malfunction or are used as space heaters, and from improperly vented woodstoves and fireplaces. Combustion of natural gas results in the emission of nitrogen dioxide ($NO_2$) and carbon monoxide (CO). Levels of $NO_2$ in the home generally are increased during the winter when ventilation is reduced to conserve energy. During the winter, average indoor concentrations of $NO_2$ in homes with gas cooking stoves are as much as twice as high as outdoor levels. Some of the highest indoor $NO_2$ levels have been measured in homes where ovens were used as space heaters.[3] Residential levels of CO generally are low. Cooking or heating with wood results in the emission of liquids (suspended droplets), solids (suspended particles), and gases such as $NO_2$ and sulfur dioxide ($SO_2$).[3] The aerosol mixture of very fine solid and liquid particles or "smoke" contains particles in the inhalable range, less than 10 μm in diameter. Few measurements of wood smoke in indoor environments in the United States have been done. In several studies, concentrations of inhalable particles were higher in homes with woodstoves, compared with homes without woodstoves. Depending on the frequency and duration of cooking or heating with wood and the adequacy of ventilation, the concentration of inhalable particles may exceed outdoor air standards. With adequate ventilation, however, operating a woodstove or fireplace may not adversely affect indoor air quality.

### Systems Affected

The mucous membranes of the eyes, nose, throat, and respiratory tract are affected.

### Clinical Effects

Exposure to high levels of $NO_2$ and $SO_2$ may result in acute muco-cutaneous irritation and respiratory effects. The relatively low water solubility of $NO_2$ results in minimal mucous membrane irritation of the upper airway; the principal site of toxicity is the lower respiratory tract.[4] In contrast, the high water solubility of $SO_2$ makes it extremely irritating to the eyes and upper respiratory tract. Whether exposure to the relatively low levels of these gases attained in houses is associated with any health effects remains to be determined.

Exposure to inhaled particles in wood smoke may result in irritation and inflammation of the upper and lower respiratory tract resulting in rhinitis, cough, wheezing, and worsening of asthma.[5-7]

Use of space heaters, kerosene lamps or heaters, and gas ovens or ranges as home heating devices should raise concerns about exposure to combustion products, particularly if there is any indication that appliances may not be properly vented to the outside or that heating equipment may be in disrepair. Burning wood indoors in a woodstove or fireplace may suggest the source of the respiratory problem.

### Diagnostic Methods

If CO poisoning is suspected, a carboxyhemoglobin level should be promptly measured (see Chapter 10).

For an indoor air pollution–related respiratory illness, a specific etiology may be difficult to establish because most respiratory signs and symptoms are nonspecific and only may occur in association with significant exposures. Effects of lower exposures may be milder and more vague. Furthermore, signs and symptoms in infants and children may be atypical. Multiple pollutants may be involved in a given situation. Establishing the environmental cause of a given respiratory illness is further complicated by the similarity of effects to those associated with allergies and respiratory infections. Clinicians should be aware of whether their patients live in mobile homes or new houses, or burn wood. The effects of exposure to CO are discussed in Chapter 10.

### Prevention of Exposure

Measures that may help to minimize exposure include periodic professional inspection and maintenance of furnaces, gas water heaters, and clothes dryers; venting such equipment directly to the outdoors; and regular cleaning and inspection of fireplaces and woodstoves. Charcoal (in a hibachi or grill) should never be burned indoors.

## Volatile Organic Compounds

### Routes and Sources of Exposure

The route of exposure to VOCs occurs through inhalation and dermal contact of surfaces where they are deposited. Many household furnishings and products off-gas VOCs.[1,2] These include chemicals such as aliphatic and aromatic hydrocarbons (including chlorinated hydrocarbons), alcohols, and ketones in products such as finishes, rug and oven cleaners, paints and lacquers, and paint strippers. Formaldehyde is found primarily in building materials and home furnishings.[1,2,8,9] Because product labels may not always specify the presence of organic compounds, the specific chemical(s) to which a product user may be exposed may be difficult to discern. Over the normal range of room temperatures, VOCs are released as gases or vapors from furnishings or consumer products. Volatile organic compound measurements in residential and nonresidential buildings show that exposure to VOCs is widespread and highly variable.[10,11] In general, VOCs are likely to be higher in recently constructed or renovated buildings compared with older buildings. Once building-related emissions decrease, consumer products are likely to remain the predominant source of exposure to VOCs. Studies have shown that indoor concentrations of VOCs (measured using a personal monitor) are greater than outdoor concentrations, breath levels correlate better with air exposures in a person's breathing zone than with outdoor air levels, and inhalation accounts for more than 99% of exposure for many VOCs.[12]

Formaldehyde is one of the most ubiquitous indoor air contaminants. It is used in hundreds of products such as urea-formaldehyde

and phenol-formaldehyde resin, used to bond laminated wood products and to bind wood chips in particle board; as a carrier solvent in
dyeing textiles and paper products; and as a stiffener, wrinkle resistant,
and water repellent in floor coverings (eg, rugs and linoleums).[1-3]
Urea-formaldehyde foam insulation, one source of formaldehyde used
in home construction until the early 1980s, is no longer used. The
addition of new furniture to a home increases formaldehyde concentrations. Mobile homes, which have small enclosed spaces, low air
exchange rates, and many particle board furnishings, may have much
higher concentrations of formaldehyde than other types of homes.[1]
Table 6.1 lists common VOCs and their uses.

## Clinical Effects

Exposure to VOCs may result in dermal, mucocutaneous, and nonspecific effects.[13]

Depending on the dominant compounds and route and level of
exposure, signs and symptoms may include upper respiratory tract
and eye irritation, rhinitis, nasal congestion, rash, pruritus, headache,
nausea, and vomiting.[14-16]

Volatile organic compounds have only recently attracted study,
and studies are ongoing to determine which VOCs are associated with
specific health effects.[17]

The effects of exposure to formaldehyde have received more attention. Exposure to airborne formaldehyde may result in conjunctival
and upper respiratory tract irritation (ie, burning or tingling sensations in eyes, nose, and throat); these symptoms are temporary and
resolve with cessation of exposure.[18,19] Formaldehyde may exacerbate
asthma in some infants and children,[20,21] and it has been linked to
nasopharyngeal cancer in occupationally exposed adults.[22]

## Diagnostic Methods

Several questions may help to identify potential exposure. These
include: Does the family live in a new home with large amounts of
pressed wood products? Is there new pressed wood furniture? Have

**Table 6.1**
**Commonly Used Volatile Organic Compounds (VOCs)**

| VOCs | Uses |
|---|---|
| 1,1,1-Trichloroethane | Used as a dry-cleaning agent, a vapor degreasing agent, and a propellant |
| 1,4-Dichlorobenzene | Used as an air deodorant and an insecticide |
| 2-Butanone | Used as a solvent, and in the surface coating industry, in manufacturing synthetic resins |
| Acetone | Used as a solvent in the production of lubricating oils and as an intermediate in pharmaceuticals and pesticides |
| Benzene | Constituent in motor fuels, solvent for fats, inks, oils, paints, plastics, and rubber; also used in the manufacturing of detergents, pharmaceuticals, explosives, and dyestuffs |
| Chlorobenzene | Used in the manufacture of dyestuffs and pesticides |
| Chloroform | Used as a solvent; widely distributed in atmosphere and water |
| Ethylbenzene | Used as a solvent and in the manufacture of styrene-related products; emitted vapors at filling stations and from motor vehicles |
| Formaldehyde | Used in particleboard, insulation (UFFI), carpeting, mobile homes, temporary classrooms, and trailers |
| m-Xylene, p-Xylene, and o-Xylene | Used as solvents, constituents of paint, lacquers, varnishes, inks, dyes, adhesives, cement, and aviation fluids; also used in the manufacture of perfumes, insect repellants, pharmaceuticals, and the leather industry |
| Perchloroethylene | Used in dry cleaning |
| Styrene | At high temperature becomes a plastic; used in the manufacture of resins, polyesters, insulators, and drugs |
| Toluene | Used in the manufacture of benzene, as a solvent for paints and coatings, and as a component of car and aviation fuels |
| Trichloroethylene | Used as a solvent in vapor degreasing, for extracting caffeine from coffee, as a dry-cleaning agent, and as an intermediate in production of pesticides, waxes, gums, resins, tars, and paints |

household members recently worked on craft or graphic materials? Are chemical cleaners used extensively? Has remodeling recently been done? Has anyone recently used paints, solvents, or sprays in the home? Do the child's symptoms clear when he is removed from the home and reappear when he returns?

### Prevention of Exposure

Prevention strategies include increasing ventilation and avoiding storage of opened containers of unused paints and similar materials within the home. If formaldehyde is thought to be the cause of the problem, the source should be identified and, if possible, removed. Measuring levels of formaldehyde in the air usually is not necessary. If it is not possible to remove the source, the exposure can be reduced by coating cabinets, paneling, and other furnishings with polyurethane or other nontoxic sealants and by increasing the amount of ventilation in the home. Formaldehyde concentrations decrease rapidly over the first year after a product is manufactured.

## Molds

### Routes and Sources of Exposure

Exposure to molds occurs via inhalation of contaminated air and dermal contact with surfaces where they are deposited. Molds are ubiquitous in the outdoor environment and can enter the home through doorways, windows, heating, ventilation systems, and air conditioning systems. Molds proliferate in environments that contain excessive moisture, such as from pet urine or leaks in roofs, walls, and plant pots. The most common indoor molds are *Cladosporium, Penicillium, Aspergillus,* and *Alternaria.*[23]

### Systems Affected

The mucous membranes of the eyes, nose, throat, and respiratory tract are affected by exposure to molds.

### Clinical Effects

The clinical effects of exposure to molds may be allergic or toxic. Some children who are exposed to molds have persistent upper respiratory tract symptoms such as rhinitis, sneezing, and eye irritation, as well as lower respiratory tract symptoms such as coughing and wheezing.[24–26]

Toxic effects of molds may be due to inhalation of mycotoxins, lipid-soluble toxins readily absorbed by the airways.[27] Species of mycotoxin-producing molds include *Fusarium, Trichoderma,* and *Stachybotrys.* Exposure to *Stachybotrys* and other molds has been associated with acute pulmonary hemorrhage among young infants in Cleveland,[28–33] Kansas City, MO,[34] and Delaware.[35] Exposure to *Trichoderma* and other molds has been associated with acute pulmonary hemorrhage in a North Carolina infant.[36]

### Diagnostic Methods

Several questions may help to identify exposure to molds. They include: Has the home been flooded? Is there any water-damaged wood or cardboard in the house? Has there been a roof or plumbing leak? Have occupants seen any mold or noticed a musty smell? Testing the environment for specific molds usually is not necessary. There currently is no diagnostic test for mycotoxins in human tissue.

### Prevention of Exposure

Prevention strategies include cleaning up water and removing all water-damaged items (including carpets) within 24 hours of a flood or leak. If this is done, toxic mold will not have the opportunity to grow. If some mold already is present, the affected area needs to be washed with soap and water, followed with a solution of 1 part bleach to 10 parts water. Protective gloves should be worn during cleanup.

## Frequently Asked Questions

Q  *What are the most important things I can do to protect my child from indoor air pollution?*

A  Do not smoke. Preventing children from being exposed to environmental tobacco smoke (ETS) is important. Keep your home dry. Woodstoves and fireplaces need to be checked yearly by a professional to make sure they are clean and running efficiently. Gas ovens should not be used to provide supplemental heat. Children should not come into contact with mothballs because they contain dangerous chemicals. Air fresheners do not improve air quality and use artificial chemicals to provide scent. Families inquiring about air fresheners should be encouraged to reconsider their use.

Q  *My child has had a persistent runny nose. Could this be due to the new carpet we installed last month?*

A  The symptom could be due to viruses, bacteria, or allergies. It also is possible that the symptoms relate to something in the child's environment such as ETS or the chemical compounds released from a new carpet. Sometimes an exact diagnosis is difficult to determine. Symptoms from colds are temporary, and symptoms from environmental irritants tend to improve once exposure to the irritant is eliminated. If possible, have the child play and sleep in another room to see if symptoms improve. It may take some time to determine the cause of the child's symptoms.

Q  *Are air fresheners dangerous?*

A  Currently no information indicates that air fresheners are dangerous. However, the long-term effects have not been studied.

Q  *My child's asthma inhaler contains chlorofluorocarbons (CFCs). Does this harm him?*

A  Using an inhaler that contains CFCs does not harm the child's health. However, CFCs harm the environment by contributing to the depletion of the stratospheric ozone layer. The EPA has mandated that CFCs be phased out.

Q *What are the effects of exposure to mothballs?*

A Two products, p-dichlorobenzene (PDCB) and naphthalene, are used as moth repellents. Reports of occupational exposure to the active ingredients of mothballs are available. Studies documenting health effects from residential exposure are limited. The active ingredient in mothballs usually is PDCB. Exposure to PDCB may cause irritation of the eyes, nose, and throat; periorbital swelling; headache; and rhinitis, which usually subside 24 hours after cessation of exposure. Prolonged occupational exposure to PDCB may result in anorexia, nausea, vomiting, weight loss, and liver damage. A case of allergic purpura induced by PDCB has been reported.

Naphthalene also may be used as a moth repellent. Exposure to large amounts of naphthalene may result in hemolytic anemia, resulting in jaundice and hemoglobinuria in children with glucose-6-phosphate dehydrogenase deficiency. Nausea, vomiting, and diarrhea also may occur.

Q *What can be done to reduce the levels of particulates from woodstoves and fireplaces?*

A Measures to reduce the levels of particulate matter from a woodstove include ensuring that the stove is placed in a room with adequate ventilation and properly vented directly to the outdoors. Newer stoves are designed to emit less particulate matter into the air.

Q *What are ionizers and other ozone-generating air cleaners? Should they be used?*

A Ion generators act by charging the particles in a room so that they are attracted to walls, floors, tabletops, draperies, or occupants. Abrasion can result in resuspension of these particles into the air. In some cases these devices contain a collector to attract the charged particles back to the unit. While ion generators may remove small particles (eg, those in tobacco smoke), they do not remove gases or odors and may be relatively ineffective in removing large particles such as pollen and house-dust allergens. Ozone generators are specifically designed to release ozone to purify the air.

Ozone is produced indirectly by ion generators and some electronic air cleaners and produced directly by ozone generators. While indirect ozone production is of concern, there is even greater concern with the direct and purposeful introduction of ozone into indoor air. No difference exists, despite the claims of some marketers, between ozone in smog outdoors and ozone produced by ozone generators. Under certain conditions, these devices can produce levels of ozone high enough to be harmful to a child. They are not recommended for use in homes or schools.

Q *Can other air cleaners help?*

A Other air cleaners include mechanical filter, electronic (eg, electrostatic precipitators), and hybrid air cleaners using 2 or more techniques. The value of any air cleaner depends on its efficiency, proper selection for the pollutant to be removed, proper installation, and appropriate maintenance. Drawbacks include inadequate pollutant removal, redispersement of pollutants, deceptive masking of the pollutant rather than its removal, generation of ozone, and unacceptable noise levels. The EPA and Consumer Product Safety Commission have not taken a position either for or against the use of these devices.

Effective control at the source of a pollutant is key. Air cleaners are not a solution but are adjunct to source control and adequate ventilation. The National Heart, Lung, and Blood Institute recommends that a good filter be installed in furnaces.

Q  *I am about to purchase a new vacuum cleaner for my home. Should I buy one with a HEPA filter?*

A  HEPA (high efficiency particulate air) filters reduce dust by trapping small particles and not rereleasing them into the air as you vacuum. Although widely advertised for use in homes in which children with asthma or allergies are living, it is not clear whether use of HEPA filters reduces symptoms or medication use in children with asthma. The use of HEPA filters should not be a substitute for other allergen-reduction methods. Some vacuum cleaners advertise HEPA filters, but that doesn't necessarily mean they have an effective air filtration system. Unless the filter is contained in a sealed, airtight chamber, dirty air can still escape from the vacuum. Look for a system that is designated as "true HEPA," a term that indicates the entire system, not just the filter, meets HEPA standards.

Q  *When I bring clothes home from the dry cleaners, are the chemicals that are released from the clothes dangerous to my child?*

A  A very small amount of the chemicals used in the dry cleaning process will be released from clothes. The quantity is probably not significant enough to cause health problems in a child. Of more concern is whether the home is located directly above or adjacent to a dry cleaning establishment. If so, the amount of daily exposure may be enough to cause health concerns.

Q  *Can carpet exposure make people sick?*

A  New carpet may emit VOCs, as do products that accompany carpet installation such as adhesives and padding. Some people report symptoms such as eye, nose, and throat irritation; headaches; skin irritation; shortness of breath or cough; and fatigue, which they may associate with new carpet installation. Carpet also can act as a "sink" for chemical and biological pollutants including pesticides, dust mites, and molds.

Anyone involved in purchasing new carpet should ask retailers for information to help them select lower VOC-emitting carpet, padding, and adhesives. Before new carpet is installed, the retailer should unroll and air out the carpet in a clean, well-ventilated area. Opening doors and windows reduces the level of chemicals released. Ventilation systems should be in proper working order and operated during installation, and for 48 to 72 hours after the new carpet is installed.

Q *Can plants control indoor air pollution?*

A Reports in the media and promotions by representatives of the decorative houseplant industry characterize plants as "nature's clean air machine," claiming that National Aeronautics and Space Administration research shows plants remove indoor air pollutants. While it is true that plants remove carbon dioxide from the air, and the ability of plants to remove certain other pollutants from water is the basis for some pollution control methods, the ability of plants to control indoor air pollution is less well established. The only available study of the use of plants to control indoor air pollutants in an actual building could not determine any benefit from the use of plants. As a practical means of pollution control, the plant removal mechanisms seem to be inconsequential when compared with common ventilation and air exchange rates. Over-damp planter soil conditions may promote growth of molds.

Q *How do I keep my fireplace safe?*

A The box lists measures to increase fireplace safety.

---

**Fireplace Safety**

1. If possible, keep a window cracked open while the fire is burning.
2. Be certain the damper or flue is open before starting a fire. Keeping the damper or flue open until the fire is out will draw smoke out of the house. The damper can be checked by looking up into the chimney with a flashlight.
3. Use dry and well-aged wood. Wet or green wood causes more smoke and contributes to soot buildup in the chimney.
4. Smaller pieces of wood placed on a grate burn faster and produce less smoke.
5. Levels of ash at the base of the fireplace should be kept to 1 inch or less because a thicker layer restricts the air supply to logs, resulting in more smoke.
6. The chimney should be checked annually by a professional. Even if the chimney is not due for cleaning, it is important to check for animal nests or other blockages that could prevent smoke from escaping.

---

Q  *What levels of mold spores in indoor air are acceptable?*

A  There are some rules of thumb for assessing the number of mold spores found in the indoor air. Some investigators have categorized mean levels of culturable fungal counts into 5 groups.[37]

Group 1:  Low (<100 colony forming units [CFUs] per cubic meter [$m^3$])

Group 2:  Medium (101–300 CFUs/$m^3$)

Group 3:  High (301–1000 CFUs/$m^3$)

Group 4:  Very high (1001–5000 CFUs/$m^3$)

Group 5:  Extremely high (>5000 CFUs/$m^3$)

## Resources

American Lung Association, phone: 800-LUNG-USA.

US Environmental Protection Agency Indoor Air Quality Information Clearinghouse, phone: 800-438-4318. Additional resources from the EPA include EPA regional offices and state and local departments of health and environmental quality. For regulation of specific pollutants, contact the EPA Toxic Substances Control Act (TSCA) Assistance Information Service, phone: 202-554-1404.

US Consumer Product Safety Commission (CPSC), phone: 800-638-CPSC. The CPSC provides information on particular product hazards.

## References

1. Spengler JD. Sources and concentrations of indoor air pollution. In: Samet JM, Spengler JD, eds. *Indoor Air Pollution. A Health Perspective.* Baltimore, MD: Johns Hopkins University Press; 1991:33–67
2. US Environmental Protection Agency. *Indoor Air Pollution: An Introduction for Health Professionals.* Washington, DC: US Environmental Protection Agency; 1994. EPA Publication 523-217/81322
3. Lambert WE, Samet JM. Indoor air pollution. In: Harber P, Schenker MB, Balmes JR, eds. *Occupational and Environmental Respiratory Disease.* St Louis, MO: Mosby; 1996:784–807
4. Samet JM, Lambert WE, Skipper BJ, et al. Nitrogen dioxide and respiratory illnesses in infants. *Am Rev Respir Dis.* 1993;148:1258–1265
5. Robin LF, Less PS, Winget M, et al. Wood-burning stoves and lower respiratory illnesses in Navajo children. *Pediatr Infect Dis J.* 1996; 15:859–865
6. Honicky RE, Osborne JS III. Respiratory effects of wood heat: clinical observations and epidemiologic assessment. *Environ Health Perspect.* 1991;95:105–109
7. Morris K, Morgenlander M, Coulehan JL, Gahagen S, Arena VC, Morganlander M. Wood-burning stoves and lower respiratory tract infection in American Indian children. *Am J Dis Child.* 1990;144:105–108
8. Wallace LA. Volatile organic compounds. In: Samet JM, Spengler JD, eds. *Indoor Air Pollution: A Health Perspective.* Baltimore, MD: Johns Hopkins University Press; 1991:252–272
9. Molhave L. Indoor air pollution due to organic gases and vapours of solvents in building materials. *Environ Int.* 1982;8:117–127

10. Wallace LA. Human exposure to environmental pollutants: a decade of experience. *Clin Exp Allergy.* 1995;25:4–9

11. Ott WR, Roberts JW. Everyday exposure to toxic pollutants. *Sci Am.* 1998;278:86–91

12. Wallace LA. Comparison of risks from outdoor and indoor exposure to toxic chemicals. *Environ Health Perspect.* 1991;95:7–13

13. Norback D, Torgen M, Edling C. Volatile organic compounds, respirable dust, and personal factors related to prevalence and incidence of sick building syndrome in primary schools. *Br J Ind Med.* 1990;47:733–741

14. Gold DR. Indoor air pollution. *Clin Chest Med.* 1992;13:215–229

15. Wieslander G, Norback D, Bjornsson E, Janson C, Boman G. Asthma and the indoor environment: the significance of emission of formaldehyde and volatile organic compounds from newly painted indoor surfaces. *Int Arch Occup Environ Health.* 1997;69:115–124

16. Norback D, Bjornsson E, Janson C, Widstrom J, Boman G. Asthmatic symptoms and volatile organic compounds, formaldehyde, and carbon dioxide in dwellings. *Occup Environ Med.* 1995;52:388–395

17. Jo WK, Weisel CP, Lioy PJ. Chloroform exposure and the health risk associated with multiple uses of chlorinated tap water. *Risk Anal.* 1990; 10:581–585

18. Wantke F, Demmer CM, Tappler P, Gotz M, Jarisch R. Exposure to gaseous formaldehyde induces IgE-mediated sensitization to formaldehyde in school-children. Clin Exp Allergy. 1996;26:276–280

19. Liu KS, Huang FY, Hayward SB, Wesolowski J, Sexton K. Irritant effects of formaldehyde exposure in mobile homes. *Environ Health Perspect.* 1991;94:91–94

20. Krzyzanowski M, Quackenboss JJ, Lebowitz MD. Chronic respiratory effects of indoor formaldehyde exposure. *Environ Res.* 1990;52:117–125

21. Smedje G, Norback D, Edling C. Asthma among secondary school children in relation to the school environment. *Clin Exp Allergy.* 1997;27:1270–1278

22. West S, Hildesheim A, Dosemeci M. Non-viral risk factors for nasopharyngeal carcinoma in the Philippines: result from a case-control study. *Int J Cancer.* 1993;55:722–727

23. American Academy of Pediatrics Committee on Environmental Health. Toxic effects of indoor molds. *Pediatrics.* 1998;101:712–714

24. Dales RE, Zwanenburg H, Burnett R, Franklin CA. Respiratory health effects of home dampness and molds among Canadian children. *Am J Epidemiol.* 1991;134:196–203

25. Jaakkola JJ, Jaakkola N, Ruotsalainen R. Home dampness and molds as determinants of respiratory symptoms and asthma in pre-school children. *J Expo Anal Environ Epidemiol.* 1993;3(suppl 1):129–142

26. Verhoeff AP, van Strien RT, van Wijnen JH, Brunekreef B. Damp housing and childhood respiratory symptoms: the role of sensitization to dust mites and molds. *Am J Epidemiol.* 1995;141:103–110

27. Croft WA, Jarvis BB, Yatawara CS. Airborne outbreak of trichothecene toxicosis. *Atmos Environ.* 1986;20:549–552

28. Dearborn DG, Smith PG, Dahms BB, et al. Clinical profile of 30 infants with acute pulmonary hemorrhage in Cleveland. *Pediatrics.* 2002;110:627–637

29. Montaña E, Etzel RA, Allan T, Horgan TE, Dearborn DG. Environmental risk factors associated with pediatric idiopathic pulmonary hemorrhage and hemosiderosis in a Cleveland community. *Pediatrics.* 1997;99:e5 Available at: http://www.pediatrics.org/cgi/content/full/99/1/e5

30. Etzel RA, Montaña E, Sorenson WG, et al. Acute pulmonary hemorrhage in infants associated with exposure to *Stachybotrys atra* and other fungi. *Arch Pediatr Adolesc Med.* 1998;152:757–762

31. Etzel RA. Indoor air pollutants in homes and schools. *Pediatr Clin North Am.* 2001;48:1153–1165

32. Update: Pulmonary hemorrhage/hemosiderosis among infants— Cleveland, Ohio, 1993–1996. *MMWR Morb Mortal Wkly Rep.* 2000; 49:180–184

33. Jarvis BB, Sorenson WG, Hintikka EL, et al. Study of toxin production by isolates of *Stachybotrys chartarum* and *Memnoniella echinata* isolated during a study of pulmonary hemosiderosis in infants. *Appl Environ Microbiol.* 1998;64:3620–3625

34. Flappan SM, Portnoy J, Jones P, Barnes C. Infant pulmonary hemorrhage in a suburban home with water damage and mold *(Stachybotrys atra).* *Environ Health Perspect.* 1999;107:927–930

35. Weiss A, Chidekel AS. Acute pulmonary hemorrhage in a Delaware infant after exposure to *Stachybotrys atra. Del Med J.* 2002;74:363–368

36. Novotny WE, Dixit A. Pulmonary hemorrhage in an infant following two weeks of fungal exposure. *Arch Pediatr Adolesc Med.* 2000;154:271–275

37. Platt SD, Martin CJ, Hunt SM, Lewis CW. Damp housing, mould growth, and symptomatic health state. *BMJ.* 1989;298:1673–1678

# 7
# Air Pollutants, Outdoor

Individual outdoor air pollutants typically exist as part of a complex mixture of multiple pollutants. The potential health risk posed by outdoor air pollution varies by the concentration and composition of this mixture, which can vary by location, time of day or year, and weather conditions. The US Environmental Protection Agency (EPA) has established national ambient (outdoor) air quality standards for 6 principal pollutants referred to as "criteria" pollutants: ozone ($O_3$), respirable particulate matter ($PM_{10}$ and $PM_{2.5}$), lead, sulfur dioxide ($SO_2$), carbon monoxide (CO), and nitrogen oxides ($NO_x$).[1] In the United States, a national monitoring network has been established for these criteria pollutants, but about 300 monitoring sites across the country provide data on some other hazardous air pollutants. From 1980 to 1999, national levels of the criteria pollutants showed general improvements in the nation's air quality.[1] However, air quality in some areas of the United States actually declined during the 1990s, and recent scientific research suggests health effects at levels of some pollutants previously considered to be "safe." Outdoor air pollutants can come from many sources, including large industrial facilities; smaller industrial operations such as dry cleaners and gas stations; natural sources such as wildfires; highway vehicles; and other sources such as aircraft, locomotives, and lawn mowers. The relative importance of these different sources varies from one community to another.

## Ozone
Ozone is one of the most pervasive outdoor air pollutants. Ozone and other photochemical oxidants, such as peroxyacetylnitrate, are secondary pollutants formed in the atmosphere from a chemical

reaction between volatile organic compounds (VOCs) and $NO_x$ in the presence of heat and sunlight. The primary sources of these precursor compounds include motor vehicle exhaust and power plants, although hydrocarbon emissions from chemical plants and refineries and evaporative emissions from gasoline and natural sources also can contribute to their formation. The atmospheric movement of these precursor pollutants can affect ozone levels hundreds of miles downwind from the sources of these pollutants. Ozone is the principal component of urban smog. Levels of ozone generally are highest on hot, dry, stagnant summer days, and increase to maximum levels in the late afternoon. Changes in weather patterns can contribute to differences in ozone levels from year to year. Indoor concentrations of ozone can vary from 10% to 80% of outdoor levels, depending on the amount of fresh air entering the building.

**Particulate Matter**
Particulate matter is a general term that refers to a mixture of solid particles and liquid droplets. The term is applied to pollutants of varying chemical composition and physical properties. Particle size is the primary determinant of where the particles will be deposited in the respiratory system. Particles larger than 10 μm in aerodynamic diameter are too large to be inhaled beyond the nasal passages. Children, however, frequently breathe through their mouths, thus bypassing the nasal clearance mechanism.

All particulate matter less than 10 μm in aerodynamic diameter is known as $PM_{10}$. Particles of this size cannot be seen with the naked eye, but their presence in the atmosphere can be seen as sooty clouds or general haze that impairs visibility. Particulates smaller than 2.5 μm in aerodynamic diameter ($PM_{2.5}$) are referred to as "fine" particles. Fine particles result from the combustion of fuels used in motor vehicles, power plants, and industrial operations, as well as the combustion of organic material such as fires and woodstoves. Particles between 2.5 μm and 10 μm in aerodynamic diameter (or even larger) are referred to as "coarse" particles. Coarse particles can include dusts that have been generated from the mechanical breakdown of solid matter (such as rocks, soil, and dust) and windblown dust. Compared with coarse particles, fine particles can remain suspended in the atmosphere for longer periods and be transported over longer distances. As a result, the concentration of fine particles tends to be more uniformly distributed over large urban areas, whereas the concentration of coarse particles tends to be more localized near particular sources. While fine and coarse particles have been linked with adverse health effects, recent evidence suggests that fine particles have stronger respiratory effects in children than coarse particles.[2]

## Lead

While paint and soil generally are the most common sources of lead exposure for children (see Chapter 19), industrial operations such as ferrous and nonferrous smelters, battery manufacturers, and other sources of lead emissions can generate potentially harmful air emissions of lead. Before the introduction of unleaded gasoline in the United States, the use of leaded gasoline in motor vehicles was an important source of lead exposure for children. In many other countries, particularly developing countries, use of leaded gasoline continues. Together with the absence of stringent controls on automotive emissions and the volume of traffic, the use of leaded gasoline in some major cities of the developing world creates the potential for serious risks to children from mobile sources of lead exposure.[3]

## Sulfur Compounds

Sulfur-containing compounds include $SO_2$, sulfuric acid aerosol ($H_2SO_4$), and sulfate particles. The primary source of $SO_2$ is from the burning of coal and sulfur-containing oil; thus major emitters of $SO_2$ include coal-fired power plants, smelters, and pulp and paper mills. Sulfuric acid aerosol is formed in the atmosphere from the oxidation of $SO_2$ in the presence of moisture. Facilities that either manufacture or use acids also can emit $H_2SO_4$. Sulfate particles are formed in the atmosphere from the chemical reaction of sulfuric acid with ammonia and may be measured as fine particles ($PM_{2.5}$). In addition to adverse short-term and long-term health effects on the respiratory system, $SO_2$ contributes to the formation of acid rain.

## Carbon Monoxide and Nitrogen Dioxide

In addition to fine particles and photochemical pollution, motor vehicle emissions also contribute to outdoor levels of CO and $NO_2$. Another important source of $NO_x$ is fuel combustion from power plants. The emissions of $NO_x$ that lead to $NO_2$ also contribute to the formation of ozone and nitrogen-bearing particles (nitrates and nitric acid). Outdoors, CO occurs in areas of heavy traffic and is primarily a problem in cold weather. Indoor sources of CO and $NO_2$ can generate higher levels of exposure indoors than those typically measured outdoors (see chapters 6 and 10).

## Toxic Air Pollutants

Toxic air pollutants, also known as air toxics or hazardous air pollutants, represent a large group of substances, including volatile organic compounds (VOCs), heavy metals, solvents, and combustion by-products (such as dioxin), that are known or suspected to cause cancer or other serious health effects. There currently are 188 substances included on the list of hazardous air pollutants subject to emission regulations under the Clean Air Act. Some toxic air pollutants, such as benzene, 1,3-butadiene, and diesel exhaust, are emitted primarily from mobile sources such as cars and trucks. Other toxic air pollutants come primarily from large, stationary industrial facilities. Smaller area sources (such as dry cleaners) and indoor sources also can release toxic air pollutants. Indoor concentrations of 11 prevalent VOCs often exceed outdoor concentrations, and obvious industrial sources (such as chemical plants) contribute a relatively small proportion to the average person's total exposure to many of these substances (see Chapter 6).

## Traffic-Related Pollutants and Diesel Exhaust

In most urban areas, traffic-related emissions are a major source of air pollution. Increased incidence of wheezing, bronchitis, and asthma hospitalizations have been linked to residence near areas of high traffic density.[4-7] Epidemiologic studies suggest that diesel exhaust may be particularly harmful to children.[6] Diesel exhaust particles may enhance allergic and inflammatory responses to antigen challenge and may facilitate development of new allergies.[8,9] Diesel exhaust exposure may worsen symptoms in children with allergic rhinitis or asthma. Most US school buses run on diesel fuel; a child riding in a school bus may be exposed to as much as 4 times the level of diesel exhaust as one riding in a car.[10]

## Odors

The chemical identity of odors sometimes can be difficult to determine. Some common sources of odorous air pollution include sewage treatment plants, landfills, livestock feed lots, composts, pulp mills, geothermal plants, waste lagoons, tanneries, and petroleum refineries, among others. The odor of some compounds can be detected at levels below those generally recognized as posing a significant health risk. However, odors can negatively impact a person's quality of life and can exacerbate health problems among persons who are particularly sensitive to odors.[11] Hydrogen sulfide ($H_2S$), a fairly prevalent odorous air pollutant, is emitted as part of a variety of industrial processes, including oil refining, wood pulp production, and wastewater treatment, as well as from concentrated animal feeding operations, geothermal plants, and landfills. Hydrogen sulfide, also known as sewer gas, has an odor similar to that of rotten eggs.

## Routes of Exposure

The primary route of exposure to air pollution is through inhalation. Substances released into the atmosphere, however, can enter the hydrologic cycle as a result of atmospheric dispersion and precipitation and thus contaminate aquatic ecosystems. Similarly, deposition of suspended particulate matter occurs in soil. Thus material that was originally released into the atmosphere can be ingested as a result of the subsequent contamination of water, soil, or vegetation or the consumption of fish from contaminated waters. Some toxic air pollutants (such as mercury, lead, polychlorinated biphenyls, and dioxins) degrade very slowly or not at all and thus persist or accumulate in soil and the sediments of lakes and streams (see chapters 14 and 27).

## Systems Affected

Most of the common outdoor air pollutants are recognized irritants to the respiratory system, with ozone being the most potent irritant. Some toxic air pollutants are known to have other systemic effects (eg, cancer and impaired neurologic development), and the specific health risks from many of these toxic compounds (lead, mercury, carbon monoxide, dioxins, VOCs) are addressed in other chapters.

## Clinical Effects

Children are considered especially vulnerable to outdoor air pollution for several reasons. Because children tend to spend more time outside than adults, often while being physically active, they have a greater opportunity for exposure to pollutants. While playing or at rest, children breathe more rapidly and inhale more pollutants per pound of body weight than adults. In addition, because airway passages in children are narrower than those in adults, irritation caused by air pollution can result in proportionally greater airway obstruction. Unlike adults, children may not cease vigorous outdoor activities when bronchospasm occurs.

From the viewpoint of toxicity, the key distinguishing features of outdoor air pollutants are their chemical and physical characteristics and concentration. It is common for air pollutants to occur together; for example, on days when ozone levels are high, outdoor air levels of fine particles and acid aerosols also may be high. The combined effects of multiple pollutants are not completely understood but could produce synergistic effects.

In children, acute health effects associated with outdoor air pollution include increased respiratory symptoms, such as wheezing and cough, transient decrements in lung function, more serious lower respiratory tract infections, and increased school absenteeism due to respiratory illness.[12,13] Because children with asthma have increased airway reactivity, the effects of air pollution on the respiratory system can be more serious for them. Increases in the number of hospital emergency department admissions have been observed when air pollution levels are elevated, which commonly occurs in major urban areas.[14,15] Children with asthma have been shown to experience more respiratory symptoms, use extra medication, produce chronic phlegm, and have more bronchitis following exposure to high levels of particulate pollution.[16–18] In addition, children with asthma whose condition is not well managed and who may have exposures to other pollutants also can be more vulnerable to asthma attacks because of poor air quality.

Most of the acute respiratory effects of outdoor air pollution, such as symptoms of cough, shortness of breath, or decrements in lung function, are thought to be reversible, but recent studies indicate that long-term exposure to outdoor air pollution, particularly ozone and related co-pollutants, is associated with decrements in lung function among children.[19,20] Some of the increases in the prevalence of chronic obstructive lung disease in adults who live in more polluted areas could be the result of exposures that occurred during childhood.

## Treatment of Clinical Symptoms
The treatment of symptoms and the use of medication should be based on the usual clinical indications. A therapeutic regimen should not be changed in response to periods of poor air quality unless there is a clear indication of a change in a patient's respiratory symptoms or

function. However, it might be advisable to recommend restriction of strenuous physical activity during periods of poor air quality.

## Prevention of Exposure

Under the Clean Air Act, the EPA has the authority to set standards for air pollutants that protect the health of people with specific sensitivities, including children and those with asthma (see Table 7.1). The current US national ambient air quality standards are shown

**Table 7.1**
**Clean Air Act Amendments**

| |
| --- |
| **Setting Guidelines for Criteria Air Pollutants**<br>A few common air pollutants are regulated by first developing health-based criteria (science-based guidelines) as the basis for setting permissible levels. One set of limits (primary standard) protects health; another set of limits (secondary standard) is intended to prevent environmental and property damage. The criteria air pollutants are ozone, carbon monoxide, particulate matter, sulfur dioxide, lead, and nitrogen dioxide. |
| **Regulating Non-attainment Areas**<br>A non-attainment area is a geographic area whose air quality does not meet federal air quality standards designed to protect public health. Non-attainment areas are classified according to the severity of the area's air pollution problem. For ozone, these classifications are marginal, moderate, serious, severe, and extreme. The EPA assigns each non-attainment area to 1 of these categories, thus triggering varying requirements the area must comply with to meet the ozone standard. Similar programs exist for areas that do not meet the federal health standards for carbon monoxide and particulate matter. |
| **Regulating Mobile Sources**<br>Cars and trucks are the source for more than half of the pollutants that contribute to ozone and up to 90% of carbon monoxide emissions in urban areas. Tighter standards were established to reduce tail-pipe emissions and control fuel quality. Reformulated gasoline was required in the cities with the worst ozone problems, and oxygenated fuel was introduced in the winter months in areas that exceeded the carbon monoxide standard. |
| **Reducing Toxic Air Pollutants**<br>Toxic air pollutants are those pollutants that are hazardous to human health or the environment but are not specifically covered under another portion of the Clean Air Act. Emissions of toxic air pollutants are to be reduced through "maximum achievable control technology" standards for each major category of emissions sources. |

in Table 7.2. Although ambient concentrations of these 6 pollutants have decreased over the past decade, large numbers of people are still exposed to potentially unhealthful levels of these pollutants.

In November 1996 the EPA proposed revisions to the national ambient air quality standards for particulate matter and ozone, citing health risks to children as a major reason. For particulate matter, the new standard retains the current annual $PM_{10}$ standard of 50 µg/m³ but establishes a new annual standard for fine particulate matter ($PM_{2.5}$) of 15 µg/m³ and a new 24-hour standard (air measurement made for 24 hours) for $PM_{2.5}$ of 65 µg/m³. For ozone, the new standard replaced the former 1-hour standard of 0.12 ppm with an 8-hour standard of 0.08 ppm. It should be noted that there are different averaging times used for each pollutant. Final standards were adopted in 1997, and the US Supreme Court has upheld the scientific basis for the revised standards.

**Table 7.2**
**National Ambient Air Quality Standards (1997)**

| Pollutant | Ambient Air Limit | Averaging Time |
|-----------|-------------------|----------------|
| Ozone | 0.08 ppm | 8 h |
| $PM_{10}$* | 50 µg/m³<br>150 µg/m³ | Annual arithmetic mean<br>24 h |
| $PM_{2.5}$† | 15 µg/m³<br>65 µg/m³ | Annual arithmetic mean<br>24 h |
| Sulfur dioxide | 0.03 ppm<br>0.14 ppm | Annual arithmetic mean<br>24 h |
| Nitrogen dioxide | 0.053 ppm | Annual arithmetic mean |
| Carbon monoxide | 9 ppm<br>35 ppm | 8 h<br>1 h |
| Lead | 1.5 µg/m³ | Quarterly |

*Particles up to 10 µm in aerodynamic diameter.
†Particles up to 2.5 µm in aerodynamic diameter.

Emission standards were developed for only a few of the hazardous air pollutants prior to the passage of the Clean Air Act amendments of 1990. These amendments gave the EPA the authority to develop technology-based emission standards for an initial list of 189 hazardous air pollutants (currently 188 pollutants). Although these standards also are designed to protect public health, they are based on the available technology to control emissions.

## Frequently Asked Questions

Q *How can I find out about the levels of air pollution in my community?*

A Most large metropolitan areas are required to regularly monitor air quality for one or more of the national ambient (outdoor) air quality standards. The result of air quality monitoring is expressed as the Pollutant Standards Index, which also is commonly known as the Air Quality Index (AQI). The AQI converts the concentrations of 5 specific pollutants (CO, ozone, $NO_2$, $SO_2$, and particulate matter) into one number, scaled from 0 to 500. The AQI value of 100 corresponds to the short-term national ambient air quality standard. Thus an AQI value above 100 indicates that the concentration of one or more pollutants exceeds its national standard. The descriptor terms associated with different AQI values are as follows: 0 to 50 = "good"; 51 to 100 = "moderate"; 101 to 150 = "unhealthy for sensitive groups"; 151 to 200 = "unhealthy"; 201 to 300 = "very unhealthy"; 301 to 500 = "hazardous." Table 7.3 gives additional information about the AQI.[21]

Information about the air quality in a community often is made available through local news media. Parents can contact their state department of environmental protection or the nearest EPA regional office for more information about air quality measurements in their community. Environmental information about a particular ZIP code area can be retrieved from the EPA Web site at http://www.epa.gov/epahome/whereyoulive.htm.

**Table 7.3**
**Air Quality Index (AQI) and Associated General Health Effects
and Cautionary Statements\***

| Index Value | AQI Descriptor | General Health Effects | General Cautionary Statements |
|---|---|---|---|
| 0–50 | Good | None for the general population. | None required. |
| 51–100 | Moderate | Few or none for the general population. Possibility of aggravation of heart or lung disease among persons with cardiopulmonary disease and the elderly with elevations of $PM_{2.5}$.[†] | Unusually sensitive people should consider limiting prolonged outdoor exertion. |
| 101–150 | Unhealthy for sensitive groups | Mild aggravation of respiratory symptoms among susceptible people. | Active children and adults and people with respiratory disease (such as asthma) and cardiopulmonary disease should avoid prolonged outdoor exertion. |
| 151–200 | Unhealthy | Significant aggravation of symptoms and decreased exercise tolerance in persons with heart or lung disease. Possible respiratory effects in the general population. | Active children and adults and people with respiratory and cardiovascular disease should avoid prolonged outdoor exertion. Everyone else, especially children, should limit prolonged outdoor exertion. |
| 201–300 | Very unhealthy | Increasingly severe symptoms and Impaired breathing likely in sensitive groups. Increasing likelihood of respiratory effects in the general population. | Active children and adults and people with respiratory and cardiovascular disease should avoid all outdoor exertion. All others should limit outdoor exertion. |
| 301+ | Hazardous | Severe respiratory effects and impaired breathing in sensitive groups, with serious risk of premature mortality in persons with cardiopulmonary disease and the elderly. Increasingly severe respiratory effects in the general population. | Elderly and persons with existing respiratory and cardiovascular diseases should stay indoors with the windows closed. Everyone should avoid outside physical exertion. |

\*From US Environmental Protection Agency (1999).
†Particles up to 2.5 μm in aerodynamic diameter.

Q *What can be done to protect my children from outdoor air pollution when they want and need to be able to play outdoors?*

A The potential harm posed by outdoor air pollution depends on the concentration of pollutants, which can vary from day to day and even during the course of a day. While exposure to outdoor air pollutants cannot be entirely prevented, it can be reduced by restricting the amount of time that children spend outdoors during periods of poor air quality, especially time spent engaged in strenuous physical activity. For example, ozone levels during the summer tend to be highest in the middle to late afternoon. On days when ozone levels are expected or reported to be high, outdoor activities could be restricted during the afternoon or rescheduled to the morning, particularly for children who have exhibited sensitivity to high levels of air pollution. In many areas, local radio stations, television news programs, and newspapers regularly provide information on air quality conditions.

Q *The recommendation to exercise in the early morning often conflicts with the reality of children's sports activity schedules. Should organized sports activities be cancelled on days when air quality is poor?*

A Children should be encouraged to participate in physical activities because of the many health benefits associated with exercise. In most instances, the health benefits of physical activity likely outweigh the potential harm posed by intermittent or moderate levels of air pollution. However, on hot summer days when temperatures as well as smog levels are high, this balance could shift and it may be advisable to shorten or cancel outdoor physical activities, especially for young children. When children have asthma, physicians aim for optimal asthma control so that the asthma remains controlled and children can participate in normal outdoor sports activities, even on days with poor air quality. When asthma is unstable, children need to taper or hold off on their physical activities until their asthma becomes controlled again. Recent evidence suggests that children who exercise heavily (participating in 3 or more sports) and who live in communities with high levels of ozone pollution may experience a higher risk of developing asthma compared with children who don't play sports.[22]

Q *My family lives in an area that places them at risk for exposure to increased levels of outdoor air pollution. How can I help my child with asthma?*

A It is very appropriate for parents to discuss their concerns about air pollution and other possible asthma triggers with their child's physician. A child's entire environment, including the home, school, and playground, should be reviewed for possible exposures to asthma triggers. Improved medical management of the child's asthma and control of exposure to allergens and irritants in the child's home may be very effective in preventing asthma exacerbations. If a parent or a physician believes that emissions from a particular facility are harmful to a child with asthma, this information should be shared with the local or state environmental agencies that have authority over operating permits and enforcement actions.

Q *Would face dust masks be effective for protecting my children when air pollution levels are high?*

A Dust masks and other forms of respiratory protection, which are sized for adults and not children, are not recommended for protection against outdoor air pollution. Not only do poor fit and uncertain compliance limit any potential benefits, but most simple dust masks do not include the materials needed to filter out harmful VOCs or ozone.

Q *What is the relationship between ozone in urban smog and stratospheric ozone?*

A These issues are unrelated. Ozone in the troposphere, or ground level, is a major component of urban smog and a respiratory health hazard. The formation of ground-level ozone is independent of ozone in the upper atmosphere, or stratosphere. Stratospheric ozone provides a protective shield absorbing harmful ultraviolet (UV) radiation. Too little stratospheric ozone increases the risk of skin cancer and eye damage from UV rays.

Q *Why is asthma on the increase?*

A Scientists and public health officials are concerned by the apparent increase in the prevalence of asthma. The explanation for the increase has not been found but seems most likely to be related to a complex combination of factors, including increased exposure to environmental allergens and irritants indoors; increased exposure to complex environmental pollutants such as environmental tobacco smoke, diesel exhaust, and irritant gases during the early postnatal period of life; delayed maturation of immune responses due to changes in exposure to infection and infectious products; dietary factors; and psychosocial factors (such as stress and poverty).[23,24] The increase in asthma does not seem to be related to outdoor air pollution.

Q *Are odors from hog farms harmful to children?*

A Odors are an indicator of the presence of chemical emissions. Emissions from hog farms include VOCs, $H_2S$, ammonia, endotoxins, and organic dusts. At sufficient concentrations over extended periods, there is ample evidence that these chemicals can cause disease. Whether the level and duration of exposures from emissions from hog farms is sufficient to cause harm to children is not known.[25] We do know, however, that odors can impact people through psychophysiological mechanisms, resulting in increased respiratory symptoms and other indicators of reduced quality of life.[11]

Q  *What air pollutants were released after the World Trade Center disaster?*

A  The destruction of the World Trade Center on September 11, 2001, released vast amounts of toxic materials into the air of New York City. These materials included

- *Asbestos.* Chrysotile asbestos was used as structural fireproofing in the North Tower up to the 40th story. Some of the asbestos had been removed in the years since the construction of the tower, but many hundreds of tons remained and were released into the air when the towers collapsed. Elevated airborne levels of asbestos were detected for the first several days after the disaster but not thereafter. Quantities of asbestos also entered some of the apartment and office buildings near the World Trade Center where they posed a potential hazard to children and other residents.

- *Airborne Particulates.* Thousands of tons of particulates were liberated by the collapse of the towers. Much of this material consisted of pulverized cement dust with a pH of 11. This material is extremely irritating. New cases of asthma and reactive airways disease as well as exacerbations of existing cases have been seen in exposed persons.

- *Polycyclic Aromatic Hydrocarbons (PAHs).* Carcinogenic PAHs were released into the atmosphere by the fires. Elevated levels of PAHs were detectable in lower Manhattan for several weeks after September 11th.

- *Volatile Organic Compounds.* Volatile organic compounds were released as combustion by-products.

- *Lead.* Many hundreds of pounds of lead were present in computers. Some of this lead was liberated. Elevated levels were detected in air samples during the first week after the collapse.

- *Dioxins and Furans.* Toxic and carcinogenic dioxins and furans were liberated as products of combustion.

In general, levels of airborne pollutants were highest on September 11th and in the first days and weeks after the collapse of the towers, and diminished thereafter. Levels of particulates remained above background in New York City until December, when the fires at the disaster site were finally extinguished. Levels of pollutants tended to be higher at night, when the air was still, and to diminish during the day.

Pediatricians advised parents and children in Manhattan in the days and weeks after September 11th to stay indoors and to minimize outdoor exercise. Pediatricians also advised parents to have apartments cleaned by properly trained contractors, certified by the EPA in the removal of asbestos.

New cases of asthma and exacerbations of existing cases have been seen in children exposed to air pollution since September 11th. The long-term health consequences, particularly of exposure to asbestos, will be ascertained only through prospective follow-up study.

## Resources

American Lung Association, phone: 212-315-8700, local associations phone: 800-LUNG-USA, Internet: www.lungusa.org

The Health Effects Institute, phone: 617-886-9330, fax: 617-886-9335, Internet: www.healtheffects.org

US Environmental Protection Agency, Air Risk Information Support Center, Office of Air Quality Planning and Standards, phone: 919-541-0888, fax: 919-541-1818, Internet: www.epa.gov/airnow/publications.html

## References

1. US Environmental Protection Agency. *National Air Quality and Emissions Trends Report, 1999.* Washington, DC: Office of Air Quality Planning and Standards; 2001. EPA Publication 454/R-01-004
2. World Health Organization. *Air Quality Guidelines.* Geneva, Switzerland: Department of Protection of the Human Environment; 1999

3. Schwartz J, Neas LM. Fine particles are more strongly associated than coarse particles with acute respiratory health effects in school children. *Epidemiology.* 2000;11:6–10

4. Edwards J, Walters S, Griffiths RK. Hospital admissions for asthma in preschool children: relationship to major roads in Birmingham, United Kingdom. *Arch Environ Health.* 1994;49:223–227

5. van Vliet P, Knape M, de Hartog J, Janssen N, Harssema H, Brunekreef B. Motor vehicle exhaust and chronic respiratory symptoms in children living near freeways. *Environ Res.* 1997;74:122–132

6. Brunekreef B, Janssen NA, de Hartog J, Harssema H, Knape M, van Vliet P. Air pollution from truck traffic and lung function in children living near motorways. *Epidemiology.* 1997;8:298–303

7. Ciccone G, Forastiere F, Agabiti N, et al. Road traffic and adverse respiratory effects in children. SIDRA Collaborative Group. *Occup Environ Med.* 1998;55:771–778

8. Diaz-Sanchez D, Garcia MP, Wang M, Jyrala M, Saxon A. Nasal challenge with diesel exhaust particles can induce sensitization to a neoallergen in the human mucosa. *J Allergy Clin Immunol.* 1999;104:1183–1188

9. Nel AE, Diaz-Sanchez D, Ng D, Hiura T, Saxon A. Enhancement of allergic inflammation by the interaction between diesel exhaust particles and the immune system. *J Allergy Clin Immunol.* 1998;102:539–554

10. Natural Resources Defense Council. *No Breathing in the Aisles: Diesel Exhaust Inside School Buses.* San Francisco, CA. National Resources Defense Council; 2001

11. Shusterman D. Odor-associated health complaints: competing explanatory models. *Chem Senses.* 2001;26:339–343

12. Bates DV. The effects of air pollution on children. *Environ Health Perspect.* 1995;103(suppl 6):49–53

13. Gilliland FD, Berhane K, Rappaport EB, et al. The effects of ambient air pollution on school absenteeism due to respiratory illnesses. *Epidemiology.* 2001;12:43–54

14. Tolbert PE, Mulholland JA, MacIntosh DL, et al. Air quality and pediatric emergency room visits for asthma in Atlanta, Georgia USA. *Am J Epidemiol.* 2000;151:798–810

15. Committee of the Environmental and Occupational Health Assembly of the American Thoracic Society. Health effects of outdoor air pollution. *Am J Respir Crit Care Med.* 1996;153:3–50, 477–498

16. Ostro B, Lipsett M, Mann J, Braxton-Owens H, White M. Air pollution and exacerbation of asthma in African-American children in Los Angeles. *Epidemiology.* 2001;12:200–208

17. White MC, Etzel RA, Wilcox WD, Lloyd C. Exacerbations of childhood asthma and ozone pollution in Atlanta. *Environ Res.* 1994;65:125–134

18. McConnell R, Berhane K, Gilliland F, et al. Air pollution and bronchitic symptoms in Southern California children with asthma. *Environ Health Perspect.* 1999;107:757–760

19. Gauderman WJ, Gilliland GF, Vora H, et al. Association between air pollution and lung function growth in southern California children: results from a second cohort. *Am J Respir Crit Care Med.* 2002;166:76–84

20. Tager IB. Air pollution and lung function growth: is it ozone? *Am J Respir Crit Care Med.* 1999;160:387–389

21. US Environmental Protection Agency. *Guidelines for Reporting of Daily Air Quality Index (AQI).* Washington, DC: US Environmental Protection Agency; 1999. EPA-454/R-99-010

22. McConnell R, Berhane K, Gilliland F, et al. Asthma in exercising children exposed to ozone: a cohort study. *Lancet.* 2002;359:386–391

23. Plopper CG, Fanucchi MV. Do urban environmental pollutants exacerbate childhood lung diseases? *Environ Health Perspect.* 2000;108:A252–A253

24. Gergen PJ. Remembering the patient. *Arch Pediatr Adolesc Med.* 2000; 154:977–978

25. Merchant JA, Kline J, Donham KJ, Bundy DS, Hodne CJ. Human health effects. In: *Iowa Concentrated Animal Feeding Operation Air Quality Study, Final Report.* Ames, IA: Iowa State University and the University of Iowa Study Group; 2002:121–145. Available at: http://www.public-health.uiowa.edu/ehsrc/CAFOstudy.htm

# 8
# Arsenic

Arsenic (As) is the 20th most abundant element in the earth's crust. Commonly referred to as a heavy metal (density >5 g/cm³), this element has been recognized for centuries as a valuable substance with many potential uses as well as a highly effective poison that is toxic to virtually all members of the animal kingdom, from insects to humans. In recent years, the scope of human exposure and the associated health consequences have led to the passage of federal rules designed to protect the public from excessive exposure to arsenic.

Children may have greater exposure to arsenic than adults. Because many aspects of organogenesis and organ maturity take place during childhood, exposure to arsenic, which has antimetabolic and carcinogenic properties, may have greater impact on children.

Arsenic exists naturally in inorganic and organic forms. Inorganic arsenic is found in trivalent (arsenite) and pentavalent (arsenate) forms. Trivalent arsenic is substantially more toxic and carcinogenic than pentavalent. Most industrial uses of arsenic employ the trivalent form.

There are several forms of organic arsenic, including methylarsonic and dimethylarsinic acids.[1] All naturally occurring forms of organic arsenic are thought to be relatively nontoxic. Organic arsenicals that have been developed as pesticides (eg, dimethylarsinic acid) are very toxic.

## Routes of Exposure

Arsenic can be ingested or inhaled. There is no significant exposure through intact skin. Arsenic can be transmitted through the placenta.

## Sources of Exposure

### *Natural*

Arsenic is distributed in the earth in discrete locations or "veins." In the United States, higher concentrations are found in the southwestern states, eastern Michigan, and parts of New England.[2] Large veins of arsenic in bedrock can create contaminated swaths adjacent to areas with little to no arsenic. Groundwater in contact with arsenic veins can produce significant concentrations of arsenic in untreated well water. Arsenic in the earth's crust leaches into ocean water where it is ingested by marine life, thus entering the food chain.

### *Anthropogenic*

Arsenic has been used industrially for many purposes, including pest control, and in the semiconductor, petroleum refining, and mining/smelting industries.[2] Its reliable toxicity contributed to arsenic's widespread use as a pesticide and antimicrobial. Before safer alternatives were found, arsenic commonly was administered to humans for treatment of syphilis, trypanosomiasis, and other infections,[3] and for skin conditions (where it was known as Fowler solution). As a pesticide, arsenic was broadly used until the ban of most arsenical pesticides by the US Environmental Protection Agency (EPA) in 1991. Until the 1991 ban, sodium arsenate (Terro®) was a common ant killer for home use. Of note, one arsenic-based pesticide that was exempt from this ban is copper chromium arsenate (CCA), a wood preservative (see Chapter 24). Pressure-treated wood is impregnated with the compound CCA to prevent termites and other pests from accelerating the decomposition of wood. Copper chromium arsenate contains 22% arsenic by weight; a 12-ft section of pressure-treated wood contains approximately 1 oz of arsenic.[4] Gallium arsenide, another form of arsenic, is a semiconductor that often is used in place of silicon.[1] Finally, arsenic may be found in alternative medications including Chinese proprietary medicines and herbal remedies.[5]

As a result of anthropogenic use, arsenic is widely distributed in the environment. For example, it has been found at 1014 of the 1598 National Priorities List sites identified by the Agency for Toxic Substances and Disease Registry and the EPA.[6]

With its widespread presence in nature, along with extensive industrial uses, human exposure to arsenic can be extensive. Industrial emissions, including incineration, can release arsenic into ambient air. Water, particularly unprocessed well water, may have significant inorganic arsenic contamination.[7] Many small water systems and private wells do not have arsenic treatment installed. Even treated water may be left with residual concentrations of arsenic, depending on the efficacy of the purification technique.

Foods, particularly seafood, can contain large quantities of organic arsenic; shellfish (eg, oysters and lobster) can have extremely large concentrations (as much as 120 ppm vs 2–8 ppm in fish).[3] Such arsenic, however, is in a much less toxic form, so there is no concern about eating these foods.

Although arsenic pesticides have been banned, foods still can be contaminated with arsenic from past use, inadvertent use, or misuse of pesticides. Pesticidal forms of arsenic are very toxic, and such food could likely be unsafe for children's consumption. The US Food and Drug Administration (FDA) estimates that a 6-year-old child consumes an average of 4.6 µg of inorganic arsenic daily in food. Exposure to inorganic arsenic in water, while highly variable, is estimated to be up to 4.5 µg daily.[4]

Soil contamination by arsenic (eg, from nearby mining, hazardous waste sites, and agricultural use) can expose children playing nearby and can contaminate clothes and be brought into the home. Pressure-treated wood may be a potential source of children's exposure to arsenic, in part because of its ubiquity and because children routinely play on these surfaces on home decks or playgrounds. Recent data suggest that arsenic in pressure-treated wood can slowly leach out of the wood over time, resulting in increased concentrations of arsenic in soil.[4] When these are sites where children play, children's exposure to arsenic by inadvertent ingestion is amplified. According to the EPA, simple rubbing of hands on the surface of pressure-treated wood can transfer small amounts of arsenic to the hands.[4] Coupled with the normal hand-to-mouth activity of children, play around pressure-treated wood has the potential to produce an increased body burden of arsenic; one environmental group has estimated that children could be exposed to many times the "safe" lifetime exposure level for cancer (1 in a million).[4] Even more exposure could be created by sawing CCA-treated wood or burning it. There is a case report of mild arsenic poisoning in a family of 8 exposed to the fumes from the burning of CCA-treated wood[8] (see Chapter 24).

## Toxicokinetics, Biological Fate

Arsenic is well absorbed after its inhalation or ingestion. In animal models, gastrointestinal absorption of arsenic is increased in the presence of iron deficiency. Once absorbed, arsenic's half-life in blood is 10 hours. Circulating arsenic crosses the placenta and can result in elevated arsenic concentrations in the newborn and even fetal demise.[1] Humans are able to detoxify absorbed inorganic arsenic by transforming it to organic species including monomethylarsenate, dimethylarsenate, or trimethylarsenate forms. Children are less able than adults to methylate arsenic, consequently having more persistent concentrations of the toxic inorganic metal.[4]

Elimination of arsenic is almost exclusively renal; only 10% is excreted in bile. The average concentration of arsenic in urine is less than 25 μg/L. Within 2 to 4 weeks after exposure, the remaining body burden of arsenic is found in hair, skin, and nails.[1]

## Systems Affected

Arsenic affects every organ. Its primary action is as an antimetabolite. The mechanism of arsenic toxicity includes its replacement of phosphate molecules in adenosine triphosphate (ATP) (arsenolysis) as well as potent inhibitory effects on key enzymes, including thiamine pyrophosphate. Arsenic recently has been shown to have endocrine-disrupting effects, inhibiting glucocorticoid-mediated transcription.[9] The clinical significance of this finding is unknown. Primary target organs for arsenic effects are the gastrointestinal tract and skin (because these are the most metabolically active tissues in the body). Arsenic exposure is associated with an increased risk of diabetes mellitus.[4,9]

## Clinical Effects

The characteristics of arsenic toxicity are different for acute versus chronic exposures. Acute, high-dose exposure to inorganic arsenic (>3–5 mg/kg) affects all major organs including the gastrointestinal tract, brain, heart, kidneys, liver, bone marrow, skin, and peripheral nervous system. Severe ingestions lead within 30 minutes to gastrointestinal injury manifested by nausea, vomiting, hematemesis, diarrhea, and abdominal cramping. Intractable shock can ensue.[10] Lower-dose exposures result in a more protracted course: initial signs of gastrointestinal upset are followed by bone marrow suppression with pancytopenia, hepatic dysfunction, myocardial depression with cardiac conduction disturbances, and a peripheral neuropathy.[11] The peripheral neuropathy of arsenic is of the sensorimotor type, typically involving the lower extremity more than upper extremity, and generally is stocking-glove in distribution. The early sign consists of ascending paresthesias quickly followed by loss of proprioception, anesthesia and weakness, a clinical picture that mimics Guillain-Barré syndrome. Severe central nervous system dysfunction is uncommon. Many of these effects can be permanent. A characteristic feature of acute arsenic exposure is the appearance of Mees lines (white, transverse creases across the fingernails).

Chronic exposure may produce generalized fatigue and malaise. Bone marrow depression, if present, is low grade. Other complications include malnutrition and inanition, and increased risk for infections, particularly pneumonia. There also may be signs of specific organ malfunction, such as neurologic or hepatic dysfunction, or skin rashes. Skin changes of arsenic poisoning include eczematoid eruptions, hyperkeratosis, and melanosis. The fingernails may contain Mees lines. Alopecia also may occur.[1,3,6,11]

Arsenic is classified as a known human carcinogen by the National Toxicology Program[12] and the International Agency for Research on Cancer.[13] Chronic exposure is associated, in a dose-response relationship, with an increased risk of bladder, lung, and skin cancers.[12] Arsenic also has been associated with an excess risk of acute myelogenous leukemia, aplastic anemia, and cancers of the kidney and liver.[1] The chronic consumption of water contaminated with arsenic in a concentration of 500 ppm ($\mu$g/L) is associated with an estimated risk of 1 in 10 people developing lung, bladder, or skin cancer. At the current federal water standard of 50 ppb ($\mu$g/L), cancer mortality is estimated to be in the range of 0.6 to 1.5 per 100, or about 1 in 100.[14] At 10 ppb, the EPA standard for drinking water to be phased in over the next few years, the risk of bladder or lung cancer is 1 to 3 per 1000. Even arsenic concentrations of 3 ppb are associated with lifetime risk for bladder and lung cancer at 4 to 10 per 10 000.[12] Given that federal standards for environmental carcinogens historically have been set at concentrations that produce a cancer risk in the range of 1 in 1 million, the allowable amount of arsenic in drinking water confers an unusually high risk.

Due to transplacental transmission of arsenic, women chronically exposed to arsenic-contaminated water are at increased risk for spontaneous abortion, stillbirth, and preterm birth.[15] While inorganic arsenic is teratogenic in animals, it has not been clearly shown to have teratogenicity in humans.[1]

## Diagnostic Methods

Because most arsenic is excreted in urine, the diagnostic test of choice is a urine collection.[11] In adult patients the concentration of arsenic in a single urine specimen is commonly measured, adjusting the concentration to the concentration of urinary creatinine. Such "spot" urine tests for arsenic have not been validated in children and are not recommended. Rather, a timed urinary collection for 8 to 24 hours is preferred. The method most commonly used for arsenic measurement in urine does not distinguish organic from more toxic inorganic forms. Therefore, in circumstances where it is important to determine the form of arsenic, the pediatrician should request that the urinary arsenic be speciated or fractionated. Alternatively, to establish a diagnosis of intoxication by inorganic arsenic, patients should abstain from ingestion of all seafood for at least 2 to 5 days prior to conducting the urine collection. Because the half-life of arsenic in blood is short, its measurement in blood is not recommended.

Hair and fingernail analyses have been used for the diagnosis of arsenic exposure. However, like hair analysis for most other environmental agents, its validity has not been proven.[11] While techniques including segmental analysis and use of pubic hair may improve the reliability of hair analysis, hair should not be the sole specimen analyzed for the diagnosis of arsenic poisoning. Similarly, fingernail analysis is not sufficiently sensitive to establish the diagnosis of arsenic poisoning. Therefore, neither hair nor nail analysis is recommended.[1,16]

## Treatment

If a diagnosis of significant arsenic exposure is established, chelation therapy may be indicated. Chelators that have been demonstrated to be effective in accelerating arsenic clearance are dimercaprol (BAL), d-penicillamine, and succimer.[7] As with all metal intoxications, chelation therapy should be undertaken only in consultation with a toxicologist.

## Prevention of Exposure

Public health policies primarily have focused on control of arsenic in water. The EPA, through the Safe Drinking Water Act, is required to regulate the concentration of water contaminants, including arsenic. Since 1947 the maximum contaminant level of arsenic in water has been 50 ppb. After recent recommendations by the Institute of Medicine to lower the acceptable standard to 10 ppb, the EPA has announced plans to implement this change. However, this change will be phased in over a number of years, more so in the case of small water systems that can make a case for financial hardship. There have been recommendations to reduce the standard to 3 ppb, although even at 3 ppb cancer mortality risk exceeds 1 in 10 000.[14] However, concentrations of arsenic in water lower than 3 ppb currently are not achievable by municipal systems at reasonable cost with existing technology.

The World Health Organization recommends a water standard of 10 ppb.[2] Other guidelines to the public include the recommendation that all drinking water wells be tested for arsenic.[7] In areas with large water systems, water will be tested for arsenic by the water company or provider. Water providers are required to inform consumers when water fails to meet drinking water standards. In areas with elevated levels of arsenic in drinking water, home water treatment devices are available; however, these have varying efficacy at removing arsenic. In addition, bottled water is an option. Boiling water and filtering water through charcoal filters will not remove arsenic.

The use of CCA in pressure-treated wood for residential uses will voluntarily cease as of December 31, 2003, as a result of an agreement between the manufacturers and EPA. However, existing structures will continue to be potential sources of concern, and wood treated by manufacturers prior to that date still may be available for sale.

**Frequently Asked Questions**

Q *What precautions should I take about my young children's exposure to the pressure-treated wood on my deck and playground structure?*

A Copper chromium arsenate is a pesticide used in pressure-treated wood to prolong its useful life. Copper chromium arsenate–treated wood commonly is used for decking, poles that are sunk in the ground, raised beds for gardens, and playground play structures. With aging of the wood and exposure to water, arsenic may be leached out and be present on the wood surface and in soil under decks or in garden beds made of CCA-treated lumber. Touching treated wood or contaminated soils and then engaging in hand-to-mouth activities may result in significant childhood exposure to arsenic, a known human carcinogen.[17,18] In several countries that have banned or severely restricted the use of CCA, as is now under way in the United States, alternative treatments are available. Currently there is limited availability of lumber treated with these chemicals in the United States.[19] Coating treated wood with a sealant at least every year (in accordance with wood manufacturers' recommendations) will reduce arsenic leaching.[20]

1. When possible use alternatives to CCA-treated wood for new outdoor structures including rot-resistant woods.
2. Keep children and pets out from under deck areas from which arsenic may have leached.
3. Do not use CCA-treated wood for raised gardens, and do not grow vegetables near CCA-treated decks.
4. Never burn CCA-treated wood.
5. Make sure that children wash their hands after playing on CCA-treated surfaces, particularly before eating.
6. Cover picnic tables that are made with treated wood with a plastic cover before placing food on the table.

Further information is available in a fact sheet from the Connecticut Department of Public Health, available at http://www.dph.state.ct.us/publications/bch/eeoh/pressurtr.pdf.

Q *What types of coatings are most effective to reduce leaching of arsenic from CCA-treated wood?*

A Some studies suggest that applying certain penetrating coatings (eg, oil-based, semitransparent stains) on a regular basis (once per year or every other year depending on wear and weathering) may reduce the migration of wood preservative chemicals from CCA-treated wood. In selecting a finish, consumers should be aware that, in some cases, "film-forming," non-penetrating stains (eg, latex semitransparent, latex opaque, and oil-based opaque stains) on outdoor surfaces such as decks and fences are not recommended because they are less durable. Talk with a hardware or paint store about appropriate coatings in your area.

Q *My child's child care center, which has a large play structure built from pressure-treated wood, was recently found to have soil arsenic concentrations of 80 ppm. Should I be concerned?*

A Cleanup standards for arsenic in soil are established by federal (EPA) and state guidelines. State guidelines are highly variable, depending on background concentrations of arsenic in soil, and range from 10 to 1000 ppm. Based on conservative risk estimates, remediation should be considered when the soil arsenic concentration in areas where children routinely play exceeds 20 to 40 ppm. Options, depending on concentration, include placement of a ground cover (eg, additional soil) or removal. If the source of arsenic is determined to be the structure, and not background activity, the child care center also should develop a plan for frequent application of a wood sealant or other barrier while plans for the structure's eventual removal are developed.

Q  *Do I need to limit my child's seafood consumption because of possible arsenic contamination? Are there ever fish advisories about arsenic like there are for mercury and polychlorinated biphenyls?*

A  The arsenic in seafood is organic, a form that has not been associated with toxicity. Therefore, there is no reason to limit your child's consumption of seafood as an arsenic avoidance measure.

## Resource

Massachusetts Department of Public Health. Pressure Treated Wood Use in Playground Equipment. Massachusetts Department of Public Health; 2000. Available at: http://www.state.ma.us/dph/beha/wood/dphptw.htm

## References

1. Dart RC. Arsenic. In: Sullivan JB, Krieger GR, eds. *Hazardous Materials Toxicology—Clinical Principles of Environmental Health.* Baltimore, MD: Williams & Wilkins; 1992:818–824

2. Breslin K. Safer sips: removing arsenic from drinking water. *Environ Health Perspect.* 1998;106:A548–A550

3. Malachowski ME. An update on arsenic. *Clin Lab Med.* 1990;10:459–472

4. Environmental Working Group. *Poisoned Playgrounds.* Washington, DC: Environmental Working Group; 2001. Available at: http://www.ewg.org/pub/home/reports/poisonedplaygrounds/

5. Espinoza EO, Mann MJ, Bleasdell B. Arsenic and mercury in traditional Chinese herbal balls. *N Engl J Med.* 1995;333:803–804

6. Agency for Toxic Substances and Disease Registry. *Arsenic.* Atlanta, GA: Agency for Toxic Substances and Disease Registry; 2001

7. Franzblau A, Lilis R. Acute arsenic intoxication from environmental arsenic exposure. *Arch Environ Health.* 1989;44:385–390

8. Peters HA, Croft WA, Woolson EA, Darcey BA, Olson MA. Seasonal arsenic exposure from burning chromium-copper-arsenate–treated wood. *JAMA.* 1984;251:2393–2396

9. Kaltreider RC, Davis AM, Lariviere JP, Hamilton JW. Arsenic alters the function of the glucocorticoid receptor as a transcription factor. *Environ Health Perspect.* 2001;109:245–251

10. Levin-Scherz JK, Patrick JD, Weber FH, Gamabedian C Jr. Acute arsenic ingestion. *Ann Emerg Med.* 1987;16:702–704

11. Landrigan PJ. Arsenic—state of the art. *Am J Ind Med.* 1981;2:5–14

12. National Toxicology Program. *10th Report on Carcinogens.* Washington, DC: US Department of Health and Human Services Public Health Service; 2002. Available at: http://ehp.niehs.nih.gov/roc/toc10.html

13. International Agency for Research on Cancer. *Overall Evaluations of Carcinogenicity.* IARC Monographs. Lyon, France: International Agency for Research on Cancer; 1987;suppl 7

14. National Research Council. *Arsenic in Drinking Water: 2001 Update.* Washington, DC: National Academies Press; 2001. Available at: http://www.nap.edu/books/0309076293/html/

15. Ahmad SA, Sayed MH, Barua S, et al. Arsenic in drinking water and pregnancy outcomes. *Environ Health Perspect.* 2001;109:629–631

16. Hall AH. Arsenic and arsine. In: Haddad L, Shannon M, Winchester J, eds. *Clinical Management of Poisoning and Drug Overdose.* 3rd ed. Philadelphia, PA: WB Saunders; 1998:784–789

17. Office of Environmental Health Hazard Assessment, California Department of Health Services. *Evaluation of Hazards Posed by the Use of Wood Preservatives on Playground Equipment.* California Department of Health Services; 1987

18. Stilwell DE, Gorny KD. Contamination of soil with copper, chromium, and arsenic under decks built from pressure treated wood. *Bull Environ Contam Toxicol.* 1997;58:22–29

19. Fields S. Caution—children at play: how dangerous is CCA? *Environ Health Perspect.* 2001;109:A262–A269

20. Exterior deck treatments test: all decked out. *Consumer Reports.* 1998;63:32–34

# 9
# Asbestos

Asbestos is a fibrous mineral product and includes 6 minerals: amosite, chrysotile, and crocidolite, and the fibrous varieties of tremolite, actinolite, and anthophyllite. Asbestos occurs naturally in rock formations in certain areas of the world and is mined and refined for commercial use. Asbestos fibers vary in length; they may be straight or curled; they can be carded, woven, and spun into cloth; and they can be used in bulk or mixed with materials such as asphalt or cement.

Asbestos is virtually indestructible. It resists heat, fire, and acid. Because of these properties, asbestos has been used in a wide range of manufactured goods, including insulation, roofing shingles, ceiling and floor tiles, paper products, asbestos cement, clutches, brakes and transmission parts, textiles, packaging, gaskets, and coatings. Between the 1920s and the early 1970s, millions of tons of asbestos were used in the construction of homes, schools, and public buildings in the United States, mainly for insulation and fireproofing.

Today in the United States, use of asbestos in new construction has come to almost a complete halt. However, large amounts of asbestos remain in place in older buildings, especially in schools, posing a hazard to children now and in the future. Large amounts of asbestos are still used in new construction in other nations, especially in certain developing countries. A major challenge to pediatricians, public health officials, and school authorities in the United States has been to develop a systematic and rational approach to dealing with asbestos in schools and other buildings to protect the health of children.

In 1980 (the last time that national statistics were compiled) the US Environmental Protection Agency (EPA) estimated that more than 8500 schools nationwide contained deteriorated asbestos, and that approximately 3 million students (as well as more than 250 000 teachers, personnel, and staff) were at risk of exposure.[1] Subsequent field studies have found that about 10% of the asbestos in schools is deteriorating and/or accessible to children and thus poses an immediate threat to health. The remaining 90% is not deteriorating or accessible to children and therefore does not pose an immediate hazard.[2]

## Routes of Exposure

Inhalation of microscopic airborne asbestos fibers is the major route of exposure. Asbestos becomes a health hazard when fibers become airborne.[3] Asbestos that is tightly contained within building materials (such as in insulation or ceiling tiles) or behind barriers poses no immediate hazard. However, when asbestos fibers are liberated into the air through deterioration, destruction, or repair/renovation of asbestos-containing materials, children and adults are at risk of inhaling airborne fibers.

Children can be exposed to asbestos from living in areas where there are naturally occurring deposits of ore containing asbestos or where mining or refining of such ore occurs. From 1924 through 1990, vermiculite ore was mined and milled from Zonolite Mountain in Libby, MT. Apparently the vermiculite was used widely in the community at residential and commercial locations. The ore from Libby was contaminated with asbestos, and radiologic evidence of adverse health effects has been noted in workers employed in Libby at the mine, mill, and refining plant. Workers in the mine and their families have experienced increased rates of asbestos-related diseases including mesothelioma.[4,5]

Gastrointestinal exposure to asbestos occurs rarely, usually in circumstances in which drinking water is transferred through deteriorating concrete-asbestos pipes. Asbestos fibers also can enter drinking water that passes through rock formations that contain naturally occurring asbestiform fibers.

## Systems Affected

The organs in which asbestos can cause cancer include the lungs, throat, larynx, and gastrointestinal tract. Malignancies caused by asbestos also are seen in the pleura and peritoneum. High-dose occupational exposure (an unlikely exposure scenario in children) can cause asbestosis, a fibrotic disease of the lungs and/or pleura.

## Clinical Effects

Asbestos produces no acute toxicity. Workers who have been heavily exposed to asbestos in industry may develop asbestosis. In its earlier stages, asbestosis neither causes symptoms nor impairs lung function. Asbestosis is not seen in children because of their much lower levels of exposure.

The main risk of asbestos to children lies in its capacity to cause cancer many years after exposure.[4] The 2 most important cancers caused by asbestos are (1) lung cancer and (2) malignant mesothelioma, a malignancy that can arise in the pleura, pericardium, or peritoneum. Asbestos also has been observed to cause cancer of the throat, larynx, and gastrointestinal tract among adults heavily exposed in industry.

The relationship between asbestos and cancer was first recognized among workers exposed occupationally as miners, shipbuilders, and insulation workers.[6] Thousands of cases of mesothelioma and lung cancer have occurred in these men and women, and cases resulting from past exposures will continue to develop into the 21st century. An estimated 300 000 US workers will eventually die of asbestos-related diseases,[7] and it is projected that 250 000 workers will die over the next 35 years in Western Europe, where adoption of protective measures was delayed.[8] Ongoing exposures in developing nations will produce a further toll of disease and death that has not yet been quantified.

### Lung Cancer

Asbestos exposure can by itself cause lung cancer. Additionally, a strongly synergistic interaction has been found between asbestos and cigarette smoking and lung cancer.[9] Adults who are exposed to asbestos, but who do not smoke, have 5 times the background rate of lung cancer. In contrast, adults who are exposed to asbestos and who also smoke have more than 50 times the background rate of lung cancer. This powerful synergistic association is one more reason why pediatricians should urge parents, children, and adolescents not to smoke.

### Mesothelioma

Malignant mesothelioma seems to arise solely as a result of exposure to asbestos. No interaction is evident between asbestos and smoking in the causation of mesothelioma. Mesothelioma is the form of cancer that is of greatest concern for children exposed to asbestos in homes and schools because it can be caused by low levels of exposure and can appear as long as 5 decades after exposure.

### Dose-Response

The degree of cancer risk associated with asbestos is dose-related, and the greater the cumulative exposure, the greater the risk.[10] However, any exposure to asbestos involves some risk of cancer; no safe threshold level of exposure has been established. For example, mesotheliomas have been observed decades after exposure in the spouses and children of asbestos workers who brought asbestos fibers home on their work clothing, in nonsmoking women who were never employed in the asbestos industry but lived their entire lives in the asbestos mining area of Quebec,[11] and in persons who lived in a town near an asbestos-cement factory in Italy.[12]

Some scientists and industry representatives have claimed that the form of asbestos used most commonly in buildings in North America (Canadian chrysotile) is harmless. However, extensive clinical, epidemiologic, and toxicologic data have consistently documented that chrysotile asbestos is carcinogenic in experimental animals and that it can cause lung cancer and mesothelioma in humans.[13] *All forms of asbestos are hazardous and carcinogenic. Exposure to all forms of asbestos must be kept to a minimum.*[14]

## Diagnostic Methods

There is no reliable method of detecting past asbestos exposure except through obtaining a history of exposure. Chest roentgenograms are not indicated for children exposed or potentially exposed to asbestos because acute radiographs provide no information on whether exposure has occurred. Past exposure to asbestos can be diagnosed by the identification of pleural plaques, raised fibrous plaques, sometimes calcified, that are radiographically evident on the pleura or pericardium. Such plaques are seen in 6.4% of US males and 1.7% of US females aged 35 to 74 years examined between 1976 and 1980 in the National Health and Nutrition Examination Survey (NHANES II). No comparable data are available for children.[15]

To determine whether children are at risk of asbestos exposure or have been exposed, an environmental inspection should be undertaken by a properly certified inspector in schools and other buildings where children live, work, and play. Bulk samples need to be obtained of insulation or other suspicious materials and examined by electron microscopy in a certified laboratory. Children may be at risk of exposure if asbestos in a building is deteriorating or it is within reach, or renovations are taking place. Air sampling is of little value in assessing a potential asbestos hazard to children in a school because airborne releases of asbestos fibers are typically intermittent and likely to be missed.

## Treatment

Because asbestos produces no acute symptoms, there is no treatment for acute exposure. There also is no treatment that removes asbestos fibers from the lungs once they are inhaled. Discussion of the meaning of risk with children who have been exposed or potentially exposed to asbestos and with their parents is very important (see Chapter 41). While no exposure is completely free of risk, parents need to be assured that the risk associated with brief, low-level exposure to asbestos is minimal.[16] The context of such a discussion provides an important "teachable moment" in which a pediatrician can reinforce warnings about tobacco smoking.

## Prevention of Exposure

The most effective approach to prevention of exposure to asbestos is to use alternative, less hazardous materials in building construction and renovation. This approach is now followed almost universally in the United States, Canada, and Western Europe, where use of asbestos in new construction is severely restricted. To prevent exposure in developing nations, where asbestos is still used widely in new construction, a call for an international ban on all new uses of asbestos has been issued by the Collegium Ramazzini, an independent group of experts in environmental and occupational medicine.[17]

Prevention of exposure to asbestos in the home is most efficiently achieved by wrapping any small areas of fraying asbestos insulation with duct tape. If more than minor repairs are needed or if asbestos is to be removed, a certified asbestos contractor always should be recruited and full EPA and state regulations obeyed. "Do-it-yourself" removal of asbestos is never recommended.

Prevention of asbestos exposure in schools requires full compliance with the provisions of the federal Asbestos Hazard Emergency Response Act (AHERA) of 1986. This act requires periodic inspection of every school—public, private, and parochial—by a certified inspector, and it establishes criteria specifying when asbestos must be removed and when it can be safely managed in place. If asbestos must be removed, removal must proceed in full compliance with state and federal law. The results of all inspections conducted under AHERA must be made available to the public by school authorities (see also Chapter 30).

## Frequently Asked Questions

Q *How will I know if there are asbestos materials in my house?*

A Asbestos is not found as commonly in private homes in the United States as in schools, apartment buildings, and public buildings. Nevertheless, asbestos is present in many homes, especially those built prior to the 1970s.

The following are locations in homes where asbestos may be found:
- Insulation around pipes, stoves, and furnaces (the most common locations)
- Insulation in walls and ceilings, especially as sprayed-on or troweled-on material
- Patching and spackling compounds and textured paint
- Roofing shingles and siding
- Older appliances such as washers and dryers

To determine if your home contains asbestos, you can take the following steps:
- Evaluate appliances and other consumer products by examining the label or the invoices to obtain the product name, model number, and year of manufacture. If this information is available, the manufacturer can supply information about asbestos content.
- Evaluate building materials. A professional asbestos manager with qualifications similar to those of managers employed in school districts may be hired. This person can inspect your home to determine whether asbestos is present and give advice on its proper management.
- Test for asbestos. State and local health departments as well as regional EPA offices have lists of individuals and laboratories certified to analyze a home for asbestos and test samples for the presence of asbestos (see Resources).

Q *If there is asbestos in my home, what should I do?*

A If asbestos-containing materials are found in your home, the same options exist for dealing with these materials as in a school. In most cases, asbestos-containing materials in a home are best left alone. If materials such as insulation, tiling, and flooring are in good condition, and out of the reach of children, there is no need to worry. However, if materials containing asbestos are deteriorating, or if you are planning renovations and the materials will be disturbed, it is best to find out beforehand if they contain asbestos and, if necessary, have them properly removed. Improper removal of asbestos may cause serious contamination by dispersing fibers throughout the area. Any asbestos removal in a home must be performed by properly accredited and certified contractors. A listing of certified contractors in your area may be obtained from state or local health departments or from the regional office of the EPA (see Resources). Many contractors who advertise themselves as asbestos experts have not been trained properly. Only contractors who have been certified by the EPA or by a state-approved training school should be hired. The contractor should be able to provide written proof of up-to-date certification.

Children should not be permitted to play in areas where there are friable asbestos-containing materials.

To obtain additional information about asbestos in the home, you can write to the EPA for the booklet "Asbestos in Your Home," which can be obtained from the Toxic Substances Control Act Assistance Information Service, Mail Code 7408M, 1200 Pennsylvania Ave NW, Washington, DC 20460, phone: 202-554-1404, e-mail: tsca-hotline@epamail.epa.gov. State or local health departments will have additional information about asbestos (see Resources).

Q  *Is there asbestos in hair dryers?*
A  In the past, asbestos was used in some electrical appliances, including hair dryers. However, hair dryers containing asbestos were recalled by the US Consumer Product Safety Commission

(CPSC) more than a decade ago, and currently manufacturers of household appliances in the United States are not allowed to use asbestos. If your hair dryer is more than 10 years old, it should be discarded. Hair dryers should not be opened and inspected.

Q  *Is there asbestos in talc?*

A  Talc, like asbestos, is a mineral product. Talc from some mines contains asbestoslike fibers, and these fibers are present in talcum powder made from that talc. Because talcum powder is not required to carry a label indicating whether it contains asbestos-like fibers, pediatricians and parents are urged not to use talc-containing products for infant and child care. A further reason to avoid talcum powder in the nursery is to prevent asphyxiation, which can result from accidental inhalation of bulk powder if a can should tip over into a baby's face.

Q  *Is there asbestos in play sand?*

A  Play sand that comes from naturally occurring sand deposits, such as sand dunes or beaches, generally does not contain asbestos. However, some commercially available play sand is produced by crushing quarried rock, and this sand has been shown to contain asbestoslike fibers. The CPSC does not require that the label on play sand indicate the source of the sand. Also, the label on sand is not required to carry any information on whether it contains asbestoslike fibers. For these reasons, pediatricians are advised to warn parents against the use of play sand unless the source of the sand can be verified or the sand is certified asbestos-free.

Q  *My spouse works with asbestos. Is there danger to my child?*

A  Any family member who works in an occupation potentially involving contact with asbestos (or similar fibers such as fiberglass or reactive ceramic fibers) is at risk of bringing fibers home on clothing, shoes, hair, skin, and in the car. These fibers can contaminate the home environment and become a source of exposure to children.[18]

Studies conducted in the homes of asbestos workers have shown that the dust in these homes can be heavily contaminated by asbestos fibers. Mesothelioma, lung cancer, and asbestosis all have been observed in the family members of asbestos workers. In many cases, these diseases have occurred years or even decades after the exposure.

Prevention of household exposure is essential. People who work with asbestos (eg, construction and demolition workers and workers who repair brakes) must scrupulously shower, change clothing, and change shoes before getting into a car and returning home. These procedures are mandated by the federal Occupational Safety and Health Act but often are not enforced. Also, workers often are not aware of their exposure. Exposure is prevented only if employees leave their contaminated shoes and clothing at the workplace.

---

Many jobs involve potential occupational exposure to asbestos. These include
- Asbestos mining and milling
- Asbestos product manufacture
- Construction trades, including sheet metal work, carpentry, plumbing, insulation work, air-conditioning, rewiring, cable installation, spackling, drywall work, and demolition work
- Shipyard work
- Asbestos removal
- Fire fighting
- Custodial and janitorial work
- Brake repair

---

Q *Is there a risk of asbestos exposure from the events of September 11,
2001?*

A The risk associated with low levels of exposure to asbestos or with
brief encounters lasting only a few days or weeks such as occurred
in September 2001 among children in communities near the
World Trade Center in New York City is not nil. However, the risk
associated with such exposure is certainly much lower than the
risk that results from continuing exposure, such as occurs among
adults in industry who have been exposed for many years.[19]

## Resources

Agency for Toxic Substances and Disease Registry, phone: 888-422-
8737, Internet: http://www.atsdr.cdc.gov

US Environmental Protection Agency, phone: 202-272-0167, Internet:
http://www.epa.gov or http://www.epa.gov/epahome/postal.htm. The
principal resources for information on asbestos in buildings are the
10 regional offices of the US EPA. Each office has an asbestos coordinator. Regional offices are located in Boston, New York City,
Philadelphia, Atlanta, Chicago, Dallas, Kansas City, Denver, San
Francisco, and Seattle. Information on asbestos identification, health
effects, abatement options, analytic techniques, asbestos in schools,
and contract documents in each region is available online at
http://www.epa.gov/opptintr/asbestos/regioncontact.html.
The EPA Asbestos Information Line is 202-554-1404. The EPA
Small Business Ombudsman's Hotline at 800-368-5888 can provide
information and documents on preventing asbestos emissions from
asbestos manufacturing, processing, removal, abatement, and disposal activities. State and local health departments also can provide
information on asbestos.

# References

1. American Academy of Pediatrics Committee on Environmental Hazards. Asbestos exposure in schools. *Pediatrics.* 1987;79:301–305

2. US Environmental Protection Agency. Asbestos-containing materials in schools: final rule and notice. *Fed Regist.* 1987;52:41826–41903

3. American Academy of Pediatrics Committee on Injury and Poison Prevention. Rodgers GC Jr, ed. *Handbook of Common Poisonings in Children.* 3rd ed. Elk Grove Village, IL: American Academy of Pediatrics; 1994

4. Agency for Toxic Substances and Disease Registry. *The Community Environmental Health Project in Libby, Montana.* Atlanta, GA: Agency for Toxic Substances and Disease Registry. Available at: http://www.atsdr.cdc.gov/HEC/HSPH/v12n1-1.html

5. US Environmental Protection Agency. *Region 8—Libby Cleanup.* Washington, DC: US Environmental Protection Agency. Available at: http://www.epa.gov/region8/superfund/libby

6. Selikoff IJ, Churg J, Hammond EC. Asbestos exposure and neoplasia. *JAMA.* 1964;188:22–26

7. Nicholson WJ, Perkel G, Selikoff IJ. Occupational exposure to asbestos: population at risk and projected mortality—1980–2030. *Am J Ind Med.* 1982;3:259–311

8. Peto J, Decarli A, LaVecchia C, Levi F, Negri R. The European mesothelioma epidemic. *Br J Cancer.* 1999;79:666–672

9. Selikoff IJ, Hammond EC, Churg J. Asbestos exposure, smoking and neoplasia. *JAMA.* 1968;204:106–112

10. Agency for Toxic Substances and Disease Registry. *Toxicological Profile on Asbestos.* Atlanta, GA: Agency for Toxic Substances and Disease Registry; 1995

11. Camus M, Siemiatycki J, Meek B. Nonoccupational exposure to chrysotile asbestos and the risk of lung cancer. *N Engl J Med.* 1998;338:1565–1571

12. Magnani C, Dalmasso P, Biggeri A, Ivaldi C, Mirabelli D, Terracini B. Increased risk of malignant mesothelioma of the pleura after residential or domestic exposure to asbestos: a case-control study in Casale Monferrato, Italy. *Environ Health Perspect.* 2001;109:915–919

13. International Agency for Research on Cancer. *The Evaluation of Carcinogenic Risks to Humans.* IARC Monographs. Lyon, France: International Agency for Research on Cancer; 1987;suppl 7:106–116

14. Landrigan PJ. Asbestos—still a carcinogen. *N Engl J Med.* 1998;338:1618–1619

15. Rogan WJ, Ragan NB, Dinse GE. X-ray evidence of increased asbestos exposure in the US population from NHANES I and NHANES II 1973–1978. National Health Examination Survey. *Cancer Causes Control.* 2000;11:441–449

16. Needleman HL, Landrigan PJ. *Raising Children Toxic Free: How to Keep Your Child Safe From Lead, Asbestos, Pesticides, and Other Environmental Hazards.* New York, NY: Farrar, Straus and Giroux; 1994

17. LaDou J, Landrigan P, Bailar JC III, Foa V, Frank A. A call for an international ban on asbestos. *CMAJ.* 2001;164:489–490

18. Chisolm JJ Jr. Fouling one's own nest. *Pediatrics.* 1978;62:614–617

19. Claudio L. Environmental aftermath. *Environ Health Perspect.* 2001;109:A528–A536

# 10
# Carbon Monoxide

Carbon monoxide (CO) is a colorless, odorless, tasteless toxic gas that is a product of the incomplete combustion of carbon-based fuels. Carbon monoxide has a vapor density slightly less than that of air. The health effects from acute CO exposure range from non-specific flulike symptoms, such as headache, dizziness, nausea, vomiting, weakness, and confusion, to coma and death from prolonged or intense exposure. Fetuses, infants, pregnant women, elderly people, and people with anemia or with a history of cardiac or respiratory disease may be particularly sensitive to CO. Evidence of delayed neuropsychological health effects and slow resolution of these sequelae from CO exposures are documented in the literature, though no definitive diagnostic or therapeutic approaches have been established. The effects of long-term, low-level exposure is another area of CO poisoning that lacks a definitive approach for diagnosis and treatment.[1-3]

Unintentional CO poisonings account for hundreds of deaths annually.[4] In a study of 3034 poisoning deaths among 10- to 19-year-olds, 38.2% were due to CO inhalation, of which 65.1% were categorized as suicide and 34.9% as unintentional. Motor vehicle exhaust accounted for 84.4% of the CO-related suicides and 65.6% of the unintentional fatal CO poisonings.[5] Death rates from fire-related CO intoxication are higher for children younger than 15 years and for the elderly than for other age groups.[6] The prevalence of unintentional nonfatal CO poisonings is difficult to estimate because the nonspecific clinical presentation of mild and severe poisoning poses a diagnostic challenge.[3,7-9] Often, the presentation can mimic influenza. In a study of 46 children presenting during winter months to the emergency department for flulike symptoms, more than half had carboxyhemoglobin (COHb) levels that exceeded 2%, and 6 of these children had levels that exceeded 10%.[7]

## Route and Sources of Exposure

The route of exposure to CO is through inhalation. Unintentional exposure to CO can be largely attributed to smoke inhalation from fires, motor vehicle exhaust, faulty or improperly vented combustion appliances (including heating appliances), and tobacco smoke. Confined, poorly ventilated spaces such as garages, campers, tents, and boats also are susceptible to elevated, often lethal, levels of CO.[1,2] Common sources of CO exposure are listed in Table 10.1. Exposure to CO may occur in and around motor vehicles when there is inadequate combustion resulting from substandard vehicle maintenance and poor ventilation. Exposure also may occur when gasoline-powered equipment such as generators, lawn mowers, snow blowers, leaf blowers, and ice rink resurfacing machines are used in poorly ventilated spaces.[1,2,6,10]

## Systems Affected

Carbon monoxide is inhaled, diffuses across the alveolar-capillary membrane, and is measurable in the bloodstream as COHb. The

**Table 10.1**
**Sources of Carbon Monoxide Exposure**

| |
|---|
| Motor vehicle exhaust |
| Unvented kerosene and propane gas space heaters |
| Leaking chimneys and furnaces |
| Backdrafting from furnaces |
| Woodstoves and fireplaces |
| Charcoal grills |
| Gas appliances: stoves, dryers, water heaters |
| Gasoline-powered generators |
| Gasoline-powered equipment: ice rink resurfacers, lawnmowers, leaf blowers, floor polishers, snowblowers, pressure washers |
| Tobacco smoke |

relative affinity of CO for hemoglobin is approximately 240 to 270 times greater than that of oxygen, resulting in decreased oxygen-carrying capacity of the blood when CO levels are elevated. Carbon monoxide in the bloodstream causes a leftward shift of the oxyhemoglobin dissociation curve, resulting in decreased oxygen delivery to the tissues. Removal from the source of CO exposure leads to dissociation of the COHb complex, resulting in excretion of CO by the lungs.[11–13]

Infants and children have an increased susceptibility to CO toxicity because of their higher metabolic rates. Fetuses are especially vulnerable. Maternal CO diffuses across the placenta and increases the levels of CO in the fetus. Fetal hemoglobin has a higher affinity for CO than does adult hemoglobin, and the elimination half-life of COHb is longer in the fetus than in the adult. The leftward shift in the normal oxyhemoglobin dissociation curve caused by CO results in a substantial decrease in oxygen delivery to the placenta and ultimately to fetal tissues.[14–16] Children with existing pulmonary or hematologic illness (eg, anemia) that compromise oxygen delivery also are more susceptible to adverse effects at lower levels of CO exposures than healthy individuals.[1,2]

Intoxication from exposure to CO results in tissue hypoxia affecting multiple organ systems. Systems with high metabolic rates and high oxygen demand are preferentially affected, with the central nervous and cardiovascular systems being primary targets.[1–3,17] Typical pathologic changes revealed in neuroimaging studies have shown bilateral necrosis in the globus pallidus and diffuse homogenous demyelination of the white matter of the cerebral hemispheres.[18] Cardiac toxicity can be manifested by ischemia on electrocardiography, arrhythmia, and infarction.[17]

Studies investigating the mechanism of toxicity from CO have been the focus of recent research. Mechanisms include tissue hypoxia due to decreased oxygen carrying capacity, but also due to decreased cardiac output secondary to myocardial dysfunction. Other mechanisms of interest that are being investigated include the production of hydroxyl radicals and nitric oxide radicals.[3]

## Clinical Effects

The clinical presentation of CO intoxication is highly variable, and the severity of the symptoms correlates poorly with the level of exposure (parts per million of CO over time) and clinical laboratory determination of poisoning (COHb blood levels). This important phenomenon is explained in part by the fact that within the body, CO can be found in 4 distinct states. In addition to binding to hemoglobin, CO also binds to myoglobin and the cytochrome p450 system and exists in its free state in the plasma at a low concentration, the latter of which is thought to play an important role in clinical toxicity. This is illustrated by animal studies that showed no clinical symptoms in animals transfused with blood containing highly saturated COHb, but minimal free CO. Low levels of COHb may be present in cases of severe poisoning.[3,7,9,11]

Symptoms of CO intoxication include headache, dizziness, fatigue, lethargy, weakness, drowsiness, nausea, vomiting, loss of consciousness, skin pallor, dyspnea on exertion, palpitations, confusion, irritability, irrational behavior, coma, and death. Severity of symptoms ranges from mild to very severe (coma, respiratory depression) and is not correlated with the magnitude of COHb levels.[17] In a series of pediatric patients treated for CO poisoning, lethargy and syncope were reported more frequently than in adult series. These symptoms also occurred at lower COHb levels than usually reported for adults.[9]

Delayed neuropsychological sequelae following CO exposure have been reported in adults and children. This usually occurs 3 to 240 days following exposure. Symptoms include cognitive and personality changes, parkinsonism, dementia, and psychosis.[1,9,13,14,17,19] The incidence of delayed neuropsychiatric sequelae varies widely, but has been estimated to occur in 10% to 30% of victims.[17] Neuropsychiatric testing is only completed on a small proportion of patients being treated for CO intoxication.[19]

## Diagnosis

A thorough history and physical examination as well as a high index of clinical suspicion are necessary to diagnose CO poisoning. Physicians should consider CO exposure when cohabitants present with similar nonspecific symptoms as previously mentioned. Clinical examination is often without findings suggestive of CO intoxication, other than the nonspecific signs and symptoms described in the previous section.

Measurement of oxygen saturation by pulse oximetry and arterial blood gas determination are not helpful in the diagnosis of CO poisoning. The pulse oximeter typically misinterprets COHb as oxyhemoglobin, resulting in an elevated oxygen saturation reading by this device.[20,21] Arterial oxygen tension ($PaO_2$) is typically normal in CO poisoning because this measures the amount of oxygen dissolved in plasma, which is unaffected in this condition. However, the blood gas determination will demonstrate metabolic acidosis in significant CO poisoning.

The measurement of COHb blood levels establishes that exposure to CO has occurred. An elevated level confirms the diagnosis of CO intoxication. Low and moderately increased levels must be interpreted with caution because the COHb level does not indicate severity of illness. Delay between exposure and laboratory measurement, treatment with oxygen, and complicating factors such as exposure to tobacco smoke should be considered when interpreting COHb results. Background levels of COHb range from 1% to 3% in nonsmokers.[17] Baseline COHb levels in smokers typically range from 3% to 8%, although higher values have been reported.[1,17,22,23]

## Treatment

Patients who have been exposed to CO should be removed from the source immediately. Therapy consists of supplemental oxygen, ventilatory support, and monitoring for cardiac dysrhythmias. Administration of 100% oxygen is required to improve the oxygen content of the blood. The elimination half-life of COHb is approximately 4 hours in room air and approximately 1 hour with the administration of 100% oxygen. Administration of hyperbaric oxygen (HBO) decreases the half-life to approximately 20 to 30 minutes.[11–13,17]

The use of HBO remains controversial.[24–26] Although some randomized controlled trials have failed to show benefit from this intervention,[24] a recent double-blind randomized trial of patients 16 years and older poisoned by CO showed fewer cognitive sequelae following 3 hyperbaric oxygen treatments within a 24-hour period.[26] This randomized trial did not enroll children younger than 16 years, so it is not known whether the results can be generalized to children. If hyperbaric oxygen therapy is being considered, the following have been used as criteria: (1) COHb of greater than or equal to 25%, (2) anginal pain or ischemia on electrocardiogram, or (3) measurable neurologic impairment.[12] The choice of treatment modalities is tailored to the patient based on the severity of the poisoning as determined by the observed clinical manifestations. When the patient poisoned by CO is cared for, consultation with a pediatric critical care specialist familiar with treatment options, including HBO therapy, is suggested.

## Prevention of Exposure

Primary prevention of CO poisoning requires limiting exposure to known sources. Proper installation, maintenance, and use of combustion appliances can help to reduce excessive CO emissions. Table 10.2 provides suggestions to prevent CO poisoning.[10]

The US Environmental Protection Agency has set significant harm levels of 50 ppm (8-hour average), 75 ppm (4-hour average), and 125 ppm (1-hour average). Exposure under these conditions could result

**Table 10.2**
**Preventing Problems With Carbon Monoxide (CO) in the Home**

| |
|---|
| **Fuel-Burning Appliances**<br>Forced-air furnaces should be checked by a professional once a year or as recommended by the manufacturer. Pilot lights can produce CO and should be kept in good working order.<br>All fuel-burning appliances (eg, gas water heaters, gas stoves, gas clothes dryers) should be checked professionally once a year or as recommended by the manufacturer.<br>Gas cooking stove tops and ovens should not be used for supplemental heat. |
| **Fireplaces and Woodstoves**<br>Fireplaces and woodstoves should be checked professionally once a year or as recommended by the manufacturer. Check to ensure the flue is open during operation. Proper use, inspection, and maintenance of vent-free fireplaces (and space heaters) are recommended as well. |
| **Space Heaters**<br>Fuel-burning space heaters should be checked professionally once a year or as recommended by the manufacturer.<br>Space heaters should be properly vented during use according to the manufacturer's specifications. |
| **Barbecue Grills/Hibachis**<br>Barbecue grills and hibachis should never be used indoors.<br>Barbecue grills and hibachis should never be used in poorly ventilated spaces such as garages, campers, and tents. |
| **Automobiles/Other Motor Vehicles**<br>Regular inspection and maintenance of the vehicle exhaust system are recommended. Many states have vehicle inspection programs to ensure this practice.<br>Never leave an automobile running in the garage or other enclosed space; CO can accumulate even when a garage door is open. |
| **Generators/Other Fuel-Powered Equipment**<br>Follow the manufacturer's recommendations when operating generators and other fuel-powered equipment.<br>Never operate a generator indoors. |

in COHb levels of 5% to 10% and cause significant health effects in sensitive individuals. The current ambient air quality standards for CO (9 ppm for 8 hours and 35 ppm for 1 hour) are intended to keep COHb levels below 2.1% to protect the most sensitive members of the general population (ie, individuals with coronary artery disease).[2]

Smoke and CO detectors, when used properly, may provide early detection and warning and prevent unintentional CO-related deaths. Carbon monoxide detectors are designed to alarm before potentially life-threatening levels of CO are reached. Carbon monoxide detectors measure the amount of CO (parts per million) that has accumulated over time and should alarm within 189 minutes when CO in the air reaches 70 ppm,[27] corresponding to a level of approximately 5% COHb in the blood. This is based on relationships between CO levels measured in air and corresponding blood levels in adults. Significant exposure to children may have occurred before the CO alarm sounds.[28]

The US Consumer Product Safety Commission (CPSC) recommends installation of a CO detector in the hallway near every separate sleeping area of the home. A residential CO detector should meet the requirements of the most recent revision of Underwriters Laboratories (UL) standard 2034. Because electric heating and cooking appliances shut down during a power failure, battery-operated detectors are recommended when gas appliances or auxiliary heating sources (eg, fireplaces) are used during periods when electrical service is disrupted. The effectiveness of CO detectors in preventing CO poisoning has not been evaluated.

## Frequently Asked Questions

Q *Is using a CO detector a good way to prevent CO poisoning?*

A Carbon monoxide detectors are widely available in stores, and you may want to consider buying one as a backup *but not as a replacement* for proper use and maintenance of fuel-burning appliances (see Table 10.2). The technology of CO detectors is still developing. There are several types on the market, and they are not generally considered to be as reliable as the smoke detectors found in homes today. Some CO detectors have been laboratory-tested, and their performance varied. Some performed well, others failed to alarm even at very high CO levels, and still others alarmed even at very low levels that do not pose any immediate health risk. With smoke detectors, you can easily confirm the cause of the alarm, but because CO is invisible and odorless, it is harder to tell if an alarm is false or a real emergency.

Organizations such as Consumers Union (publisher of *Consumer Reports*), the American Gas Association, and UL have published guidance for consumers. Look for UL certification on any CO detector. Carbon monoxide detectors always have been and still are designed to alarm before potentially life-threatening levels of CO are reached. The UL standard 2034 (1998 revision) has stricter requirements that the detector/alarm must meet before it can sound. As a result, the possibility of nuisance alarms is decreased.

Q *Should I purchase a CO detector for my motor home or other recreational vehicles?*

A The CPSC notes that CO detectors are available for boats and recreational vehicles and that they should be used, and that the Recreational Vehicle Industry Association requires CO detectors in motor homes and in towable recreational vehicles that have a generator or are prepped for a generator.

Q *What do I do if my CO detector alarms?*

A Never ignore an alarming CO detector/alarm. If the CO detector goes off

- Make sure it is your CO detector and not your smoke detector.
- Check to see if any member of the household is experiencing symptoms of poisoning.
- If they are, get them out of the house immediately and call 911. Seek medical attention at an emergency department. Tell the doctor that you suspect CO poisoning.
- If no one is feeling symptoms, ventilate the home with fresh air, turn off all potential sources of CO, including oil or gas furnace, gas water heater, gas range, oven, gas dryer, gas or kerosene space heater, and any vehicle or small engine.

- Have a qualified technician inspect your fuel-burning appliances and chimneys to make sure they are operating correctly and that there is nothing blocking the fumes from being vented out of the house. Checking appliances and other possible CO sources should be done before they are turned back on.

Q *What sort of things can I do to help limit my family's exposure to CO?*

A Table 10.2 lists recommendations for preventing CO problems in the home.[10]

Q *I recently found out that my furnace has been leaking CO, even though I feel fine. Are there any long-term effects?*

A There are no data that show chronic CO exposure produces any long-term sequelae. The long-term effects, such as the neuropsychiatric sequelae, only have been described in patients who have had documented evidence of a severe, acute CO poisoning. Even though you feel fine, it is *imperative* that you and your family vacate the premises and have the furnace problem evaluated and fixed *immediately.* Ignoring this problem could prove fatal to you and your family.

## Resources

Undersea and Hyperbaric Medical Society, phone: 301-942-2980, Internet: http://uhms.org

Underwriters Laboratories, phone: 847-272-8800, Internet: http://www.ul.com

US Consumer Product Safety Commission, phone: 800-638-2772, Internet: http://www.cpsc.gov

US Environmental Protection Agency Indoor Air Quality Information Clearinghouse, phone: 800-438-4318, Internet: http://www.epa.gov/iaq/iaqinfo.html

# References

1. US Environmental Protection Agency. *Air Quality Criteria for Carbon Monoxide.* Research Triangle Park, NC: Office of Health and Environmental Assessment, Office of Research and Development; 1991. EPA Publication 600/8-90/045F

2. US Environmental Protection Agency. *Air Quality Criteria for Carbon Monoxide.* Research Triangle Park, NC: Office of Health and Environmental Assessment, Office of Research and Development; 2000. EPA Publication 600/P-99/001F

3. Raub JA, Mathieu-Nolf M, Hampson NB, Thom SR. Carbon monoxide poisoning—a public health perspective. *Toxicology.* 2000;145:1–14

4. Mah JC. *Non-Fire Carbon-Monoxide Deaths and Injuries Associated With the Use of Consumer Products: Annual Estimates—October 2000.* Bethesda, MD: US Consumer Product Safety Commission; 2001. Available at: http://www.cpsc.gov/library/co00.pdf

5. Shepherd G, Klein-Schwartz W. Accidental and suicidal adolescent poisoning deaths in the United States, 1979–1994. *Arch Pediatr Adolesc Med.* 1998;152:1181–1185

6. Cobb N, Etzel RA. Unintentional carbon monoxide-related deaths in the United States, 1979 through 1988. *JAMA.* 1991;266:659–663

7. Baker MD, Henretig FM, Ludwig S. Carboxyhemoglobin levels in children with nonspecific flu-like symptoms. *J Pediatr.* 1988;113:501–504

8. Heckerling PS, Leikin JB, Terzian CG, Maturen A. Occult carbon monoxide poisoning in patients with neurologic illness. *J Toxicol Clin Toxicol.* 1990;28:29–44

9. Crocker PJ, Walker JS. Pediatric carbon monoxide toxicity. *J Emerg Med.* 1985;3:443–448

10. American Thoracic Society. Environmental controls and lung disease. *Am Rev Respir Dis.* 1990;142:915–939

11. Vreman HJ, Mahoney JJ, Stevenson DK. Carbon monoxide and carboxyhemoglobin. *Adv Pediatr.* 1995;42:303–334

12. Piantadosi CA. Diagnosis and treatment of carbon monoxide poisoning. *Respir Care Clin North Am.* 1999;5:183–202

13. Thom SR, Keim LW. Carbon monoxide poisoning: a review epidemiology, pathophysiology, clinical findings, and treatment options including hyperbaric oxygen therapy. *J Toxicol Clin Toxicol.* 1989;27:141–156

14. Koren G, Sharev T, Pastuszak A, et al. A multicenter prospective study of fetal outcome following accidental carbon monoxide poisoning in pregnancy. *Reprod Toxicol.* 1991;5:397–404

15. Longo LD. The biological effects of carbon monoxide on the pregnant woman, fetus, and newborn infant. *Am J Obstet Gynecol.* 1977;129:69–103

16. Kopelman AE, Plaut TA. Fetal compromise caused by maternal carbon monoxide poisoning. *J Perinatol.* 1998;18:74–77

17. Ernst A, Zibrak JD. Carbon monoxide poisoning. *N Engl J Med.* 1998;339:1603–1608

18. Bianco F, Floris R. MRI appearances consistent with haemorrhagic infarction as an early manifestation of carbon monoxide poisoning. *Neuroradiology.* 1996;38(suppl 1):S70–S72

19. Seger D, Welch L. Carbon monoxide controversies: neuropsychologic testing, mechanism of toxicity, and hyperbaric oxygen. *Ann Emerg Med.* 1994;24:242–248

20. Barker SJ, Tremper KK. The effect of carbon monoxide inhalation on pulse oximetry and transcutaneous $PO_2$. *Anesthesiology.* 1987;66:677–679

21. Buckley RG, Aks SE, Eshom JL, Rydman R, Schaider J, Shayne P. The pulse oximetry gap in carbon monoxide intoxication. *Ann Emerg Med.* 1994;24:252–255

22. Hausberg M, Somers VK. Neural circulatory responses to carbon monoxide in healthy humans. *Hypertension.* 1997;29:1114–1118

23. Hee J, Callais F, Momas I, et al. Smokers' behaviour and exposure according to cigarette yield and smoking experience. *Pharmacol Biochem Behav.* 1995;52:195–203

24. Scheinkestel CD, Bailey M, Myles PS, et al. Hyperbaric or normobaric oxygen for acute carbon monoxide poisoning: a randomized controlled clinical trial. *Med J Australia.* 1999;170:203–210

25. Juurlink DN, Stanbrook MB, McGuigan MA. Hyperbaric oxygen for carbon monoxide poisoning. *Cochrane Database Syst Rev.* 2000; 2:CD002041

26. Weaver LK, Hopkins RO, Chan KJ, et al. Hyperbaric oxygen for acute carbon monoxide poisoning. *N Engl J Med* 2002; 347:1057–1067

27. Underwriters Laboratories. *UL2034: Standard for Single and Multiple Station Carbon Monoxide Detectors.* Northbrook, IL: Underwriters Laboratories; 1992. Revised standard available at: http://ulstandardsinfonet.ul.com/scopes/2034.html

28. Etzel RA. Indoor air pollutants in homes and schools. *Pediatr Clin North Am.* 2001;48:1153–1165

# 11
# Electric and Magnetic Fields

Electric and magnetic fields (EMFs) are invisible lines of force created by electric charges that surround power lines, electrical appliances, and other electrical equipment. Humans have always been exposed to EMFs from natural sources, including the earth's magnetic field. Electric and magnetic fields also are emitted by living organisms, including humans. The advent of electricity 120 years ago led to expanding usage for heating, lighting, communications, and other uses.[1] The most common form of electricity is alternating current (AC), which reverses direction 60 times per second in the United States.[2] The unit that denotes the frequency of alternation is called a hertz (Hz).

Electrical charges create electric fields when the charges stand still, and magnetic fields when the charges are in motion.[2] The strength or intensity of magnetic fields is commonly measured in units called gauss (1 gauss equals 1000 milligauss) or tesla. One tesla equals 1 million microtesla; 1 milligauss is the same as 0.1 microtesla.[2]

The EMFs associated with electric power are extremely low-frequency or power-frequency (50 Hz or 60 Hz) field levels. Cellular telephones and towers emit and receive radio-frequency and microwave-frequency EMFs, involving a much higher frequency range (800–900 and 1800–1900 megahertz [MHz; 1 MHz = 1 million Hz]) than power lines or many electrical appliances.[2]

## Sources of Exposure
Electricity is produced from coal or other sources at power plants, then sent through long-distance high-power transmission lines to substations, where the current is stepped down.[2] The lower levels of electrical current are then transmitted to homes, schools, workplaces, and other locations via distribution lines. In addition to power lines, other sources

of EMF exposure to children are from electrical appliances held close to the body (including hair dryers, heating pads, and electric blankets) and others to which children are exposed at varying distances (including televisions, microwave ovens, and arcade games).[2] Electric and magnetic field levels are reduced dramatically by increasing distance from the source, with magnetic field levels reduced to background levels at distances as short as a few feet from most electrical appliances (see Table 11.1), approximately 100 ft from a distribution line and 300 ft to 500 ft from a transmission line.[2]

Typical median magnetic field levels for children are slightly under 0.1 microtesla based on studies of children who carried computerized meters taking measurements every 30 seconds while at home or away from home over the course of 24 hours.[3] Population surveys confirm the results from measurement studies of children.[4] The sources of children's EMF exposure vary with age. Most of the magnetic field exposure to younger children is related to power lines near their homes, and to a much lesser extent exposures away from home, whereas only about 40% of the exposure to older children comes from power lines near their homes and 60% from other sources away from home.[4]

The primary sources of radio-frequency and microwave-frequency exposures to children currently are from microwave ovens and, more recently, handheld cellular telephones.[5,6] To date children's typical exposure to radio-frequency fields has not been measured using meters as described previously for power-frequency exposures. The average number of years of exposure to radio-frequency field sources and the mean number of minutes of exposure to children by day, week, month, or year have not been examined.

## Energy Levels of EMFs

The 60-Hz extremely low-frequency fields deliver low "packets" of energy not strong enough to break chemical bonds to cause irreversible changes to molecules, such as deoxyribonucleic acid (DNA), or to body tissue.[2] The low-energy packets from microwaves cannot

**Table 11.1**
**Median 60-Hz Magnetic Field Exposure Level (in Microtesla) From Household Appliances According to Distance From the Appliance**

| Major Category | Specific Type | Distance | | | |
|---|---|---|---|---|---|
| | | 6 in | 1 ft | 2 ft | 4 ft |
| Bathroom | Hair dryer | 30 | 0.1 | —* | — |
| | Electric shaver | 10 | 2 | — | — |
| Kitchen | Blender | 7 | 1 | 0.2 | — |
| | Can opener | 60 | 15 | 2 | 0.2 |
| | Coffee maker | 0.7 | — | — | — |
| | Dishwasher | 2 | 1 | 0.4 | — |
| | Food processor | 3 | 0.6 | 0.2 | — |
| | Microwave oven† | 20 | 0.4 | 1 | 0.2 |
| | Mixer | 10 | 1 | 0.1 | — |
| | Electric oven | 0.9 | 0.4 | — | — |
| | Refrigerator | 0.2 | 0.2 | 0.1 | — |
| | Toaster | 1 | 0.3 | — | — |
| Living/family room | Ceiling fan | NM‡ | 0.3 | — | — |
| | Window air conditioner | NM | 0.3 | 0.1 | — |
| | Color TV | NM | 0.7 | 0.2 | — |
| | Black/white TV | NM | 0.3 | — | — |
| Laundry/utility room | Electric dryer | 0.3 | 0.2 | — | — |
| | Washing machine | 2 | 0.7 | 0.1 | — |
| | Iron | 0.8 | 0.1 | — | — |
| | Vacuum cleaner | 30 | 6 | 1 | 0.1 |
| Bedroom | Digital clock | NM | 0.1 | — | — |
| | Analogue (dial-face) clock | NM | 1.5 | 0.2 | — |
| | Baby monitor | 0.6 | 0.1 | — | — |
| Workshop | Battery charger | 3 | 0.3 | — | — |
| | Drill | 15 | 3 | 0.4 | — |
| | Power saw | 20 | 4 | 0.5 | — |
| Office | Video display terminal (color monitor) | 1.4 | 0.5 | 0.2 | — |
| | Electric pencil sharpener | 20 | 7 | 2 | 0.2 |
| | Fluorescent lights | 4 | 0.6 | 0.2 | — |
| | Fax machine | 0.6 | — | — | — |
| | Copy machine | 9 | 2 | 0.7 | 0.1 |
| | Air cleaner | 18 | 3.5 | 0.5 | 0.1 |

*—, magnetic field levels at background level or lower.

† For microwave ovens the range of 60-Hz magnetic field levels (in microtesla) according to distance are: at 6 in (10–30), at 1 ft. (0.1–20), at 2 ft. (0.1–3), and at 4 ft (0–2).

‡ NM, not measured.

break up DNA, but the electric charges on water molecules "wiggle" in response to the oscillations of the microwaves.[5,6] The friction generated by the wiggling generates heat by the same basic principle that allows microwave ovens to heat food. Radio-frequency fields from radio and television transmitters or cellular telephones alternate millions of times per second, compared with extremely low-frequency or power-frequency fields that alternate only 60 times per second.[1,5,6] At high power levels, microwave- or radio-frequency radiation can heat body tissues or create electric currents that might interfere with a cardiac pacemaker or the normal cardiac conduction system when a person is very near the source.[5]

There are no federal standards limiting occupational or residential exposure to 60-Hz EMFs, but several states have set standards for transmission line electric fields.[1] Interference with cardiac pacemakers and implantable defibrillators from sources producing lower-frequency exposures (such as power lines, rail transportation, and welding equipment), as well as higher-frequency sources (such as cellular telephones, paging transmitters, citizen band radios, wireless computer links, microwave signals, and radio and television transmitters) is currently an area of active research. Although a federal radio-frequency protection guide for workers was issued in 1971, it is advisory and not regulatory. The radio-frequency exposure safety limits adopted by the Federal Communications Commission in 1996 are based on criteria quantified according to the specific absorption rate, a measure of the rate at which the body absorbs radio-frequency energy.[6] These exposure limits have been derived to avoid the adverse biological effects at high power levels, such as heating of body tissues or creation of electric currents that can interfere with pacemakers.

Power levels associated with handheld cellular telephones are low, and it is unlikely that such exposures cause consequential heating of brain tissue.[7] Similarly, the exposure to the general public from radio waves emanating from cellular transmitting towers is very low at distances greater than several meters from the antenna.[6] The 60-Hz fields similarly do not have enough energy to break chemical bonds or to heat body tissues.[2] Some physicists have indicated that the weak electric currents produced in the human body by 60-Hz AC magnetic fields in a typical living room are thousands of times weaker than the physiological currents occurring in normal nerve cells.[8] Even fields 10 to 50 times stronger than that would deposit energies equivalent to a whisper in the "hurricane of Brownian molecular movement" in the body. For this reason, many physicists have argued that physiological or pathological effects of AC magnetic fields below 10 microtesla are theoretically impossible.[8,9] Other physicists, however, have argued that there may be an array of molecules or interconnected cells that could sort out the weak "signal" from the "noise."

## Epidemiology Results

### *Extremely Low-Frequency Magnetic Field Exposures*

There is some epidemiologic evidence suggesting an association between occupational exposures to magnetic fields and breast cancer in men (a very rare condition),[10,11] adult leukemia,[12] and adult brain cancer.[13] The greatest public concern, however, is based on epidemiologic studies showing an association between childhood cancer and proximity to power lines. A recent review[1] and update of the literature from 1979 to 2001, including approximately 20 epidemiologic studies, suggests little evidence of an association of residential magnetic field exposures and childhood brain tumors. In general, childhood leukemia is not associated with residential magnetic field exposures under 0.4 microtesla, but a 2-fold increase in risk of childhood leukemia is associated with exposures of 0.4 microtesla or higher.[1,14] The epidemiologic studies suggesting an association between residential magnetic field exposures and childhood leukemia estimated exposure in a variety of ways, including (1) distance of residences from power lines; (2) "wire codes," a system of classification based on type of power line (transmission lines or distribution lines) and distance from the lines; (3) measurements (including spot or 30-second measurements, 24- and 48-hour residential measurements, and personal measurements) of children's estimated exposure to the magnetic field obtained after diagnosis; and (4) estimates of the magnetic field around the time of diagnosis based on historical records of current flows and the distance of the lines from the home.[1]

Five studies have evaluated risks of childhood leukemia or brain and nervous system tumors associated with use of electrical appliances.[1] Associations with childhood leukemia have been observed in 2 or 3 of these studies, including small increases in risk linked with prenatal and postnatal use of electric blankets, hair dryers, and televisions. An extensive body of literature evaluating adult occupational (but not residential) exposures to extremely low-frequency magnetic field exposures suggests that there may be modest increases in risk of brain tumors and chronic lymphocytic leukemia.[1,12,13] Some epidemiologic evidence has suggested that male, and to a lesser extent female, breast cancer may be linked with occupational (but not residential) exposure to extremely low-frequency EMFs, but the evidence is inconsistent.[1,10,11] Several studies have evaluated the relationship of residential EMF exposures and occurrence of adult brain tumors, leukemia, and breast cancer; there is no consistent evidence of association.[1,15]

In summary, a 2-fold excess risk of childhood leukemia is associated with residential magnetic field exposures of 0.4 microtesla or higher, but risks of childhood leukemia are not increased with lower magnetic field levels nor are risks of brain tumors linked with residential magnetic fields based on results of a pooled analysis of major studies.[16] Reasons are unknown for the elevated risk of childhood leukemia in relation to high residential magnetic field exposures.[17] Findings have been inconsistent for childhood leukemia and brain tumors in relation to prenatal or postnatal exposures to electrical appliances.

### Radio-Frequency and Microwave-Frequency Exposures

There have been no epidemiologic studies assessing the relation between radio-frequency or microwave-frequency exposures and serious children's diseases. A comprehensive and critical review of epidemiologic studies of radio-frequency exposures and human cancers published in 1999 reported that a few positive associations have been identified, but the results are inconsistent and no type of cancer has been consistently found to be increased.[14] Since then, 4 recent case-control studies have shown no clear evidence of significantly elevated risk overall or a dose-response relationship between the use of hand-held cellular telephones and occurrence of brain tumors in adults.[18] However, the studies reported to date have not included sufficient numbers of long-term heavy users to rule out the possibility of risks subsequent to long-term induction.

## Laboratory Results

### Extremely Low-Frequency Magnetic Field Exposures

Because the 60-Hz and radio-frequency fields usually present in the environment do not ionize molecules or heat tissues, it was believed that they have no effect on biological systems.[8] During the mid-1970s, a variety of laboratory studies on cell cultures and animals demonstrated that biological changes could be produced by these fields when applied in intensities of hundreds or thousands of microtesla. A series of comprehensive studies reported during 1997 to 2001, however, have shown no consistent evidence of an association between extremely low-frequency magnetic field exposures and risk of leukemia or lymphoma in rodents based on long-term (up to 2.5 years) bioassays, initiation/promotion studies, investigations in transgenic models, and tumor growth studies. Three large-scale chronic bioassays of carcinogenesis in rats or mice exposed to magnetic fields for 2 years revealed no increase in mammary cancer, resulting in a general consensus that power-frequency magnetic fields do not act as a complete carcinogen in the rodent.[9]

Inconsistent findings from one laboratory, suggesting that magnetic fields may stimulate mammary carcinogenesis in rats treated with a chemical carcinogen, could not be replicated in 2 other laboratories.[9] A specific concern in relation to breast cancer was that extremely low-frequency magnetic field exposures might mediate occurrence of breast cancer through melatonin.[4,19] To date the experimental literature has shown relatively little support for the melatonin hypothesis.[9]

In studies undertaken to investigate alterations in cellular processes associated with magnetic field exposures previously reported in the literature, regional EMF exposure facilities established to investigate these reports, which were provided with experimental protocols, cell lines, and relevant experiment details, generally found no effects of magnetic fields on gene expression, particularly those genes that may be involved in cancer; killing of cells cultured from patients with ataxia-telangiectasia, which are highly sensitive to genotoxic chemicals; gap junction intercellular communication; the influx of calcium ions across the plasma membrane of cells or the intracellular calcium concentration; activity of ornithine decarboxylase (an enzyme implicated in tumor promotion); or other in vitro processes that may be related to carcinogenesis.[9] Therefore, the preponderance of the evidence suggests that EMFs are not genotoxic or carcinogenic.[9]

### Radio-Frequency and Microwave-Frequency Exposures

Radio-frequency field sources in the home include microwave ovens, cellular telephones, burglar alarms, video display units, and television sets. Although some experimental studies suggest that radio-frequency fields may accelerate the development of certain tumors, including one demonstrating an increase in lymphoma incidence in transgenic mice,[20] overall data from more than 100 studies conducted in frequency ranges from 800 to 3000 MHz indicate that these exposures are not directly mutagenic nor do they act as cancer initiators. Adverse effects from exposure of organisms to high radio-frequency exposure levels are predominantly the result of hyperthermia, although some studies suggest an effect on intracellular levels of ornithine decarboxylase.[21-23]

## Frequently Asked Questions

*Q  I am about to buy a house, but there is a power line (or transformer) near the home. Should I buy it?*

A  This is a decision only a parent can make. Reasonable people, when they think of the uncertainty of the hazard, the low individual risk, and the comparable environmental risks (eg, traffic hazards) in other locations, may make the purchase. Obtaining magnetic field measurements in the home sometimes will show that field levels are at about the average level despite proximity to the power line.

*Q  Our child has leukemia and was exposed to power lines or an electric appliance. Could this have caused the leukemia?*

A  It is important to find out why the parents suspect the power lines as the cause of leukemia and whether they are blaming themselves for the exposure or considering litigation. Be attentive to the feelings related to the question and deal with those. From an objective viewpoint, pinpointing the cause of a particular case of childhood leukemia is currently beyond the ability of science. Even when there is scientific consensus that a factor such as ionizing radiation can cause childhood leukemia, it is impossible to be certain whether a particular case of leukemia was due to radiation. It is even more problematic for EMFs, for which evidence of an association is weak.

*Q  Have any states or countries set standards for EMFs?*

A  Lack of knowledge has constrained scientists from recommending any health-based regulations. Despite this, several states have adopted regulations governing transmission line–generated 60-Hz fields. The initial concern was the risk of electric shock from strong electric fields (measured in kilovolts per meter). More recently, some states, such as Florida and New York, have adopted regulations that preclude new lines from exceeding the fields at the edge of the current right of way. These standards are in the hundreds of milligauss. The California Department of Education requires that new schools be built at certain distances from transmission lines. These distances, 100 ft for 100 kV lines and 250 ft for 345 kV power lines, were chosen based on the estimate that electric fields would have reached the background level at these distances. All of the current regulations relate to transmission lines, and no state has adopted regulations that govern distribution lines, substations, appliances, or other sources of EMFs.

Q *Is it all right for my child or teenager to use a cellular telephone?*

A Epidemiologic studies have not been conducted to assess the risk of cellular telephone use by children. The level of energy absorption in children while using cellular telephones is comparable to the levels in adults; however, due to the larger number of ions contained in the tissue of children, the specific tissue absorption rate may be higher.[24] Experts in some countries have suggested that widespread use of cellular telephones by children be discouraged.[25] Special devices involving use of earplugs could reduce children's exposures, depending on where the antenna of the cell phone is located. Therefore, use of these devices may be helpful if the antenna is kept away from the brain, the genitals, or other sensitive organs.

Q *I understand the uncertainty in the science, but I believe that it is prudent to avoid magnetic fields when possible. What low- and no-cost measures of avoidance can I take?*

A For most people, their highest magnetic field exposures come from using household appliances with motors, transformers, or heaters.[26] The easily avoidable exposures would come from these appliances. If a parent is concerned about EMF exposure from appliances, the major sources of exposure could be identified and the parent could limit the child's time near such appliances.[2] Manufacturers have reduced magnetic field exposures from electric blankets (since 1990) and from computers (since the early

1990s). Because magnetic fields decline rapidly with increasing distance, an easy measure is to increase the distance between the child and the appliance.

## Resources

National Institute of Environmental Health Sciences, phone: 919-541-3345, Internet: http://www.niehs.nih.gov. Available publications include *Questions and Answers About EMF* and *Assessment of Health Effects from Exposure to Power-Line Frequency Electric and Magnetic Fields,* both available at: http://www.niehs.nih.gov/emfrapid/booklet/home.htm.

National Research Council, phone: 800-624-6242. Available publications include *Possible Health Effects of Exposure to Residential Electric and Magnetic Fields.*

US Federal Communications Commission (FCC), Internet: http://www.fcc.gov. The FCC licenses communications systems that use radio-frequency and microwave-frequency EMF (available at: http://www.fcc.gov/oet/info/documents/bulletins/#56).

US Food and Drug Administration (FDA), phone: 888-INFO-FDA (888-463-6332), Internet: http://www.fda.gov. Information about cellular telephones can be found at: http://www.fda.gov/cellphones.

## References

1. Ahlbom IC, Cardis E, Green A, Linet M, Savitz D, Swerdlow A. Review of the epidemiologic literature on EMF and Health. *Environ Health Perspect.* 2001;109(suppl 6):911–933
2. EMF RAPID Program. *Questions and Answers About EMF.* Research Triangle Park, NC; National Institute of Environmental Health Sciences, National Institutes of Health; 2002. Available at: http://www.niehs.nih.gov/emfrapid/booklet/home.htm
3. Friedman DR, Hatch EE, Tarone R, et al. Childhood exposure to magnetic fields: residential area measurements compared to personal dosimetry. *Epidemiology.* 1996;7:151–155

4. Zaffanella L. *Survey of Residential Magnetic Field Sources. Volume 1: Goals, Results and Conclusions. Volume 2: Protocol, Data Analysis, and Management.* Palo Alto, CA: EPRI; 1993:224–248. Report Nos. TR-102759-V1 and TR-102759-V2

5. Electromagnetic fields (300 Hz to 300 GHz). Geneva, Switzerland: World Health Organization; 1993

6. Cleveland RF Jr, Ulcek JL. *Questions and Answers About Biological Effects and Potential Hazards of Radiofrequency Electromagnetic Fields.* 4th ed. Washington, DC: Federal Communications Commission; 1999:9–17. OET Bulletin #56

7. Dimbylow PJ, Mann SM. Characterisation of energy deposition in the head from cellular phones. *Radiat Prot Dosim.* 1999;83:139–141

8. American Physical Society. APS council adopts statement on EMFs and public health. *APS News Online.* 1995;4. Available at: http://www.aps.org/apsnews/july95.html

9. Moulder JE. The electric and magnetic fields research and public information dissemination (EMF-RAPID) program. *Radiat Res.* 2000;153:613–616

10. Tynes T, Andersen A. Electromagnetic fields and male breast cancer. *Lancet.* 1990;336:1596

11. Matanoski GM, Breysse PN, Elliott EA. Electromagnetic field exposure and male breast cancer. *Lancet.* 1991;337:737

12. Kheifets LI, Afifi AA, Buffler PA, Zhang ZW, Matkin CC. Occupational electric and magnetic field exposure and leukemia. A meta-analysis. *J Occup Environ Med.* 1997;39:1074–1091

13. Kheifets LI. Electric and magnetic field exposure and brain cancer: a review. *Bioelectromagnetics.* 2001;suppl 5:S120–S131

14. Elwood JM. A critical review of epidemiologic studies of radiofrequency exposure and human cancers. *Environ Health Perspect.* 1999;107 (suppl 1):155–168

15. Davis S, Mirick DK, Stevens RG. Residential magnetic fields and the risk of breast cancer. *Am J Epidemiol.* 2002;155:446–454

16. Ahlbom A, Day N, Feychting M, et al. A pooled analysis of magnetic fields and childhood leukaemia. *Br J Cancer.* 2000;83:692–698

17. Hatch EE, Kleinerman RA, Linet MS, et al. Do confounding or selection factors of residential wiring codes and magnetic fields distort findings of electromagnetic fields studies? *Epidemiology.* 2000;11:189–198

18. Frumkin H, Jacobson A, Gansler T, Thun MJ. Cellular phones and risk of brain tumors. *CA Cancer J Clin.* 2001;51:137–141

19. Stevens RG, Wilson BW, Anderson LE, eds. *The Melatonin Hypothesis: Breast Cancer and Use of Electric Power.* Columbus, OH: Battelle Press; 1997

20. Repacholi M, Basten A, Gebski V, et al. Lymphomas in E-Pim1 transgenic mice exposed to pulsed 900 MHz electromagnetic fields. *Radiation Res.* 1997;147:631–640

21. Brusick D, Albertini R, McRee D, et al. Genotoxicity of radiofrequency radiation. DNA/Genetox Expert Panel. *Environ Mol Mutagen.* 1998;32:1–16

22. Repacholi MH. Health risks from the use of mobile phones. *Toxicol Lett.* 2001;120:323–331

23. Michaelson SM, Lin JC. *Biological Effects and Health Implications of Radiofrequency Radiation.* New York, NY: Plenum Press; 1987

24. Schonbonn F, Burkhardt M, Kuster N. Differences in energy absorption between heads of adults and children in the near field sources. *Health Physics.* 1998;74:160–168

25. Independent Expert Group on Mobile Phones. *Mobile Phones and Health.* Independent Expert Group on Mobile Phones; 2001. Available at http://www.iegmp.org.uk

26. National Radiological Protection Board. *ELF Electromagnetic Fields and the Risk of Cancer. Report of an Advisory Group on Non-Ionising Radiation.* Chilton, UK: National Radiological Protection Board; 2001

# 12
# Endocrine Disruptors

Endocrine disruptors are exogenous synthetic or natural chemicals that can mimic or modify the action of endogenous hormones. Although initially applied to substances with estrogenic effects, use of the term has widened to include those that interfere with thyroid hormone, insulin and androgen activity, and complex hormonal processes involving multiple hormones, such as pubertal growth and development.

The idea that pesticides could interfere with endocrine processes in vertebrates goes back to the observation that dichlorodiphenyl-trichloroethane (DDT) decreased the hatchability of the eggs of pelagic birds.[1] Dichlorodiphenyltrichloroethane and other pesticides, such as methoxychlor and chlordecone,[2] as well as industrial chemicals such as specific polychlorinated biphenyls (PCBs), can act as estrogens in laboratory assays. Although there are few documented studies in humans, specific chemicals have been identified as disrupting hormonal events in wildlife, with male alligators in Florida being feminized by exposure to a spill of the pesticide dicofol[3] and Great Lakes birds having failed to reproduce because of high body burdens of DDT.[1]

In addition to the synthetic chemicals, there also are many naturally occurring phytoestrogens in plants that can occur at sufficiently high concentrations to be active as estrogens in animals consuming them. Some ecologists postulate that such phytoestrogens may have evolved to protect the plants by interfering with reproduction in grazing animals.

## Routes of Exposure

The primary route of exposure is ingestion, with the fetus being exposed transplacentally.

## Systems Affected and Clinical Effects

A wide variety of chemicals have estrogenic activity in some biological systems, with the most widely used being a yeast with a human estrogen receptor and a reporter gene.[4] (Reporter genes are nucleic acid sequences encoding easily assayed proteins. Reporter genes can "report" many different properties and events.) A listing of chemicals that have been tested for estrogenicity is available from the National Academy of Sciences.[4] Although estrogenicity is the most familiar of the hormonelike activity of exogenous chemicals, one form of dichlorodiphenyldichloroethene (DDE) is an anti-androgen,[5] some pesticides and congeners of PCBs can occupy thyroid hormone receptors,[6] and other agents produce symptoms (such as infertility in workers in contact with chlordecone and dibromochloropropane) that are plausibly the result of interference with normal endocrine function, even if a hormonal basis has yet to be established.

Secular trends in sperm counts,[7] rates of testicular cancer,[8] undescended testicles,[9] hypospadias,[10] and the ratio of male to female births in the general population[11] have been attributed to endocrine disruption by synthetic environmental agents, although no studies are available in which the specific outcome and the responsible chemical have been measured in the same individuals or groups. A number of studies of breast cancer reveal no consistent relationship between body stores of DDT or PCBs and the risk of breast cancer.[12]

Table 12.1 shows pediatric studies of plausible endocrine outcomes in which an environmental chemical has either been measured or in which exposure can be reasonably inferred. In the United States, at background exposures to PCBs and DDE, the higher the prenatal exposure to DDE, the taller and heavier the boys were at age 14 years.[13] There was no effect on the ages at which pubertal stages

**Table 12.1**
**Listing of Pediatric Studies**

| Chemical | Outcome | Age/Route of Exposure | Comments |
|---|---|---|---|
| Polychlorinated biphenyls | ↑ weight in adolescent females; no effect on pubertal development | Prenatal | Prospective study, 300 females[13] |
| | Changes in thyroid economy | Mostly prenatal | Inconsistent results from several studies[14] |
| Dichlorodiphenyl-trichloroethane | ↑ weight in adolescent males; no effect on pubertal development | Prenatal | Prospective study, 300 males[13] |
| | ↓ duration of lactation | Maternal exposure to food supply in US and Mexico | Prospective studies in the US, 800 females,[15] and Mexico, 230 females[16] |
| Polychlorinated biphenyls/ polychlorinated dibenzofurans | ↓ penis size at adolescence ↓ height in adolescent females | Prenatal-maternal poisoning from contaminated cooking oil | Prospective study 25 males, 104 females[17] |
| | ↓ sperm motility | | Prospective study, 12 exposed males[18] |
| Dioxin | ↓ in number of male births | Preconception, to the father, from an industrial explosion | Historical cohort— 239 males, 298 female parents with 328 males, 346 female children[19] |
| Soy isoflavones | Altered cholesterol metabolism in infants | Infant formula | Clinical trial, 7 infants[20] |
| | Minor menstrual irregularities in 20–34-year-olds | | Follow-up of a clinical trial, 128 females[21] |
| Polybrominated biphenyls | Early menarche | Prenatal | Survey of 327 5- to 24-year-old female offspring of participants in an exposure registry[22] |
| Phthalate esters | Early thelarche | Concurrent body burden | Case-control study with 41 cases[23] |

were attained. Postnatal (ie, lactational) exposures to DDE had no apparent effects; neither did exposure to PCBs. Girls with the highest transplacental PCB exposures were 5.4 kg heavier for their heights than other girls by age 14 years, but the difference was significant only if the analysis was restricted to whites. While there was some evidence that the girls with the highest PCB exposure reached the early stages of puberty sooner, the numbers were small, and age at menarche seemed unaffected.[13] In 2 studies of background exposure to PCBs and child development, hypotonia at birth was related to prenatal exposure to PCBs[24] or to a history of consuming PCB-contaminated fish.[25] The hypotonia suggested an effect on thyroid hormone. Polychlorinated biphenyls were known to be toxic to the developing thyroid gland.[26] Subsequently, hypotonia was shown to be accompanied by higher thyroid-stimulating hormone levels in one study,[27] and now there are comparable data from 5 studies.[14] In general, associations among a variety of measures of thyroid hormone status have been weak, inconsistent, or absent. The hypothesis has a very reasonable basis in laboratory evidence, though, and is probably worth further innovative study. An estrogenlike effect of DDE (ie, shortened duration of lactation) was seen in 2 studies, one in North Carolina, the other in Mexico.[16]

In Taiwan, adolescent males who had been exposed in utero to high levels of PCBs and polychlorinated dibenzofurans when their mothers were poisoned[28] had normal progression through the Tanner stages but smaller penises than a comparison group. Puberty in girls was unaffected.[17] This is a complicated effect, not obviously an estrogenic one, and its mechanism is unknown. In a different study of the same cohort, the prenatally exposed adolescents had decreased sperm motility compared with a comparison group.[18]

There was a clear excess of female births in the Seveso region of Italy, where an explosion had released large quantities of 2,3,7,8-tetrachlorodibenzodioxin, a toxic halogenated hydrocarbon, but the effect was seen only when the father was exposed and so far has no laboratory confirmation.[19]

Soybeans contain very large amounts of estrogenic isoflavones. In a clinical trial in which postmenopausal women ate soy foods or their regular diets, vaginal smears showed some estrogen effect, but all other physiological measures, including sex hormone–binding globulin, were unaffected.[29] In a clinical trial in which infants were either fed cow milk or soy-based formulas, the infants absorbed and excreted the estrogenic isoflavones, and their cholesterol synthesis patterns were modified in association with isoflavone excretion.[20] The only follow-up study available is one of 128 women fed soy formula as infants who filled out a mailed questionnaire at 20 to 34 years old; the only differences plausibly related to estrogenicity of their formula are longer duration of menstrual bleeding and more pain with their menstrual periods.[21] This study is useful but small, and more work is needed in this area.

Maternal exposure to polybrominated biphenyls, which had occurred during a statewide food contamination episode in Michigan in the mid-1970s, was associated in one study with earlier menarche,[22] and Puerto Rican girls with premature thelarche had higher serum levels of phthalate plasticizers.[23]

What role, if any, environmental chemicals have in morbidity due to endocrine disruption remains unclear. Many studies of endometriosis, testicular cancer, puberty, neonatal estrogenization, and other plausible end points are under way. Currently, however, endocrine disruption of humans by environmental pollution still is mainly extrapolation of laboratory evidence and speculation.

## Regulation

In 1996 Congress enacted legislation to be implemented in 1998, requiring the US Environmental Protection Agency to screen and test chemicals in food and water for estrogenic and possibly other hormonal activity. Most likely, such testing would serve to select agents for more intense study. It would not replace more traditional tests for general toxicity and carcinogenicity.

## Frequently Asked Questions

Q *Could my child's undescended testicle or hypospadias be due to my exposure to a pollutant chemical during pregnancy?*

A No controlled studies show such associations. Some evidence exists that these conditions have perhaps been increasing, but even if they are increasing, the cause of such an increase is unclear.

Q *My daughter started her menstrual period when she was 10 years old. Could this be because of chemical exposure?*

A Since about 1840, menarche has been starting earlier among white, northern European girls, perhaps due to better nutrition. There has been no abrupt change in age at menarche in the United States recently, although the standards have been changed to reflect the inclusion of black girls and their generally younger age at menarche.

## References

1. Fry DM. Reproductive effects in birds exposed to pesticides and industrial chemicals. *Environ Health Perspect.* 1995;103(suppl 7):165–171
2. Boylan JJ, Egle JL, Guzelian PS. Cholestyramine: use as a new therapeutic approach for chlordecone (kepone) poisoning. *Science.* 1978;199:893–895
3. Guillette LJ Jr, Gross TS, Mason GR, Matter JM, Percival HF, Woodward AR. Developmental abnormalities of the gonad and abnormal sex hormone concentrations in juvenile alligators from contaminated and control lakes in Florida. *Environ Health Perspect.* 1994;102:680–688
4. National Research Council. *Hormonally Active Agents in the Environment.* National Academies Press: Washington, DC; 1999
5. Kelce WR, Stone CR, Laws SC, Gray LE, Kemppainen JA, Wilson EM. Persistent DDT metabolite p,p'-DDE is a potent androgen receptor antagonist. *Nature.* 1995;375:581–585
6. Rickenbacher U, McKinney JD, Oatley SJ, Blake CC. Structurally specific binding of halogenated biphenyls to thyroxine transport protein. *J Med Chem.* 1986;29:641–648

7. Swan SH, Eilkin EP, Fenster L. The question of declining sperm density revisited: an analysis of 101 studies published 1934–1996. *Environ Health Perspect.* 2000;108:961–966

8. Liu S, Semenciw R, Waters C, Wen SW, Mery LS, Mao Y. Clues to the aetiological heterogeneity of testicular seminomas and non-seminomas: time trends and age-period-cohort effects. *Int J Epidemiol.* 2000;29:826–831

9. James WH. Secular trends in monitors of reproductive hazard. *Hum Reprod.* 1997;12:417–421

10. Paulozzi LJ, Erickson JD, Jackson RJ. Hypospadias trends in two US surveillance systems. *Pediatrics.* 1997;100:831–834

11. Davis DL, Gottlieb MB, Stampnitzky JR. Reduced ratio of male to female births in several industrial countries: a sentinel health indicator? *JAMA.* 1998;279:1018–1023

12. Laden F, Collman G, Iwamoto K, et al. 1,1-Dichloro-2,2-bis(p-chlorophenyl)ethylene and polychlorinated biphenyls and breast cancer: combined analysis of five US studies. *J Natl Cancer Inst.* 2001;93:768–776

13. Gladen BC, Ragan NB, Rogan WJ. Pubertal growth and development and prenatal and lactational exposure to polychlorinated biphenyls and dichlorodiphenyl dichloroethene. *J Pediatr.* 2000;136:490–496

14. Brouwer A, Longnecker MP, Birnbaum LS, et al. Characterization of potential endocrine-related health effects at low-dose levels of exposure to PCBs. *Environ Health Perspect.* 1999;107(suppl 4):639–649

15. Rogan WJ, Gladen BC, McKinney JD, et al. Polychlorinated biphenyls (PCBs) and dichlorodiphenyl dichloroethene (DDE) in human milk: effects on growth, morbidity, and duration of lactation. *Am J Public Health.* 1987;77:1294–1297

16. Gladen BC, Rogan WJ. DDE and shortened duration of lactation in a northern Mexican town. *Am J Public Health.* 1995;85:504–508

17. Guo YL, Lai TJ, Ju SH, Chen YC, Hsu CC. Sexual developments and biological findings in Yucheng children. In: Fiedler H, Frank H, Hutzinger O, Parzefall W, Riss A, Safe S, eds. *Organohalogen Compounds.* 14th ed. Vienna, Austria: Federal Environmental Agency; 1993:235–238

18. Guo YL, Hsu PC, Hsu CC, Lambert GH. Semen quality after prenatal exposure to polychlorinated biphenyls and dibenzofurans. *Lancet.* 2000;356:1240–1241

19. Mocarelli P, Gerthoux PM, Ferrari E, et al. Paternal concentrations of dioxin and sex ratio of offspring. *Lancet.* 2000;355:1858–1863

20. Cruz ML, Wong WW, Mimouni F, et al. Effects of infant nutrition on cholesterol synthesis rates. *Pediatr Res.* 1994;35:135–140

21. Strom BL, Schinnar R, Ziegler EE, et al. Exposure to soy-based formula in infancy and endocrinological and reproductive outcomes in young adulthood. *JAMA.* 2001;286:807–814

22. Blanck HM, Marcus M, Tolbert PE, et al. Age at menarche and Tanner stage in girls exposed in utero and postnatally to polybrominated biphenyl. *Epidemiology.* 2000;11:641–647

23. Cólon I, Caro D, Bourdony CJ, Rosario O. Identification of phthalate esters in the serum of young Puerto Rican girls with premature breast development. *Environ Health Perspect.* 2000;108:895–900

24. Rogan WJ, Gladen BC, McKinney JD, et al. Neonatal effects of transplacental exposure to PCBs and DDE. *J Pediatr.* 1986;109:335–341

25. Jacobson JL, Jacobson SW, Fein GG, Schwartz PM, Dowler JK. Prenatal exposure to an environmental toxin: a test of the multiple effects model. *Dev Psychol.* 1984;20:523–532

26. Collins WT Jr, Capen CC. Fine structural lesions and hormonal alterations in thyroid glands of perinatal rats exposed in utero and by the milk to polychlorinated biphenyls. *Am J Pathol.* 1980;99:125–142

27. Koopman-Esseboom C, Morse DC, Weisglas-Kuperus N, et al. Effects of dioxins and polychlorinated biphenyls on thyroid hormone status of pregnant women and their infants. *Pediatr Res.* 1994;36:468–473

28. Rogan WJ, Gladen BC, Hung KL, et al. Congenital poisoning by polychlorinated biphenyls and their contaminants in Taiwan. *Science.* 1988;241:334–346

29. Baird DD, Umbach DM, Lansdell L, et al. Dietary intervention study to assess estrogenicity of dietary soy among postmenopausal women. *J Clin Endocrinol Metab.* 1995;80:1685–1690

# 13
# Environmental Tobacco Smoke and Smoking Cessation

Environmental tobacco smoke (ETS) and smoking cessation are uniquely linked in the pediatric setting because a significant source of ETS exposure is parental smoking inside the home. Environmental tobacco smoke, also known as secondhand smoke, is exhaled smoke or smoke released from the smoldering end of cigarettes, cigars, and pipes. It contains more than 4000 different chemical compounds, many of which are poisons.[1] Cigarette smoking is the most important factor determining the level of particulate matter in the indoor air, and concentrations of particulates less than 2.5 μm (a size that reaches the lower airways) can be 2 to 3 times higher in homes with smokers than in homes without smokers.[2–4] In 1992 the US Environmental Protection Agency (EPA) declared ETS as a Group A carcinogen*, the most dangerous class of carcinogens.[5]

## Route and Sources of Exposure

The route of exposure to ETS is through inhalation. Most children exposed to ETS are exposed in their own homes, and because many young children spend a large proportion of their time indoors with their families, the exposure to ETS may be significant.[6] Twenty-three percent of US adults are cigarette smokers.[7] From 1988 to 1994, 38% of children aged 2 months through 5 years lived in homes in which cigarettes were smoked on a daily basis.[8] These percentages may be much higher outside of the United States, in countries in which

---

*A US District Court decision vacated several chapters of an EPA scientific risk assessment document that served as the basis for the EPA's classification of secondhand smoke as a Group A carcinogen. The ruling was largely based on procedural grounds, and the EPA is appealing the decision. None of the court's findings concerning the serious health effects of secondhand smoke were challenged.

smoking is more prevalent and people may be less aware of the dangers of ETS exposure. Other settings in which children are exposed to ETS include child care settings, relatives' homes, smoking areas of restaurants, bars, airports, and motor vehicles.

## Clinical Effects

In adult nonsmokers, the effects of ETS exposure include increased risk of lung cancer,[5] causing approximately 3000 lung cancer deaths each year in the United States,[5] and increased risk of coronary heart disease.[9,10] Evidence for other effects in adults exposed to ETS is growing.

The effects of exposing children to ETS are well established, with some researchers suggesting that developing lungs are even more susceptible to ETS than adult lungs.[11] Short-term effects are primarily respiratory[12] and include increased upper and lower respiratory infections,[5] incidence of otitis media with effusion,[12–14] incidence of sudden infant death syndrome (SIDS),[15–17] and incidence of asthma exacerbations.[5,18–20] Each year in the United States, ETS exposure causes an estimated 1900 to 2700 deaths from SIDS, 136 to 212 deaths from acute lower respiratory illness in children up to 18 months, 700 000 to 1.6 million physician office visits for otitis media, 8000 to 26 000 new cases of asthma as well as 400 000 to 1 million asthma exacerbations, and 150 000 to 300 000 cases of bronchitis or pneumonia in children aged 18 months and younger (of which 7500 to 15 000 require hospitalization).[10,21] There is a growing body of evidence for long-term effects of ETS exposure during childhood, especially early childhood, including decreased lung function,[22,23] increased incidence of asthma,[24] and increased incidence of cancer.[5,25] Children exposed to ETS are more likely to have respiratory complications when undergoing general anesthesia.[26–29] Passive smoking is also associated with pediatric dental caries.[30] Among children aged 4 to 16 years, ETS exposure is significantly associated with 6 or more days of school absence in the past year.[18] Children living in households with smokers are

at greater risk for injury and death due to fires.[12] Cigarettes are responsible for about 25% of deaths from residential fires, causing some 1000
fire-related deaths and 3300 injuries each year.[31]

## Prevention of Exposure

### *Counseling of Parents by Pediatricians*

Parental smoking cessation may be the most effective means of ensuring
decreased exposure of children to ETS, and pediatricians are in a good
position to provide smoking cessation counseling to parents. Pediatricians often are the only physicians many parents of young children
visit,[32] and may be the primary source of health information for the
family. Pediatricians therefore may have an important role in efforts to
reduce the exposure of children to ETS. Just as pediatricians counsel
parents on diet and safety, it is appropriate for pediatricians to counsel
parents about ways to reduce exposure of children to ETS. Messages
about risks to children from ETS may become an important factor in
a parent's decision to quit smoking. Many "teachable moments" occur
when a child has a medical condition exacerbated by ETS exposure,
such as asthma or recurrent otitis media. Despite the similarity between
counseling about smoking and counseling about other parental behaviors that affect children, many pediatricians express concerns about
their role in counseling parents in smoking cessation. Some of the concerns are fear of alienating the parent by asking the parent to change
their behavior, but a survey of parents found that more than 50%
agreed that it is the pediatrician's job to advise parents to quit smoking,
and 52% of the current smokers surveyed responded they would welcome advice to quit smoking.[33] In a recent study of parents of children
hospitalized for an illness that could be exacerbated by exposure to
tobacco smoke, all parents who smoked and participated in the study
believed that pediatricians should offer parents who smoke the chance
to participate in a smoking-cessation program.[34] Other barriers to
counseling parents in smoking cessation include time, lack of training,
and lack of reimbursement.[35,36]

### *Discussions of Smoking Outside the Home*

While quitting is best, not all parents may be ready to quit. An intermediate step toward quitting may be smoking only outside the home. The success of counseling parents to smoke outside has not been well studied,[37] but at least 3 studies have shown that repeated counseling of mothers to smoke only outside the home reduced exposure of children to ETS.[38–41] Beeber[42] recommends the following stages in the path to quitting:

1. Never smoke while holding, bathing, or feeding a child; in the car with a child; or in the child's room.
2. Smoke only in one room in the home.
3. Smoke only outside the home.
4. Smoke only when away from the home and the child.
5. Quit smoking.

## The Process of Quitting

At baseline, without counseling or any other intervention, about 4% to 9% of smokers quit each year.[43] Success increases with each attempt to quit, and interventions such as counseling, nicotine replacement products, and bupropion (a medication also used as an antidepressant) approximately double the odds of success for each quit attempt.[44] Approximately 10% of all smokers who receive counseling from a physician stop smoking.[44] Although this rate may not seem significant within the context of an individual practice, it reflects a tremendous public health impact at the population level. If there were a 10% rate of cessation in patients in all physician practices in the United States, 2 million smokers would quit each year.[45,46] Over time, advice from physicians also may influence family members to quit smoking completely, reduce the numbers of cigarettes they smoke, or change the venue of smoking (ie, from indoors to outdoors).

### Treating Adult Tobacco Use and Dependence

The US Public Health Service updated their clinical practice guideline on smoking cessation counseling in 2000.[44] Counseling by physicians and pharmacotherapy were found to increase quit rates in adult smokers coming to physicians for their own health care. Although smoking cessation counseling provided by pediatricians to parents has not been as well studied, the guideline recommends that counseling also be offered to parents. In addition to a comprehensive review of the efficacy of various smoking cessation strategies, the guideline recommends that all health care professionals routinely assess the smoking status of their patients at every medical visit, regardless of the reason for the visit. Health care professionals are urged to provide counseling at each visit and assess the eligibility of their patients for pharmaceutical products.[44] See Strategies for Counseling Parents and Caregivers in Smoking Cessation for further information on counseling.

---

**Strategies for Counseling Parents and Caregivers in Smoking Cessation**

*The "Five As"*

The clinical practice guideline suggests a "5 As" smoking cessation educational program, which includes the following components: (1) *Ask* about smoking at every appropriate opportunity, and assess smoking status with specific attention to the patient's motivation and barriers to change; (2) *Advise* the smoker to quit smoking; (3) *Assess* by determining the smoker's readiness to quit within the next 2 to 4 weeks; (4) *Assist* the smoker with change; and (5) *Arrange* follow-up.[47] Although these steps are fairly brief, concern is frequently expressed about the limited time available for smoking cessation counseling during a health care visit. Even brief advice from pediatricians in the context of well-child care may have a positive impact on reducing maternal smoking and relapse rates.

---

| Strategies for Counseling Parents and Caregivers in Smoking Cessation, *continued* |
|---|
| *Pharmacotherapies* Because nicotine is so highly addictive, the role of pharmacotherapies in smoking cessation is extremely important. While we believe that it is not the role of pediatricians to prescribe medications to parents and other caregivers, it is important for pediatricians to understand the use and role of nicotine replacement products, especially those available over-the-counter, and bupropion (Zyban®). There are many resources available explaining the role of pharmacotherapies in smoking cessation (see Resources). |

### Billing for Counseling of Parents in Smoking Cessation

Unfortunately, there is no reimbursement or *Physicians' Current Procedural Terminology* code for the counseling of parents in smoking cessation at this time. Despite these barriers, counseling parents effectively in the context of a busy practice is possible because the intervention can be very brief. The simple statement, "you should quit smoking," when delivered by a member of the health care team increased the quit attempts and success of those quit attempts in adults.[44] Because the consequences of ETS exposure are so great, and the intervention can be so brief, even a busy pediatrician can deliver smoking cessation counseling.

### Strategies for Adolescents

Most smokers started when they were teenagers, and prevention of smoking initiation is an important goal for pediatricians. The American Academy of Pediatrics Committee on Substance Abuse has addressed the issue in 2 statements: "Tobacco's Toll: Implications for the Pediatrician"[48] and "Tobacco, Alcohol, and Other Drugs: The Role of the Pediatrician in Prevention and Management of Substance Abuse,"[49] and a chapter in *Substance Abuse: A Guide for*

*Health Professionals.*[50] The reader is referred to these sources for a more complete discussion of adolescent smoking.

It is important to note the role of the media in smoking initiation and maintenance. Advertisements for tobacco products, including chewing tobacco, cigars, and snuff, are pervasive in the United States[51] despite the 1998 ban on youth-targeted tobacco advertisements (http://www.naag.org/issues/issue-tobacco).

Early identification of the adolescent who is at risk for tobacco use is important, and the US Surgeon General has identified 4 categories of risk factors for adolescent use of tobacco.[48]

- *Personal*—belief that use of tobacco will make the teenager fit better into the social scene
- *Behavioral*—lack of strong educational goals, lack of attachment to school and social clubs
- *Socioeconomic*—low socioeconomic status
- *Environmental*—use of cigarettes by peers and/or parents, exposure to tobacco products and advertisements

The effectiveness of physicians' counseling of teenagers who smoke is much less well established than it is with adult smokers. The guideline recommends using the same kinds of counseling with teenagers that have been shown to be effective with adults, with the message tailored to the teenager. Delivering messages about the effects of ETS exposure to children and teenagers also may be useful in reducing their exposure and the rate that their parents quit.[44] Messages can focus on the short-term effects of smoking, such as high cost, bad breath, smelly clothes, decreased physical performance, and social unacceptability. Additionally, it may be useful to raise teenagers' awareness of attempts by tobacco companies to "hook" teenagers on smoking through seductive advertising campaigns.

Because there is no evidence that pharmacotherapies are harmful for children or teenagers, use of nicotine replacement products and bupropion SR may be considered. When doing so, pediatricians must determine how many cigarettes are smoked, the degree of dependence, the presence of any contraindications, body weight, and the teenaged smoker's intent to quit.[44] Confidentiality often is an issue, especially when pharmacotherapies are prescribed for teenagers. Because most insurance companies do not reimburse for smoking cessation counseling, and some do not reimburse for prescription smoking cessation

**Table 13.1**
**Steps to Help Teenagers Stop Using Tobacco***

| |
|---|
| 1. Ask teenagers to consider that most adults who smoke started when they were teenagers, and wish that they had quit as teenagers. Mention that tobacco companies actively solicit teenagers to try smoking. |
| 2. Ask teenagers to make a list of reasons why someone might want to quit, then talk about any that could apply to them. |
| 3. If the teenager has not been smoking too long or is not yet smoking more than 10 cigarettes a day, point out that it is easier to quit before the body is more addicted. |
| 4. Ask teenagers who are not willing to discontinue use to promise that they will not increase the amount they smoke. |
| 5. Ask teenagers who insist that tobacco is not a problem for them, "At what point would tobacco become a problem for you?" |
| 6. Ask teenagers who insist that they are not addicted to enter into a verbal contract with you to avoid tobacco for a week. Follow up by telephone. |
| 7. Once the teenager has made a commitment to stop, the pediatrician's task is to encourage and educate. Suggest that teenagers who are determined to give up tobacco do the following: <br> • Consider the logical arguments in favor of cessation, including health hazards. <br> • Learn about ways to quit. <br> • Think about how and why they use tobacco. <br> • Develop a plan to cope with (or avoid) situations where the urge to use is great. <br> • Make the commitment. <br> • Get the help they need (eg, nicotine patch or gum, bupropion, cessation clinics, quitting partners). <br> • Decide on a cessation plan and stay with it. <br> • Anticipate and prepare for occasional urges to smoke long after discontinuing use. |

*Adapted from Heyman RB.[52]

pharmacotherapies, cost can be a concern. Table 13.1 identifies steps to help teenagers stop using tobacco.

## Strategies for Preadolescents

It is important to begin delivery of the "don't start smoking" message as early as possible and to engage parents during this stage, even parents who smoke. One powerful message that can be delivered by a parent who smokes is that "quitting is hard, and I wish I had never started smoking." Teenagers whose parents smoke are more likely to smoke themselves. The process of smoking initiation follows a Stages of Change pattern.

- *Preparation*—stage during which the preteenager or teenager develops knowledge, beliefs, and expectations about nicotine use and the functions it can serve (eg, a perception that smoking will result in a more glamorous image, maturity, independence, etc). "Don't start" messages at this stage include discussions about the declining numbers of people who smoke, because youth often overestimate the prevalence of smoking, and about the tobacco companies' attempts to encourage smoking among youth.
- *Initial trying*—the first 2 or 3 attempts to smoke, typically occurring with friends. Messages at this stage can focus on the unpleasantness of these first attempts and how bad smoke must be to make the "tryer" nauseated, lightheaded, and cough.
- *Experimentation*—involves irregular use over an extended period, often several years. Discussions can emphasize the ease of quitting during this stage but that the smoker can easily become addicted because addiction often occurs insidiously.
- *Regular use*—stage during which youth use tobacco on a regular basis (ie, on weekends, going to school, after school, etc). Although many regular users are not daily users, signs of nicotine dependence and addiction begin during this stage. Discussions can emphasize that quitting at this stage is still easier than when the smoker is smoking a pack a day or more.

- *Nicotine dependence or addiction*—stage defined by the development of an internally regulated need for nicotine. Messages similar to those presented to smoking parents may be effective, especially if the discussion is tailored to the concerns of the young smoker.

Effective prevention techniques have been found, with evidence supporting multipronged approaches that include school-based prevention programs, antismoking media messages, smoking restrictions in the home and public places, restrictions on access to tobacco products, tax policies, and health care system support for smoking cessation attempts.[50]

## The Pediatrician's Office and Smoking

Reinforcement of the antitobacco message is important, and the office setting and office staff can play important roles in delivering the message.[53,54] It is helpful to record tobacco use and exposure at every visit in a standard place on the patient's chart using a vital signs stamp or medical record flow sheet[55] (see Table 13.2).

## Frequently Asked Questions From Parents

Q  *If I smoke, should I breastfeed?*

A  Breast milk is the best food for infants, regardless of whether you smoke. However, for the same reasons we highly recommend that pregnant women don't smoke, breastfeeding mothers shouldn't smoke because nicotine and other toxicants may be transferred through the breast milk to the infant. If you do continue to smoke, never breastfeed while smoking because a high concentration of ETS will be in close proximity to your infant.

Q  *When visitors come to my home, they ask if they can smoke in another room. What should I tell them?*

A  Children's homes should be completely smoke-free. Even if smokers smoke in a separate room, smoke-filled air is spread throughout the home, exposing everyone in the house to ETS. Ask your visitors to smoke outside.

**Table 13.2**
**Office Intervention**

| |
|---|
| 1. **Set an example.** The pediatrician should serve as a role model and should not smoke, particularly in the presence of patients and office staff. The office should have signs stating the no-smoking policy. Remove magazines that contain cigarette advertisements from the waiting room. |
| 2. **Systematically assess parents' smoking status and children's ETS exposure.** Systematic strategies for identifying smokers, such as stickers on the medical chart as reminders or a vital sign form that includes smoking status, should be implemented. The goal is to prompt all health care professionals who have contact with patients or parents who smoke to provide information about smoking cessation. In the context of a pediatric visit, it is important to ask about the smoking status of parents and household members as part of the child's health assessment. The issue of parents or household members smoking should be placed on a problem list and addressed at each office visit. |
| 3. **Involve several staff members in providing information about smoking cessation.** Educating additional office staff (eg, a nurse or health educator) in smoking cessation counseling can extend the physician's efforts and provide parental support. |
| 4. **Serve as an "agenda setter."** The pediatrician may serve as a catalyst for a parent to quit smoking. The pediatrician may initiate the process and provide referrals to specialists in smoking cessation and maintenance of a smoke-free lifestyle. |
| 5. **Provide patient education materials.** Materials can be obtained free or at low cost from many organizations (see Resources) and on the Web. |
| 6. **Use local resources.** Local resources are available in most cities. Physician referrals should include a specific agency or program, telephone number, and description of what to expect. Self-help materials also are available from many agencies. The makers of nicotine gum and other nicotine replacement therapies offer self-help smoking cessation programs as adjuncts to these products. |

*Adapted from Fiore MC, Bailey WC, Cohen SJ, et al.[44]

Q  *I can't stop smoking right now. How can I reduce my child's exposure to ETS?*

A  Because your child will be exposed to ETS if you smoke in any part of your home, be sure that you only smoke outside the house, and never smoke in your car or any vehicle in which an infant rides. Choose a smoke-free child care setting, and avoid taking your child to places where smoking is permitted, such as bars, smoking areas of restaurants, airport smoking lounges, etc.

Q *How strong is the evidence that smoking causes asthma?*

A Dozens of studies have shown a strong association between exposure to ETS and asthma or wheezing.

## Frequently Asked Questions From Clinicians

Q *How do I counsel anyone in the context of a busy practice?*

A Even the briefest of statements, such as, "You should quit smoking," have been shown to effectively increase the number and success of quit attempts. Most pediatricians already make these or similar statements to parents when treating a patient with asthma or other respiratory illness. Tailoring the message to the parent's readiness to quit adds only a few minutes and can make the message much more effective.

Q *How can a pediatrician be expected to counsel when counseling is not reimbursed by most insurance plans?*

A Unfortunately, many insurance companies do not reimburse for preventive services counseling. The consequences of ETS exposure to the health of children and their families are so great, and the time needed to deliver a brief "stop smoking" message so short, that many pediatricians find the time to provide this important service.

## Resources

Agency for Health Care Research and Quality, phone: 800-358-9295

American Academy of Pediatrics, phone: 866-843-2271, Internet: http://www.aap.org

American Cancer Society, phone: 800-ACS-2345, Internet: http://www.cancer.org, and for quitting smoking: http://www.cancer.org/docroot/ped/content/ped_10_13X_quitting_smoking.asp?sitearea=ped

American Lung Association, Environmental Health, phone: 800-LUNG-USA or 202-785-3355, Internet: http://www.lungusa.org/tobacco

Asthma and Allergy Foundation of America, phone: 800-7-ASTHMA or 800-727-8462 or 202-466-7643, Internet: http://www.aafa.org

LUNGLINE/National Jewish Hospital, phone: 800-222-5864

National Cancer Institute, phone: 800-4-CANCER or 800-422-6237, Internet: http://www.nci.nih.gov

Nicotine Anonymous, phone: 415-750-0328, Internet: http://www.nicotine-anonymous.org

Office on Smoking and Health at the Centers for Disease Control and Prevention, phone: 800-CDC-1311 or 770-488-5701, Internet: http://www.cdc.gov/tobacco

US Environmental Protection Agency Indoor Air Quality Information Clearinghouse, phone: 800-438-4318 or 703-356-4020, Internet: http://www.epa.gov/iaq/pubs

## References

1. National Research Council. *Environmental Tobacco Smoke: Measuring Exposures and Assessing Health Effects.* Washington, DC: National Academies Press; 1986:28
2. Spengler JD, Dockery DW, Turner WA, et al. Long-term measurements of respirable sulfates and particles inside and outside homes. *Atmos Environ.* 1981;15:23–30
3. Dockery DW, Spengler JD. Indoor-outdoor relationship of respirable sulfates and particles. *Atmos Environ.* 1981;15:335–344
4. Lefcoe NM, Inculet II. Particulates in domestic premises. I. Ambient levels and central air filtration. *Arch Environ Health.* 1971;22:230–238
5. US Environmental Protection Agency. *Respiratory Health Effects of Passive Smoking: Lung Cancer and Other Disorders.* Research Triangle Park, NC: US Environmental Protection Agency, Office of Research and Development, Office of Air and Radiation, 1992. EPA Publication 600/6-90/006F
6. Schwab M, McDermott A, Spengler JD. Using longitudinal data to understand children's activity patterns in an exposure context: data from the Kanawha County Health Study. *Environ Int.* 1992;18:173–189

7. Centers for Disease Control and Prevention. State-specific prevalence of current cigarette smoking among adults and the proportion of adults who work in a smoke-free environment—United States, 1999. *MMWR Morb Mortal Wkly Rep.* 2000;49:978–982

8. Gergen PJ, Fowler JA, Maurer KR, Davis WW, Overpeck MD. The burden of environmental tobacco smoke exposure on the respiratory health of children 2 months through 5 years of age in the United States: Third National Health and Nutrition Examination Survey, 1988 to 1994. *Pediatrics.* 1998;101:e8. Available at: http://www.pediatrics.org/cgi/content/full/101/2/e8

9. Centers for Disease Control and Prevention, Office on Smoking and Health. *The Health Consequences of Involuntary Smoking: A Report of the Surgeon General.* Rockville, MD: Public Health Service; 1986. DHHS Publication (CDC) 87-8398

10. California Environmental Protection Agency. *Health Effects of Exposure to Environmental Tobacco Smoke.* Sacramento, CA: California Environmental Protection Agency, Office of Environmental Health Hazard Assessment; 1997

11. Wiencke JK, Thurston SW, Kelsey KT, et al. Early age at smoking initiation and tobacco carcinogen DNA damage in the lung. *J Natl Cancer Inst.* 1999;91:614–619

12. DiFranza JR, Lew RA. Morbidity and mortality in children associated with the use of tobacco products by other people. *Pediatrics.* 1996;97:560–568

13. American Academy of Pediatrics Committee on Environmental Health. Environmental tobacco smoke: a hazard to children. *Pediatrics.* 1997;99:639–642

14. Etzel RA, Pattishall EN, Haley NJ, Fletcher RH, Henderson FW. Passive smoking and middle ear effusion among children in day care. *Pediatrics.* 1992;90:228–232

15. Mitchell EA, Ford RP, Stewart AW, et al. Smoking and sudden infant death syndrome. *Pediatrics.* 1993;91:893–896

16. Schoendorf KC, Kiely JL. Relationship of sudden infant death syndrome to maternal smoking during and after pregnancy. *Pediatrics.* 1992;90:905–908

17. Klonoff-Cohen HS, Edelstein SL, Lefkowitz ES, et al. The effect of passive smoking and tobacco exposure through breast milk on sudden infant death syndrome. *JAMA.* 1995;273:795–798

18. Mannino DM, Moorman JE, Kingsley B, Rose D, Repace J. Health effects related to environmental tobacco smoke exposure in children in the United States: data from the Third National Health and Nutrition Examination Survey. *Arch Pediatr Adolesc Med.* 2001;155:36–41

19. Chilmonczyk BA, Salmun LK, Megathlin KN, et al. Association between exposure to environmental tobacco smoke and exacerbations of asthma in children. *N Engl J Med.* 1993;328:1665–1669

20. Martinez FD, Cline M, Burrows B. Increased incidence of asthma in children of smoking mothers. *Pediatrics.* 1992;89:21–26

21. Davis RM. Exposure to environmental tobacco smoke: identifying and protecting those at risk. *JAMA.* 1998;280:1947–1949

22. Berkey CS, Ware JH, Dockery DW, Ferris BG Jr, Speizer FE. Indoor air pollution and pulmonary function growth in preadolescent children. *Am J Epidemiol.* 1986;123:250–260

23. Corbo GM, Agabiti N, Forastiere F, et al. Lung function in children and adolescents with occasional exposure to environmental tobacco smoke. *Am J Respir Crit Care Med.* 1996;154:695–700

24. Larsson ML, Frisk M, Hallstrom J, Kiviloog J, Lundback B. Environmental tobacco smoke exposure during childhood is associated with increased prevalence of asthma in adults. *Chest.* 2001;120:711–717

25. Sandler DP, Everson RB, Wilcox AJ, Browder JP. Cancer risk in adulthood from early life exposure to parents' smoking. *Am J Public Health.* 1985;75:487–492

26. Skolnick ET, Vomvolakis MA, Buck KA, Mannino SF, Sun LS. Exposure to environmental tobacco smoke and the risk of adverse respiratory events in children receiving general anesthesia. *Anesthesiology.* 1998;88:1144–1153

27. Koop CE. Adverse anesthesia events in children exposed to environmental tobacco smoke and the risk of adverse respiratory events in children receiving general anesthesia. *Anesthesiology.* 1998;88:1141–1142

28. Lakshmipathy N, Bokesch PM, Cowen DE, Lisman SR, Schmid CH. Environmental tobacco smoke: a risk factor for pediatric laryngospasm. *Anesth Analg.* 1996;82:724–727

29. Lyons B, Frizelle H, Kirby F, Casey W. The effect of passive smoking on the incidence of airway complications in children undergoing general anaesthesia. *Anaesthesia.* 1996;51:324–326

30. Aligne CA, Moss ME, Auinger P, Weitzman M. Association of pediatric dental caries with passive smoking. *JAMA.* 2003;289:1258–1264

31. Miller AL. *The US Smoking-Material Fire Problem Through 1990: The Role of Lighted Tobacco Products in Fire.* Quincy, MA: National Fire Protection Association; 1993

32. Perry CL, Silvis GL. Smoking prevention: behavioral prescriptions for the pediatrician. *Pediatrics.* 1987;79:790–799

33. Frankowski BL, Weaver SO, Secker-Walker RH. Advising parents to stop smoking: pediatricians' and parents' attitudes. *Pediatrics*. 1993;91:296–300

34. Winickoff JP, Hibberd PL, Case B, Sinha P, Rigotti NA. Child hospitalization: an opportunity for parental smoking intervention. *Am J Prev Med*. 2001;21:218–220

35. Perez-Stable EJ, Juarez-Reyes M, Kaplan C, Fuentes-Afflick E, Gildengorin V, Millstein S. Counseling smoking parents of young children: comparison of pediatricians and family physicians. *Arch Pediatr Adolesc Med*. 2001;155:25–31

36. Christakis DA. Parental smoking cessation counseling: it's about time. *Arch Pediatr Adolesc Med*. 2001;155:15–16

37. Hovell MF, Zakarian JM, Wahlgren DR, Matt GE. Reducing children's exposure to environmental tobacco smoke: the empirical evidence and directions for future research. *Tob Control*. 2000;9(suppl 2):II40–II47

38. Hovell MF, Zakarian JM, Matt GE, Hofstetter CR, Bernert JM, Pirkle J. Effect of counselling mothers on their children's exposure to environmental tobacco smoke: a randomised controlled trial. *BMJ*. 2000;321 (7257):337–342

39. Wahlgren DR, Hovell MF, Meltzer SB, Hofstetter CR, Zakarian JM. Reduction of environmental tobacco smoke exposure in asthmatic children. A 2-year follow-up. *Chest*. 1997;111:81–88

40. Hovell MF, Meltzer SB, Zakarian JM, et al. Reduction of environmental tobacco smoke exposure among asthmatic children: a controlled trial. *Chest*. 1994;106:440–446

41. Emmons KM, Hammond SK, Fava JL, Velicer WF, Evans JL, Monroe AD. A randomized trial to reduce passive smoke exposure in low-income households with young children. *Pediatrics*. 2001;108:18–24

42. Beeber SJ. Parental smoking and childhood asthma. *J Pediatr Health Care*. 1996;10:58–62

43. US Department of Health and Human Services. *Reducing Tobacco Use: A Report of the Surgeon General*. Washington, DC: US Department of Health and Human Services, Centers for Disease Control and Prevention, National Center for Chronic Disease Prevention and Health Promotion, Office on Smoking and Health; 2000

44. Fiore MC, Bailey WC, Cohen SJ, et al. *Treating Tobacco Use and Dependence*. Clinical Practice Guideline. Washington, DC: US Department of Health and Human Services, Public Health Service; 2000

45. Ockene JK. Physician-delivered interventions for smoking cessation: strategies for increasing effectiveness. *Prev Med*. 1987;16:723–737

46. Kottke TE, Battista RN, DeFriese GH, Brekke ML. Attributes of successful smoking cessation interventions in medical practice. A meta-analysis of 39 controlled trials. *JAMA*. 1988;259:2883–2889

47. Glynn TJ, Manley MW. *How to Help Your Patients Stop Smoking: A National Cancer Institute Manual for Physicians.* Bethesda, MD: National Cancer Institute, US Department of Health and Human Services, Public Health Service, National Institutes of Health; 1990. Publication NIH 90-3064

48. American Academy of Pediatrics Committee on Substance Abuse. Tobacco's toll: implications for the pediatrician. *Pediatrics.* 2001;107:794–798

49. American Academy of Pediatrics Committee on Substance Abuse. Tobacco, alcohol, and other drugs: the role of the pediatrician in prevention and management of substance abuse. *Pediatrics.* 1998;101:125–128

50. Heyman RB. Tobacco use and abuse. In: Schydlower M, ed. *Substance Abuse: A Guide for Health Professionals.* 2nd ed. Elk Grove Village, IL: American Academy of Pediatrics; 2002:277–291

51. Strasburger VC, Donnerstein E. Children, adolescents, and the media in the 21st century. *Adolesc Med.* 2000;11:51–68

52. Heyman RB. Tobacco: prevention and cessation strategies. *Adolesc Health Update.* 1997;9:1–8

53. Stein RJ, Haddock CK, O'Byrne KK, Hymowitz N, Schwab J. The pediatrician's role in reducing tobacco exposure in children. *Pediatrics.* 2000;106:e66. Available at: http://www.pediatrics.org/cgi/content/full/106/5/e66

54. Fiore MC, Hatsukami DK, Baker TB. Effective tobacco dependence treatment. *JAMA*. 2002;288:1768–1771

55. Task Force on Community Preventive Services. Recommendations regarding interventions to reduce tobacco use and exposure to environmental tobacco smoke. *Am J Prev Med.* 2001;20:10–15

# 14
# Food Contaminants

This chapter focuses on a variety of contaminants in foods, including microbes, prions, pesticides, certain food additives, and mycotoxins. Lead and mercury are described in detail in chapters 19 and 20, respectively.

## Pathogenic Hazards

Although the US food supply is among the safest in the world, there are 76 million food-borne illnesses every year in the United States and an estimated 325 000 hospitalizations and 5000 deaths per year, mostly among the elderly and the very young.[1] The 2003 *Red Book*® describes the diagnosis and treatment of illnesses caused by food-borne pathogens.[2] Contaminants in foods include

- Viruses such as hepatitis A and caliciviruses including Norwalk virus
- Bacteria such as *Salmonella, Shigella, Campylobacter, Escherichia coli, Vibrio cholerae, Yersinia enterocolitica,* and *Listeria*
- Toxins from bacteria including *Staphylococcus aureus, Bacillus cereus, Clostridium perfringens, Clostridium botulinum,* and *E coli* O157:H7
- Toxins from molds such as aflatoxins and vomitoxin
- Parasites such as *Toxoplasma gondii, Cryptosporidium parvum, Cyclospora, Giardia lamblia, Taenia,* and *Trichinosis*
- Aquatic microorganisms such as *Pfiesteria piscicida* that elaborate toxins
- Products accumulated in the food chain of fish and shellfish, such as scombrotoxin, saxitoxin, ciguatera toxin, and domoic acid
- Prions, the agents of mad cow disease and other transmissible spongiform encephalopathies

The American Medical Association, Centers for Disease Control and Prevention (CDC), Food Safety and Inspection Service (FSIS), and US Food and Drug Administration (FDA) have produced a primer for physicians that describes the diagnosis and management of these food-borne illnesses.[3]

Infectious organisms are ubiquitous in the environment and can enter the food supply in a multitude of ways. Chickens infected with *Salmonella* species can excrete these organisms into the eggs before the shells are formed or excrete the organisms in feces that can contaminate the shells. Shellfish and other seafood can become contaminated by pathogens, such as the hepatitis A virus in manure runoff and sewage overflows and *Anisakis simplex* (herring worm, a roundworm) in sushi. Animal feces can contaminate foods via polluted irrigation water, unsafe handling of manure, and unsanitary production and processing activities. Food can become contaminated in retail facilities, institutional settings, and homes because of inappropriate food handling. The major nonhuman use of antibiotics is in food animal production, and millions of pounds are used annually at nontherapeutic doses in healthy animals, contributing to increased antibiotic resistance in humans (see Chapter 39).

The food production system is becoming more centralized and global, adding to the complexity of food-borne pathogen exposures. For example, in the United States there have been large outbreaks of infection due to *Cyclospora* associated with raspberry consumption.[4,5] Extensive investigation identified the source as *Cyclospora*-contaminated irrigation water in Guatemalan raspberry fields. Severe outbreaks of hemolytic-uremic syndrome and death due to *E coli* O157:H7-contaminated hamburger meat have involved the transport and blending of meats from various parts of the country, often with distribution to regions quite remote from the source of the contamination.[6,7]

Many pathogens are particularly virulent for children. *Salmonella, Listeria, Cyclospora, Cryptosporidium, E coli* O157:H7, *Shigella,* and *Campylobacter* are among many food-borne pathogens that pose risks to young children.[1] Standards for pathogens are established for meat, poultry, and egg products by the FSIS and for all other foods by the FDA. State public health agencies monitor the incidence of food-borne illness, along with local public health officers, and the US Environmental Protection Agency (EPA) regulates the discharge of pollutants into waters that may later contaminate food.

Powdered infant formula is not a sterile product and may be contaminated with bacteria. During 2001 powdered formula contaminated with *Enterobacter sakazakii* caused an epidemic of illnesses, including a fatal case of neonatal meningitis in Tennessee.[8]

The prion, the agent responsible for transmissible spongiform encephalopathies, is neither a virus nor a bacteria, but an abnormal form of a normal glycoprotein. Prion diseases include bovine spongiform encephalopathy (mad cow disease), scrapie in sheep, chronic wasting disease in deer and elk, and Creutzfeldt-Jakob disease and variant Creutzfeldt-Jakob disease in humans.[9] In the United Kingdom, an epidemic of variant Creutzfeldt-Jakob disease has followed the epidemic of bovine spongiform encephalopathy.[10] Although one case of variant Creutzfeldt-Jakob disease has been reported in the United States, the patient was born in the United Kingdom in 1979 and moved to the United States in 1992.[11]

**Toxic Hazards**

Toxic chemicals in food can be grouped into the following broad categories

- Residues of pesticides deliberately applied to food crops or to stored or processed foods
- Colorings, flavorings, and other chemicals deliberately added to food during processing (direct food additives) and substances used

in food-contact materials including adhesives, dyes, coatings, paper, paperboard, and polymers (plastics) that may come into contact with food as part of packaging or processing equipment but are not intended to be added directly to food (indirect food additives)

- Chemicals that inadvertently enter the food supply, such as aflatoxins, nitrites, polychlorinated biphenyls (PCBs), dioxins, heavy metals including mercury, persistent pesticide residues such as dichlorodiphenyltrichloroethane (DDT), and vomitoxin

### Pesticides

The diet is a major route of exposure of children to pesticides; exposure by other routes is described in Chapter 24.

Pesticides are applied extensively to food crops around the world. More than 400 different pesticidal active ingredients, formulated into thousands of products, are registered for use on agricultural products in the United States. Pesticides are used at all stages of food production to protect against pests in the field and in shipping and storage. In 1997 nearly a billion pounds of pesticides were used in the United States.[12] The EPA sets standards called tolerances for allowable levels of pesticides on food. The FDA and FSIS monitor the food supply for pesticide residues.

In 1993 the National Research Council (NRC) published a report titled "Pesticides in the Diets of Infants and Children,"[13] which assessed health implications of pesticides on food and made numerous recommendations for improving assessment and regulation of pesticides. The report concluded that the government has provided inadequate attention to prenatal and postnatal developmental toxic effects and the unique food consumption patterns of children, and thus is not providing an adequate level of protection to children in establishing standards for pesticides on food. As a result, many changes are under way in the pesticide food safety area, and legislation enacted in 1996 incorporates a number of the recommendations of the NRC. The Food Quality Protection Act (FQPA) of 1996 requires that when the risks for children are uncertain, the EPA will provide an additional margin of safety, referred to as an uncertainty factor, to ensure that children are adequately protected. Consumption studies can fail to capture the dietary patterns of small children. Significant features of the FQPA are shown in Table 14.1. (See also the FQPA sidebar in Chapter 24.)

Pesticide residues on individual commodities may be extremely variable. In the past the EPA established residue levels to ensure that average levels were safe. However, in 1992 the EPA discovered that it is possible for individual food items (eg, potatoes and bananas) to have high enough levels to make a child acutely ill, even when

**Table 14.1**
**Food Quality Protection Act of 1996: Provisions Related to Protection of Infants and Children**

| |
|---|
| **Health-based standard:** A new standard of a "reasonable certainty of no harm" that prohibits economic considerations when children are at risk. |
| **Additional margin of safety:** Requires that the US Environmental Protection Agency (EPA) use an additional 10-fold margin of safety when setting standards for pesticides on food to protect children. Less than a 10-fold margin of safety may be used when there are adequate data to assess prenatal and postnatal developmental risks. |
| **Account for children's diets:** Requires the use of age-appropriate estimates of dietary consumption in establishing allowable levels of pesticides on food to account for children's unique dietary patterns. |
| **Account for all exposures:** In establishing acceptable levels of a pesticide on food, the EPA must now account for exposures that may occur via other routes, such as drinking water and residential application of the pesticide. |
| **Cumulative effects:** The EPA must now consider the cumulative effects of all pesticides that share a common mechanism of action. |
| **Tolerance reassessments:** All existing pesticide food standards must be reassessed over a 10-year period to ensure that they meet the new standard to protect children. |
| **Endocrine disruptor testing:** The EPA must screen and test all pesticides and pesticide ingredients for estrogen effects and other endocrine disruptor activity. |
| **Registration renewal:** Establishes a 15-year renewal process for all pesticides to ensure that they have up-to-date science evaluations over time. |

the average level for the crop is within EPA standards. Such illnesses would be expected to be sporadic, and thus not detectable by disease surveillance efforts.[14] Since the enactment of the FQPA, the EPA has reassessed approximately 3600 of the 9721 food pesticide standards that existed in 1996. This process will be completed by 2006 and involves a number of intensive studies of the pesticides on food commonly eaten by children.

### Food Additives

Some food additives may cause adverse reactions in children. Tartrazine (also known as FD&C—food dye and coloring—yellow No. 5) is a dye used in some foods and beverages. Cake mixes, candies, canned vegetables, cheese, chewing gum, hot dogs, ice cream, orange drinks, salad dressings, seasoning salts, soft drinks, and catsup may contain tartrazine. In those who are sensitive to it, tartrazine may cause urticaria and asthma exacerbations.

Monosodium glutamate (MSG) is associated with the so-called Chinese restaurant syndrome of headache, nausea, diarrhea, sweating, chest tightness, and a burning sensation along the back of the neck. It seems to be linked to the consumption of large amounts of MSG, not only in Chinese food, but also in any other food in which a large concentration of MSG is used as a flavor enhancer.

Sulfites are used to preserve foods and sanitize containers for fermented beverages. They may be found in soup mixes, frozen and dehydrated potatoes, dried fruits, fruit juices, canned and dehydrated vegetables, processed seafood products, jams and jellies, relishes, and some bakery products. Some beverages, such as hard cider, wine, and beer, also contain sulfites. Because sulfites can cause asthma exacerbations in sulfite-sensitive patients, the FDA has ruled that packaged foods be labeled if they contain more than 10 ppm of sulfites.

Indirect food additives are substances that enter the food supply through contact with food in manufacturing, packing, packaging, transporting, or holding, even though that substance is not intended to have any technical effects on the food. More than 3000 of such substances are recognized by the FDA. One category is called "food contact substances"; these include packaging materials (adhesives and compounds of coatings, paper and paperboard products, polymers, adjuvants, and production aids) as well as a wide array of other materials. Recently certain plasticizer substances have come under increased scrutiny as food contact items. One is bisphenol A, which is used in certain hard plastics. Another is a class of plasticizers called phthalates, which are used in soft plastics.[15] Bisphenol A acts as a weak estrogen and phthalates are weak estrogens/anti-androgen (androgen blocking) chemicals. Some phthalates are suspected to cause cancer. Bisphenol A has been found in hard plastic baby bottles, water bottles, and many other food containers. The extent of exposure is unknown. The FDA has approved these uses; however, new scientific data on bisphenol A is accumulating. Phthalates have numerous industrial uses (in industrial plastics, inks, and dyes and adhesives in food packaging), consumer uses (eg, in cosmetics and vinyl clothing), and medical uses (as a softener in polyvinyl chloride intravenous tubing, blood bags, and dialysis equipment). Over the years, phthalate compounds were used in pacifiers, baby bottle nipples, and teething toys, and then removed from these uses by the US Consumer Product Safety Commission. The FDA allows the use of phthalates in food contact items, and in the past has found that exposures are very low. However, there has not been a recent review of their toxicities and the potential for exposures via this use. The CDC has started to track trends of phthalates in the human population.

### Mycotoxins

Mycotoxins, toxins produced by certain molds, are present in many agricultural products, such as peanuts and corn.[16] The best known mycotoxin, aflatoxin, is produced by the *Aspergillus* fungus, but others include patulin, citrinin, zearalenone, vomitoxin, and the trichothecenes. The principal human exposure to aflatoxins is from food. The International Agency for Research on Cancer has concluded that aflatoxin is a carcinogen.[17] Aflatoxin $B_1$ is an important risk factor for hepatocellular carcinoma in humans, based on studies conducted in areas with a high incidence of hepatocellular carcinoma, such as Asia, where the incidence of chronic hepatitis B viral infections also is high.[18–20]

Vomitoxin, a frequent contaminant of corn and wheat products, can lead to epidemics of vomiting within hours of consuming contaminated food. The disease usually is self-limiting.[21]

### *Dioxins and PCBs*

Dioxins and furans are inadvertently produced in manufacture of certain chemicals and by incineration. Polychlorinated biphenyls were manufactured for use as fire retardants and in electrical transformers and capacitors. Dioxins and PCBs are persistent and bioaccumulative chemicals and are found at highest levels in fish in contaminated areas. They can enter the food supply via animal feed as well. In the United States in 1998 and in Belgium in 1999 there were episodes where a large proportion of the food supply (chickens, eggs, and catfish in the United States and chicken and eggs in Belgium) became contaminated by dioxins due to adulteration of animal feeds.[22,23] In 2001 the European Commission established a tolerable weekly intake of dioxins and dioxinlike PCBs in the diet.[24] There is no regulatory standard for these compounds in food in the United States (see Chapter 25).

### Prevention of Food Contamination

Care must be taken during food production and preparation to prevent the introduction of pathogens and other contaminants into the food supply. When used in the manufacturing process, these methods are referred to as Hazard Analysis and Critical Control Point (HACCP) systems. These HACCP systems require that food manufacturers identify points at which contamination is likely to occur and implement control processes to prevent it. Also important are efforts to prevent antibiotic resistance, control use of pesticides and food additives, prevent environmental contamination of food, consumer education on proper preparation and storage of foods, pasteurization, irradiation of food, protection of animal health, prevention of discharge of pathogens and nitrogen into water bodies, and numerous other efforts to ensure that pathogens and other contaminants are not introduced into the food supply.

Food contamination is best prevented by application of appropriate agricultural and manufacturing practices. Integrated pest management, which uses information about pest biology to control pests, is a means to reduce the risks and use of pesticides (see Chapter 24).

Enforcement of food safety laws is important in prevention at all levels. Regulation and enforcement involve a complex network of federal, state, and local laws and regulations. Some enforcement efforts involve routine monitoring and surveillance of the food supply; other efforts are in response to reports of problems and incidents. Child health care professionals have an important role in reporting food-borne illnesses to local and state public health agencies. For example, physician reports of outbreaks of hemolytic-uremic syndrome caused by *E coli* O157:H7 led to stronger enforcement efforts to ensure that foods such as hamburger meat and apple juice are safe for consumption. Table 14.2 lists some steps to reduce the likelihood of food-borne illness resulting from pathogens.

## Food Biotechnology

Food engineered through biotechnology is now common in our food supply. Through genetic engineering, unique traits can be inserted into the genes of plants and animals, thereby causing the organism to predictably express the new trait. This technology has proven very controversial. Many argue that the newly expressed traits are harmless, and that selecting desirable traits has gone on for centuries. Others

**Table 14.2**
**Steps to Reduce the Likelihood of Food-borne Illness Resulting From Pathogens in Food**

- Thorough washing of fruits and vegetables with water removes some pathogens as well as many pesticide residues. Wash before you peel. Don't peel anything you wouldn't normally peel. It is unnecessary to use soap or chemicals when washing food.
- Raw eggs, fish, and meat should not be eaten, and unpasteurized milk products should not be consumed.
- Thoroughly cook meat, poultry, and eggs to ensure that pathogens are killed. For hamburgers, a thermometer inserted into the center should read 160°F.
- After poultry is prepared, hands, cutting boards, and any implements that were used on the raw poultry should be washed with soap and hot water. Cook stuffings for poultry separately rather than inside the birds.
- Store food appropriately. Refrigeration of prepared food prevents growth of many microorganisms responsible for food poisoning.
- Use of disinfectants and sterilants in the home is not necessary to prevent transmission of pathogens from food. At this time, incorporation of chemical agents into high-chair trays and cutting boards, use of disinfectants on kitchen floors and sinks, and similar practices do not have a role in preventing food-borne infections. It also is unnecessary to use chemical disinfectants for washing hands in the home; soap and water are quite effective.

argue that there are too many uncertainties, and the regulatory science is inconclusive.

While the debate continues, genetically engineered food likely will be maintained in the United States as new products are developed and approved. Currently genetically modified foods include corn, soybeans, rice, potatoes, milk, and a dozen or so other products. Before genetically modified food products are commercialized, the FDA, EPA, and US Department of Agriculture (USDA) conduct scientific reviews to help ensure the safety of these products. Specifically, the FDA conducts a premarket notification and safety review of bioengineered foods to ensure they meet the safety standards in the Federal Food, Drug, and Cosmetic Act. If products have been genetically modified to express a pesticide for insect or disease control, the EPA is responsible for conducting a rigorous scientific review process to ensure the product will not cause unreasonable adverse effects on people or the environment. To ensure that the new technology does not jeopardize existing plants or animals, the USDA conducts premarket reviews.

As the government regulatory process and the science underlying biotechnology are evolving and improving, questions still remain on the safety of these products. It is important that the government and scientific and medical communities remain vigilant to monitor possible adverse effects from and ensure the safety of biotechnology foods.

## Frequently Asked Questions

Q  *Are pesticides found on fresh vegetables in the store?*

A  Pesticides commonly are found on fruits and vegetables in the store. Because no labeling is required, parents cannot tell which fruits and vegetables contain pesticides. Even organically grown fruits and vegetables are not necessarily pesticide-free. Parents should be advised to scrub all fruits and vegetables under running water to remove superficial particle residues. Fruits and vegetables are good for children because they provide vitamins, minerals, and roughage. Because of these health benefits, children should continue to consume a wide variety of fruits and vegetables, particularly those in season.

Q  *Is store-bought baby food safe?*

A  Yes. Processed foods generally contain lower residues of pesticides than fresh fruits and vegetables, in part because federal standards are stricter for processed foods. Some makers of baby foods voluntarily make their products free of all pesticide residues, although they do not advertise this action.

Q  *Could cancer develop in my child because of exposure to pesticides?*

A  Many factors contribute to cancer, including genetics, contact with viruses, and diet. More research is needed to determine how and why cancers develop during childhood. No causal relationship between exposure to chemicals in foods and cancer has been proven. A number of pesticides can cause tumors in laboratory animals and are associated with cancer in some farmworkers exposed to very high doses.

Q *Are organic foods safer than other foods?*

A It is not known whether organic foods are safer than other foods. However, under the recently adopted organic foods standard, organic foods must meet additional requirements. They must be grown without pesticides or chemical fertilizers and they must not use biotechnology-bred plants. There should be lower levels of pesticide residues on foods marketed as organic. (This was true even before the standards were in place.)

Q *What is the concern about peanut butter?*

A There have been 3 concerns about peanut butter. The first is that peanuts can contain higher levels of carcinogenic aflatoxins. In the United States, there are standards for aflatoxins; however, peanut butter is not frequently monitored. The second concern is that many children are allergic to peanuts. Peanuts are among the most potent of food allergens; for some individuals even a minute amount of peanuts can cause serious or even fatal allergic responses. Therefore, it is important that children who have allergies to peanuts strictly avoid peanut butter; this avoidance sometimes means that other children in close contact with such a child should not have peanut butter (or other foods containing peanuts) because children often share foods. Finally, there have been past concerns with arsenical pesticides used for other crops getting into peanut fields and thus into peanut butter. In the United States today stricter enforcement of pesticide laws has addressed this practice.

Q *Are pesticides in foods 10 times more hazardous for children than adults?*

A Many scientists recognize that children may respond differently to pesticides and other chemicals. To account for this difference, standards for pesticides in foods must be set such that it is assumed that children are 10 times more sensitive than adults.

Q *I heard that hot dogs can cause brain cancer in children. Should my children avoid hot dogs?*

A Sodium nitrite prevents the growth of *Clostridium botulinum* in meat products. In the early 1990s consumption of nitrite-cured hot dogs was reported to be associated with brain cancer in a group of children in California. Although more research needs to be done to confirm this association, manufacturers have been working to reduce the amount of nitrite in their cured meat products. Children should eat a balanced diet, and an occasional hot dog may be a part of that diet.

Q *What can I do to prevent my children from eating products contaminated with prions (the agents of mad cow disease)?*

A Avoid consumption of brains or any food containing nervous tissue. Although there have been no cases of bovine spongiform encephalopathy (mad cow disease) reported in the United States, there have been confirmed cases of chronic wasting disease, a spongiform encephalopathy of deer and elk, in the western and midwestern states. Avoid feeding children products made with deer or elk from areas known to have chronic wasting disease.

Q *Are there simple tests readily available to determine if food has been bioengineered?*

A It depends on the exact food. For example, there are simple and inexpensive testing procedures available for genetically modified corn; however, there are not simple tests available for many other biotechnology food products. Because the genetic modifications vary according to trait, the testing regimen can require identification of exact gene sequences and sophisticated equipment. To expand the testing capacity, there are a variety of products under development (eg, strip tests) that will detect the presence of genetically modified material.

Q *Are bioengineered food products required to be labeled?*

A No. The FDA does not require labeling to indicate whether a food or food ingredient is a bioengineered product. Currently the FDA has guidance available for companies that wish to voluntarily label their bioengineered food products.

## Resource

US Department of Agriculture, Internet: http://www.usda.gov, Meat and Poultry Hotline: 800-535-4555

## References

1. Mead PS, Slutsker L, Dietz V, et al. Food-related illness and death in the United States. *Emerg Infect Dis.* 1999;5:607–625
2. American Academy of Pediatrics. Pickering LK, ed. *Red Book®: 2003 Report of the Committee on Infectious Diseases.* 26th ed. Elk Grove Village, IL: American Academy of Pediatrics; 2003
3. American Medical Association, Centers for Disease Control and Prevention, Food and Drug Administration, Food Safety and Inspection Service. *Diagnosis and Management of Foodborne Illnesses: A Primer for Physicians.* Chicago, IL: American Medical Association; 2001
4. Herwaldt BL, Ackers ML. An outbreak in 1996 of cyclosporiasis associated with imported raspberries. The Cyclospora Working Group. *N Engl J Med.* 1997;336:1548–1556
5. Ho AY, Lopez AS, Eberhart MG, et al. Outbreak of cyclosporiasis associated with imported raspberries, Philadelphia, Pennsylvania, 2000. *Emerg Infect Dis.* 2002;8:783–788
6. Slutsker L, Ries AA, Maloney K, Wells JG, Greene KD, Griffin PM. A nationwide case-control study of *Escherichia coli* O157:H7 infection in the United States. *J Infect Dis.* 1998;177:962–966
7. Tuttle J, Gomez T, Doyle MP, et al. Lessons from a large outbreak of *Escherichia coli* O157:H7 infections: insights into the infectious dose and method of widespread contamination of hamburger patties. *Epidemiol Infect.* 1999;122:185–192
8. Centers for Disease Control and Prevention. *Enterobacter sakazakii* infections associated with the use of powdered infant formula—Tennessee, 2001. *MMWR Morb Mortal Wkly Rep.* 2002;51:297–300

9. Whitley RJ, MacDonald N, Asher DM, American Academy of Pediatrics Committee on Infectious Diseases. Technical report: transmissible spongiform encephalopathies: a review for pediatricians. *Pediatrics.* 2000;106:1160–1165

10. Spencer MD, Knight RS, Will RG. First hundred cases of variant Creutzfeldt-Jakob disease: retrospective case note review of early psychiatric and neurological features. *BMJ.* 2002;324:1479–1482

11. Centers for Disease Control and Prevention. Probable variant Creutzfeldt-Jakob disease in the US resident—Florida, 2002. *MMWR Morb Mortal Wkly Rep.* 2002;51:927–929

12. Aspelin AL, Grube AH. *Pesticide Industry Sales and Usage: 1996 and 1997 Sales and Usage.* Washington, DC: US Environmental Protection Agency, Office of Prevention, Pesticides and Toxic Substances; 1999

13. National Research Council. *Pesticides in the Diets of Infants and Children.* Washington, DC: National Academies Press; 1993

14. Goldman LR. Children—unique and vulnerable. Environmental risks facing children and recommendations for response. *Environ Health Perspect.* 1995;103(suppl 6):13–18

15. Shea KM, American Academy of Pediatrics Committee on Environmental Health. Pediatric exposure and potential toxicity of phthalate plasticizers. *Pediatrics.* 2003;111:1467–1474

16. Morgan MR, Fenwick GR. Natural foodborne toxicants. *Lancet.* 1990;336:1492–1495

17. International Agency for Research on Cancer. *Aflatoxins: Naturally Occurring Aflatoxins (Group 1). Aflatoxin M1 (Group 2B).* IARC Monographs. Lyon, France: International Agency for Research on Cancer; 1993;56

18. Alpert ME, Hutt MS, Wogan GN, Davidson CS. Association between aflatoxin content of food and hepatoma frequency in Uganda. *Cancer.* 1971;28:253–260

19. Yeh FS. Aflatoxin consumption and primary liver cancer: a case control study in the USA. *J Cancer.* 1989;42:325–328

20. Yeh FS, Yu MC, Mo CC, Luo S, Tong MJ, Henderson BE. Hepatitis B virus, aflatoxins, and hepatocellular carcinoma in southern Guangxi, China. *Cancer Res.* 1989;49:2506–2509

21. Etzel RA. Mycotoxins. *JAMA.* 2002;287:425–427

22. Bernard A, Hermans C, Broeckaert F, DePoorter G, DeCock A, Houins G. Food contamination by PCBs and dioxins. *Nature.* 1999;401:231–232

23. Hayward DG, Northrup D, Gardner A, Clower M Jr. Elevated TCDD in chicken eggs and farm-raised catfish fed a diet with ball clay from a Southern United States mine. *Environ Res.* 1999;81:248–256

24. Dioxin in food. Byrne welcomes adoption by council of dioxin limits in food [press release]. Brussels, Belgium: European Commission; 2001

# 15
# Gasoline and Its Additives

Gasoline is a complex mixture of volatile hydrocarbons derived by distillation from crude petroleum. Gasoline contains as many as 1000 different chemical substances,[1] including alkanes, alkenes, and aromatics. The composition of gasoline varies depending on the source of crude oil, refining process, geographic region, season of the year, and performance requirements (octane rating). More than 100 billion gallons of gasoline are consumed annually in the United States,[2] (approximately 40% of consumption worldwide),[3] and gasoline combustion is an important contributor to ambient air pollution and global warming.[4] This chapter reviews the health effects of gasoline and its additives. The hazards associated with exposure to automotive exhaust, including diesel exhaust, are considered in Chapter 7.

Important toxic and carcinogenic constituents of gasoline include benzene; 1,3-butadiene; 1,2-dibromoethane; toluene; ethyl benzene; antiknock agents; and oxygenates.[1] Benzene, a polycyclic aromatic hydrocarbon that causes leukemia and probably causes multiple myeloma,[5-7] comprises up to 4% of gasoline by weight, except in Alaska, where it comprises 5% by weight.[5]

Tetraethyl lead was the principal antiknock agent used in gasoline in the United States until its phase-out in the years 1976 to 1990. Tetraethyl lead is still used in gasoline in many nations, especially developing countries.[8] Its phase-out in the United States led to a 90% reduction in blood lead levels.[9] Average blood lead levels among children in nations that still use leaded gasoline are 10 to 15 µg/dL higher than those in US children.[8] Further discussion of these issues is found in Chapter 19.

Methylcyclopentadienyl manganese tricarbonyl (MMT) has been proposed as a replacement for tetraethyl lead as an antiknock agent.[10]

Occupational exposure to manganese is a known cause of parkinsonism.[11] The available scant data suggest that community exposures to manganese resulting from combustion of MMT in gasoline may be associated with subclinical neurologic impairment.[12,13] A further discussion of MMT and manganese can be found in Chapter 21.

Oxygenates are added to gasoline, especially in the winter months, to reduce carbon monoxide emissions.[14] Methyl tertiary butyl ether (MTBE) is the oxygenate most widely used in the United States, and is added to gasoline at concentrations up to 15% by volume.[15] Combustion of MTBE produces acrid emissions, including formaldehyde, and has been linked to respiratory irritation and asthma attacks in children.[14,16] It has leaked into groundwater in many areas of the United States, creating an unpleasant taste that can render the water undrinkable. In California, a maximum contaminant level of 5 ppb was set for MTBE in drinking water based on taste and odor.[17] Methyl tertiary butyl ether was not subjected to toxicologic testing prior to its commercial introduction.[18] It subsequently has been shown in experimental animal studies to cause lymphatic tumors and testicular cancer.[19] In view of these findings, the governor of California ordered MTBE to be completely phased out of gasoline in California by December 31, 2002.[20]

Ethanol also is used as an oxygenate in the United States, and is added at concentrations of up to 10% by volume. People are briefly exposed to low levels of known carcinogens and other potentially toxic compounds while pumping gasoline, regardless of whether the gasoline is oxygenated.[21,22]

## Routes and Sources of Exposure

### *Inhalation*

Children can inhale volatile gasoline vapors at service stations, along highways, and in communities near petroleum processing and gasoline transfer facilities. Children can inhale gasoline engine exhaust. Engine exhaust includes uncombusted gasoline and toxic gasoline combustion products such as polyaromatic hydrocarbons.[23] If tetraethyl lead or MMT have been added to gasoline, exhaust will contain lead or manganese. Children's exposure to components of gasoline exhaust such as carbon monoxide, oxides of nitrogen, and respirable particulates can cause health problems. These issues are considered in detail in Chapter 7 and Chapter 10. Children can be exposed acutely to high doses of gasoline vapor through gasoline "sniffing."[24]

### Dermal Absorption

Gasoline is lipophilic and can be absorbed through the skin.

### Ingestion

Children can inadvertently ingest gasoline. A common scenario is that a child will swallow gasoline that has been stored in an attractive container, such as a soda bottle. Severe toxicity can result. Children can be exposed to certain components of gasoline, such as MTBE and benzene, through consumption of contaminated water and through showering.

## Systems Affected

Severe ingestion can result in any or all of 3 acute systemic syndromes: (1) pneumonitis, (2) central nervous system (CNS) toxicity, or (3) visceral involvement, which may include hepatotoxicity, cardiomyopathy, renal toxicity, or hepatosplenomegaly.[25] Chronic exposure to gasoline and certain of its components is carcinogenic.

### Lungs

Ingestion of liquid gasoline is followed by chemical pneumonitis.[26,27] Aspiration seems to be the principal route of pulmonary exposure, and therefore vomiting should not be induced following gasoline ingestion, except in very special circumstances (see Treatment). Symptoms of dyspnea, gagging, and fever may appear within 30 minutes of exposure. Cyanosis appears in 2% to 3% of patients. Symptoms typically worsen over 48 to 72 hours after ingestion, but then resolve in 5 days to 1 week. Death occurs in fewer than 2% of cases.

Pathologic changes in the lungs in gasoline pneumonitis include interstitial inflammation, edema, and intra-alveolar hemorrhage. The pathophysiology is incompletely understood but probably involves direct injury to pulmonary tissue as well as disruption of the surfactant layer.[27] Radiographic changes include increased perihilar markings, basilar infiltrates, and consolidation, and these changes appear in 50% to 90% of patients. X-ray changes do not correlate well with severity of clinical symptoms. Radiographic changes can persist for many weeks after resolution of symptoms. Long-term follow-up of survivors shows occasional cases of bronchiectasis and pulmonary fibrosis and a high prevalence (82%) of asymptomatic minor abnormalities on pulmonary function tests.[28]

### Central Nervous System

Acute exposure to gasoline vapors in high concentrations is narcotic and can produce dizziness, excitement, anesthesia, and loss of consciousness.[29] Seizures and coma are reported in a small percentage of cases. Death has followed exposure to high concentrations of gasoline vapors for periods as brief as 5 minutes.[30]

### Liver

High-dose exposure can cause hepatocellular damage and hepatosplenomegaly.[5,17]

### Heart

Arrhythmias and cardiomyopathy can occur after high-dose gasoline ingestion or gasoline sniffing, but are uncommon. In fatal cases, cardiac arrhythmias coupled with CNS toxicity may be the immediate cause of death.

### Kidneys

High-dose exposure can cause renal tubular injury.[5,17]

## Carcinogenicity

Chronic occupational exposure to gasoline seems to be associated with renal cell carcinoma and nasal cancer.[1,30] This may be an important finding for public health given the widespread exposure to gasoline vapors in retail service stations and rising rates of kidney cancer in the United States. An association between gasoline exposure and kidney cancer also is seen in experimental studies.[1,31]

Several components of gasoline are proven or probable carcinogens.

| Chemical | Associated Cancers | Certainty of Causal Association |
|----------|--------------------|--------------------------------|
| Benzene | Leukemias, multiple myeloma | Leukemia proven, myeloma probable[6,7] |
| 1,3-Butadiene | Lymphomas, leukemias, myeloid metaplasia | Probable[32] |
| MTBE | Testicular, lymphatic cancers | Strongly positive in animal studies,[19] no human data |

It is important to note the inherent limitations of epidemiologic studies examining the human carcinogenicity of gasoline and its components. These limitations include (1) the absence of complete information on past exposure levels to gasoline vapor or on concurrent exposures to other substances such as gasoline or diesel engine exhaust, (2) the constantly changing composition of gasoline, and (3) the need to wait for a long period, frequently many years, between exposure to a constituent of gasoline and the subsequent appearance of disease because of the long latency that may be required between exposure and illness. For these reasons, epidemiologic studies tend to underestimate the strength of associations between toxic exposures and disease. Toxicologic studies in experimental animals are a necessary complement to epidemiologic investigations.

## Diagnosis

Acute, high-dose exposure to gasoline is diagnosed by history and by detecting the odor of gasoline on exhaled breath. Methyl tertiary butyl ether and its breakdown product, butyl alcohol, can be measured in exhaled air, blood, and urine. Benzene can be measured in exhaled air and blood. Certain metabolites of benzene, such as phenol, can be measured in the urine. However, this test is not a quantitative indicator of the level of benzene exposure because phenol is present in urine from other sources such as diet.[33] It should be noted that these tests for the metabolites of MTBE and benzene are most appropriately used in the context of epidemiologic studies and generally will be available in academic medical research centers, but not in community hospitals.

Assessment of levels of exposure to gasoline and its constituents in community air or in groundwater requires expert air or water sampling by a certified environmental scientist or government agency such as a state or county health department or department of environmental protection. An important source of data on community exposures is the US Environmental Protection Agency's (EPA) Toxic Release Inventory (www.scorecard.org).

## Treatment

Treatment of chemical pneumonitis caused by acute high-dose exposure to gasoline begins with clinical assessment of the severity of illness and evaluation of the amount of gasoline ingested. Because most cases involve only small amounts of gasoline, and symptoms are not severe, outpatient evaluation with close follow-up (depending on the reliability of the family) is usually sufficient. More severe cases require hospital admission, possibly to the pediatric intensive care unit.

Whether to employ gastric emptying is the subject of long-standing debate. In most cases, gastric emptying is contraindicated because of the danger of aspiration. Rarely, however, it may be indicated if, for example, the amount of gasoline ingested is very large or the gasoline has been used to dissolve another chemical toxicant (as in a suicide attempt).[27]

Steroids seem to offer little benefit in gasoline pneumonitis. Antibiotics are indicated if bacterial superinfection develops. Debate is long-standing and unresolved as to whether prophylactic antibiotics are warranted.

In the most severe cases with advanced respiratory distress, mechanical ventilation may be required. Positive end-expiratory pressure (PEEP) ventilation has been employed, as well as high-frequency jet ventilation using very high respiratory rates (220–260/min). Extracorporeal membrane oxygenation has been employed when all other options failed.[27]

## Prevention of Exposure

Exposure of children and adolescents to gasoline and its vapors should be minimized to prevent occurrence of delayed health consequences, especially cancer. Young children should not pump self-service gasoline or work in retail service stations.

Gasoline should never be stored in soft-drink bottles or in other containers that are accessible and attractive to young children.

Community exposures to gasoline vapors near refineries, transfer stations, and other petroleum-handling facilities may require concerted community action for their amelioration, including the development of partnerships among community residents, pediatricians, and environmental agencies.

Prevention of exposures to gasoline and its additives in groundwater requires either installation of activated charcoal filters at the tap or switching to bottled water. Prevention of exposure to the most toxic additives to gasoline, such as tetraethyl lead, MMT, MTBE, or benzene, is best achieved by governmental regulation or phasing out of these compounds.[9,20]

## Frequently Asked Questions

Q  *What is the risk to a child of brief exposure to gasoline vapors when a parent brings the family car to a service station for fueling?*

A  The risk is minimal, but still should be kept as brief as possible to minimize risk of delayed consequences, especially leukemia caused by inhalation of benzene vapor.

Q  *What is the responsibility of a pediatrician who lives in a community where the leaking underground storage tank of a gasoline station is contaminating ground water?*

A  Strong state and federal regulations developed in recent years require monitoring and abatement of leaking underground storage tanks. A pediatrician should inform the state environmental agency and/or US EPA of the problem. Families who may drink water from a gasoline-contaminated source should be advised to install activated charcoal filters to their water tap or switch to bottled water. These measures should be taken when there is an unknown source of contamination, when contaminant levels are rising even though levels still may be below drinking water standards, or when levels of contaminants are steady but higher than drinking water standards. (See Chapter 27 for drinking water standards.)

Q  *What are the long-term risks of gasoline sniffing to children and adolescents?*

A  Mental deterioration and chronic injury to the nervous system are the principal dangers.[24,34] Renal damage may occur. Gasoline sniffing usually is symptomatic of a very disturbed and unhappy child in very deleterious social circumstances.

Q *Should pediatricians be concerned about proposals to add MMT to gasoline as antiknock agents?*

A Yes. Manganese is a known neurotoxin. It currently is not used in US gasoline. It has been used in Canadian gasoline since 1976 as an antiknock agent and to improve octane rating. Neurotoxic effects have been seen at high- and low-dose exposures and span the range from overt symptomatic parkinsonism at high exposures to subclinical neurobehavioral impairment. To permit addition of MMT to the US gasoline supply would not be prudent. It could increase risk of widespread subclinical neurotoxicity.

Q *What can pediatricians do to reduce gasoline consumption and thus prevent global climate change?*

A Pediatricians should support campaigns to develop safe, efficient mass transportation that will reduce atmospheric emissions and risk of automotive injury to children. Children should be encouraged, where possible, to walk or bike to school and to play activities, and pediatricians should take the lead in encouraging construction of community walkways and bikeways. Reduction of obesity among children will be an added benefit of this strategy. Pediatricians should take the lead in their communities in land-use planning that results in reduced dependence on driving and that fosters walking, bicycle riding, and use of mass transportation.

## References

1. Dement JM, Hensley L, Gitelman A. Carcinogenicity of gasoline: a review of epidemiological evidence. *Ann N Y Acad Sci.* 1997;837:53–76

2. US Department of Energy, Energy Information Administration. *Estimated Consumption of Vehicle Fuels in the United States, 1992–2002.* Available at: http://www.eia.doe.gov/cneaf/alternate/page/datatables/table10.html

3. Ad Hoc Committee on Environmental Stewardship. *Green Facts for the United States at the World at Large.* Atlanta, GA: Emory University. Available at: http://www.environment.emory.edu/green/world.shtml

4. Intergovernmental Panel on Climate Change. *Climate Change 2001: The Scientific Basis.* Geneva, Switzerland: Intergovernmental Panel on Climate Change; 2001

5. Agency for Toxic Substances and Disease Registry. *Toxicological Profile for Benzene.* Available at: http://www.atsdr.cdc.gov/toxprofiles/tp3.html

6. Rinsky RA, Smith AB, Hornung R, et al. Benzene and leukemia. An epidemiologic risk assessment. *N Engl J Med.* 1987;316:1044–1050

7. International Agency for Research on Cancer. *The Evaluation of Carcinogenic Risk to Humans: Occupational Exposures in Petroleum Refining: Crude Oil and Major Petroleum Fuels.* IARC Monographs. Vol. 45. Lyon, France: International Agency for Research on Cancer; 1989

8. Landrigan PJ, Boffetta P, Apostoli P. The reproductive toxicity and carcinogenicity of lead: a critical review. *Am J Ind Med.* 2000;38:231–243

9. Centers for Disease Control and Prevention. Update: blood lead levels—United States, 1991–1994. *MMWR Morb Mortal Wkly Rep.* 1997; 46:141–146

10. Needleman HL, Landrigan PJ. Toxins at the pump. *New York Times.* March 13, 1996; Op-Ed, A19

11. Gorell JM, Johnson CC, Rybicki BA, et al. Occupational exposures to metals as risk factors for Parkinson's disease. *Neurology.* 1997;48:650–658

12. Mergler D. Neurotoxic effects of low level exposure to manganese in human population. *Environ Res.* 1999;80:99–102

13. Mergler D, Baldwin M, Belanger S, et al. Manganese neurotoxicity, a continuum of dysfunction: results from a community based study. *Neurotoxicology.* 1999;20:327–342

14. Mehlman MA. Dangerous and cancer-causing properties of products and chemicals in the oil refining and petrochemical industry—Part XXII: health hazards from exposure to gasoline containing methyl tertiary butyl ether: study of New Jersey residents. *Toxicol Ind Health.* 1996;12:613–627

15. Ahmed FE. Toxicology and human health effects following exposure to oxygenated or reformulated fuel. *Toxicol Lett.* 2001;123:89–113

16. Joseph PM, Weiner MG. Visits to physicians after the oxygenation of gasoline in Philadelphia. *Arch Environ Health.* 2002;57:137–154

17. Office of Environmental Health Hazard Assessment. *Water—Public Health Goals* [memorandum]. Available at: http://www.oehha.org/water/phg/ 399MTBEa.html

18. Mehlman MA. MTBE toxicity. *Environ Health Perspect.* 1996;104:808

19. Belpoggi F, Soffritti M, Maltoni C. Methyl-tertiary-butyl ether (MTBE)— a gasoline additive—causes testicular and lymphohaematopoietic cancers in rats. *Toxicol Ind Health.* 1995;11:119–149

20. Schremp G. *Staff Findings: Timetable for the Phaseout of MTBE From California's Gasoline Supply.* California Energy Commission; 1999. Available at: http://www.energy.ca.gov/mtbe/documents/1999-06-18_ findings_ppt/index.htm

21. Backer LC, Egeland GM, Ashley DL, et al. Exposure to regular gasoline and ethanol oxyfuel during refueling in Alaska. *Environ Health Perspect.* 1997;105:850–855

22. Moolenaar RL, Hefflin BJ, Ashley DL, Middaugh JP, Etzel RA. Blood benzene concentration in workers exposed to oxygenated fuel in Fairbanks, Alaska. *Int Arch Occup Environ Health.* 1997;69:139–143

23. International Agency for Research on Cancer. *Diesel and Gasoline Engine Exhausts and Some Nitroarenes.* IARC Monographs. Vol 46. Lyon, France: International Agency for Research on Cancer; 1989

24. Cairney S, Maruff P, Burns C, Currie B. The neurobehavioural consequences of petrol (gasoline) sniffing. *Neurosci Biobehav Rev.* 2002; 26:81–89

25. Reese E, Kimbrough RD. Acute toxicity of gasoline and some additives. *Environ Health Perspect.* 1993;101(suppl 6):115–131

26. Eade NR, Taussig LM, Marks MI. Hydrocarbon pneumonitis. *Pediatrics.* 1974;54:351–357

27. Shih RD. Hydrocarbons. In: Goldfrank L, ed. *Goldfrank's Toxicologic Emergencies.* 6th ed. Stamford, CT: Appleton & Lange; 1998:1383–1398

28. Gurwitz D, Kattan M, Levinson H, Culham JA. Pulmonary function abnormalities in asymptomatic children after hydrocarbon pneumonitis. *Pediatrics.* 1978;62:789–794

29. Burbacher TM. Neurotoxic effects of gasoline and gasoline constituents. *Environ Health Perspect.* 1993;101(suppl 6):133–141

30. Lynge E, Andersen A, Nilsson R, et al. Risk of cancer and exposure to gasoline vapors. *Am J Epidemiol.* 1997;145:449–458

31. Mehlman MA. Dangerous and cancer-causing properties of products and chemicals in the oil refining and petrochemical industry: Part I. Carcinogenicity of motor fuels: gasoline. *Toxicol Ind Health.* 1991;7:143–152

32. Landrigan PJ. Critical assessment of epidemiological studies on the carcinogenicity of 1,3-butadiene and styrene. In: Sorsa M, Peltonen K, Vainio H, Hemminki K, eds. *Butadine and Styrene: Assessment of Health Hazards.* Lyon, France: International Agency for Research on Cancer; 1993:375–388. IARC Scientific Publication No. 127

33. Agency for Toxic Substances and Disease Registry. *ToxFAQs.* Available at: http://www.atsdr.cdc.gov/toxfaq.html

34. Burns TM, Shneker BF, Juel VC. Gasoline sniffing multifocal neuropathy. *Pediatr Neurol.* 2001;25:419–421

# 16
# Herbs, Dietary Supplements, and Other Remedies

A dietary supplement can be defined as a product (other than tobacco) that contains one or more of the following ingredients: a vitamin, a mineral, an herb or other botanical, an amino acid; a dietary substance for use by humans to supplement the diet by increasing the total dietary intake; or a concentrate, metabolite, constituent, extract, or combination of the above ingredients (see Table 16.1).[1]

## Prevalence and Trends

The use of herbs and dietary supplements by Americans is growing. In 1997 a telephone survey of adults found that an estimated 15 million US adults (1 in 5 adults who responded that they were taking prescription medicine) took prescription medications concurrently with herbal remedies and/or high-dose vitamins.[2] Estimated out-of-pocket expenditures for high-dose vitamins rose from $0.9 billion in 1990 to $3.3 billion in 1997.[2] Americans spent more than $5.1 billion on herbal products and $1.7 billion on dietary supplements in 1997.[2] Such products are now being marketed to parents for the treatment of their children. In one survey, 11% of 1911 families using the clinics of the University of Montreal sought alternative therapies for their children's medical conditions.[3] A recent study of 348 Washington, DC, families interviewed in pediatricians' offices revealed 21% of parents used alternative therapies for their children's health problems. Of these, 25% used nutritional supplements or diets and 40% used herbal therapies for their children.[4]

Families whose children have chronic conditions, such as autism or cystic fibrosis, may be particularly likely to use dietary supplements as part of their treatment regimen. The American Academy of Pediatrics

**Table 16.1**
**Categories of Dietary Supplements***

| The term "dietary supplement" means |
|---|
| 1. A product (other than tobacco) intended to supplement the diet that bears or contains one or more of the following dietary ingredients:<br>• Vitamin<br>• Mineral<br>• Herb or other botanical<br>• Amino acid<br>• Dietary substance for use by people to supplement the diet by increasing the total dietary intake<br>• Concentrate, metabolite, constituent, extract, or combination of any ingredients described in the previous entries |
| 2. A product that is<br>• Intended for ingestion<br>• Not represented for use as a conventional food or as a sole item of a meal in the diet |

*Definition taken from Food and Drug Administration, Center for Food Safety and Applied Nutrition.[1]

Committee on Children With Disabilities has issued guidelines for discussing such issues with parents.[5]

A "natural" product is advertised as such to imply that it is not synthetic in origin; however, consumers frequently confuse "natural" with "safe." "Natural" strychnine, extracted from the nut of the plant *Strychnos nux-vomica,* still has the same potentially life-threatening toxicity. The definition of "natural" is ambiguous because the term is used in different contexts by food and dietary supplement manufacturers, consumers, scientists, and policy makers. Chemical structures do not change, regardless of their origin. Synthesized ascorbic acid has the same structure as ascorbic acid found in orange juice or rose hips. Farmers, in their use of "natural," may intend to certify that a food or herb was grown without the use of commercial fertilizers or pesticides. Marketers of herbs in the form of pills or capsules may use terms like "safe" or "natural" to mislead consumers. A survey of dietary supplements advertised in popular health and bodybuilding magazines showed that no human toxicology data were available in the peer-reviewed scientific literature for approximately 60% of ingredients in the products advertised.[6] Herbals containing caffeine or ephedra also are marketed as "safe" ecstasy alternatives; "safe" dietary aids; and as a source of energy, improved alertness, and a "natural high." Student athletes may be influenced by the performance-enhancing claims of the purveyors of herbs and dietary supplements that contain ingredients such as caffeine, ephedra, amino acids, proteins, or creatine. Adolescents and young adults are particularly easy targets for such promoting tactics.

## Definitions

Herbs used for medicinal purposes come in a variety of forms. Active parts of a plant may include leaves, flowers, stems, roots, seeds and/or berries, and essential oils.[7] They may be taken internally as liquids, capsules, tablets, or powders; dissolved into tinctures or syrups; or brewed in teas and decoctions. Although few products are available as rectal suppositories, a wide variety of substances, in particular herbal products, are used in solutions for "therapeutic enemas." Table 16.2 lists terms used in the context of herbal therapy that are useful to know.

## Therapeutic Efficacy

To give better advice to patients and their families, the pediatrician should read what is known about how the active ingredients in the herb work pharmacologically and what animal or human studies demonstrate the herb's effectiveness.[8] In clinical studies some herbs have shown promising results. For example, *Artemesia* spp have compared favorably with chloroquine in the treatment of some types of malaria,[9] *Astragalus membranaceus* extracts enhanced the antibody response in immunosuppressed mice,[10] and the use of herbal teas containing chamomile seemed to have a salubrious effect on infantile colic.[11]

**Table 16.2**
**Definitions and Types of Preparations**

| Preparation | Definition |
|---|---|
| Abortifacient | Agent that induces an abortion. |
| Aromatherapy | Inhalation of volatile oils in the treatment of certain health conditions. |
| Carminative | Agent that aids in expelling gas from the gastrointestinal tract. |
| Carrier oil | Fixed oils (non-volatile long-chain fatty acids such as safflower oil) into which are put a few drops of the potent, essential oils to dilute them for topical uses. |
| Decoction | A dilute aqueous extract prepared by boiling an herb in water and straining and filtering the liquid, similar to an infusion. |
| Discipline of signatures | Historical term suggesting that the appearance of a plant gives a clue as to its medical value (eg, the extract of St John's wort is red, thus it is restorative for conditions involving the blood). |
| Elixir | A clear sweetening hydro-alcoholic solution for oral use. |
| Emmenagogue | Agent that influences menstruation. |
| Essential oil | Class of volatile oils composed of complex hydrocarbons (often terpenes, alkaloids, and other large molecular weight compounds) extracted from a plant. |
| Excipient | Other ingredients, such as binders and fillers, used to make a supplement product. |
| Extract | A concentrated form of a natural substance, which can be a powder, liquid, or tincture. The concentration varies from 1:1 in a fluid extract to 1:0.1 in a tincture. |
| "Natural" product | The term natural defies accurate definition because, strictly speaking, everything is derived from nature. In common usage it is intended to imply a substance that is not synthetic or is not grown using pesticides or other chemicals. |
| Poultice | Salve used in a preparation that is applied to skin, scalp, or mucous membrane. |
| Resin | Solid or semisolid organic substance found in plant secretions and applied topically in a cream or ointment. |
| Rubifacient | Agent that warms and reddens the skin by local cutaneous vasodilation. |

## Ethnic Remedies

Pediatricians should be culturally competent in their approach to the diagnosis and treatment of children in families from diverse ethnic backgrounds, whose health beliefs and practices may be different than those of Western practices. For example, *empacho*, described as an illness in which food, saliva, or other matter becomes "stuck" to the intestines, is accepted among some Latino people as the etiology of gastrointestinal symptoms and treated with a variety of home-based remedies, as well as visits to a physician and/or a traditional healer.[12] More than half the Southeast Asian patients using one Seattle, WA, primary care clinic used one or more traditional practices such as moxibustion (cupping), coining, aromatic oils, or massage.[13] The formation of the therapeutic alliance between physician, parent, and child requires a sensitivity to the family's background and interests, with the goals of optimizing communications and facilitating a partnership in the clinical care of the child. For example, ethnomedical remedies practiced by the Puerto Rican community may hold some medical risks, but also considerable benefits in decreasing the symptoms of asthma.[14] *Cao gio*, or coin rubbing of the skin to alleviate symptoms of illness, is an innocuous traditional Vietnamese practice that has unfortunately been confused by some Western physicians as traumatic abuse, leading to instances of distrust and avoidance of health care.[15] Certain Afro-Caribbean and Latino practices, such as the exposure to vapors of elemental mercury, may have risks of toxicity.[16] Some treatments for *empacho*, such as greta or azarcon, are contaminated by significant amounts of lead. Table 16.3 lists some of the common folk remedies that can produce toxic effects. Authorities recommend an approach of education and community outreach to effect changes in such potentially harmful practices. Pediatricians can be helpful in assessing the traditional practices families may be using to treat their children, supporting their involvement in building a therapeutic alliance, and counseling them about possible harmful side effects.

## Adverse Effects

Products that are natural are frequently promoted to consumers as having no side effects; however, many potent drugs are derived from natural products (eg, ergot alkaloids, opiates, digitalis, and estrogen), and other natural substances and plants are poisonous (eg, aconite, certain types of mushrooms, snake venom, and hemlock). On occasion, foragers who seek herbal remedies will mistakenly collect one plant confusing it with another. This can be a lethal error if, for example, water hemlock is mistakenly harvested and eaten after being identified as wild ginseng.[29] Tables 16.3 and 16.4 reference other examples of some of the potent chemicals present in certain herbs and ethnic remedies and the toxic effects they can produce.

**Table 16.3**
**Examples of Toxicity of Some Ethnic Remedies and Dietary Supplements**

| Product/Remedy | Toxic Agent | Adverse Effects | References |
|---|---|---|---|
| Ayurvedic remedies | Lead, arsenic | Plumbism, arsenic poisoning (wt loss, myalgias, neuro-pathy, shock, death) | 17 |
| Azarcon | Lead | Plumbism | 18 |
| GHB | $\gamma$-hydroxybutyrate | Coma, respiratory failure | 19,20 |
| Ghasard, bala goli, kandu | Lead | Plumbism | 21 |
| Glycerite asafoetida | Terpenes, undifferentiated | Methemoglobinemia | 22 |
| Greta | Lead | Plumbism | 18 |
| Pay-loo-ah | Lead, arsenic | Plumbism, arsenic poisoning | 23 |
| Santeria, palo, voodoo, espiritismo | Mercury | Rash, neuropathy, seizures | 24 |
| Tryptophan | Excipient | Eosinophilia-myalgia syndrome | 25–28 |

**Table 16.4**
**Examples of Known Herbal Ingredients and Their Associated Toxic Effects**

| Herbal Product | Toxic Chemicals | Effect or Target Organ | References |
|---|---|---|---|
| Chamomile<br>*Matricaria chamomilla*<br>*Anthmis noblis* | Allergens:<br>*Compositae*<br>plant species | Anaphylaxis, contact<br>dermatitis | 30 |
| Chaparral<br>*Larrea divericata*<br>*Larrea tridentata* | Nordihydroguaiaretic<br>acid | Nausea, vomiting,<br>lethargy<br>Hepatitis | 31,32 |
| Cinnamon oil<br>*Cinnamomum spp* | Cinnamaldehyde | Dermatitis, abuse<br>syndrome | 33,34 |
| Coltsfoot<br>*Tussilago farfara* | Pyrrolizidines | Hepatic veno-occlusive<br>disease (HVOD) | 35–39 |
| Comfrey<br>*(Symphytum officinale)* | Pyrrolizidines | HVOD | 35–39 |
| *Crotalaria* spp | Pyrrolizidines | HVOD | 35–39 |
| Echinacea<br>*Echinacea augustifolia*<br>  *(Compositae* spp) | Polysaccharides | Asthma, atopy, ana-<br>phylaxis, urticaria,<br>angioedema | 40 |
| Eucalyptus<br>*Eucalyptus globulus* | 1,8 cineole | Drowsiness, ataxia,<br>seizures, coma<br>Nausea, vomiting,<br>respiratory failure | 41–43 |
| Garlic<br>*Allium sativum* | Allicin | Dermatitis, chemical<br>burns | 44 |
| Germander<br>*Teucrium chamaedrys* |  | Hepatotoxicity | 45 |
| Ginseng<br>*Panax Ginseng* | Ginsenoside | Ginseng abuse<br>syndrome: diarrhea,<br>insomnia, anxiety,<br>hypertension | 46 |
| Glycerated asafetida | Oxidants | Methemoglobinemia | 22 |
| Groundsel<br>*Senecio longilobus* | Pyrrolizidines | HVOD | 35–39 |
| Heliotrope, turnsole<br>*Heliotropium spp*<br>*Crotalaria fulva*<br>*Cynoglossum officinale* | Pyrrolizidines | HVOD | 35–39 |

**Table 16.4**
**Examples of Known Herbal Ingredients and Their Associated Toxic Effects,**
*continued*

| Herbal Product | Toxic Chemicals | Effect or Target Organ | References |
|---|---|---|---|
| Jin bu huan<br>*Stephania* spp<br>*Corydalis* spp | L-Tetrahydro palmitin | Hepatitis, lethargy, coma | 47–49 |
| Kava kava<br>*Piper methysticum* | Kawain, methysticine | Hepatic failure, "kawaism," neurotoxicity | 50–51 |
| Laetrile | Cyanide | Coma, seizures, death | 52 |
| Licorice<br>*Glycyrrhiza glabra* | Glycyrrhetic acid | Hypertension, hypo-kalemia, cardiac arrhythmias | 53 |
| Ma huang<br>*Ephedra sinica* | Ephedrine | Cardiac arrhythmias, hypertension, seizures, stroke | 54,55 |
| Monkshood<br>*Aconitum napellus*<br>*Aconitum columbianum* | Aconite | Cardiac arrhythmias, shock, seizures, weakness, coma, paresthesias, vomiting | 56,57 |
| Nutmeg<br>*Myristica fragrans* | Myristicin, eugenol | Hallucinations, emesis, headache | 58,59 |
| Nux vomica | Strychnine | Seizures, abdominal pain, respiratory arrest | 60 |
| Pennyroyal<br>*Mentha pulegium* or<br>*Hedeoma* spp | Pulegone | Centrilobular liver necrosis, shock Fetotoxicity, seizures, abortion | 61–63 |
| Ragwort (Golden)<br>*Senecio jacobaea*<br>*(Senecio aureus*<br>*or Echium)* | Pyrrolizidines | HVOD | 35–39 |
| Wormwood | Thujone | Seizures, dementia, tremors, headache | 64,65 |

The concentration of active ingredients as well as other chemicals in plants varies by the part of the plant harvested and sold as a remedy, the maturity of the plant at the time of harvest, and the time of year during harvest. The geography and soil conditions where the plant is grown; soil composition and its contaminants; and year-to-year variations in soil acidity, water, and weather conditions and other growth factors also can affect the concentration of the herb's active ingredients. Because of this variability in herbal product ingredients, the actual dose of active ingredients being consumed often is variable, unpredictable, or simply unknown. Children are particularly susceptible to such dosage considerations by virtue of their smaller size and different capacity for detoxifying chemicals compared with adults. For some herbs, such as those containing pyrrolizidine alkaloids, there may be no safe dose for children. The duration of use is another consideration, with longer courses of herbal therapy exposing the patient to a higher risk of acute and cumulative or chronic adverse effects.

Adverse effects resulting from consumption of dietary supplements may involve one or more organ systems. In some cases a single ingredient can have multiple adverse effects. More than one dietary supplement product may be consumed concurrently, and many products may contain more than one physiologically active ingredient. Plants have complex mixtures of terpenes, sugars, alkaloids, saponins, and other chemicals. For example, more than 100 different chemicals have been identified in tea tree oil.[66] Certain herbs and dietary supplements can cause unexpected reactions when used with medications. Effects on a drug's pharmacokinetics may be pronounced and lead either to toxicity or therapeutic ineffectiveness. St John's wort induces hepatic cytochromes and may decrease blood levels of medications such as indinavir,[67] digoxin,[68] and cyclosporin[69] with a loss of their effectiveness.

Contaminants and adulterants of herbal products can be pharmacologically active and responsible for unexpected toxicity. Herbal plants may be harvested from contaminated soils or cleaned improperly such that they contain illness-producing microorganisms or soil contaminants. Contaminated ayurvedic medications have been known to cause lead poisoning in children. (Ayurvedic medicine, or "ayurveda," is a system of health that has been practiced in India for more than 5000 years.) Asian patent remedies contain drugs such as phenylbutazone, barbiturates, benzodiazepines, or coumadinlike chemicals and contaminants such as lead, cadmium, or arsenic. An analysis of 260 imported traditional Chinese medicines by the California health department found high levels of contaminants in almost half of them.[70]

Parents may be tempted to give the herbs to children, based on product advertising or information from a magazine or Web site or advice from friends or relatives, without any guidance from a knowledgeable source. Such experimentation can be expensive and risks exposure of the child to adverse effects. Herbal products are misused in excessive doses or in combinations without any known rationale. Some products are sold as mixtures of 10 or more different plants, vitamins, minerals, etc. The "stacking" of many different herbs increases the risk of toxicity from any of them or from their interactions. Some toxic reactions may be unforeseen until the remedy has seen widespread use.

The allergic potential of plants is well known. Infants and young children may be particularly sensitive to their first introduction to chemicals in herbs and dietary supplements. Manifestations may include dermatitis, wheezing, rhinitis, conjunctivitis, itchy throat, and other allergic manifestations. In infants, allergies also may cause nonspecific effects such as irritability, colic, poor appetite, or gastrointestinal disturbances. Angelica and rue, which contain psoralen-type furocoumarins, and hypericin, the active ingredient in St John's wort, are capable of photosensitization.[71]

Children differ from adults in their absorption and detoxification of some substances. However, they also have developing nervous and immune systems that may make them more sensitive to the adverse effects of herbs. For example, some herbs, such as buckthorn, senna, and aloe, are known cathartics, and some herbal teas and juniper oil contain powerful diuretic compounds.[71,72] Their actions may cause clinically significant dehydration and electrolyte disturbances quickly in an infant or young child, whereas adults would more easily make up such fluid losses.

While the chemicals in herbs may have carcinogenic effects, this concern has not been adequately investigated. Some chemicals found in plants are known carcinogens, for example, pyrrolizidines (Comfrey, Colt's Foot, Senecio), safrole (Sassafras), aristolochic acids (Wild Ginger), and catechin tannins (Betel nuts).[72] Whether such chemicals pose a threat for children who, by virtue of their longer lives, are particularly vulnerable to those chemicals with a long latency to tumor induction is unknown.

Toxic effects of herbs on the male or female reproductive systems are of concern, but have not been adequately investigated. Some essential oils, for example, have cytotoxic properties or cause cellular transformation in in vitro cell culture studies.[73] The effects of herbs on the embryo and fetus are not known in many cases. It is possible that herbal chemicals may be transported through the placenta to cause toxic effects on the sensitive growing fetus. For example, Roulet and associates[38] reported the case of a newborn whose mother drank senecionine-containing herbal tea daily for the duration of her pregnancy. The infant was born with hepatic vaso-occlusive disease and died; senecionine is one of the pyrrolizidine alkaloids associated with hepatic venous injury. Animal studies have confirmed the teratogenicity of some herbs (eg, the popular Eastern European herb *plectranthus fruticosus*).[74] The excretion of herbs into breast milk is a concern to pediatricians because some have lipophilic chemicals that might be expected to concentrate in breast milk, although there are little data to confirm or refute this.

While alert clinicians should be aware of the cultural heritage and practices of patients, lack of a unique cultural identity should not dissuade them from inquiring into the use of these products.

## Regulation and Adverse Effect Reporting

Clinicians can play an important role in identifying, reporting, and preventing adverse effects from dietary supplements. Unfortunately, gaps exist in the regulation of herbal products and dietary supplements. Congress has passed legislation, the Dietary Supplement Health and Education Act of 1994, which does not include consumer protections that are applied to medications used in the treatment of health problems. Pharmacologically active substances such as melatonin, ephedrine, and dehydroepiandrosterone can be marketed as dietary supplements provided no therapeutic claims are made for them.

There are no international conventions in naming plants, and many confusing synonyms exist. The common names of plants and herbal remedies can be archaic and variable depending on the geographical region. For example *cohosh* can refer to several different species of plants depending on where a person lives. There is little regulation of the manufacture, quality, purity, concentration, or labeling claims of herbal remedies and dietary supplements. Errors in labeling may be inadvertent; however, intentional mislabeling also has been problematic. For example, one study revealed that products sold as ginseng actually contained such substitutes as scopolamine and reserpine.[75]

A special segment of the MedWatch program, administered by the US Food and Drug Administration (FDA), has been targeted to adverse events involving such products. To report adverse reactions to the FDA, the MedWatch telephone number is 800-FDA-1088 or the fax number is 800-FDA-0178. Consumers can report adverse events to the FDA Consumer Hotline at 888-INFO-FDA. Local or regional poison control centers also are a valuable resource for information on the adverse effects of dietary supplements and can be reached at 800-222-1222.

---

**Dietary Supplement Health and Education Act of 1994**

- Premarketing testing or oversight protections of the US Food and Drug Administration (FDA) licensing process for an herbal remedy or dietary supplement are not required.
- The use of child-resistant containers or safe packaging for herbs or dietary supplements is not mandated.
- Nutritional support claims made in the labeling or marketing of an herb or dietary supplement do not require FDA approval.
- Pharmacologically active substances can be marketed as dietary substances provided no unsubstantiated claims concerning the cure of specific illnesses or conditions are made for them.
- The secretary of the US Department of Health and Human Services is empowered to act to remove a dietary supplement only when it "poses an imminent hazard to public health or safety."
- There is no regulatory provision for mandatory reporting of adverse health effects associated with the use of herbs or dietary supplements.

---

## Advice to Parents

Pediatricians will develop strategies in their practice of medicine that are adapted to the needs of their patients and families. The assessment of children whose parents may be seeking complementary and alternative medicine (CAM) options also requires the use of strategies that promote the therapeutic interaction among physician, parent, and child to the benefit of the patient. Physicians and other health professionals should ask questions about use of dietary supplements, minerals, vitamins, or herbs as well as the reasons or health conditions for which these products are used.[76] Eisenberg[77] suggests some guidelines for practitioners in the assessment of a patient whose parents also may be seeking medical solutions involving CAM, modified here to make them more specific to the needs of pediatricians.

- Carry out a thorough medical evaluation.
- Explore conventional therapeutic options—establish a dialogue with the parents about what in your opinion is the best treatment for the condition as well as what may be established or untested alternatives. Keep an open mind and research what beliefs the parents may bring to the assessment.
- Ask the unasked question—find out about the current beliefs of the parents and any current alternative therapies, herbs, or other remedies in use by the family and given to children. In one study, up to 50% of families using CAM did not reveal this to their primary care physician.[3]
- Obtain consultations as needed—for example, if the child has frequent unresolved ear infections, suggest that the parents follow up on your referral of the child to an otolaryngologist before trying herbs.
- Document CAM requests or therapeutic refusals/exhaustion in the medical record.
- If you disagree with the plan, discuss why and document your disagreement in the record.

The best interests of the child are always paramount. When the pediatrician disagrees with the family's intended actions, such disagreement should be voiced along with the reasons behind it. In other circumstances, the pediatrician can and should support the parents' decision to pursue herbal remedies or dietary supplements when the risk of harm is low, the possibility of benefit is backed by scientific evidence, and the parents can be engaged in an integrative approach to the child's care.

## Frequently Asked Questions

Q *Conventional medications have many side effects. Shouldn't I worry more about the known side effects?*

A Conventional pharmaceutical products have been through extensive testing for safety and efficacy by manufacturers and through FDA approval processes. Many of the known side effects in adults have been documented and studied. None of this is true for dietary supplements.

Q *Does my child need extra vitamins/food supplements? Won't they help my child grow, eat, and study better?*

A A diet that provides enough calories and is balanced in all the major food groups should provide adequate nutrition for an otherwise healthy growing child. Additional supplements are rarely necessary for children. Certain kinds of birth defects are known to occur more frequently when the diet is deficient in folic acid. Therefore, women in their reproductive years, including teenagers who may become pregnant, should consume 0.4 mg of folic acid daily.

Q *Doesn't the FDA approve food additives and dietary supplements?*

A No. Legislation enacted in 1994 made dietary ingredients exempt from FDA premarket approval for food additives. Manufacturers no longer must prove that an ingredient is safe. The FDA needs to prove the ingredient is hazardous if it believes there is a risk. The 1994 law also allows companies to make medical claims for dietary supplements that in the past would have been regulated as drugs.

Q *Is it OK to give my child chamomile or spearmint tea?*

A Weak teas made from the leaves and flowers of chamomile or spearmint probably pose a negligible threat of an adverse effect, although there is little evidence of clear therapeutic benefits on children's health from such teas. Parents should keep in mind that children as well as adults might experience allergic reactions to any plant-derived products such as mint (*Mentha* species) and chamomile (*Compositae* species).

Q *Is zinc of any value in the treatment of colds?*

A Zinc is an essential metal for good health, and zinc deficiencies can reduce immunocompetence. Zinc supplementation was recently found to improve the survival of infants who were small for their gestational age. Its value in the treatment of childhood upper respiratory infections has yet to be shown in carefully controlled studies.

Q *Are over-the-counter herbs of any value in treating my child's colds?*

A Many laboratory or animal-based studies of certain herbs, such as echinacea or astralagus, have shown them to have remarkable effects on the immune system. However, such results may not be extrapolated to imply necessarily a benefit in the management of the ill child. Investigations of the use of echinacea to treat colds in adult volunteers showed mixed results: some studies implied a benefit whereas others could not detect a significant difference from controls. There have been no controlled studies of the medicinal use of echinacea for upper respiratory infections in children, although several such trials are planned. Parents should be warned that some herbal remedies, such as camphor or eucalyptus oil, may be soothing if inhaled, but also can have harmful effects, including seizures or coma, if ingested by children.

## Resources

American Botanical Council:
    http://www.herbalgram.org
Center for Food Safety & Applied Nutrition:
    http://vm.cfsan.fda.gov/~dms/dietsupp.html
Center for Holistic Pediatric Education & Research (CHPER) Children's Hospital:
    http://www.childrenshospital.org/holistic
Center for Pediatric Integrative Medical Education at Children's Hospital:
    http://www.holistickids.org

Consumer Federation of America:
http://www.quackwatch.org
Dr Duke's Phytochemical & Ethnobotanical Databases:
http://www.ars-grin.gov/duke
Herb Research Foundation:
http://www.herbs.org
Longwood Herbal Task Force:
http://www.mcp.edu/herbal
National Center for Complementary and Alternative Medicine:
http://www.nccam.nih.gov
National Certification Commission for Acupuncture and Oriental
Medicine:
http://www.nccaom.org
National Council Against Health Fraud:
http://www.ncahf.org
US Department of Agriculture Food & Nutrition Information Center:
http://www.nal.usda.gov/fnic

## References

1. Dietary Supplement Health and Education Act of 1994. Available at:
http://vm.cfsan.fda.gov/~dms/dietsupp.html
2. Eisenberg DM, Davis RB, Ettner SL, et al. Trends in alternative medicine
use in the United States, 1990–1997: results of a follow-up national survey.
*JAMA.* 1998;280:1569–1575
3. Spigelblatt L, Laine-Ammara G, Pless IB, Guyver A. The use of alternative
medicine by children. *Pediatrics.* 1994;94:811–814
4. Ottolini MC, Hamburger EK, Loprieato JO, et al. Complementary and
alternative medicine use among children in the Washington, DC area.
*Ambul Pediatr.* 2001;1:122–125
5. American Academy of Pediatrics Committee on Children With Disabilities. Counseling families who choose complementary and alternative
medicine for their child with chronic illness or disability. *Pediatrics.*
2001;107:598–601
6. Philen RM, Ortiz DI, Auerbach SB, Falk H. Survey of advertising for
nutritional supplements in health and bodybuilding magazines. *JAMA.*
1992;268:1008–1011

7.  Woolf A. Essential oil poisoning. *J Toxicol Clin Toxicol.* 1999;37:721–727

8.  Angell M, Kassirer JP. Alternative medicine—the risks of untested and unregulated remedies. *N Engl J Med.* 1998;339:839–841

9.  White NJ, Waller D, Crawley J, et al. Comparison of artemether and chloroquine for severe malaria in Gambian children. *Lancet.* 1992;339:317–321

10. Zhao KS, Mancini C, Doria G. Enhancement of the immune response in mice by *Astragalus membranaceus* extracts. *Immunopharmacology.* 1990;20:225–233

11. Weizman Z, Alkrinawi S, Goldfarb D, Bitran C. Efficacy of herbal tea preparation in infantile colic. *J Pediatr.* 1993;122:650–652

12. Pachter LM. Culture and clinical care. Folk illness beliefs and behaviors and their implications for health care delivery. *JAMA.* 1994;271:690–694

13. Buchwald D, Panwala S, Hooton TM. Use of traditional health practices by Southeast Asian refugees in a primary care clinic. *West J Med.* 1992;156:507–511

14. Pachter LM, Cloutier MM, Bernstein BA. Ethnomedical (folk) remedies for childhood asthma in a mainland Puerto Rican community. *Arch Pediatr Adolesc Med.* 1995;149:982–988

15. Yeatman GW, Dang VV. Cao gio (coin rubbing). Vietnamese attitudes toward health care. *JAMA.* 1980;244:2748–2749

16. Forman J, Moline J, Cernichiari E, et al. A cluster of pediatric metallic mercury exposure cases treated with meso-2,3 dimercaptosuccinic acid (DMSA). *Environ Health Perspect.* 2000;108:575–577

17. Moore C, Adler R. Herbal vitamins: lead toxicity and developmental delay. *Pediatrics.* 2000;106:200–202

18. Risser A, Mazur LJ. Use of folk remedies in a Hispanic population. *Arch Pediatr Adolesc Med.* 1995;149:978–981

19. Dyer JE. Gamma-hydroxybutyrate: a health-food product producing coma and seizure-like activity. *Am J Emerg Med.* 1991;9:321–324

20. Centers for Disease Control and Prevention. Gamma hydroxy butyrate use—New York and Texas, 1995–1996. *MMWR Morb Mortal Wkly Rep.* 1997;46:281–283

21. Centers for Disease Control. Lead poisoning-associated death from Asian Indian folk remedies—Florida. *MMWR Morb Mortal Wkly Rep.* 1984;33:638–664

22. Kelly KJ, Neu J, Camitta BM, Honig GR. Methemoglobinemia in an infant treated with the folk remedy glycerited asafoetida. *Pediatrics.* 1984;73:717–719

23. Centers for Disease Control. Folk remedy-associated lead poisoning in Hmong children—Minnesota. *MMWR Morb Mortal Wkly Rep.* 1983;32:555–556

24. Riley DM, Newby CA, Leal-Almeraz TO, Thomas VM. Assessing elemental mercury exposure from cultural and religious practices. *Environ Health Perspect.* 2001;109:779–784

25. Philen RM, Posada M. Toxic oil syndrome and eosinophilia-myalgia syndrome: May 8–10, 1991, World Health Organization meeting report. *Semin Arthritis Rheum.* 1993;23:104–124

26. Belongia EA, Hedberg CW, Gleich GH, et al. An investigation of the cause of eosinophilia-myalgia syndrome associated with tryptophan use. *N Engl J Med.* 1990;323:357–365

27. Kamb ML, Murphy JJ, Jones JL, et al. Eosinophilia-myalgia syndrome in L-tryptophan-exposed individuals. *JAMA.* 1992;267:77–82

28. Hertzman PA, Blevins WL, Mayer J, et al. Association of the eosinophilia-myalgia syndrome with the ingestion of tryptophan. *N Engl J Med.* 1990;322:868–873

29. Centers for Disease Control and Prevention. Water hemlock poisoning—Maine, 1992. *MMWR Morb Mortal Wkly Rep.* 1994;43:229–231

30. Benner MH, Lee HJ. Anaphylactic reaction to chamomile tea. *J Allergy Clin Immunol.* 1973;53:307–308

31. Grant KL, Boyer LV, Erdman BE. Chaparral-induced hepatotoxicity. *Integrative Med.* 1998;1:83–87

32. Centers for Disease Control and Prevention. Chaparral-induced toxic hepatitis—California and Texas. *MMWR Morb Mortal Wkly Rep.* 1992;41:812–814

33. Miller RL, Gould AR, Bernstein ML. Cinnamon-induced stomatitis venenata. *Oral Surg Oral Med Oral Pathol.* 1992;73:708–716

34. Perry PA, Dean BS, Krenzelok EP. Cinnamon oil abuse by adolescents. *Vet Hum Toxicol.* 1990;32:162–164

35. Huxtable RJ. Herbal teas and toxins: novel aspects of pyrrolizidine poisoning in the United States. *Perspect Biol Med.* 1980;24:1–14

36. Ridker PM, Ohkuma S, McDermott WV, Trey C, Huxtable RJ. Hepatic veno-occlusive disease associated with the consumption of pyrrolizidine-containing dietary supplements. *Gastroenterol.* 1985;88:1050–1054

37. Mattocks AR. Toxicity of pyrrolizidine alkaloids. *Nature.* 1968; 217:723–728

38. Roulet M, Laurini R, Rivier L, Calame A. Hepatic veno-occlusive disease in the newborn infant of a woman drinking herbal tea. *J Pediatr.* 1988; 112:433–436

39. Bach N, Thung SN, Schaffner F. Comfrey herb tea-induced hepatic veno-occlusive disease. *Am J Med.* 1989;87:97–99

40. Mullins RJ, Heddle R. Adverse reactions associated with echinacea: the Australian experience. *Ann Allergy Asthma Immunol.* 2002;88:42–51

41. Spoerke DG, Vandenberg SA, Smolinske SC, et al. Eucalyptus oil: 14 cases of exposure. *Vet Hum Toxicol.* 1989;31:166–168

42. Tibbalis J. Clinical effects and management of eucalyptus oil ingestion in infants and young children. *Med J Aust.* 1995;163:177–180

43. Webb NJR, Pitt WR. Eucalyptus oil poisoning in childhood: 41 cases in south-east Queensland. *J Paediatr Child Health.* 1993;29:368–371

44. Tarty BZ. Garlic burns. *Pediatrics.* 1993;91:658–659

45. Larrey D, Vial T, Pauwels A, et al. Hepatitis after germander (Teucrium chamaedrys) administration: another instance of herbal medicine hepatotoxicity. *Ann Intern Med.* 1992;117:129–132

46. Siegel RK. Ginseng abuse syndrome. Problems with the panacea. *JAMA.* 1979;241:1614–1615

47. Jin bu huan toxicity in children—Colorado 1993. *MMWR Morb Mortal Wkly Rep.* 1993;42:633–635

48. Horowitz RS, Feldhaus K, Dart RC, Stermitz FR, Beck JJ. The clinical spectrum of Jin Bu Huan toxicity. *Arch Int Med.* 1996;156:899–903

49. Woolf GM, Petrovic LM, Rojter SE, et al. Acute hepatitis associated with the Chinese herbal product Jin Bu Huan. *Ann Int Med.* 1994;121:729–735

50. Russman S, Lauterburg BH, Helbling A. Kava hepatotoxicity. *Ann Intern Med.* 2001;135:68

51. Escher M, Desmeules J, Giostra E, Mentha G. Hepatitis associated with Kava, a herbal remedy for anxiety. *BMJ.* 2001;322:139

52. Hall AH, Linden CH, Kulig KW, et al. Cyanide poisoning from laetrile ingestion: role of nitrite therapy. *Pediatrics.* 1986;78:269–272

53. Walker BR, Edwards CRW. Licorice-induced hypertension and syndromes of apparent mineralocorticoid excess. *Endocrinol Metab Clin North Am.* 1994;23:359–377

54. Samenuk D, Link MS, Homoud MK, et al. Adverse cardiovascular events temporally associated with Ma Huang, an herbal source of ephedrine. *Mayo Clin Proc.* 2002;77:12–16

55. Haller CA, Benowitz NL. Adverse cardiovascular and central nervous system events associated with dietary supplements containing ephedra alkaloids. *N Engl J Med.* 2000;343:1833–1838

56. Fatovich DM. Aconite: a lethal Chinese herb. *Ann Emerg Med.* 1992; 21:309–311

57. Chan TYK, Tse LKK, Chan JCN, Chan WWM. Aconitine poisoning due to Chinese herbal medicines: a review. *Vet Human Toxicol.* 1994;36:452

58. Abernathy MK, Becker LB. Acute nutmeg intoxication. *Am J Emerg Med.* 1992;10:429–430

59. Brenner N, Frank OS, Knight E. Chronic nutmeg psychosis. *J Roy Soc Med.* 1993;86:179–180

60. Katz J, Prescott K, Woolf AD. Strychnine poisoning from a traditional Cambodian remedy. *Am J Emerg Med.* 1996;14:475–477

61. Sullivan JB Jr, Rumack BH, Thomas H Jr, Peterson RG, Bryson P. Pennyroyal oil poisoning and hepatotoxicity. *JAMA.* 1979;242:2873–2874

62. Anderson IB, Mullen WH, Meeker JE, et al. Pennyroyal toxicity: measurement of four metabolites in two cases and review of the literature. *Ann Intern Med.* 1996;124:726–734

63. Gordon WB, Forte AJ, McMurtry RJ, et al. Hepatotoxicity and pulmonary toxicity of pennyroyal oil and its constituent terpenes in the mouse. *Toxicol Appl Pharmacol.* 1982;65:413–424

64. Arnold WN. Vincent van Gogh and the thujone connection. *JAMA.* 1988;260:3042–3044

65. Weisbord SD, Soule JB, Kimmel PL. Poison on line-acute renal failure caused by oil of wormwood purchased through the Internet. *N Engl J Med.* 1997;337:825–827

66. Carson CF, Riley TV. Toxicity of the essential oil of Melaleuca alternifolia or tea tree oil. *J Toxicol Clin Toxicol.* 1995;33:193–194

67. Piscitelli SC, Burstein AH, Chaitt D, Alfaro RM, Falloon J. Indinavir concentrations and St John's wort. *Lancet.* 2000;355:547–548

68. Johne A, Brockmoller J, Bauer S, Maurer A, Langheinrich M, Roots I. Pharmacokinetic interaction of digoxin with an herbal extract from St John's wort (*Hypericum perforatum*). *Clin Pharmacol Ther.* 1999; 66:338–345

69. Ruschitzka F, Meier PJ, Turina M, Luscher TF, Noll G. Acute heart transplant rejection due to Saint John's wort. *Lancet.* 2000;355:548–549

70. Kaltsas HJ. Patent poisons. *Altern Med.* November, 1999:24–28

71. Toxic reactions to plant products sold in health food stores. *Med Lett Drugs Ther.* 1979;21:29–32

72. Saxe TG. Toxicity of medicinal herbal preparations. *Am Fam Physician.* 1987;35:135–142

73. Pecevski J, Savkovic D, Radivojevic D, Vuksanovic L. Effect of oil of nutmeg on the fertility and induction of meiotic chromosome rearrangements in mice and their first generation. *Toxicol Lett.* 1981;7:239–243

74. Pages N, Salazar M, Chamorro G, et al. Teratological evaluation of Plectranthus fruticosus leaf essential oil. *Planta Med.* 1988;54:296–298
75. Siegel R. Kola, ginseng, and mislabeled herbs. *JAMA.* 1978;237:25
76. Ang-Lee MK, Moss J, Yuan CS. Herbal medicines and perioperative care. *JAMA.* 2001;286:208–216
77. Eisenberg DM. Advising patients who seek alternative medical therapies. *Ann Intern Med.* 1997;127:61–69

## Further Reading

American Botanical Council. *Herbalgram* quarterly journal

Blumenthal M, et al. *Therapeutic Monographs on Medicinal Plants for Human Use.* German Commission E Monographs. Austin, TX: American Botanical Council; 1998

Ernst E. The risk-benefit profile of commonly used herbal therapies: ginkgo, St John's wort, ginseng, echinacea, saw palmetto, and kava. *Ann Intern Med.* 2002;136:42–53

Gardiner P, Kemper K. Herbs in pediatric and adolescent medicine. *Pediatr Rev.* 2000;21:44–57

Kemper KJ. *The Holistic Pediatrician: A Parent's Comprehensive Guide to Safe and Effective Therapies for the 25 Most Common Childhood Ailments.* 2nd ed. New York, NY: Harper Perennial Press; 2002

Lippincott JB, Co. *The Lawrence Review of Natural Products.* Quarterly monograph series

National Institutes of Medicine, Office of Alternative Medicine. *Alternative Medicine: Expanding Medical Horizons.* Washington, DC: US Government Printing Office

*PDR for Herbal Medicines.* 2nd ed. Montvale NJ: Medical Economics Co; 2001

Snodgrass WR. Herbal products: risks and benefits of use in children. *Curr Ther Res Clin Exp.* 2001;62:724–737

# 17
# Ionizing Radiation (Including Radon)

Radiation includes energy transmitted by waves through space or some type of medium, such as light seen as colors, infrared rays perceived as heat, and audible radio waves amplified through radio and television. We cannot similarly perceive radiation with shorter wavelengths: ultraviolet rays, x-rays, and gamma rays. Radiation with the shortest wavelengths, x-rays and gamma rays, possess immense quantities of energy and penetrate solid objects. This energy may cause ionization in tissue, which drives outer electrons from their orbits around atoms. The free electrons created can react with other molecules in living organisms and cause tissue damage. Figure 17.1 shows wavelengths for different types of radiation.

## Sources of Exposure
Exposures to radiation can be from external sources (radon and x-ray machines) or from internal emitters (radioactive fallout, ingested or inhaled, or medical radioisotopes). The transfer of energy in sufficient doses from the environment to individuals can adversely affect their health.[1] X-rays transfer energy along thin paths, whereas neutrons have greater mass and transfer energy along wider paths. The units of measure of energy absorbed by x-rays and gamma rays were the rad (radiation absorbed dose) and the rem (roentgen equivalents man), with the latter measurement based on the greater relative biological effectiveness (RBE) of doses from particulate radiation, such as neutrons. Thus rem = (rad) x (RBE). The RBE of gamma radiation is 1, and if the RBE of neutrons is 10, exposure to 100 rad of each is (100 x 1) + (100 x 10) = 1100 rem. The rad and rem have been replaced by the gray (1 Gy = 100 rad) and the sievert (1 Sv = 100 rem) in accordance with the International System (SI) of Units. The unit of activity for radiation emission from a radionuclide (a radioactive element) is curie (Ci), or in SI, the becquerel (Bq).

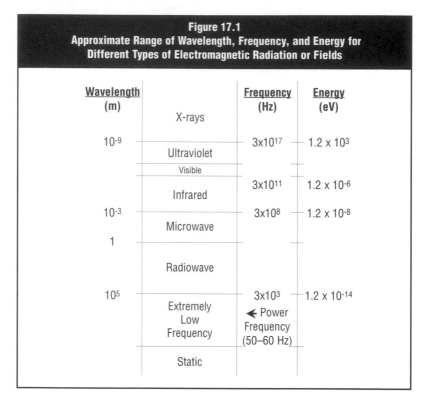

**Figure 17.1**
**Approximate Range of Wavelength, Frequency, and Energy for Different Types of Electromagnetic Radiation or Fields**

On average, the annual effective dose equivalent of ionizing radiation to a person in the United States is 0.0036 Sv (0.36 rem), 55% of which is from radon, 27% from other natural sources, 11% from medical x-rays, and 7% from other man-made sources (see Figure 17.2).[2] Doses from radiological examinations vary with the operator, procedure, and machine over time, so tables for typical exposures have not been published.

Radiation exposure may be instantaneous (atomic bomb), chronic (uranium miners), fractionated (radiotherapy), or partial-body. For a given dose, whole-body exposure is more harmful than partial-body exposure. Radioisotopes decay with time into stable elements and

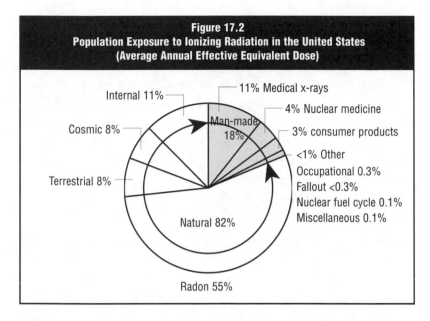

**Figure 17.2**
**Population Exposure to Ionizing Radiation in the United States**
**(Average Annual Effective Equivalent Dose)**

Internal 11%

Cosmic 8%

Terrestrial 8%

11% Medical x-rays

4% Nuclear medicine

Man-made 18%

3% consumer products

<1% Other
Occupational 0.3%
Fallout <0.3%
Nuclear fuel cycle 0.1%
Miscellaneous 0.1%

Natural 82%

Radon 55%

have physical half-lives of various lengths, from fractions of a second to millions of years. They also have biological half-lives related to the rate at which they are excreted from the body.

## Biological Processes and Clinical Effects

Atoms or molecules that become ionized attain stability again by forming substances that may alter molecular processes within a cell or its environment. Ionizing radiation, in colliding with a cell, can cause changes in its constituents, including deoxyribonucleic acid (DNA). Such damage, if unrepaired, may disable or kill the cell.

## Acute Effects

Ionizing radiation produces the same reactions regardless of the type of particle or ray emitted. Differences are quantitative, not qualitative. Prompt effects of overexposure include acute radiation sickness (nausea, vomiting, diarrhea, declining white blood cell count, and thrombocytopenia), epilation (loss of hair), and death. Table 17.1 shows the sequence of these effects and doses at which they occur.

## Delayed Effects

In general, the best estimates of dose-related delayed effects of ionizing radiation come from studies of the Japanese atomic bomb survivors who experienced a single, instantaneous whole-body exposure, possibly affected by other adverse influences such as malnutrition in war-torn Japan. Delayed effects largely are due to mutagenesis, teratogenesis, and carcinogenesis. The smaller the exposure, the less likely that late effects will be found.

### Mutagenesis

Ionizing radiation is a germ-cell mutagen in plants and experimental animals, and is assumed to affect humans too. Studies of children who were conceived after one or both parents were exposed to the atomic bomb have as yet shown no excess of genetic effects. The studies started with clinical observations, and then included cytogenetic, biochemical, and molecular studies as soon as laboratory procedures were developed.[4] Two-dimensional electrophoresis examination of 30 serum and

**Table 17.1**
**Estimated Threshold Doses for Effects Following Acute Radiation Exposure\***

| Health Effect | Organ | Absorbed Dose (rad) |
|---|---|---|
| Temporary sterility | Testes | 15 |
| Blood formation depressed | Bone marrow | 50 |
| Nausea and vomiting in 10% of people within 48 hrs | Gastrointestinal | 100 |
| Permanent sterility, female | Ovaries | 250–600 |
| Temporary alopecia | Skin | 300–500 |
| Permanent sterility, male | Testes | 350 |
| Skin erythema | Skin | 500–600 |

\*From the National Council on Radiation Protection and Measurements.[3]

erythrocyte proteins from about 16 000 children were made. Among 1.2 million locus tests, 3 apparent mutations were observed in the parent-exposed group and 4 mutations were observed in the (one-third smaller) parent-unexposed group. Deoxyribonucleic acid studies are now in progress in the search for germline mutations through study of stored samples on the child and both parents.

Ionizing radiation causes chromosome breaks in somatic cells (eg, lymphocytes and skin fibroblasts) that are detectable decades after exposure,[5] and presumably account for the increased rates of cancer observed after exposure in childhood or adulthood. In the studies of atomic bomb survivors, differential color staining of 4 chromosomes was initiated as soon as it was developed, and staining of all 23 chromosome pairs, as recently reported, greatly improves detection of small translocations.[6]

### *Teratogenesis*

Intrauterine exposure to ionizing radiation may cause small head size alone or with severe mental retardation. Susceptibility to severe mental retardation is greatest at 8 to 15 weeks of gestational age, with some occurring during the 16th to 25th week. The lowest dose that caused severe mental retardation from atomic bomb exposure was 0.6 Sv, far above diagnostic exposures in medical radiology. The lowest dose that caused small head size without mental retardation was 0.10 to 0.19 Sv among conceptuses exposed at 4 to 17 weeks of gestational age. Mental retardation is apparently due to interruption in the proliferation and migration of neurons from near the cerebral ventricles to the cortex.[7]

### *Carcinogenesis*

#### Diagnostic Radiation

In a series of reports from 1956 to 1975, Bithell and Stewart[8] described and expanded on their report of a 1.5-fold excess of almost every type of cancer in children younger than 10 years after maternal exposure to diagnostic abdominal x-rays during pregnancy. These reports led to near-elimination of diagnostic x-rays during pregnancy and ended the possibility of future studies along the same lines. The development of new laboratory techniques can, of course, be applied to new or stored specimens from the Japanese A-bomb survivors exposed in utero.

There is disagreement about the interpretation of the available data on diagnostic x-ray exposures. One group claims that any form of childhood cancer can be induced,[9] and the other claims this is biologically implausible given what is known about diversity in the genesis of these cancers in the general population.[10] Among them, for example, was lymphoma, which has not been linked to radiation exposure at any age. It is reasonable to believe that leukemia, other than the chronic lymphocytic form, can be radiation induced by in utero exposure because leukemia can be induced at any age.

## Atomic Bomb Exposure

Among the 807 Japanese atomic bomb survivors exposed in utero, no excess of childhood cancer was observed.[11] Because the increase in the number of cases of leukemia after childhood exposure ended about 30 years after exposure, more cases are unlikely among the in utero cohort. An excess in breast cancer after childhood exposure was not found until the cohort became 30 years old (ie, the usual age for early-onset breast cancer in the general population).[12] No cases have been observed yet among the in utero group. An excess of thyroid cancer occurred in children exposed to the atomic bomb beginning at 11 years of age,[8] but because of its rarity, no cases are expected among the group exposed in utero.

After childhood exposure to ionizing radiation, increased frequencies of cancers in adulthood are expected if the exposure and sample size are large enough. Among all atomic bomb survivors, the lowest dose at which an excess of cancer was found was 0.05 Sv (5 rem).[13] Intrauterine exposures to as little as 0.01 Sv (well below the minimal carcinogenic dose detectable epidemiologically) for medical diagnosis during pregnancy have been the basis of litigation concerning children with severe mental retardation or parental fear of childhood cancer.

## Radon

The US population is constantly exposed to radon, which accounts for 55% of background radiation (average exposure, 0.002 Sv [0.2 rem] per person per year). Radon gas comes from radioactive decay of radium, a product of ubiquitous uranium deposits in rocks and soil. When inhaled, radon decay products (also known as radon daughters or radon progeny) caused an increase in rates of lung cancer in uranium miners. Radon enters homes through cracks in the foundation, porous cinderblocks, and granite walls.[14] Thus radiation exposures in basements may be higher than those on the first-floor level. Extrapolation downward from the dose-response curve for lung cancer among uranium miners indicates that about 10% of lung cancer in the United States is attributable to radon exposure.[15] Most of these cancers occur in cigarette smokers. Until recently there were insufficient data to detect an increased risk of lung cancer after life-long residential radon exposure. A summary analysis (meta-analysis) has now been made of 8 epidemiologic studies, the results of which are consistent with low-dose effects found in other studies of humans and animals.[16] These results indicate a linear dose-response relationship detectable down to 4 pCi/L, the level at which remedial action should be taken according to the US Environmental Protection Agency (EPA) and the US Department of Health and Human Services.

For more information, see the EPA Web site on radon for an overview, a chart for the risk of developing lung cancer (much higher in smokers) as exposure mounts (http://www.epa.gov/iaq/radon/riskcht.html), a map of exposures from the earth and rocks in the United States (http://www.epa.gov/iaq/radon/zonemap.html), and publications (http://www.epa.gov/iaq/radon/pubs/index.html). Also, see the Executive Summary of BEIR VI, an authoritative volume on radon by the Committee on the Biological Effects of Ionizing

Radiation of the National Research Council (http://www.epa.gov/iaq/
radon/beirvi.html). The EPA Radon Hotline is 800-767-7236.

## Special Susceptibility and Epidemics

### Special Susceptibility

Children with ataxia-telangiectasia (AT) are prone to the development
of lymphoma and, when treated with conventional doses of radiotherapy, suffer an acute radiation reaction that may result in death.[17,18] A
DNA repair defect in patients with AT interferes with the repair of
cells damaged by radiation. This catastrophic reaction has been seen
when AT was not diagnosed prior to radiotherapy because some
young children had only ataxia. Ocular telangiectasia, which develops
at about age 6 years, was not yet apparent.

### Epidemics

Gamma rays (external radiation) and radioisotopes (internal emitters)
in fallout have caused epidemics of delayed radiation effects after in
utero or childhood exposure: (1) developmental effects and cancer
were caused by exposure to the atomic bomb, (2) thyroid ablation in
2 infants and thyroid neoplasia in the Marshall Islanders were due to
fallout from nuclear weapons tests, and (3) hundreds of cases of thyroid cancer in children in the Ukraine and Belarus were attributed
to fallout from the Chernobyl accident.[19] A small cluster of cases of
leukemia and lymphoma in children near the Sellafield nuclear facility
in England was associated with paternal radiation exposure during the
6 months before conception, although this is controversial.[20]

### Diagnostic Methods

Radiation-induced diseases are indistinguishable from those that
occur in the general population. The role of radiation can be implicated only by epidemiologic studies (1) that show a dose-response
effect, (2) after alternative explanations have been excluded (eg, cigarette smoking), and (3) that show the link between exposure and
the effect is biologically plausible. Biological dosimetry can estimate

exposures above 0.2 Gy (20 rad) by such methods as painting chromo-somes for the detection of chromosomal translocations and by the glycophorin A test for somatic cell mutations of red blood cells.

## Treatment of Clinical Symptoms

For acute radiation sickness caused by the Chernobyl accident, blood counts of those affected were sustained through the use of combined treatment with cytokines, such as stem-cell factors and colony-stimulating factors that produce rapid and delayed hemato-poietic responses from surviving progenitor cells. Otherwise the treat-ment was symptomatic. For delayed radiation effects, treatment of the disease was the same as that when radiation exposure was not involved. Drugs to prevent radiation sickness have substantial side effects, or are not yet known to be safe or effective. For details see Mettler and Voelz[21] and Moulder.[22]

## Prevention of Exposure

### External Radiation

The risk of cancer associated with most diagnostic radiation is low, and use of radiation should not be restricted when needed for cor-rect diagnosis. Any medical procedure has a risk, and diagnostic radi-ography is no exception. Limitation of radiation, shielding sensitive body parts such as the thyroid, and ensuring a nonpregnant state are components of good medical practice. Computed tomography (CT) scans require radiation exposures that are projected in one authorita-tive report to induce cancer later in life: 500 cases among an estimated 600 000 children exposed annually.[23] More active reduction in CT exposure settings was recommended. *Radiation Risks and Pediatric Computed Tomography: A Guide for Health Care Providers,*[24] issued by the National Cancer Institute in summer 2002, shows that by lowering the milliampere settings, CT scan doses to the head can be cut by 50% and to the stomach by 75% (see Table 17.2).

Special populations, such as infants with extremely low birth weight, may undergo multiple radiological examinations during a short period. Fluoroscopy and CT scan should be used sparingly for premature infants, particularly when other imaging techniques are available. Table 17.2 shows that the exposure for a PA/lateral chest x-ray is only 0.01 to 0.15 mSv compared with 30 mSv for a CT scan of the head.[24] Limiting exposures will keep the cumulative dose low, the better to endure future unavoidable exposures. Pediatricians should make sure that the most conservative procedures are used.

**Table 17.2**
**Dose Comparisons of Examination Types on Relevant Organs***

| Examination Type | Relevant Organ | Approximate Equivalent Dose to Relevant Organ (mSv)[†] |
|---|---|---|
| Pediatric head computed tomography (CT) scan *unadjusted* settings[‡] (200 mAs,[§] neonate) | Brain | 60 |
| Pediatric head CT scan *adjusted* settings[‡] (100 mAs, neonate) | Brain | 30 |
| Pediatric abdominal CT scan *unadjusted* settings (200 mAs, neonate) | Stomach | 25 |
| Pediatric abdominal CT scan *adjusted* settings (50 mAs, neonate) | Stomach | 6 |
| Chest x-ray (PA/lateral) | Lung | 0.01–0.15 |
| Screening mammogram | Breast | 3 |

*From National Cancer Institute, Society for Pediatric Radiology.[25]
† For comparison, the lowest equivalent doses for which increased cancer risks were observed in atom-bomb survivors were in the range from 50 to 200 mSv (5 to 20 rem).
‡ Unadjusted refers to using the same settings as for adults. Adjusted refers to settings adjusted for body weight.
§ mAs, milliamperes.

## Radon

The EPA recommends that homes be tested for radon. Radon can be measured by 2 methods: (1) $\alpha$-track detectors can be placed in the home for at least 3 months to obtain a time-integrated measurement of the radon level, or (2) charcoal canisters can be exposed to the air in the home for 4 days.[14] These canisters are extremely sensitive and humidity dependent but are appropriate as a screening device. However, the $\alpha$-track detector, used for a long period, gives a better estimate of exposure than does the charcoal canister because the $\alpha$-track detector averages out daily fluctuations in indoor radon levels. Radon exposure can be reduced by increasing ventilation and by reducing the influx of radon in the home. Several methods of reducing exposure include sealing cracks in the foundation, creating negative pressure under the basement floor, and prohibiting the use of building materials containing excessive radium. When levels of radon higher than 4 pCi/L are found, repairs should be made to reduce the radon level. Information about home radon abatement measures is available from the EPA at http://www.epa.gov/iaq/radon/pubs/consguid.html. Pediatricians should advise families about the hazards of radon exposure and should point out that cigarette smoking adds to the radon-induced risk of lung cancer.

Water also may be a source of exposure to radon. In a limited number of studies, radon exposure has been linked to gastrointestinal cancers.

## Fallout (Internal Emitters)

Radioisotopes can be inhaled or ingested. People in exposed areas should avoid drinking fresh milk in particular. Foods are edible if they were harvested or prepared before the fallout occurred and were not exposed to it. Radioiodines are expected to be released after a malfunction or terrorist event occurring at a nuclear power plant or after the detonation of a nuclear weapon. Potassium iodide

(KI) should be administered promptly to protect the thyroid from radioiodines. The Nuclear Regulatory Commission (NRC) recommends that state and local governments consider providing KI to all citizens living within 10 miles of a nuclear power plant as a supplement to plans for evacuation and sheltering.[26] In December 2001 the NRC wrote to the 31 states that had or were within 10 miles of a plant to offer 2 KI pills for every person living within the 10-mile radius.[27] In November 2001 the US Food and Drug Administration (FDA) issued a Center for Drug Evaluation and Research Guidance Document and Recommendations for the use of KI in radiation emergencies.[28] The guidance is aimed at federal agencies and state and local governments responsible for radiation emergencies. It is based primarily on data accumulated after the accident at the Chernobyl nuclear power plant on April 26, 1986. This disaster resulted in the massive release of [131]I and other radioiodines, some with very short half-lives. The short-lived radioiodines are believed to increase the risk of thyroid cancer in children more than [131]I. Many people, including pregnant women and children, were exposed to radioactive fallout primarily through ingesting contaminated fresh cow milk (from cows grazing on contaminated fields) and from consuming contaminated vegetables.

Because the protective effect of KI lasts about 24 hours, daily dosing provides optimum prophylaxis until a significant risk from inhalation or ingestion no longer exists. Because early action is crucial, KI optimally should be administered before exposure, on notification of an emergency. Potassium iodide may have a protective effect even if taken 3 to 4 hours after exposure. See Table 17.3 for KI dosage by age.

In 2002 the FDA issued instructions on how to prepare KI tablets as a fluid for infants and children[29] (see Tables 17.4 and 17.5). The instructions state that, "The mixture of potassium iodide with raspberry syrup disguises the taste of potassium iodide best. The mixtures of potassium iodide with low fat chocolate milk, orange juice, and flat soda (for example, cola) generally have an acceptable taste. Low fat white milk and water did not hide the salty taste of potassium iodide." Three KI products are approved by the FDA for over-the-counter (OTC) use as a thyroid-blocking agent in radiation emergencies. These are Thyro-Block (MedPointe Inc, Somerset, NJ), IOSAT (Anbex Inc, Palm Harbor, FL), and ThyroSafe (Recip US, Honey Brook, PA). IOSAT can be obtained by calling 866-283-3986 and through the Internet at www.nukepills.com; Thyro-Block can be obtained by calling 800-804-4147 and at www.nitro-pak.com; and Thyro-Safe can be obtained by calling 610-942-8972 and at www.thyrosafe.com. Potassium iodide also can be ordered from Anbex Inc by calling 727-784-3483 and at www.anbex.com.[29] Potassium iodide approved by the FDA is also carried by some pharmacies. Detailed information about radiation disasters can be found in the 2003 American Academy of Pediatrics policy statement "Radiation Disasters and Children."[29]

## Regulations

Recommendations concerning radiation protection are made by the National Commission on Radiation Protection and Measurements and the International Commission on Radiological Protection. The NRC regulates and monitors nuclear facilities and the medical/research uses of radioisotopes.

**Table 17.3. Guidelines for Potassium Iodide (KI) Administration\*†**

| Patient | Exposure, Gy (rad) | KI dose (mg) |
|---|---|---|
| >40 years of age | >5 (500) | 130 |
| 18 through 40 years of age | ≥0.1 (10) | 130 |
| Adolescents 12 through 17 years of age‡ | ≥0.05 (5) | 65 |
| Children 4 through 11 years of age | ≥0.05 (5) | 65 |
| Children 1 month through 3 years of age§ | ≥0.05 (5) | 32 |
| Birth through 1 month of age | ≥0.05 (5) | 16 |
| Pregnant or lactating women | ≥0.05 (5) | 130 |

\*From US Food and Drug Administration, Center for Drug Evaluation and Research.[27]

† KI is useful for exposure to a radioiodine only. KI is given once only to pregnant women and neonates unless other protective measures (evacuation, sheltering, and control of the food supply) are unavailable. Repeat dosing should be on the advice of public health authorities.

‡ Adolescents weighing more than 70 kg should receive the adult dose (130 mg).

§ KI from tablets or as a freshly saturated solution may be diluted in water and mixed with milk, formula, juice, soda, or syrup. Raspberry syrup disguises the taste of KI the best. KI mixed with low-fat chocolate milk, orange juice, or flat soda (eg, cola) has an acceptable taste. Low-fat white milk and water did not hide the salty taste of KI.


**Table 17.4.**
**Guidelines for Home Preparation of Potassium Iodide (KI) Solution Using 130-mg Tablet\***

| |
|---|
| • Put one 130-mg KI tablet in a small bowl and grind into a fine powder with the back of a spoon. The powder should not have any large pieces.<br>• Add 4 tsp (20 mL) of water to the KI powder. Use a spoon to mix them together until the KI powder is dissolved in the water.<br>• Add 4 tsp (20 mL) of milk, juice, soda, or syrup (eg, raspberry) to the KI/water mixture. The resulting mixture is 16.25 mg of KI per teaspoon (5 mL).<br>• Age-based dosing guidelines<br>  – Newborn through 1 month of age: 1 tsp<br>  – 1 month through 3 years of age: 2 tsp<br>  – 4 years through 17 years of age: 4 tsp (if child weighs more than 70 kg, give one 130-mg tablet) |
| **How already prepared KI mixture should be stored**<br>Potassium iodide mixed with any of the recommended drinks will keep for up to 7 days in the refrigerator. |
| The US Food and Drug Administration recommends that the KI drink mixtures be prepared fresh weekly; unused portions should be discarded. |

\*Adapted from US Food and Drug Administration, Center for Drug Evaluation and Research.[28]

**Table 17.5.**
**Guidelines for Home Preparation of Potassium Iodide (KI) Solution Using 65-mg Tablet\***

- Put one 65-mg KI tablet in a small bowl and grind into a fine powder with the back of a spoon. The powder should not have any large pieces.
- Add 4 tsp (20 mL) of water to the KI powder. Use a spoon to mix them together until the KI powder is dissolved in the water.
- Add 4 tsp (20 mL) of milk, juice, soda, or syrup (eg, raspberry) to the KI/water mixture. The resulting mixture is 8.125 mg of KI per teaspoon (5 mL)
- Age-based dosing guidelines
  - Newborn through 1 month of age: 2 tsp
  - 1 month through 3 years of age: 4 tsp
  - 4 years through 17 years of age: 8 tsp or one 65-mg tablet (if child weighs more than 70 kg, give two 65-mg tablets)

**How already prepared KI mixture should be stored**
Potassium iodide mixed with any of the recommended drinks will keep for up to 7 days in the refrigerator.

The US Food and Drug Administration recommends that the KI drink mixtures be prepared fresh weekly; unused portions should be discarded.

*Adapted from US Food and Drug Administration, Center for Drug Evaluation and Research.[28]

## Frequently Asked Questions

Q  *Should I test for radon in my home?*

A  The EPA recommends that all homes be checked. An inexpensive home-testing kit should be used, and the sample obtained should be sent to a certified laboratory for analysis. If the level of radon exceeds 4 pCi/L, the cracks through which radon enters the house, as in the basement, should be sealed. Further information can be obtained from the booklet *Radon Reduction Methods: A Home-owner's Guide,* published by the EPA. See Resources for the hotline and information telephone number.

Q  *How many x-rays are safe for my child?*

A  As many as your child's physicians think necessary for diagnosis and follow-up, taking into account the benefit weighed against the (very small) risk. Because the radiation doses from certain diagnostic procedures (ie, CT scans) are high, pediatricians are urged to request radiologic procedures only when necessary and to check to ensure that CT operators use settings appropriate for children.

Q *Will x-ray examinations of my child affect future grandchildren?*

A No genetic effects of radiation from the atomic bombs in Japan have been demonstrable in a series of studies, most recently involving effects on DNA. Mutations must have occurred, as in all living organisms, but have not as yet been demonstrated in survivors. In evaluating the feasibility of studying the offspring of military veterans, an expert committee of the Institute of Medicine noted that exposures of fathers to fallout from weapons tests, as in the South Pacific, seldom exceeded 0.005 rem (0.5 Sv).[30] The committee noted that at the maximum relative risk (0.2% increase in adverse reproductive outcomes), a sample size of 212 million exposed children would be needed to detect a statistically significant excess compared with unexposed children. Or, the frequency of such effects among the 500 000 children of veterans exposed to the atomic bomb would have to be increased 150-fold to be detected.

Q *Is my child's leukemia due to past radiation exposures?*

A There is no way to determine this for an individual patient. Illnesses induced by radiation cannot be distinguished from illnesses in the general population. The relationship can only be established by large epidemiologic studies showing a higher incidence in a radiated group (such as atomic bomb survivors) supported by other evidence.

## Resources

National Cancer Institute, Radiation Epidemiology Branch, phone: 301-496-6600, fax: 301-402-0207

National Council on Radiation Protection, phone: 301-657-2652, fax: 301-907-8768

US Environmental Protection Agency, Internet: http://www.epa.gov/iaq/radon/pubs/consguid.html. Radon Hotline: 800-767-7236

## References

1. Mettler FA Jr, Upton AC. *Medical Effects of Ionizing Radiation.* 2nd ed. Philadelphia, PA: WB Saunders Co; 1995
2. Committee on the Biological Effects of Ionizing Radiation (BEIR V). *Health Effects of Exposure to Low Levels of Ionizing Radiation.* Washington, DC: National Academies Press; 1990;352–370
3. National Council on Radiation Protection and Measurements. *Management of Terrorist Events Involving Radioactive Material.* Bethesda, MD: National Council on Radiation Protection and Measurements; 2001: 257. NCRP Report No. 138
4. Weiss KM, Schull WJ. Perspectives fulfilled: the work and thought of J. V. Neel (1915–2000). *Perspect Biol Med.* 2002;45:46–64
5. Kodama Y, Pawel D, Nakamura N, et al. Stable chromosome aberrations in atomic bomb survivors: results from 25 years of investigation. *Radiat Res.* 2001;156:337–346
6. Nakano M, Kodama Y, Ohtaki K, et al. Detection of stable chromosome aberrations by FISH in A-bomb survivors: comparison with previous solid Giemsa staining data on the same 230 individuals. *Int J Radiat Biol.* 2001;77:971–977
7. Miller RW. Delayed effects of external radiation exposure: a brief history. *Radiat Res.* 1995;144:160–169
8. Bithell JF, Stewart AM. Pre-natal irradiation and childhood malignancy: a review of British data from the Oxford Survey. *Br J Cancer.* 1975; 31:271–287
9. Doll R, Wakeford R. Risk of childhood cancer from fetal irradiation. *Br J Radiol.* 1997;70:130–139
10. Boice JD Jr, Miller RW. Childhood and adult cancer after intrauterine exposure to ionizing radiation. *Teratology.* 1999;59:227–233
11. Miller RW. Discussion: severe mental retardation and cancer among atomic bomb survivors exposed in utero. *Teratology.* 1999;59:234–235
12. Land CE. Studies of cancer and radiation dose among atomic bomb survivors. The example of breast cancer. *JAMA.* 1995;274:402–407
13. Pierce DA, Preston DL. Radiation-related cancer risks at low doses among atomic bomb survivors. *Radiat Res.* 2000;154:178–186

14. US Environmental Protection Agency. *Home Buyer's and Seller's Guide to Radon.* Washington, DC: Office of Air and Radiation, Office of Radiation and Indoor Air; 2000. 402-K-00-008. Available at: http://www.epa.gov/iaq/radon/pubs/hmbyguid.html

15. Committee on Health Risks of Exposure to Radon (BEIR VI) National Research Council. *The Health Effects of Exposure to Indoor Radon.* BEIR VI. Washington, DC: National Academies Press; 1998. Executive summary available at: http://www.epa.gov/iaq/radon/beirvi1.html

16. Lubin JH, Boice JD Jr. Lung cancer risk from residential radon: meta-analysis of eight epidemiologic studies. *J Natl Cancer Inst.* 1997;89:49–57

17. Cunlift PN, Mann JR, Cameron AH, Roberts KD, Ward HN. Radiosensitivity in ataxia-telangiectasia. *Br J Radiol.* 1975;48:374–376

18. Becker-Catania SG, Gatti RA. Ataxia-telangiectasia. *Adv Exp Med Biol.* 2001;495:191–198

19. Tronko MD, Bogdanova TI, Komissarenko IV, et al. Thyroid carcinoma in children and adolescents in Ukraine after the Chernobyl nuclear accident: statistical data and clinicomorphologic characteristics. *Cancer.* 1999; 86:149–156

20. Doll R, Evans HJ, Darby SC. Prenatal exposure not to blame. *Nature.* 1994;367:678–680

21. Mettler FA Jr, Voelz GL. Major radiation exposure—what to expect and how to respond. *N Engl J Med.* 2002;346:1554–1561

22. Moulder JE. Report on an interagency workshop on the radiobiology of nuclear terrorism. Molecular and cellular biology dose (1–10 Sv) radiation and potential mechanisms of radiation protection (Bethesda, Maryland, December 17–18, 2001). *Radiat Res.* 2002;158:118–124

23. Brenner D, Elliston C, Hall E, Berdon W. Estimated risks of radiation-induced fatal cancer from pediatric CT. *AJR Am J Roentgenol.* 2001; 176:289–296

24. National Cancer Institute, Society for Pediatric Radiology. *Radiation and Pediatric Computed Tomography: A Guide for Health Care Providers.* Bethesda, MD: National Cancer Institute; Summer 2002. Available at: http://www.cancer.gov/cancerinfo/causes/radiation-risks-pediatric-CT

25. US Nuclear Regulatory Commission. *Frequently Asked Questions about Potassium Iodide.* Washington, DC: US Nuclear Regulatory Commission; 2002. Available at: http://www.nrc.gov/what-we-do/regulatory/emer-resp/emer-prep/ki-faq.html

26. American Thyroid Association. *American Thyroid Association Endorses Potassium Iodide for Radiation Emergencies.* Falls Church, VA: American Thyroid Association; 2001. Available at: http://www.thyroid.org/ professionals/publications/statements/ki/02_04_09_ki_endrse.html

27. US Food and Drug Administration, Center for Drug Evaluation and Research. *Guidance Document Potassium Iodide as a Thyroid Blocking Agent in Radiation Emergencies.* Rockville, MD: US Food and Drug Administration; Drug Information Branch, HFD-210. Available at: http://www.fda.gov/cder/guidance/4825fnl.htm

28. US Food and Drug Administration, Center for Drug Evaluation and Research. Home Preparation Procedure for Emergency Administration of Potassium Iodide Tablets for Infants and Small Children. 2002. Available at: http://www.fda.gov/cder/drugprepare/kiprep.htm

29. American Academy of Pediatrics Committee on Environmental Health. Radiation disasters and children. *Pediatrics.* 2003;111:1455–1466. Available at: http://www.aap.org/policy/radiationdisastersandchildren.pdf

30. Committee to Study the Feasibility of, and Need for, Epidemiologic Studies of Adverse Reproductive Outcomes in Families of Atomic Veterans. *Adverse Reproductive Outcomes in Families of Atomic Veterans: The Feasibility of Epidemiologic Studies.* Washington, DC: National Academies Press; 1995

# 18
# Irradiation of Food

Food irradiation is a process by which food is exposed to a controlled source of ionizing radiation to prolong shelf life and reduce food losses, improve microbiological safety, and/or reduce the use of chemical fumigants and additives. It can be used to reduce insect infestation of grain, dried spices, and dried or fresh fruits and vegetables; inhibit sprouting in tubers and bulbs; retard postharvest ripening of fruits; inactivate parasites in meats and fish; eliminate spoilage microbes from fresh fruits and vegetables; extend shelf life in poultry, meats, fish, and shellfish; decontaminate poultry and beef; and sterilize foods and feeds.[1]

The dose of the ionizing radiation determines the effects of the process on foods. Food generally is irradiated at levels from 50 Gy to 10 kGy (1 kGy = 1000 Gy), depending on the goals of the process. Low-dose irradiation (up to 1 kGy) primarily is used to delay ripening of produce, or kill or render sterile insects and other higher organisms that may infest fresh food. Medium-dose irradiation (1–10 kGy) reduces the number of pathogens and other microbes on food and prolongs shelf life. High-dose irradiation (>10 kGy) sterilizes food.[2]

In the United States, the most common irradiation source for food is cobalt 60, a gamma radiation emitter that is produced by exposing naturally occurring cobalt 59 to neutrons in a nuclear reactor.[3] Cesium 137, a by-product of other nuclear technologies, is the other gamma source approved for food irradiation in the United States, but it is less commonly used on food. In a gamma facility, food is sent via an automated conveyor system through a maze of stainless steel rods that contain the radiation source. The speed at which the conveyor operates determines the dose received by the food. Gamma irradiation penetrates deeply into food, making it useful in many different food types and for virtually all food processing goals. X-ray food irradiation up to a maximum of 5 million electron volts also is permitted by law and can penetrate deeply as well, but it is too expensive currently to be commercially viable. Food also may be irradiated by machine-generated accelerated electrons up to a maximum of 10 million electron volts. This process has fewer applications because the irradiation only penetrates the surface layers of the food.

Food irradiation is considered a "process" by many nations. The US Congress explicitly included sources of irradiation as "food additives" under the 1958 Food Additives Amendment to the Federal Food, Drug, and Cosmetic Act of 1938.[4] This designation places food irradiation under the same regulatory umbrella of the US Food and Drug Administration (FDA) as other food additives. Thus irradiated food is defined as adulterated and illegal to market unless irradiation conforms to specified federal rules. All petitioners for FDA approval of food irradiation must satisfy technical requirements that limit dose and specify conditions under which the food will be irradiated. The technical effect on the food, dosimetry, and environmental controls must be defined and in compliance with the Federal Food, Drug, and Cosmetic Act. Facilities also must pass an environmental impact study to comply with the National Environmental Policy Act of 1969. Nutritional adequacy, as well as radiologic, toxicologic, and microbiological safety, must be ensured under FDA regulations. In addition, the US Department of Agriculture (USDA) has regulatory responsibilities for some types of foods irradiated for defined purposes. For example, as part of its inspection services, the USDA regulates irradiation when used as a quarantine procedure for fruits. Under federal meat and poultry inspection laws, the USDA has responsibility for ensuring safety and wholesomeness of irradiated meat, poultry, and eggs.

All irradiated food sold in the United States must be labeled with the international sign of irradiation, the radura (Figure 18.1). Current

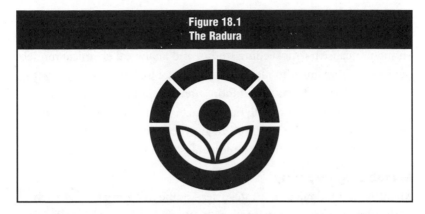

**Figure 18.1
The Radura**

labeling rules do not require that the dose of the irradiation or the purpose of the irradiation be specified.[5] Thus it is not possible for consumers to know if food has been treated to reduce pathogen loads or merely to prolong shelf life. Furthermore, current rules do not require food services to identify irradiated foods they serve.

### Radiologic Safety

Neither the food nor the packaging materials become radioactive as a result of food irradiation.[6] The sources of radiation approved for use in food irradiation are limited to those producing energy too low to induce formation of radioactive compounds or radioactive atomic species.

### Toxicologic Safety

Studies have not identified any unusual toxicity after foods have been irradiated. Radiation absorbed by food causes a host of chemical reactions proportional to the dose of radiation applied. The desired reactions involve disrupting the deoxyribonucleic acid (DNA) of spoilage and disease-causing microbes and pests. Undesired reactions could involve creation of toxic compounds. A number of approaches involving hundreds of studies have been employed over decades to determine whether such toxic compounds are created during irradiation, and, if created, whether they are unique to the irradiation process (versus canning, freezing, drying, etc) or created in amounts large enough to cause harm. Feeding studies and analytical chemical modeling studies have failed to identify any unusual toxicity associated with irradiation.[7] In fact, irradiated food often contains fewer changed molecules (also called radiolytic products) than food processed in conventional ways. For example, heat processed foods can contain 50 to 500 times more changed molecules than irradiated foods.[3]

## Microbiological Safety

Microbes in food fall into 3 categories.[2] Some microorganisms, such as those that produce fermentation, create desirable changes in foods. Spoilage microorganisms change the color, odor, and texture of food, rendering it unpalatable, but they do not cause human illness. Pathogens cause human disease and include invasive and toxigenic bacteria, toxigenic molds, viruses, and parasites. All food production techniques from the farm to the table are concerned with minimizing spoilage, eliminating pathogens, and prolonging shelf life. Irradiation kills microbes primarily by fragmenting DNA. The sensitivity of organisms increases with the complexity of the organism. Thus viruses are most resistant to destruction by irradiation, and insects and parasites are most sensitive. Spores, cysts, toxins, and prions are quite resistant to the effects of irradiation because they contain little DNA and are in highly stable resting states. The conditions under which irradiation takes place (ie, temperature, humidity, and atmospheric content) can affect the dose required to achieve the food processing goal. Regardless, the quality of the food to be irradiated must be high, without heavy microbial contamination, for irradiation to achieve food processing goals at any level. Even when applied under optimal circumstances, when non-sterilizing doses of ionizing radiation are applied to food, the possibility of differential response of bacteria and molds exists and merits examination.

Gram-negative spoilage bacteria (bacteria that alter the color, flavor, texture, or smell of food but do not cause human disease) tend to be more sensitive to radiation than pathogens (bacteria that cause human disease), whereas gram-positive spoilage bacteria can be more resistant to radiation than pathogens. The range of radiation sensitivities, however, is narrow.[8] Initial counts of spoilage bacteria are much higher in foods than are counts of pathogens. At approved maximum levels of irradiation, surviving bacteria are significantly more likely to be spoilage types than pathogenic types. Thus irradiated food would most likely spoil long before becoming pathogenic.[9]

There is some concern regarding irradiation and sporulating toxin-producing bacteria. These may thrive in nonacidic, perishable, high-protein foods and are about 10 times more resistant to radiation than are non-spore formers. For example, *Clostridium botulinum* type E, which is found in fish and seafood, can survive non-sterilizing doses of irradiation intended to extend shelf life. When refrigerated long enough at 10°C or higher, toxin formation can occur. Thus it may be possible for food to become toxic with botulinum toxin before it is obviously spoiled.[10] Conditions that allow for toxin formation before spoilage, such as inadequate refrigeration, are well understood, and regulations can be designed to mitigate against such occurrences. This concern also applies to other non-sterilizing food processing technologies, such as heat, to which spore-forming bacteria also are relatively resistant.

Similar concerns exist about mycotoxins. Experimental data are conflicting, but some studies show an increase in mycotoxin formation after irradiation. One theory is that the higher radioresistance of molds and yeasts compared with bacteria results in a loss of competitive inhibition of mold and yeast growth. Other explanations include the possibility that more nutrients are made available for fungi by irradiation. This is an area in which additional study would be useful.[11]

## Nutritional Value

As with any food processing technique, irradiation can have a negative impact on some nutrients. These changes in nutritive value are similar to those from cooking, canning, and other heat processing of foods. It does not significantly damage carbohydrates or proteins, nor does it change the bioavailability or quantity of minerals or trace elements in foods. Slight loss of essential polyunsaturated fatty acids does occur with irradiation, but fats and oils that are major dietary sources of these nutrients tend to become rancid when irradiated and are not good candidates for this kind of treatment.[12]

Vitamin loss is the largest nutritional concern when foods are irradiated. Vitamin losses are most dramatic when studied in pure solutions. Whole foods exert a protective effect on vitamins because most of the radiation dose is absorbed by macromolecules (proteins, carbohydrates, and fats). Losses can be minimized by irradiating at low temperatures, at low doses, and by excluding oxygen and light.[2] When studied in pure solution, the water-soluble vitamins most sensitive to irradiation are thiamin ($B_1$), pyridoxine ($B_6$), and riboflavin ($B_2$). Vitamin C undergoes chemical conversion after irradiation, but normal vitamin C activity is maintained. Vitamin $B_{12}$, niacin, and pantothenic and folic acids are resistant to irradiation. Of the fat-soluble vitamins, E and A are sensitive. Plant carotenes are relatively resistant, and vitamins D and K are quite resistant to irradiation.[3]

More than 50% of thiamin (found in meats, milk, whole grains, and legumes) can be lost after irradiation under some conditions in some foods. Suboptimal irradiation and storage conditions can enhance this loss.[3] If all sources of thiamin come from irradiated products, a deficiency condition could develop, but this is unlikely in the United States. Irradiation losses of pyridoxine (found in meat, whole grains, corn, and soybeans) are not as severe as with thiamin, and deficiency states are less likely to develop. The biological availability of riboflavin (found in meat, milk, eggs, green vegetables, whole grains, and legumes) can be paradoxically increased after irradiation by shortening required cooking time for some foods, such as legumes.[3]

Of the fat-soluble vitamins, vitamin E loss can be significant after irradiation, especially in conjunction with cooking.[3] Many of the sources of vitamin E, cereal grains, seed oils, peanuts, soybeans, milk fat, and turnip greens, are unlikely to be treated with radiation and should provide for adequate alternative sources in a balanced and varied diet. Vitamin A, found primarily in milk fat and eggs, also is radiosensitive. Thus far only eggs are approved for irradiation. Plant carotenes found in dark green and yellow vegetables are relatively resistant to irradiation and are converted by the body into vitamin A. While a few vitamins are significantly affected by irradiation, in general irradiated food is quite nutritious. As long as a diet is balanced and food choices are varied, deficiency states are unlikely to develop.

## Palatability

Taste, texture, color, and smell are all components of palatable foods. Some foods, particularly foods with high fat content, suffer unacceptable changes in these qualities when irradiated. Modified conditions such as excluding oxygen from the atmosphere, lowering the temperature, excluding light, reducing water content, or lowering the radiation dose can minimize or eliminate these changes. A welcome consequence of modifying irradiation conditions to preserve palatability is that the same modifications also can minimize vitamin loss.

## Conclusion

Irradiation is increasingly suggested as an important adjunct to improving food safety and availability. Current approvals by the FDA are listed in Table 18.1.[1] Irradiated food is safe and nutritious and produces no unusual toxicity as long as best management practices are followed. It can be used safely as part of a balanced and varied diet. It is important to remember, however, that irradiation of food does not substitute for careful food handling from farm to fork.[13]

Table 18.1
US Food and Drug Administration Rules for Food Irradiation*

| Food | Purpose of Irradiation | Dose Permitted, kGy | Date of Rule |
|---|---|---|---|
| Spices, dry vegetable seasoning | Decontamination/disinfest insects | 30 (maximum) | 7/15/63 |
| Wheat, wheat powder | Disinfest insects | 0.2–0.5 | 8/21/63 |
| White potatoes | Extend shelf life | 0.05–0.15 | 11/1/65 |
| Dry or dehydrated enzyme preparations | Control insects and microorganisms | 10 (maximum) | 6/10/85 |
| Pork carcasses or fresh non-cut processed cuts | Control *Trichinella spiralis* | 0.3 (minimum)– 1.0 (maximum) | 7/22/85 |
| Fresh fruit | Delay maturation | 1 | 4/18/86 |
| Dry or dehydrated enzyme preparations | Decontamination | 10 | 4/18/86 |
| Dry or dehydrated aromatic vegetable substances | Decontamination | 30 | 4/18/86 |
| Poultry | Control pathogens | 3 | 5/2/90 |
| Red meat | Control pathogens and prolong shelf life | 4.5 (fresh)– 7 (frozen) | 12/3/97 |
| Fresh shell eggs | Control *Salmonella* species | 3.0 | 7/12/00 |

*US Department of Agriculture rules may have a different timeline.

Widespread use of food irradiation would necessitate construction of irradiation facilities in the United States and other countries. The benefits of expanding this technology and the risks involved must be thoroughly debated. Pediatricians should participate in the dialogue. As with any technology, unforeseen consequences are possible, therefore, careful monitoring and continuous evaluation of this and all food processing techniques are prudent precautions.

## Frequently Asked Questions

Q  *Can I safely feed my children rare hamburger if it has been irradiated?*

A  No. You must cook all ground beef to 160°F to ensure elimination of bacterial pathogens. There is no guarantee pathogens will be completely eliminated by irradiation under current FDA-approved rules. Furthermore, the label is not required to specify the dose of irradiation used or the purpose for use, so irradiated food can be legally labeled as such when it has received very low-dose irradiation designed only to prolong shelf life but not to reduce pathogen loads. Irradiation can never replace careful food handling from farm to fork.

Q  *Doesn't irradiation create toxic chemicals in food that are dangerous to children?*

A  During early reviews of the safety of irradiated foods, the FDA coined the term "unique radiolytic products" to describe the theoretical possibility that molecules unique to the process of food irradiation could be generated.[14] This term has been abandoned because no radiolytic products have been identified that have not eventually been found in foods processed in more conventional ways. The process of irradiation, like heat processing, essentially adds energy to food. As such, many radiolytic products are generated, but in very small numbers because the energy added is small. Heat processing forms the same general types of molecules, but in larger numbers because the amount of energy added to foods by heat processing often is greater than with irradiation.

Q  *Can irradiation be used to hide the fact that food has spoiled and allow bad food to be sold to the public?*

A  Spoiled food has undergone irreversible changes in texture, flavor, smell, and color. Irradiation cannot mask these.

Q *When food is irradiated in the package, do chemicals from the packaging get into the food? Is that dangerous for children?*

A One great advantage of irradiation is that it can be accomplished after foods are packaged, preventing recontamination during subsequent handling. Breakdown products of packaging do migrate into food as a result of irradiation. Components that migrate into food from packaging are classified by the FDA as indirect food additives. Toxicological testing of indirect food additives is required if anticipated exposure levels exceed a regulatory limit.[15] These exposure levels are calculated for adults and may not be safe for infants and children. Additionally, indirect food additives after irradiation were evaluated based on packaging materials available 10 to 30 years ago. Studies of the effects of irradiation on foods packaged in modern materials are ongoing.

Q *How much irradiated food is actually consumed in the United States?*

A Very little, so far. There are fewer than a half dozen commercial food irradiators in the United States. As of January 2000, fewer than 10% of the spices consumed in the United States were irradiated, and less than 0.002% of fruits and vegetables or poultry consumed were irradiated.[16] Irradiated meat, poultry, and fruits are available in a few retail stores in Florida and several midwestern states. The major purchasers of irradiated meat and poultry are hospitals, nursing homes, and other food services. Of note, food services are not required to disclose the irradiation status of the food they serve.

Q *Can increased use of food irradiation create resistant or mutant bacteria and viruses that could cause human disease?*

A Induction of radiation-resistant microbial populations occurs when cultures are experimentally exposed to repeated cycles of radiation.[17,18] Mutations in bacteria and other organisms develop with any form of food processing; ionizing radiation does not produce mutations by unique mechanisms. Mutations from any cause can result in greater, less, or similar levels of virulence or pathogenicity from parent organisms. Although it remains a theoretical risk, several major international reviews cite no reports of the induction of novel pathogens attributable to food irradiation.[19,20]

Q *Is irradiated food more expensive than regular food?*
A Yes. According to recent estimates, meat and poultry would be 3 to 8 cents more per pound and fruits and vegetables 2 to 3 cents more per pound than nonirradiated equivalents.[16] These estimates are subject to error because costs currently are subsidized by industry and research funding, and it is difficult to project the scale on which the technology may be applied.

Q *How dangerous is the technology of food irradiation to the public?*
A The potential dangers differ with the radiation source. X-ray and electron beam involve ionizing radiation that is machine generated. When the power is turned off, the radiation disappears and no radioactive waste is generated. Ensuring safety requires careful engineering of the facilities and compliance with appropriate regulations and safety procedures. Gamma source irradiation technology requires production and transport of the gamma source and storage or recharge of spent source rods. While in use, gamma facilities must be equipped with redundant safety systems and comply with Nuclear Regulatory Commission rules. No radioactivity is released into the environment during gamma irradiation and no human exposure occurs when all systems are used properly. Cobalt 60 degrades to nickel with a half life of 5 years. Cesium 137 degrades to barium with a half life of 30 years. Both are classified as low-level nuclear waste, and storage or recharge is the responsibility of the source rod production companies. To date, there have been no accidents in the United States involving gamma food irradiation facilities.[3]

Q  *Are the benefits of food irradiation worth the risks of the technology?*
A  This is the central issue that is debated by proponents and detrac tors of the technology.[21,22] In the United States, there are sufficient alternatives to food production, handling, storage, and preparation to make irradiation unnecessary for most foods, and for most people in the population. Individuals who are opposed to nuclear technologies can easily and safely avoid consumption of irradiated foods.

Q  *Will irradiation eliminate food-borne illness?*
A  No. Most food-borne illness (approximately 67%) is caused by viruses, which are not killed by irradiation of food. Among all illnesses attributable to food-borne transmission, only about 30% are caused by bacteria and about 3% are caused by parasites. Thus an estimated 33% of food-borne illness (those attributable to bacteria and parasites) may have the potential of prevention by food irradiation.[23]

Q  *Will irradiation kill prions?*
A  No. Irradiation does not kill prions, the agents of bovine spongi form encephalopathy.

## Resources

Gateway to Government Food Safety Information: Food Irradiation, Internet: http://www.foodsafety.gov/~fsg/irradiat.html

International Atomic Energy Agency, Internet: http://www.iaea.org/programmes/nafa/d5/index.html; facts about food irradiation: http://www.iaea.org/icgfi/documents/foodirradiation.pdf

Iowa State University, Internet: http://www.extension.iastate.edu/ foodsafety/rad/irradhome.html

## References

1. Shea KM, American Academy of Pediatrics Committee on Environmental Health. Technical report: irradiation of food. *Pediatrics.* 2000; 106:1505–1510

2. Murano EA, ed. *Food Irradiation: A Source Book.* Ames, IA: Iowa State University Press; 1995

3. Diehl J. *Safety of Irradiated Food.* 3rd ed. New York, NY: Marcel Dekker; 1999

4. Derr DD. International regulatory status and harmonization of food irradiation. *J Food Prot.* 1993;56:882–886, 892

5. US Department of Health and Human Services, Food and Drug Administration. Irradiation of the production, processing and handling of food. *Federal Register.* 1999;64:7834–7837

6. Urbain WM. *Food Irradiation.* Orlando, FL: Academic Press Inc; 1986

7. World Health Organization. *High-Dose Irradiation: Wholesomeness of Food Irradiated With Doses Above 10 kGy. Report of a Joint FAO/IAEA/WHO Study Group.* Geneva, Switzerland: World Health Organization; 1999. WHO Technical Report Series No. 890

8. Monk JD, Beuchat LR, Doyle MP. Irradiation inactivation of food-borne microorganisms. *J Food Prot.* 1995;58:197–208

9. US Department of Health and Human Services, Food and Drug Administration. Irradiation in the production, processing, and handling of food. *Federal Register.* 1997;62:64107–64121

10. Farkas J. Microbiological safety of irradiated foods. *Int J Food Microbiol.* 1989;9:1–15

11. Thayer DW. Food irradiation: benefits and concerns. *J Food Quality.* 1990;13:147 169

12. World Health Organization. *Safety and Nutritional Adequacy of Irradiated Food.* Geneva, Switzerland: World Health Organization; 1994

13. World Health Organization. *WHO Golden Rules for Safe Food Preparation.* Available at: http://www.who.int/fsf/goldenrules.htm

14. Lagunas-Solar MC. Radiation processing of foods: an overview of scientific principles and current status. *J Food Prot.* 1995;58:186–192

15. US Food and Drug Administration Center for Food Safety and Applied Nutrition Office of Premarket Approval. *Guidance for Submitting Requests Under 21 CFR 170.39. Threshold of Regulation for Substances Used in Food-Contact Articles.* Washington, DC: US Department of Health and Human Services; 1996. Available at: http://vm.cfsan.fda.gov/~dms/opa-gg2.html

16. US General Accounting Office. *Report to Congress. Food Irradiation: Available Evidence Indicates That Benefits Outweigh Risks.* Washington, DC: US General Accounting Office; 2000. Publication GAO/RCED 00-217

17. Corry JE, Roberts TA. A note on the development of resistance to heat and gamma radiation in Salmonella. *J Appl Bacteriol.* 1970;33:733–737

18. Davies R, Sinskey AJ. Radiation-resistant mutants of *Salmonella typhimurium* LT2: development and characterization. *J Bacteriol.* 1973;113:133–144

19. World Health Organization. *Wholesomeness of Irradiated Food. Report of a Joint FAO/IAEA/WHO Study Group.* Geneva, Switzerland: World Health Organization; 1981. WHO Technical Report Series No. 659

20. Frank JF, Barnhart HM. Food and dairy sanitation. In: Last JM, Wallace RB, eds. *Macy-Rosenau-Last Public Health and Preventive Medicine.* 13th ed. Norwalk, CT: Appleton & Lange; 1992:606–607

21. Tauxe RV. Food safety and irradiation: protecting the public from food-borne infections. *Emerg Infect Dis.* 2001;7(suppl 3):516–521

22. Louria DB. Food irradiation: perceptions of a qualified opponent. *Infect Dis Clin Pract.* 1993;2:313–316

23. Etzel RA. Epidemiology of foodborne illness—role of food irradiation. In: Loaharanu P, Thomas P, eds. *Irradiation for Food Safety and Quality.* Lancaster PA: Technomic Publishing Co; 2001:50–54

# 19
# Lead

Childhood lead toxicity has been recognized for at least 100 years. With the accumulation of better epidemiologic and toxicologic data, understanding of the nature of the condition has steadily changed. As recently as the 1940s, many believed that children with lead poisoning who did not die during the acute toxic episode had no residual effects. After pediatricians recognized the high prevalence of learning and behavior disorders in children who recovered from acute toxicity, many believed that only children with frank symptoms suffered neurobehavioral deficits. In the 1970s and 1980s studies worldwide demonstrated that some asymptomatic children with elevated levels of lead had lower IQ scores, more language difficulties, attention problems, and behavior disorders.[1,2]

With better epidemiologic studies, the definition of a harmful level of lead has changed dramatically. As recently as 1970, children with blood lead levels less than 60 μg/dL were considered healthy. As new data emerged over subsequent years, effects were seen at lower and lower levels. As of 2003 there is as yet no reliable threshold for these long-lasting effects of lead exposure on cognitive test scores.[3] In 2 independent meta-analyses of prospective studies from several countries,[3,4] damage has been documented beginning at a blood lead concentration of 10 μg/dL. A relationship between blood lead concentration at the time of testing and decreased scores on reading and arithmetic tests is apparent even in children 6 to 16 years old, including among those whose blood lead concentrations by then are less than 5 μg/dL.[5] Canfield et al[6] recently reported that among 172 children followed prospectively with measurements of blood lead concentration, 101 had never had a blood lead level greater than 10 μg/dL, and there was still a strong negative relationship between blood lead concentration and IQ when the children were 3 to 5 years of age.

Since the removal of lead from gasoline and paint 3 decades ago, fatal lead encephalopathy has all but disappeared and symptomatic lead poisoning is now rare. The continued exposure, however, of thousands of children to lead-laden dust in deteriorating housing mars what would otherwise be a public health triumph. Such low-level lead exposure produces cognitive impairment without identifiable clinical symptoms, and it is this asymptomatic cognitive impairment that constitutes most lead poisoning in the United States. The focus has thus shifted from the care of symptomatic children to the prevention of unacceptably high exposures and prevention of further exposure. Although much of the management of children at risk for lead poisoning is nonclinical, pediatricians commonly find themselves participating in or even directing these activities.[7]

### Routes and Sources of Exposure

Children most often are exposed to lead through the unintentional ingestion of lead-containing particles, such as dust from paint or soil, or from water or foreign bodies. Lead can be absorbed from the pulmonary tract if inhaled as fumes or respirable particles.

Lead (Pb) is an element and occurs naturally, but blood lead levels are low in the absence of industrial activities.[8] In the United States, there were 2 major sources of industrially derived lead for children: airborne lead, mostly from the combustion of gasoline containing tetraethyl lead, and leaded chips and dust, mostly from deteriorating lead paint.

The years since 1980 have witnessed a steep decline in childhood exposure to airborne lead in the United States. Federal legislation in the 1970s removed lead from gasoline and reduced smokestack emissions from smelters and other sources, causing blood lead levels in children to fall. From 1976 to 1980, before the regulations had their full impact, US children aged 1 to 5 years had a median blood lead level of 15 µg/dL; 85% of them were above 10 µg/dL.[9] From 1988 to 1991 the median was 3.6 µg/dL, with 9% above 10 µg/dL[10]; in 1999 the median was 2.0 µg/dL.[11] Although levels have declined in all children, black children and poor children continue to have relatively high blood lead levels. Airborne lead should no longer be a source of exposure in most US communities. However, residual lead in the soil in areas heavily affected by airborne lead, such as around smelters, continues to be a problem even decades after closure of the worst sites.[12] Individual children may be exposed to lead fumes or respirable dust resulting from sanding or heating old paint, burning or melting automobile batteries, or melting lead for use in a hobby or craft.

The source for most lead-poisoned children now is the dust and chips from deteriorating lead paint on interior surfaces. Children living in homes with deteriorating lead paint can achieve blood lead levels up to at least 20 µg/dL without frank pica. This exposure commonly arises from normal, developmentally appropriate hand-to-mouth behavior in an environment that is contaminated with lead dust. Children can ingest lead-laden dust with their cereal, for example, by dropping dry cereal on the floor at mealtime and then hunting it down and eating it later, or with their banana by squishing the fruit through their dust-laden hands in preparation for consumption.[13] Children can ingest lead from mouthing contaminated toys.

The use of leaded paint on interior surfaces finally ceased in the United States by the mid-1970s. However, in 1998, of the 16.4 million homes with one or more children younger than 6 years, 27% still had significant lead paint hazards (lead-based paint in such a deteriorated condition that exposure is likely).[14] Dust also is a final resting place for old airborne lead from gasoline, and lead in urban dust can recontaminate cleaned houses.[15]

Uncommon sources of exposure include cosmetics, folk remedies, pottery glaze, old or imported cans with soldered seams, and contaminated vitamin supplements.

Table 19.1 lists risk factors for lead poisoning and prevention strategies.

## Systems Affected

For the lead exposure now seen in the United States, subclinical effects on the central nervous system (CNS) are the most common effects. The best studied effect is cognitive impairment, measured by IQ tests.

**Table 19.1**
**Risk Factors for Lead Exposure and Prevention Strategies**

| Risk Factor | Prevention Strategy |
| --- | --- |
| **Environmental** | |
| Paint | Identify, evaluate, and remediate. |
| Dust | Control sources. |
| Soil | Restrict play in area, plant groundcover. |
| Drinking water | 2-min flush of water faucet in the morning; use of cold water for cooking and drinking especially if tap water used for preparing formula. |
| Folk remedies | Avoid use. |
| Cosmetics (ie, kohl or surma) | Avoid use. |
| Old ceramic or pewter cookware, old urns/kettles | Avoid use. |
| Some imported cosmetics, toys, crayons | Avoid use. |
| Parental occupations | Shower and remove work clothing and shoes before leaving work. |
| Hobbies | Proper use, storage, and ventilation. |
| Home renovation | Proper containment, ventilation. |
| Buying or renting a new home | Inquire about lead hazards, look for deteriorated paint before occupancy, hire certified lead risk assessor to evaluate hazard and recommend control options. |
| **Host** | |
| Hand-to-mouth activity (or pica) | Control sources. |
| Inadequate nutrition | Adequate iron and calcium. |
| Developmental disabilities | Enrichment programs as available. |

The strength of this association and its time course are characteristic, and have been similar in multiple studies in several countries.[5] In most countries including the United States, blood lead levels peak at about age 2 years, and then fall without intervention. That peak blood lead level at age 2 years is associated with lower IQ scores as IQ becomes reliably testable, at about age 4 years. The strength of the association is similar from study to study—as blood lead levels in 2-year-olds increase by 10 µg/dL, the IQ at age 4 years and older declines by 2 to 3 points. A reliable threshold has not been established for these effects,[2] nor have they been shown to diminish as the child gets older. There are similar but usually weaker associations between IQ and blood lead level at the time of IQ testing. Based on these data, the Centers for Disease Control and Prevention (CDC)[2] and American Academy of Pediatrics (AAP)[7] currently use 15 µg/dL as the level of concern in an individual child, which, when detected, should prompt a search for sources of lead exposure and their removal. Many children above 10 µg/dL in a community should prompt a search for community sources and their removal.

Other aspects of CNS function also may be affected by lead, but they are less well documented. Subclinical effects on hearing[16] and balance[17] may occur at commonly encountered blood lead levels. Some studies have used tooth or bone lead, which are thought to represent integrated, possibly lifetime, exposure, as exposure measures. Teachers reported that students with elevated tooth lead levels were more inattentive, hyperactive, disorganized, and less able to follow directions.[18,19] Further follow-up of the Massachusetts children[18] showed higher rates of failure to graduate from high school, reading disabilities, and greater absenteeism in the final year of high school.[20] Elevated bone lead concentrations were associated with increased attentional dysfunction, aggression, and delinquency.[21]

Although there are reasonable animal models of low-dose lead exposure and cognition and behavior,[22] the mechanisms by which lead affects CNS function are not known. Lead alters very basic nervous system functions, like calcium modulated signaling, at very low concentrations in vitro.[23] The age of 2 years, when lead levels peak, is the same age at which a major reduction in dendrite connections occurs, among other events crucial to development. It is thus plausible that lead exposure at that time interferes with a critical development process in the CNS, but what that process is has not been identified.

Lead interferes with heme synthesis beginning at blood lead levels of about 25 μg/dL.[24] Both δ-aminolevulenate dehydratase, an early step enzyme, and ferrochelatase, which closes the heme ring, are inhibited. Ferrochelatase inhibition is the basis of an erstwhile screening test for lead poisoning that measured erythrocyte protoporphyrin, the immediate heme precursor. Because it is insensitive to the lower levels of blood lead that are of concern now, the test is now obsolete for that use. A recent cross-sectional study suggests that environmental exposure to lead may delay growth and pubertal development in African American and Mexican American girls.[25]

Although lead can cause abdominal colic, peripheral neuropathy, and renal disease in adults with occupational exposures, these are rare in children.

### Clinical Effects

Children with blood lead levels greater than 60 μg/dL may complain of headaches, abdominal pain, loss of appetite, and constipation, and display clumsiness, agitation, or decreased activity and somnolence. These are premonitory symptoms of CNS involvement that may rapidly proceed to vomiting, stupor, and convulsions.[26] Symptomatic lead toxicity should be treated as an emergency.

### Diagnostic Measures

The diagnosis of lead poisoning or increased lead absorption depends on the measurement of blood lead. This is best done in a venous sample, because it is difficult to collect finger-stick samples without contamination. Most initial blood lead measurements are now done as screening tests because children meet some general eligibility criteria or because of parental concern rather than because children have symptoms suggestive of lead poisoning.

While children who developed lead encephalopathy in the past often had chips of lead paint visible on abdominal plain films, today most children with lead poisoning show no evidence of lead chips on radiographs.

### Screening

Until 1997 the AAP and CDC recommended that virtually all children have at least one measurement of blood lead beginning at age 12 months, with a retest at age 24 months, if possible. Earlier and more frequent screenings were recommended for high-risk children. Because the prevalence of elevated blood lead levels has fallen so much, a shift toward targeted screening has begun, and the criteria for and implementation of targeted screening continue to develop. As of early 2003 all children enrolled in Medicaid must be screened at ages 12 and 24 months or at ages 36 to 72 months if they have not previously been screened.[27] Most children with elevated blood lead levels are Medicaid eligible, and, currently, most of them are not screened.[28] No state is exempt from this requirement. The US Department of Health and Human Services (HHS) Advisory Committee on Childhood Lead Poisoning Prevention has proposed criteria by which a state might become exempt, but they have not yet been accepted by HHS.

The approach to screening children who are not on Medicaid is less clear. There is a personal risk questionnaire (Table 19.2), which is used to identify children at higher risk of lead poisoning, but this questionnaire has not yet been validated. State and regional criteria proposed in 1997 were dependent on census data and have not been updated.[29] Thus, although targeted screening may be desirable, the tools with which to achieve it are not yet in place. For children who

**Table 19.2**
**A Basic Personal-Risk Questionnaire***

| |
|---|
| 1. Does your child live in or regularly visit a house or child care facility that was built before 1950? |
| 2. Does your child live in or regularly visit a house or child care facility built before 1978 that is being or has recently been renovated or remodeled (within the last 6 months)? |
| 3. Does your child have a sibling or playmate who has or did have lead poisoning? |

*Adapted from Centers for Disease Control and Prevention.[29]

Note: If the answers to the questions are "no," then a screening test is not required, although the pediatrician should explain why the questions were asked to reinforce anticipatory guidance. If the answer to one or more questions is "yes" or "not sure," a screening test should be considered. The state or local health department may recommend alternative or additional questions based on local conditions.

are not on Medicaid, health care providers should consult city, county, or state health departments to determine the appropriate screening recommendations for their jurisdiction.

There is anecdotal evidence that children who are recent immigrants, refugees, or adoptees have an increased prevalence of elevated, sometimes very elevated, blood lead levels, and thus should be screened when the opportunity to do so arises.[30,31]

## *Diagnostic Testing*

Some experienced clinicians measure the blood lead level in children with growth retardation, speech or language dysfunction, anemia, and attentional or behavioral disorders, especially if the parents have a specific interest in lead or in health effects from environmental chemicals. However, persistent elevation of blood lead levels into school age is unusual, even if peak blood lead at age 2 years was high and the child's housing has not been abated. Thus a relatively low blood lead level in a school-aged child does not rule out earlier lead poisoning. If the question of current lead poisoning arises, however, the only reliable way to make a diagnosis is with blood lead measurement. Hair lead gives no useful information and should not be done.[32]

## Management of Clinical and Low-Level Lead Toxicity

Currently a blood lead concentration of 20 µg/dL requires a medical evaluation (see Table 19.3). Proper management includes finding and eliminating the source of the lead, instruction in proper hygienic measures (personal and household), optimizing the child's diet, and close follow-up (see Tables 19.4 and 19.5). Most such children live in or visit regularly a home with deteriorating lead paint.

Successful therapy depends on eliminating the child's exposure to lead. Any treatment regimen that does not control environmental exposure to lead is considered inadequate. Pediatricians should refer poisoned children to local public health offices for environmental assessment of the child's residence(s). Public health staff should conduct a thorough investigation of the child's environment and family lifestyle for sources of lead.

Deteriorated lead paint is the most common source of exposure. However, other factors also should be evaluated including tableware, cosmetics such as surma and kohl, home remedies, dietary supplements of calcium, tap water, and parental occupation. Some children will have persistently elevated blood lead levels without access to lead paint. Their exposure may come from any of the sources listed in Table 19.1. Blood lead levels should fall as the child passes age 2 years or so, and a stable or increasing blood lead level past that age is likely to be due to ongoing exposure. In children who have spent prolonged periods in a leaded environment, blood lead levels will fall more slowly after exposure ceases,[34] probably because bone stores are greater.

The Advisory Committee on Childhood Lead Poisoning Prevention issued case management guidelines for children with lead poisoning in March 2002.[33] These guidelines should be consulted as needed.

Specific attention also should be paid to treating iron deficiency and ensuring adequate calcium and zinc intake.

Chelation therapy for children with blood lead levels of 20 to 44 µg/dL can be expected to lower blood lead levels but has not been

**Table 19.3**
**Recommended Follow-up Actions, According to Blood Lead Level (BLL)\***

| BLL (μg/dL) | Actions |
|---|---|
| <10 | No action required. Continued surveillance. |
| 10–14 | Obtain a confirmatory venous BLL within 1 month; if still within this range<br>• Provide education to decrease lead exposure.<br>• Repeat BLL test within 3 months. |
| 15–19 | Obtain a confirmatory venous BLL within 1 month; if still within this range<br>• Take a careful environmental history.<br>• Provide education to decrease lead exposure and to decrease lead absorption.<br>• Repeat BLL test within 2 months. |
| 20–44 | Obtain a confirmatory venous BLL within 1 week; if still within this range<br>• Conduct a complete medical history (including an environmental evaluation and nutritional assessment) and physical examination.<br>• Provide education to decrease lead exposure and lead absorption.<br>• Either refer the patient to the local health department or provide case management that should include a detailed environmental investigation with lead hazard reduction and appropriate referrals for support services.<br>• Chelation not currently recommended for BLLs <45 μg/dL. |
| 45–69 | Obtain a confirmatory venous BLL within 2 days; if still within this range<br>• Conduct a complete medical history (including an environmental evaluation and nutritional assessment) and a physical examination.<br>• Provide education to decrease lead exposure and lead absorption.<br>• Either refer the patient to the local health department or provide case management that should include a detailed environmental investigation with lead hazard reduction and appropriate referrals for support services.<br>• Begin chelation therapy in consultation with clinicians experienced in lead toxicity therapy. |
| ≥70 | Hospitalize the patient and begin medical treatment, including parenteral chelation therapy, immediately in consultation with clinicians experienced in lead toxicity therapy.<br>• Obtain a confirmatory BLL immediately.<br>• The rest of the management should be as noted for management of children with BLLs between 45 and 69 μg/dL. |

\*Adapted from Centers for Disease Control and Prevention.[29]

**Table 19.4**
**Clinical Evaluation***

| |
|---|
| **Medical History**<br>Ask about<br>• Symptoms<br>• Developmental history<br>• Mouthing activities<br>• Pica<br>• Previous blood lead level measurements<br>• Family history of lead poisoning |
| **Environmental History**<br>Paint and soil exposure<br>• What is the age and general condition of the residence?<br>• Is there evidence of chewed or peeling paint on woodwork, furniture, or toys?<br>• How long has the family lived at that residence?<br>• Have there been recent renovations or repairs in the house?<br>• Are there other sites where the child spends significant amounts of time?<br>• What is the character of indoor play areas?<br>• Do outdoor play areas contain bare soil that may be contaminated?<br>• How does the family attempt to control dust/dirt? |
| **Relevant Behavioral Characteristics of the Child**<br>• To what degree does the child exhibit hand-to-mouth activity?<br>• Does the child exhibit pica?<br>• Are the child's hands washed before meals and snacks? |
| **Exposures to and Behaviors of Household Members**<br>• What are the occupations of adult household members?<br>• What are the hobbies of household members? (Fishing, working with ceramics or stained glass, and hunting are examples of hobbies that involve risk for lead exposure.)<br>• Are painted materials or unusual materials burned in household fireplaces? |
| **Miscellaneous Questions**<br>• Does the home contain vinyl miniblinds made overseas and purchased before 1997?<br>• Does the child receive or have access to imported food, cosmetics, or folk remedies?<br>• Is food prepared or stored in imported pottery or metal vessels? |

**Table 19.4**
**Clinical Evaluation\*, *continued***

| Nutritional History |
| --- |
| • Take a dietary history. |
| • Evaluate the child's iron status using appropriate laboratory tests. |
| • Ask about history of food stamps or Special Supplemental Nutrition Program for Women, Infants, and Children program participation. |
| **Physical Examination** |
| • Pay particular attention to the neurological examination and to the child's psychosocial and language development. |

\*Adapted from Centers for Disease Control and Prevention.[33]

**Table 19.5**
**Schedule for Follow-up Blood Lead Level (BLL) Testing\***

| Venous BLL (µg/dL) | Early Follow-up (first 2–4 tests after identification) | Late Follow-up (after BLL begins to decline) |
| --- | --- | --- |
| 10–14 | 3 months | 6–9 months |
| 15–19 | 1–3 months | 3–6 months |
| 20–24 | 1–3 months | 1–3 months |
| 25–44 | 2 weeks–1 month | 1 month |
| ≥45 | As soon as possible | Chelation with subsequent follow-up |

\*Adapted from Centers for Disease Control and Prevention.[33]

Note: Seasonal variation of BLLs exists and may be more apparent in colder climate areas. Greater exposure in the summer months may necessitate more frequent follow-ups. Some clinicians may choose to repeat blood lead tests on all new patients within a month to see whether their BLL level is rising more quickly than anticipated.

shown to reverse or diminish cognitive impairment or other behavioral or neuropsychological effects of lead based on follow-up for 3 years post-chelation.[35] Succimer, the oral drug used in that trial, is labeled for children with blood lead levels greater than 45 µg/dL. There are no data supporting its use below that level.

If the blood lead level is greater than 45 µg/dL and the exposure has been controlled, treatment with succimer should begin. A pediatrician experienced in managing children with lead poisoning should be consulted—these can be found through the AAP Committee on Environmental Health, at the hospitals that participated in the clinical trial of succimer,[35] or at the Pediatric Environmental Health Specialty Units. Baseline hepatocellular enzymes and a complete blood count and differential should be obtained, the first dose of succimer should be given while the parent observes the procedure, and the parent should administer the subsequent 3 doses of succimer under physician supervision. The capsules are emptied into palatable foods such as flavored gelatin, peanut butter, or applesauce. Hepatocellular enzymes and a complete blood count should be obtained on the fourth day after the initial dose and at the conclusion of the course of therapy.

The most common side effects of succimer listed on the label are abdominal distress, a transient rash, elevated hepatocellular enzyme levels, and neutropenia. If side effects occur, the drug treatment should be stopped and then cautiously resumed after the side effects abate. If the side effects do not recur, treatment may be completed. In the largest clinical trial (390 children given succimer), the most common drug-related adverse event was nonspecific evidence of trauma, an unusual side effect that has not been confirmed. The drug is very unpleasant to administer because of the strong rotten egg smell, and 40% of the families on active drug compared with 26% on placebo found the drug difficult to administer.[36] The succimer label provides dosages calculated by body surface area and by weight, but the equivalent dose by both methods would occur in a child about 5 years old. For the younger children typically given the drug, body surface area calculations give higher doses, which are the recommended ones.[37]

Children with symptoms, with higher blood lead levels, or who are allergic or react to succimer will need parenteral therapy and hospitalization. Children with an uncontrolled source of exposure in their homes also are candidates for hospitalization or some form of residential care. Guidelines for these circumstances are beyond the scope here, but the previously mentioned consultation is recommended. Detailed treatment guidelines were published by the AAP in 1995.[38]

## Frequently Asked Questions

Q  *We have imported ceramic dishes. Is it safe to use them?*

A  Some imported ceramic dishes contain lead. Such dishes should not be used to serve acidic substances because the acids can leach large amounts of lead from the dishes into the food.

Q  *We have vinyl miniblinds. Should I get rid of them?*

A  In the mid-1990s, some imported, non-glossy vinyl miniblinds were found to contain lead. Sunlight and heat can break down the blinds and may release lead-contaminated dust. Children who touch these miniblinds and put their fingers in their mouths may ingest small amounts of lead. If you purchase new miniblinds, look for products with labels that say "new formulation" or "nonleaded formula." Older ones must be discarded if they have begun to chalk or deteriorate.

Q  *Is there still lead in canned food?*

A  Cans with soldered seams can add lead to foods. In the United States, soldered cans have largely been replaced by seamless aluminum containers, but some imported canned products and large commercial-sized cans still have lead-soldered seams.

Q  *What about testing for lead in water?*

A  If you have an infant and are using tap water to reconstitute infant formula, you may want to know whether your water contains lead. To help determine whether your water might contain lead, call either the US Environmental Protection Agency Safe Drinking Water Hotline at 800-426-4791 or your local health department to find out about testing your water.

## Resources

National Lead Information Center, phone: 800-532-3394

Office of Healthy Homes and Lead Hazard Control, Department of Housing and Urban Development, Internet: http://www.hud.gov/offices/lead

Pediatric Environmental Health Specialty Units, Internet: http://ehpnet1.niehs.nih.gov/children/pehsu.html

US Environmental Protection Agency federal plan for eliminating childhood lead poisoning, Internet: http://yosemite.epa.gov/ochp/ochpweb.nsf/content/whatwe_tf_proj.htm

## References

1. National Research Council, Committee on Measuring Lead in Critical Populations. *Measuring Lead Exposure in Infants, Children and Other Sensitive Populations.* Washington, DC: National Academies Press; 1993
2. Centers for Disease Control and Prevention. *Preventing Lead Poisoning in Young Children.* Atlanta, GA: US Department of Health and Human Services, Centers for Disease Control and Prevention; 1991
3. Schwartz J. Low-level lead exposure and children's IQ: a meta-analysis and search for a threshold. *Environ Res.* 1994;65:42–55
4. Pocock SJ, Smith M, Baghurst P. Environmental lead and children's intelligence: a systematic review of the epidemiological evidence. *BMJ.* 1994;309:1189–1197
5. Lanphear BP, Dietrich K, Auinger P, Cox C. Cognitive deficits associated with blood lead concentrations <10 microg/dL. US children and adolescents. *Public Health Rep.* 2000;115:521–529
6. Canfield RL, Henderson CR Jr, Cory-Slechta DA, Cox C, Jusko TA, Lanphear BP. Intellectual impairment in children with blood lead concentrations below 10 µg per deciliter. *N Engl J Med.* 2003; 348:1517–1526
7. American Academy of Pediatrics Committee on Environmental Health. Screening for elevated blood lead levels. *Pediatrics.* 1998;101:1072–1078
8. Patterson CC. *Natural Levels of Lead in Humans.* Chapel Hill, NC: Institute for Environmental Studies, University of North Carolina at Chapel Hill; 1982

9. Mahaffey KR, Annest JL, Roberts J, Murphy RS. National estimates of blood lead levels: United States, 1976–1980: association with selected demographic and socioeconomic factors. *N Engl J Med.* 1982;307:573–579

10. Pirkle JL, Brody DJ, Gunter EW, et al. The decline in blood lead levels in the United States. The National Health and Nutrition Examination Surveys (NHANES). *JAMA.* 1994;272:284–291

11. Centers for Disease Control and Prevention. Blood lead levels in young children—United States and selected states, 1996–1999. *MMWR Morb Mortal Wkly Rep.* 2000;49:1133–1137

12. US Environmental Protection Agency Region 10. *Superfund Fact Sheet. Bunker Hill-Kellogg, Idaho. Spring Update.* Washington, DC: US Environmental Protection Agency; 1999. Available at: http://www.epa.gov/r10earth/offices/oec/newbunk.pdf

13. Freeman NC, Sheldon L, Jimenez M, Melnyk L, Pellizzari E, Berry M. Contribution of children's activities to lead contamination of food. *J Expo Anal Environ Epidemiol.* 2001;11:407–413

14. Jacobs DE, Clickner RP, Zhou JY, et al. The prevalence of lead-based paint hazards in US housing. *Environ Health Perspect.* 2002;110:A599–A606

15. Farfel MR, Chisolm JJ Jr. An evaluation of experimental practices for abatement of residential lead-based paint: report on a pilot project. *Environ Res.* 1991;55:199–212

16. Schwartz J, Otto D. Lead and minor hearing impairment. *Arch Environ Health.* 1991;46:300–305

17. Bhattacharya A, Shukla R, Bornschein RL, Dietrich KN, Keith R. Lead effects on postural balance of children. *Environ Health Perspect.* 1990;89:35–42

18. Needleman HL, Gunnoe C, Leviton A, et al. Deficits in psychologic and classroom performance of children with elevated dentine lead levels. *N Engl J Med.* 1979;300:689–695

19. Sciarillo WG, Alexander G, Farrell KP. Lead exposure and child behavior. *Am J Public Health.* 1992;82:1356–1360

20. Needleman HL, Schell A, Bellinger D, Leviton A, Allred EN. The long-term effects of exposure to low doses of lead in childhood. An 11-year follow-up report. *N Engl J Med.* 1990;322:83–88

21. Needleman HL, Riess JA, Tobin MJ, Biesecker GE, Greenhouse JB. Bone lead levels and delinquent behavior. *JAMA.* 1996;275:363–369

22. Rice DC. Behavioral effects of lead: commonalities between experimental and epidemiologic data. *Environ Health Perspect.* 1996;104(suppl 2): 337–351

23. Markovac J, Goldstein GW. Picomolar concentrations of lead stimulate brain protein kinase C. *Nature.* 1988;334:71–73

24. McIntire MS, Wolf GL, Angle CR. Red cell lead and γ-amino levulinic acid dehydratase. *Clin Toxicol.* 1973;6:183–188

25. Selevan SG, Rice DC, Hogan KA, Euling SY, Pfahles-Hutchens A, Bethel J. Blood lead concentration and delayed puberty in girls. *N Engl J Med.* 2003; 348:1527–1536

26. Chisolm JJ Jr, Kaplan E. Lead poisoning in childhood—comprehensive management and prevention. *J Pediatr.* 1968;73:942–950

27. Advisory Committee on Childhood Lead Poisoning Prevention. Recommendations for blood lead screening of young children enrolled in Medicaid: targeting a group at high risk. *MMWR Morb Mortal Wkly Rep.* 2002;49:1–13. Available at: http://www.cdc.gov/mmwr/PDF/RR/RR4914.pdf

28. Centers for Disease Control and Prevention. Recommendations for blood lead screening of young children enrolled in Medicaid: targeting a group at high risk. *MMWR Morb Mortal Wkly Rep.* 2000;49:1–24

29. Centers for Disease Control and Prevention. *Screening Young Children for Lead Poisoning: Guidance for State and Local Health Officials.* Atlanta, GA: Centers for Disease Control and Prevention; 1997:32. Available at: http://www.cdc.gov/nceh/lead/guide/guide97.htm

30. Geltman PL, Brown MJ, Cochran J. Lead poisoning among refugee children resettled in Massachusetts, 1995 to 1999. *Pediatrics.* 2001;108:158–162

31. Centers for Disease Control and Prevention. Elevated blood lead levels among internationally adopted children—United States, 1998. *MMWR Morb Mortal Wkly Rep.* 2000;49:97–100

32. Esteban E, Rubin CH, Jones RL, Noonan G. Hair and blood as substrates for screening children for lead poisoning. *Arch Environ Health.* 1999;54:436–440

33. Centers for Disease Control and Prevention. *Managing Elevated Blood Lead Levels Among Young Children: Recommendations from the Advisory Committee on Childhood Lead Poisoning Prevention.* Atlanta, GA: Centers for Disease Control and Prevention; 2002. Available at: http://www.cdc.gov/nceh/lead/CaseManagement/caseManage_main.htm

34. Manton WI, Angle CR, Stanek KL, Reese YR, Kuehnemann TJ. Acquisition and retention of lead by young children. *Environ Res.* 2000;82:60–80

35. Rogan WJ, Dietrich KN, Ware JH, et al. The effect of chelation therapy with succimer on neuropsychological development in children exposed to lead. *N Engl J Med.* 2001;344:1421–1426

36. Safety and efficacy of succimer in toddlers with blood lead levels of 20–44 microg/dL. Treatment of Lead-Exposed Children (TLC) Trial Group. *Pediatr Res.* 2000;48:593–599

37. Rhoads GG, Rogan WJ. Treatment of lead-exposed children. *Pediatrics.* 1996;98:162–163

38. American Academy of Pediatrics Committee on Drugs. Treatment guidelines for lead exposure in children. *Pediatrics.* 1995;96:155–160. Available at: http://www.aap.org/policy/00868.html

# 20
# Mercury

Mercury (Hg) occurs in 3 forms: the metallic element ($Hg^0$, quicksilver or elemental mercury), inorganic salts ($Hg^{1+}$, or mercurous salts, and $Hg^{2+}$, or mercuric salts), and organic compounds (methylmercury, ethylmercury, and phenylmercury). Solubility, reactivity, biological effects, and toxicity vary among these forms. Mercury has been used for more than 3000 years in medicine and industry.

Naturally occurring mercury sources include cinnabar (ore) and fossil fuels, such as coal and petroleum. Environmental contamination has resulted from mining, smelting, and industrial discharges. Mercury in lakes and stream sediments can be converted by bacteria into organic mercury compounds (eg, methylmercury) that accumulate in the food chain and are biomagnified as they ascend the food chain. The result is that certain predator fish (eg, shark, tuna, swordfish) can contain substantial quantities of mercury. Consumption of fish with high levels of methylmercury by pregnant women in Minamata Bay, Japan, in the 1950s resulted in at least 30 cases of infantile cerebral palsy.[1] To prevent this from occurring, several states have issued advisories about consumption of fish from contaminated waters (see Chapter 27). Large ocean fish, such as tuna, swordfish, king mackerel, tilefish, and shark, may have increased methylmercury content owing to exposure from naturally occurring and industrial sources of mercury pollution.

Elemental mercury is used in sphygmomanometers, thermometers, and thermostat switches. Dental amalgams contain mercury as well as silver and other metals. Fluorescent light bulbs (usually 2–4 ft tubes) and disc ("button") batteries also contain mercury. Indiscriminate disposal of these items is a major source of environmental mercury contamination when they are buried in landfills or burned in waste incinerators rather than recycled. Elemental mercury also is used in some folk remedies, such as those of Santeria, practiced by some groups of Hispanic Americans.[2,3]

Methylmercury has been used as a fungicide on seed grains and is an industrial waste product. When grain in Iraq treated with a mercury fungicide was accidentally eaten by people in Iraq between 1959 and 1972, mercury poisoning occurred in thousands of people.[4]

## Routes of Exposure

### *Elemental Mercury*

Elemental mercury is a liquid at room temperature and readily volatilizes to a colorless and odorless vapor. When inhaled, elemental mercury vapor easily passes through pulmonary alveolar membranes and enters the blood, where it distributes primarily into red blood cells and the central nervous system (CNS). In contrast, less than 0.1% of elemental mercury is absorbed from the gastrointestinal tract after ingestion, and only minimal absorption occurs with dermal exposure.[5]

### *Inorganic Mercury*

Inorganic mercury salts are poorly absorbed after ingestion, although mercuric salts tend to be extremely caustic. Dermal exposure has resulted in toxic effects in animals.

### *Organic Mercury*

In general, organic mercury compounds are lipid soluble and are well absorbed from the gastrointestinal tract. Methylmercury is essentially 100% absorbed after ingestion, contributing to concern about consumption of methylmercury-contaminated fish.[3] Methylmercury passes through the placenta and is excreted into breast milk. This form of mercury also is well absorbed after inhalation. Phenylmercury is well absorbed after ingestion and dermal contact. In contrast to other organic mercury compounds, the carbon-mercury chemical bond of phenylmercury is relatively unstable, resulting in the release of elemental mercury that can be inhaled and absorbed across pulmonary membranes.

Ethylmercury is found in thimerosal, an antiseptic and preservative for vaccines and other drug therapies. Thimerosal contains 49.6% mercury by weight. Before fall 1999 there was 12.5 to 25 μg of mercury in each dose of most diphtheria and tetanus toxoids and acellular pertussis, *Haemophilus influenzae* type b, influenza, meningococcal, pneumococcal, and rabies vaccines. In 1999, recognizing the potential for excessive exposure, the American Academy of Pediatrics (AAP), along with the American Academy of Family Physicians, the Advisory Committee on Immunization Practices, and the US Public Health Service, issued a joint recommendation that thimerosal be removed from vaccines as quickly as possible.[6,7] Currently all routinely recommended vaccines manufactured for administration to infants in the United States are available in thimerosal-free formulation.

## Systems Affected and Clinical Effects

### Elemental Mercury

At high concentrations, mercury vapor inhalation produces an acute necrotizing bronchitis and pneumonitis, which can lead to death due to respiratory failure.[8] Fatalities have resulted from heating elemental mercury in inadequately ventilated areas.[9]

Long-term exposure to mercury vapor primarily affects the CNS. Early nonspecific signs include insomnia, forgetfulness, loss of appetite, and mild tremor and may be misdiagnosed as psychiatric illness. Continued exposure leads to progressive tremor and erethism, characterized by red palms, emotional lability, and memory impairment.[10–12] Salivation, excessive sweating, and hemoconcentration are accompanying autonomic signs. Mercury also accumulates in kidney tissues. Renal toxicity includes proteinuria or nephrotic syndrome, alone or in addition to other signs of mercury exposure.[13,14] Isolated renal effects may be immunologic in origin.

Mercury exposure from dental amalgams has provoked concerns about subclinical or unusual neurologic effects, ranging from such subjective complaints as chronic fatigue to demyelinating neuropathies including multiple sclerosis.[15] Although dental amalgams are a source of mercury exposure and are associated with slightly higher urinary mercury excretion, there is no scientific evidence for any measurable clinical toxic effects other than rare hypersensitivity reactions.[16–18] The US Public Health Service concluded that dental amalgams do not pose a health risk and should not be replaced merely to reduce mercury exposure.[19]

### *Inorganic Mercury*

Mercuric bichloride ($Hg^{2+}$) is well described by its common name, corrosive sublimate. Ingestions usually are inadvertent or with suicidal intent, and gastrointestinal ulceration or perforation and hemorrhage are rapidly produced, followed by circulatory collapse. Breakdown of intestinal mucosal barriers leads to extensive mercury absorption and distribution to the kidneys. Acute renal toxic effects consist of proximal tubular necrosis and anuria.

Acrodynia, or childhood mercury poisoning, was frequently reported in the 1940s among infants exposed to calomel teething powders containing mercurous chloride.[20,21] Cases also have been reported in infants exposed to phenylmercury used as a fungicidal diaper rinse[22] and in children exposed to phenylmercuric acetate from interior latex paint.[23] Children's individual susceptibility to develop acrodynia is poorly understood, but a maculopapular rash, swollen and painful extremities, peripheral neuropathy, hypertension, and renal tubular dysfunction develop in affected children.

### *Organic Mercury*

Organic mercury toxicity occurs with long-term exposure and affects the CNS. Signs progress from paresthesias to ataxia, followed by generalized weakness, visual and hearing impairment, tremor and muscle spasticity, and then coma and death. Organic mercury also is a potent teratogen, causing disruption of the normal patterns of neuronal migration and nerve cell histology in the developing brain. In the Minamata Bay disaster, with contaminated fish, and the Iraq epidemic, with contaminated seed grain, mothers who were asymptomatic or showed mild toxic effects gave birth to severely affected infants. Typically, the infants seemed normal at birth, but psychomotor retardation, blindness, deafness, and seizures developed over time.[24]

Because the fetus and infant are more susceptible to the neurotoxic effects of methylmercury, investigators have looked for subclinical effects among children whose mothers' diets include large amounts of fish or marine mammals containing methylmercury and whose blood mercury levels are higher than those commonly seen in the United States. There are 2 such longitudinal studies—one in the Seychelles (islands in the Indian Ocean about 1000 miles off the east coast of Africa), the other in the Faroes (islands off the coast of Iceland). Among 917 Faroese children evaluated at 7 years of age, higher maternal hair mercury levels were associated with deficits in language, attention, and memory.[25] However, despite similar exposures, these deficits were not seen among 711 children examined at 66 months of age in the Seychelles.[26] Further research is necessary before the clinical and public health implications of these findings are clear.

The National Academy of Sciences (NAS) has reviewed methylmercury toxicity to determine a reference dose for mercury. A reference dose is a dosage of a chemical that has been determined to be safe on the basis of available toxicity information; it is used to provide a basis for establishing safety standards and guidelines. The NAS concluded that the reference dose for mercury, based on the development of neurobehavioral toxicity, should be established at 0.1 µg/kg per day.[27]

Ethylmercury, although it may have similar toxicity to methylmercury, has been less well studied. Very high exposures to thimerosal-containing products have resulted in toxicity, including acrodynia, chronic mercury toxicity, renal failure, and neuropathy.[28–32] Merthiolate used to irrigate the external auditory canals in a child with tympanostomy tubes caused fatal mercury poisoning.[33]

There has been concern that organic mercury exposure from thimerosal-containing vaccines and other sources has played a role in the growing incidence of autism. The NAS has reviewed this issue and determined that there currently is no significant scientific evidence for or against such a causal relationship.[34]

## Diagnostic Methods

Diagnosis of mercury poisoning usually is made by history and physical examination. In addition, laboratory tests may demonstrate elevated mercury levels. Normal blood mercury levels, however, do not exclude mercury poisoning.

### Elemental Mercury

Increased mercury vapor concentrations can be measured in exhaled air from persons with dental amalgams, but the biological significance is uncertain. Also unclear is the significance of the slight increase in urinary mercury excretion detected after dental amalgams are placed.

### Inorganic Mercury

Inorganic mercury exposure can be measured by urinary mercury determination, preferably using a 24-hour urine collection. Results greater than 10 to 20 µg/L are evidence of excessive exposure, and neurologic signs may be present at values greater than 100 µg/L. However, the urinary mercury concentration does not necessarily correlate with chronicity or severity of toxic effects, especially if the mercury exposure has been intermittent or variable in intensity. Whole blood mercury can be measured, but values tend to return to normal (<0.5–1.0 µg/dL) within 1 to 2 days after the exposure to metallic mercury vapor ends.

### Organic Mercury

Organic mercury compounds concentrate in red blood cells, so whole blood may be used to diagnose excessive exposure. In a 1999 to 2000 sample of the US population, the geometric mean blood mercury levels were 0.34 µg/L for children 1 to 5 years old and 1.02 µg/L for women 16 to 49 years old.[35] Blood mercury levels rarely exceed more than 1.5 µg/dL in the unexposed population, and a blood concentration of 5 µg/dL or greater is considered the threshold for symptoms of toxicity. Methylmercury also distributes into growing hair, thus providing a noninvasive means to estimate body burden and blood concentration over time. In the general population, the mercury level in hair is usually 1 ppm or less.[36–39] Collection of blood or hair specimens for mercury analysis requires special mercury-free collection materials and rigorous control of contamination. Such testing is usually conducted in a research setting.

## Treatment

The most important and most effective treatment is to identify the mercury source and end the exposure.

### Elemental and Inorganic Mercury

Mercury accumulates in blood and CNS and renal tissues and is very slowly eliminated. Chelating agents have been used to enhance mercury elimination, but whether chelation reduces toxic effects or speeds recovery in people who have been poisoned is unclear. Dimercaprol (BAL in oil) has been used for severe cases of inorganic mercury poisoning and can be administered to patients in renal failure because it is eliminated by hepatic excretion. d-Penicillamine is an oral chelator that enhances urinary excretion of inorganic mercury but has a 10% to 30% rate of adverse drug reactions. Newer derivatives of BAL, such as dimercaptosuccinic acid (DMSA, succimer) and 2,3-dimercapto-propane-1-sulfonate (DMPS, dimaval) have been more effective than BAL in experimental studies.[40–42] Succimer, an oral chelating agent for the treatment of childhood lead poisoning, increases urinary mercury excretion, but its efficacy is uncertain and it must be considered experimental therapy for mercury poisoning. Mercury poisoning should be treated in consultation with a physician experienced in managing children with mercury poisoning.

### Organic Mercury

There is no chelating agent approved by the US Food and Drug Administration (FDA) that is effective for methylmercury poisoning. Dimercaprol may increase the mercury concentration in the brain and should not be used in cases of methylmercury poisoning.[43] Succimer has been used for the treatment of severe organic mercury poisoning.[44] Recent data also have identified a role for N-acetylcysteine in the chelation therapy of methylmercury poisoning.[45]

Children who have had mercury poisoning should undergo periodic follow-up neurologic examinations by a pediatrician.

### Prevention of Exposure

Many mercury compounds are no longer sold in the United States. Electronic equipment has replaced many mercury-containing oral thermometers and sphygmomanometers in medical settings. Medicinal mercurials now have limited use although thimerosal still is available. Recently the American Hospital Association agreed to phase out mercury use by all its members. The purpose of this initiative is to prevent additional pollution resulting from mercury emissions from medical waste incinerators. Additionally, because the costs of abatement after a mercury spill (even a spill as seemingly trivial as a broken sphygmomanometer) can be very expensive, elimination of mercury has significant cost savings. The AAP has recommended that pediatricians eliminate their use of mercury devices, including thermometers, and that families be encouraged to do the same.[46] Local programs for the safe disposal of mercury thermometers may be available.

Organic mercury fungicides, including phenylmercury (once used in latex paints), are no longer licensed for commercial use. Newer enclosed methods for preparing mercury amalgams have reduced the likelihood of mercury spillage and exposure during dental amalgam preparation.

The amount of mercury in thermometers is small and usually insufficient to produce clinically significant exposure. If a mercury thermometer breaks, the bead of elemental mercury should be carefully rolled onto a sheet of paper and then put in a jar or an airtight container for appropriate disposal. Use of a vacuum cleaner should be avoided because it causes elemental mercury to vaporize in the air, creating greater health risks.[47] In the event of a larger elemental mercury spill, consultation with a certified environmental cleaning company is advised. They often are listed in the telephone directory yellow pages under "environmental or ecological services."

Most regulatory standards or advisories pertain to the workplace. Nonoccupational standards have been established by the US Environmental Protection Agency for drinking water (2 µg/L) and by the FDA for fish (1 ppm) and bottled drinking water (2 µg/L).

The FDA has set advisory limits for methylmercury in commercial fish of 1 ppm (1 µg/g).[48] In March 2001 the FDA recommended that pregnant women, women of childbearing age, nursing mothers, and young children should avoid consumption of shark, king mackerel, swordfish, and tilefish. For other types of fish, including tuna, the FDA has advised that consumption by children, pregnant women, and those who may become pregnant be kept below 12 ounces per week. The risks of exposure to methylmercury from fish have to be balanced with the health benefits of eating fish. Fish is a source of high-quality protein as well as unsaturated fatty acids and other beneficial nutrients. For some populations, locally caught fish may be the only good alternative for a nutritious diet. If fish with lower mercury levels are available, then it is prudent to substitute these rather than eat fish that have methylmercury advisories or commercial fish, such as swordfish and tuna, which are known to have higher mercury levels.

Although the levels of mercury in commercial fish are regulated by the FDA, the federal government does not regulate the levels of mercury in fish caught for sport. Because of the potential for mercury contamination, 41 states have issued advisories recommending public limits or the avoidance of consuming certain fish caught for sport from specific bodies of water. In some areas of the United States, certain freshwater species (eg, walleye, pike, muskie, and bass) have levels of mercury that would result in substantial mercury intakes from a meal of fish. Most state health agencies advise limiting intake of freshwater sport fish having mercury concentrations of more than 0.2 to 1 ppm. Current state fish consumption advisories can be found on the EPA Web site (http://www.epa.gov/OST/fish/).

Although there are no regulatory standards for home air, the Agency for Toxic Substances and Disease Registry suggests that acceptable residential air mercury levels should not exceed 0.5 µg/cubic meter.[49]

## Frequently Asked Questions

Q *Will toxic effects result after ingesting mercury from an oral thermometer?*

A Elemental mercury in these thermometers is poorly absorbed from the gastrointestinal tract. No treatment is needed. (The fragments of broken glass are of greater concern.) Because mercury vapor can be absorbed, sporadic cases of acrodynia have resulted from children playing on a carpet contaminated by metallic mercury. Therefore, children should not play with mercury from a broken thermometer.

Q *Should pregnant women or women planning pregnancy avoid eating fish?*

A There is no known risk that outweighs the benefit of eating commercially caught fish. However, the consumption of shark, king mackerel, tilefish, and swordfish should be avoided by women who are pregnant or nursing, and by young children.[48] For fish that are caught from local waters, check with your state health department to find out whether pregnant women should limit their fish intake (see Chapter 27).

Q *Should my child have nonmercury fillings? or Should the mercury fillings be replaced?*

A Mercury amalgams are a durable material for filling dental caries. There is no scientific evidence that this commonly used dental material is a health hazard, although mercury exposure may occur from the presence of dental amalgams. It is not necessary to replace amalgams just because of the mercury content; furthermore, the removal process may weaken the tooth.

Q *Is it true that latex paint containing mercury can be hazardous to a child's health?*

A Before 1991 it was permissible to add phenylmercuric acetate to interior latex paint as a preservative. This is no longer permitted. Therefore, paints produced in the United States since 1991 for indoor use should not contain mercury compounds.

Q *Someone spilled some mercury at my child's school. How should it be cleaned up?*

A It is necessary to enlist a specialist's help to clean up even small mercury spills in schools. The janitor should not vacuum it up because this may spread the mercury aerosol. The local health department can provide the names of local environmental companies with expertise in mercury cleanup. School children should not play with the spilled mercury or take it home from the school.

## Resources

Regional poison control centers may be resources for clinical and therapeutic information about mercury poisoning. Phone: 800-222-1222.

State and local public health and environmental agencies. They may be of assistance if a mercury spill occurs, if clinically significant poisoning is suspected, or to evaluate possible environmental exposure sources.

US Environmental Protection Agency, Internet: www.epa.gov/OST/fish

# References

1. Study Group of Minamata Disease. *Minamata Disease.* Kumamato, Japan: Kumamato University; 1968
2. Ozuah PO. Folk use of elemental mercury: a potential hazard for children? *J Natl Med Assoc.* 2001;93:320–322
3. Zayas LH, Ozuah PO. Mercury use in espiritismo: a survey of botanicas. *Am J Public Health.* 1996;86:111–112
4. Bakir F, Damluji SF, Amin-Zaki L, et al. Methylmercury poisoning in Iraq. *Science.* 1973;181:230–241
5. Clarkson TW. The pharmacology of mercury compounds. *Annu Rev Pharmacol.* 1972;12:375–406
6. American Academy of Pediatrics Committee on Infectious Diseases, Committee on Environmental Health. Thimerosal in vaccines—an interim report to clinicians. *Pediatrics.* 1999;104:570–574
7. American Academy of Family Physicians, American Academy of Pediatrics, Advisory Committee on Immunization Practices, Public Health Service. Summary of the joint statement on thimerosal in vaccines. *MMWR Morb Mortal Wkly Rep.* 2000;49:622, 631
8. Jaffe KM, Shurtleff DB, Robertson WO. Survival after acute mercury vapor poisoning. *Am J Dis Child.* 1983;137:749–751
9. Kanluen S, Gottlieb CA. A clinical pathologic study of four adult cases of acute mercury inhalation toxicity. *Arch Pathol Lab Med.* 1991;115:56–60
10. Taueg C, Sanfilippo DJ, Rowens B, Szejda J, Hesse JL. Acute and chronic poisoning from residential exposures to elemental mercury—Michigan, 1989–1990. *J Toxicol Clin Toxicol.* 1992;30:63–67
11. Fawer RF, deRibaupierre Y, Guillemin MP, Berode M, Lob M. Measurement of hand tremor induced by industrial exposure to metallic mercury. *Br J Ind Med.* 1983;40:204–208
12. Smith PJ, Langolf GD, Goldberg J. Effect of occupational exposure to elemental mercury on short term memory. *Br J Ind Med.* 1983;40:413–419
13. Agner E, Jans H. Mercury poisoning and nephrotic syndrome in two young siblings. *Lancet.* 1978;2:951
14. Tubbs RR, Gephardt GN, McMahon JT, et al. Membranous glomerulonephritis associated with industrial mercury exposure. Study of pathogenetic mechanisms. *Am J Clin Pathol.* 1982;77:409–413
15. Mortensen ME. Mysticism and science: the amalgam wars. *J Toxicol Clin Toxicol.* 1991;29:vii–xii

16. Clarkson TW, Friberg L, Hursh JB, Nylander M. The prediction of intake of mercury vapor from amalgams. In: Clarkson TW, Friberg L, Nordberg GF, Sager PR, eds. *Biological Monitoring of Toxic Metals*. New York, NY: Plenum Press; 1988:247–264

17. Eley BM. The future of dental amalgam: a review of the literature. Part 4: mercury exposure hazards and risk assessment. *Br Dent J*. 1997;182:373–381

18. Eley BM. The future of dental amalgam: a review of the literature. Part 6: possible harmful effects of mercury from dental amalgam. *Br Dent J*. 1997;182:455–459

19. Weiner JA, Nylander M, Berglund F. Does mercury from amalgam restorations constitute a health hazard? *Sci Total Environ*. 1990;99:1–22

20. Cheek DB. Acrodynia. In: Kelley V, ed. *Brenneman's Practice of Pediatrics*. Vol I. New York, NY: Harper and Row Publishers; 1977;17D:1–12

21. Warkany J. Acrodynia—postmortem of a disease. *Am J Dis Child*. 1966;112:147–156

22. Gotelli CA, Astolfi E, Cox C, Cernichiari E, Clarkson TW. Early biochemical effects of an organic mercury fungicide on infants: "dose makes the poison." *Science*. 1985;227:638–640

23. Agocs MM, Etzel RA, Parrish RG, et al. Mercury exposure from interior latex paint. *N Engl J Med*. 1990;323:1096–1101

24. Amin-Zaki L, Majeed MA, Elhassani SB, Clarkson TW, Greenwood MR, Doherty RA. Prenatal methylmercury poisoning. Clinical observations over five years. *Am J Dis Child*. 1979;133:172–177

25. Grandjean P, Weihe P, White RF, et al. Cognitive deficit in 7-year-old children with prenatal exposure to methylmercury. *Neurotoxicol Teratol*. 1997;19:417–428

26. Davidson PW, Myers GJ, Cox C, et al. Effects of prenatal and postnatal methylmercury exposure from fish consumption on neurodevelopment: outcomes at 66 months of age in the Seychelles Child Development Study. *JAMA*. 1998;280:701–707

27. National Academy of Sciences. *Methylmercury, Toxicological Effects of Methylmercury*. Washington, DC: National Academies Press; 2000

28. Axton JH. Six cases of poisoning after a parenteral organic mercurial compound (Merthiolate). *Postgrad Med J*. 1972;48:417–421

29. Fagan DG, Pritchard JS, Clarkson TW, Greenwood MR. Organ mercury levels in infants with omphaloceles treated with organic mercurial antiseptic. *Arch Dis Child*. 1977;52:962–964

30. Lowell JA, Burgess S, Shenoy S, Peters M, Howard TK. Mercury poisoning associated with hepatitis-B immunoglobulin. *Lancet.* 1996;347:480

31. Matheson DS, Clarkson TW, Gelfand EW. Mercury toxicity (acrodynia) induced by long-term injection of gammaglobulin. *J Pediatr.* 1980;97:153–155

32. Pfab R, Muckter H, Roider G, Zilker T. Clinical course of severe poisoning with thiomersal. *J Toxicol Clin Toxicol.* 1996;34:453–460

33. Rohyans J, Walson PD, Wood GA, MacDonald WA. Mercury toxicity following Merthiolate ear irrigations. *J Pediatr.* 1984;104:311–313

34. Stratton K, Gable A, McCormick MC, eds. *Immunization Safety Review: Thiomersal-Containing Vaccines and Neurodevelopmental Disorders.* Washington, DC: National Academies Press, 2001

35. Schober SA, Sinks TH, Jones RL, et al. Blood mercury levels in US children and women of childbearing age, 1999–2000. *JAMA.* 2003;289:1667–1674

36. Dickman MD, Leung CK, Leong MK. Hong Kong male subfertility links to mercury in human hair and fish. *Sci Total Environ.* 1998;214:165–174

37. Batista J, Schuhmacher M, Domingo JL, Corbella J. Mercury in hair for a child population from Tarragona Province, Spain. *Sci Total Environ.* 1996;193:143–148

38. Saeki K, Fujimoto M, Kolinjim D, Taksukawa R. Mercury concentrations in hair from populations in Wau-Bulolo area, Papua, New Guinea. *Arch Environ Contam Toxicol.* 1996;30:412–417

39. Katz SA, Katz RB. Use of hair analysis for evaluating mercury intoxication of the human body: a review. *J Appl Toxicol.* 1992;12:79–84

40. Garza-Ocanas L, Torres-Alanis O, Pineyro-Lopez A. Urinary mercury in twelve cases of cutaneous mercurous chloride (calomel) exposure: effect of sodium 2,3-dimercaptopropane-1-sulfate (DMPS) therapy. *J Toxicol Clin Toxicol.* 1997;35:653–655

41. Hohage H, Otte B, Westermann G, et al. Elemental mercurial poisoning. *South Med J.* 1997;90:1033–1036

42. Gonzalez-Ramirez D, Zuniga-Charles M, Narro-Juarez A, et al. DMPS (2,3-dimercaptopropane-1-sulfonate, dimaval) decreases the body burden of mercury in humans exposed to mercurous chloride. *J Pharmacol Exp Ther.* 1998;287:8–12

43. Agency for Toxic Substances and Disease Registry. Mercury toxicity. *Am Fam Physician.* 1992;46:1731–1741

44. Bates BA. Mercury. In: Haddad LM, Shannon MW, Winchester JF, eds. *Clinical Management of Poisoning and Drug Overdose.* 3rd ed. Philadelphia, PA: WB Saunders; 1998:750–756

45. Ballatori N, Lieberman MW, Wang W. N-acetylcysteine as an antidote in methylmercury poisoning. *Environ Health Perspect.* 1998;106:267–271

46. Goldman LR, Shannon MW, American Academy of Pediatrics Committee on Environmental Health. Technical report: mercury in the environment: implications for pediatricians. *Pediatrics.* 2001;108:197–205

47. Bonhomme C, Gladyszacak-Kholer J, Cadou A, Ilef D, Kadi Z. Mercury poisoning by vacuum-cleaner aerosol. *Lancet.* 1996;347:115

48. Center for Food Safety and Applied Nutrition, US Food and Drug Administration. An important message for pregnant women and women of childbearing age who may become pregnant about the risks of mercury in fish. Washington, DC: US Food and Drug Administration; 2001. Available at: http://vm.cfsan.fda.gov/~dms/admehg.html

49. Agency for Toxic Substances and Disease Registry. *Preliminary Health Assessment, Olin Chemical Co, Charleston, TN.* Atlanta, GA: Agency for Toxic Substances and Disease Registry; 1988

# 21
# Nickel, Manganese, and Chromium

## Chromium

Chromium (Cr), a lightweight metal, is the sixth most abundant element in the earth's crust. As an essential human nutrient, it serves as a cofactor for insulin action[1]; dietary supplements often include large amounts of chromium. However, its greatest use has been in industry, where it played a key role for more than 100 years. Chromium is considered a high production volume chemical, being made or imported in amounts exceeding 1 million pounds annually. There is no significant mining of chromium in the United States; American use relies totally on its importation.[1] Extremely versatile, chromium is added to pigments; the distinctive yellow paint of traffic markings is a lead chromate pigment.[2] Other industrial uses include glassware cleaning, metal surface plating, leather tanning, and textile production.[3] Chromium's powerful anticorrosive/antirust properties are widely exploited in energy plants and other industry sites where activity involves regular contact between metals and water.

The toxicity of chromium is dependent on its valence state. The 3 most common forms are metallic ($Cr^0$), trivalent ($Cr^{+3}$), and hexavalent ($Cr^{+6}$). Elemental chromium does not exist naturally and has little industrial use. Nutritional chromium is the trivalent form. Hexavalent chromium, the species used in industry, is extremely toxic.

### Routes of Exposure

Chromium can be ingested, inhaled, and absorbed through the skin. Hexavalent chromium crosses the placenta and passes into breast milk.

### Sources of Exposure

Chromium is naturally found in many foods and beverages (eg, green beans, broccoli, seafood, and high-bran breakfast cereals). The estimated daily intake of dietary chromium is 50 to 100 μg. The recommended daily allowance is 50 to 200 μg (20–60 μg in infants).[1] Chromium deficiency is associated with a syndrome of elevated insulin concentration, hyperglycemia, and reduced fertility.[1]

Chromium enters the soil, air, and water primarily as a result of industry emissions of the trivalent and hexavalent forms. Typical concentrations of chromium in soil are 400 ppm[2] but can range from 1 to 2000 ppm.[1] Because of its widespread use, chromium is a contaminant at more than half of all National Priorities List Superfund hazardous waste sites as well as in many landfills.[2] In the air chromium is found as fine dust particles, which can settle in soil and water.[2] Most atmospheric chromium results from fossil fuel combustion and steel production.[1] Estimated chromium concentrations in the atmosphere are 0.01 μg/m[3] in rural areas and 0.01 to 0.03 μg/m[3] in urban areas.[2] Chromium contamination of water can be extensive. In water chromium can move as a "bloom" to areas distant from the original site of contamination.[2] Typical concentrations of chromium in tap water are 0.4 to 8.0 ppb (μg/L), while those in rivers and lakes typically fall between 1 and 30 ppb.[1,2] In the infamous Pacific Gas and Electric Company mass exposure (popularized by the movie *Erin Brockovich*), concentrations of hexavalent chromium in water were 580 ppb, far in excess of the state limit of 50 ppb.[2]

Childhood exposure to hexavalent chromium most commonly occurs via ingestion of contaminated water or play near a hazardous waste site.[4] Chromium-laden dust also can be found in house dust in areas where there is significant local contamination. Adults who work in industries using chromium can bring significant amounts of it, along with other hazardous materials, into the home.

### *Biological Fate*
After exposure, the absorption of chromium is dependent on the route of exposure and the form of the element. After inhalation, elemental and trivalent chromium are poorly absorbed; in contrast the hexava-

lent form, being more water soluble, is well absorbed from the lungs. After ingestion trivalent chromium salts are poorly absorbed (<2%); in contrast, up to 50% of the hexavalent form can be absorbed from the gastrointestinal tract. However, a significant proportion of ingested hexavalent chromium is converted to the less soluble trivalent form in the gut, considerably limiting its absorption. After dermal contact, hexavalent chromium is well absorbed through intact skin while elemental and trivalent forms are not.[3]

Hexavalent chromium is transported across the placenta and into breast milk. Chromium is stored in all body tissues, although retention does not seem to be prolonged; the kidneys excrete approximately 60% of a chromium dose within 8 hours of ingestion.[1] An estimated 80% of chromium is excreted by the kidneys; bile and sweat are minor routes of excretion.

### Systems Affected

Acute exposure to chromium may affect several organ systems including the skin, gastrointestinal tract, kidneys, and lungs. Hexavalent chromium is a carcinogen.

### Clinical Effects

#### Acute and Short-term Effects

Hexavalent chromium is the most toxic of the 3 forms, having immediate and long-term effects after exposure. Even short-term skin exposure can result in significant irritation as well as sensitization, producing allergic contact dermatitis with subsequent exposures. Chromium is considered second only to nickel in being the most allergenic metal to which humans are regularly exposed.[2] Once found in significant concentration in detergents and bleaches, chromium was thought to be the cause of the once common "housewives' eczema."[3] "Blackjack disease" was a term describing the eczematous dermatitis found in card players exposed to chromium in felt. Ingestion of high-dose hexavalent chromium produces gastrointestinal upset (nausea, vomiting, hematemesis), which can be severe. Large ingestions can produce acute renal failure. High-dose inhalation can produce acute pneumonitis. Other acute toxicities include effects on the nasal mucosa, with the appearance of runny nose, sneezing, nosebleeds, and, with repeated exposures, nasal septum ulcers.[2]

## Chronic/Long-term Effects

Chronic inhalation of hexavalent chromium is associated with an increased risk of lung cancer among adults.[3] First noted in the 1920s, a number of studies have shown that those who work in industries using chromium have elevated rates of lung and nasal cancer.[2] The International Agency for Research on Cancer, the US National Toxicology Program, the World Health Organization, and the US Environmental Protection Agency (EPA) have all concluded that hexavalent chromium is a human carcinogen.[4] The risk of lung cancer increases with duration of exposure, having a latency ranging from 13 to 30 years (although cases have appeared following as few as 5 years of exposure).[1] Observed declines in the incidence of cancer as exposures fall among chromium workers suggest a threshold effect for the carcinogenic potential of hexavalent chromium.[1] Carcinogenicity has not been observed from exposure to metallic or trivalent chromium salts.

While there is evidence suggesting that hexavalent chromium increases the risk of other cancers among adults (cancers of bone, stomach, and prostate; lymphoma and leukemia), there are insufficient data to confirm this.

Hexavalent chromium has a number of other toxicities. Low birth weight, birth defects, and other reproductive toxicities have been observed in experimental models of chronic hexavalent chromium exposure.[2] In animal models exposure to chromium significantly disturbs spermatogenesis.[1]

Type IV hypersensitivity skin reactions with contact dermatitis or frank eczema are common consequences of long-term dermal exposure. For example, chromium sensitivity occurs in as many as 8% to

9% of cement workers; among workers exposed to chromium in the automotive repair industry, sensitivity has been reported in as many as 24%.[1] Finally, chronic inhalational exposure to chromium can produce chronic lung disease (pneumoconiosis).

### Diagnosis

Chromium can be measured in serum or urine. Normal concentrations in serum have been reported as 0.052 to 0.156 µg/L. Because only hexavalent chromium penetrates erythrocytes, red cell chromium may be a better indicator of exposure to that particular form rather than serum chromium, which reflects exposure to all species.[1] Urine measurement of chromium generally reflects absorption over the previous 1 to 3 days; the typical range of concentration in urine is 0 to 40 µg/L. Chromium also can be measured in hair, although reference values are not available. Samples of breast milk may have an average concentration of 0.3 ppb chromium. Because of species interconversion, no biological specimen has sufficient sensitivity to identify exposure to one particular form (eg, hexavalent).[2] Diagnosis therefore relies largely on historical evidence and environmental documentation of exposure, supplemented by biological monitoring.

### Treatment

There are no known chelators of chromium. However, given its rapid and apparently complete elimination, chelation should not be needed. Ascorbic acid (vitamin C) is considered a valuable treatment after hexavalent chromium ingestions because of its ability to reduce hexavalent to less soluble trivalent chromium.

### Prevention of Exposure

Exposure to chromium can be prevented by fencing hazardous land sites and prohibiting children from playing in soils near sites where chromium may have been discarded. Because of possible chromium contamination of well water, specific analysis for chromium in well drinking water should be considered before that water is consumed.

The EPA has set a limit of 100 ppb total chromium (not hexavalent specifically) in water. Chromium concentrations in air are not regulated, although control measures are being enacted; environmental rules that help to reduce exposure from ambient atmospheric pollution are needed.

Ingestions of chromium also should be minimized. Reference (maximum recommended) doses for chromium are 1 mg/kg per day for the trivalent chromium and 5 µg/kg per day for hexavalent chromium.[1] Finally, although trivalent chromium is an essential nutrient, there is concern about the extent of human in situ conversion to the hexavalent form; therefore, excess daily doses from dietary supplements should be avoided,[4] particularly in children.

## Manganese

Taking its name from a Greek word for magic, manganese (Mn) is ubiquitous in the environment, making up approximately 0.1% of the earth's crust.[5] Like chromium, it is a metal used for its light weight and durability. A very hard and brittle metal, manganese is a valuable constituent of steel alloys.[5,6] Uses of inorganic manganese include battery production, as a catalyst for the chlorination of organic compounds; glass and ceramics production; incendiaries; and fungicides. Permanganates (manganese oxides) are used as disinfectants and in metal cleaning, bleaching, flower preservation, and photography. Organic manganese compounds are used as gasoline and fuel oil additives and as fungicides.

Manganese is an essential human nutrient. It is a cofactor for the enzymes hexokinase, superoxide dismutase, and xanthine oxidase. Additionally, there are several metalloenzymes that require manganese, including pyruvate carboxylase, arginase, and the neuron-specific enzyme glutamine synthetase.[7]

Manganese is present in the environment in inorganic and organic forms. Of the inorganic forms there are 7 species, ranging in valence from 0 to 7+; heptavalent manganese includes the permanganates, which are potent oxidizing agents. The primary organomanganese compound is methylcyclopentadienyl manganese tricarbonyl (MMT), an antiknock gasoline additive.

### Routes of Exposure

Manganese can be ingested and inhaled.

### Sources of Exposure

Foods and beverages are significant sources of manganese, providing daily intakes ranging from 2 to 9 mg. Dietary intake is much higher among vegetarians, approaching 20 mg daily.[5] Foods high in manganese include whole barley, rye, and wheat; pecans; almonds; and leafy green vegetables. The highest amounts are found in nuts. Tea is a high-source beverage. Soy-based infant formula can contain up to 200 times more manganese than breast milk.[8] Dietary supplements and alternative medicines also can contain significant amounts of manganese; cases of manganese toxicity from the use of a Chinese herbal remedy have been reported.[9]

Major sources of non-dietary manganese exposure to children result from its pollution of air, water, and soil.[6] Typical manganese concentrations in ambient (outdoor) air range from 0.01 to 0.07 µg/cubic meter.[5] Sources of atmospheric manganese include the combustion of fossil fuels (20%) and emissions from industry (80%).

Methylcyclopentadienyl manganese tricarbonyl (25.2% manganese) was introduced into gasoline in the 1970s, replacing lead as an antiknock compound. It was added to reduce carbon monoxide emissions from auto exhausts by boosting octane rating and was present in more than 40% of gasoline sold in the United States until its use was drastically curtailed in 1978 by the Clean Air Act. Despite EPA efforts to prohibit its use until additional safety data were available, in 1995 a court decision allowed the re-introduction of MMT (although some states [eg, California] have specifically banned MMT). However, there have been persistent concerns about the value of the compound, both because it increases hydrocarbon emissions and because of its potential to significantly increase human exposure to manganese.[10] According to a risk analysis by the EPA, if all gasoline contained MMT in a concentration of 30 to 35 mg/gal, a significant segment of the population would be exposed to quantities that exceed the current ambient air reference concentration of 0.05 µg/cubic meter.[5] Methylcyclopentadienyl manganese tricarbonyl has been a fuel additive in Canada since 1976. In the United States, recent data indicate that less than 0.05% of gasoline manufacturers are currently using MMT. The American Automo-bile Manufacturer's Association has advised consumers not to use MMT because it may damage automobile combustion systems.[11] The manganese emitted from MMT combustion is in the form of inorganic phosphate and sulfate salts.[7]

Another potential source of excess manganese exposure is water contamination. Freshwater typically contains manganese in a range of 1 to 200 µg/L. Well water contamination (natural and anthropogenic) is relatively common, with concentrations as much as an order of magnitude greater (up to 2000 µg/L).

Soil can have high concentrations of manganese, naturally and from surface pollution. Concentrations of manganese in soil average 40 to 900 ppm (milligrams per kilogram) with an average of 330 ppm; concentrations near industry can approach 7000 ppm.[5] In a pattern similar to that observed when lead was added to gasoline, the concentration of manganese in soil decreases with the distance from heavily traveled roads.[12]

### Biological Fate

Manganese absorption from the gut is highly regulated via homeostatic mechanisms. Iron and manganese share the same mucosal transport system. Average absorption of dietary manganese averages 3% to 5%.[5] Children have less well developed homeostatic mechanisms for regulating manganese absorption and elimination. Iron deficiency and low protein intake are associated with increased oral manganese absorption while high dietary calcium or phosphate decrease its absorption. There also seems to be extensive genetic modulation of manganese absorption from the gut, mediated by the highly prevalent hemochromatosis gene. Women typically absorb more manganese than men, presumably because of their lower iron stores. Once absorbed, manganese is transported by plasma proteins (including the β-1 globulin transmanganin)[13] and within the erythrocyte. The plasma protein transferrin also is important in manganese transport. Excretion of manganese is primarily biliary; renal excretion of the metal is negligible. Its biological half-life is approximately 40 days. Animal data suggest that the elimination of manganese from the central nervous system (CNS) is slower than in other tissues.

Manganese is transmitted across the placenta and in breast milk. Infant formulas contain significantly more manganese than breast milk.

Unlike ingested manganese, inhaled manganese is completely absorbed; through this route it can be transported directly to the CNS without hepatic first-pass clearance.[10]

### Systems Affected

Acute exposure to manganese can affect the lungs and skin. Chronic exposure may result in neurotoxicity, pulmonary disease, and reproductive toxicity.

### Clinical Effects

#### Acute Effects

Acute exposure to manganese oxides can produce a syndrome known as metal fume fever or manganese pneumonitis.[6] This syndrome includes flulike complaints such as fever, cough, congestion, and malaise. This illness most commonly occurs in the industrial setting with processes such as welding or metal cutting. Permanganate solutions can be extremely corrosive. Another significant consequence of acute manganese poisoning is hepatic injury.[5] There is no reported acute CNS toxicity from manganese; CNS symptoms require long-term exposure.

Chronic/Long-term Effects

Central nervous system effects of manganese were first described in the 1800s where the term "manganese madness" was first coined.[5] Initial symptoms of manganese toxicity are psychiatric, characterized by emotional lability, hallucinations, asthenia, irritability, and insomnia. Chronic manganese intoxication (manganism) is best known for inducing neurological injury that mimics Parkinson disease, with masklike facies, cogwheel rigidity, tremor, and clumsiness. This syndrome typically appears after 2 to 25 years of excess manganese exposure but also has been observed within several months of heavy exposure.[5] Manganese-induced neurotoxicity can be progressive, worsening after exposure has ended.[5] The cellular mechanism of neurotoxicity is unclear. Manganese can displace iron from transferrin; the neurotoxicity of manganese may therefore be related to increases in iron-induced oxidative injury to neurons.[14] Experimental models in animals suggest that neonates have greater transport of manganese into the CNS, a lower threshold for manganese-induced neurotoxicity, and greater retention of manganese in the brain compared with older animals.[7] Iron deficiency is associated with increased CNS concentrations of manganese. Therefore, infants, children, and menstruating women are at greater risk of manganese neurotoxicity. Iron excess also increases the risk of manganese neurotoxicity. Pathologic changes include deterioration of the globus pallidus and corpus striatum as well as decreased activity of catecholamines (particularly dopamine) and serotonin in the corpus striatum.[13] Interestingly, unlike Parkinson disease, manganese toxicity is associated with preservation of nigro-striatal dopaminergic pathways.[7] Although manganese-induced neurotoxicity is most commonly found after chronic inhalation, ingestion of manganese-contaminated water also has been associated with neurotoxicity. Cohort studies in which contaminated well water (containing 0.08–14 mg/L) was ingested have reported the appearance of neurodevelopmental injury.[13] In one pediatric study, long-term manganese exposure in drinking water was associated with poor school performance and decrements in neurobehavioral performance.[15] In animal models, prenatal exposure to manganese also is associated with significant neurotoxicity among the progeny.

Chronic inhalation of manganese dust can lead to pulmonary disease, manifested by chronic respiratory tract inflammation.[6]

Male reproductive toxicities also can occur with chronic manganese exposure. Decreased spermatogenesis occurs in animal models; epidemiological studies have shown a significant decrease in the number of children born to workers exposed to manganese dust.[16] Birth defects, including stillbirth, cleft lip, imperforate anus, cardiac defects, and deafness, have been reported in populations chronically exposed to excessive manganese.[6]

### Diagnosis

Biological monitoring for manganese exposure includes blood and urine. The reference range for manganese in whole blood is 4 to 15 µg/L in adults.[5,6] Because manganese is bound to red blood cells, serum manganese concentrations are much lower, averaging 0.9 to 2.9 µg/L. Blood concentrations reflect recent exposure and cannot be used to identify past manganese exposures. Urinary measurements similarly do not reflect past exposure to manganese. Normal urinary manganese concentrations are less than 10 µg/L. According to the third National Health and Nutrition Examination Survey, the 95th percentile for urinary manganese was 3.33 µg/L.[5] Manganese also can be measured in hair; however, hair concentrations do not correlate with degree of exposure or symptoms.[13] When breast milk has been measured, concentrations average 7 to 120 µg/L.[13]

### Treatment

Treatment of excess manganese exposure may include chelation therapy. $CaNa_2EDTA$ increases urinary excretion and may provide clinical improvement in select cases of severe manganese intoxication.

## *Prevention of Exposure*

Prevention of manganese exposure includes environmental actions to reduce ambient pollution and close monitoring of water supplies, particularly well water. The EPA has calculated a reference ambient air concentration of manganese, based on changes in neuropsychological function, to equal 0.05 µg/cubic meter.[5] The current EPA limit for manganese in water is 50 µg/L; all efforts should be made to ensure that drinking water remains below this concentration. Recommended daily intakes from diet include an EPA reference dose of 0.14 mg/kg per day, based on the risk of the appearance of neurobehavioral toxicity. The National Research Council's recommended daily allowance for manganese is 0.3 to 1.0 mg/day for children up to 1 year, 1 to 2 mg/day for children up to 10 years, and 2 to 5 mg/day for all those older than 10 years. These allowances should not be exceeded.[10] Finally, with other means of increasing the octane rating of gasolines, use of MMT in gasoline should be severely limited or prohibited.

## Nickel

Nickel (Ni) is a white magnetic metal commonly used in alloys with copper, chromium, iron, and zinc. These alloys are used in fuel production, making jewelry, clothing fasteners, metallic coins, domestic utensils, medical prostheses, heat exchangers, valves, and magnets.

Nickel salts are used in electroplating, pigments, ceramics, batteries, and as a catalyst in food production. Nickel compounds are present in environmental tobacco smoke (ETS), especially nickel carbonyl ($Ni[CO]_4$), which is a potent carcinogen.

Nickel occurs naturally in the earth's crust and may be emitted from volcanoes and in rock dust. It is a natural constituent of soil and is transported in streams and waterways.[17,18] Nickel has been reported in Montreal snow at 200 to 300 ppb.[19]

Anthropogenic emissions include industrial sources from mining and recycling, steel production, and municipal incineration. Power plants fueled by peat, coal, natural gas, and oil are sources of nickel compound emissions. Nickel accumulates along roadways from abrasion of metal parts of vehicles and the use of gasoline containing nickel. Industrial waste has been disposed of by land spreading, land filling, ocean dumping, and incineration. Emissions by aerosols can be transported far from the source.[20]

### Routes of Exposure
Nickel can enter the body through inhalation, ingestion, or the skin.

### Sources of Exposure
Children are exposed to nickel through air, especially when it contains ETS. They are exposed through food, possibly through drinking water, and by dermal absorption. There is a potential for iatrogenic exposure through dialysis and through dental and surgical prostheses.[18] Nickel has been found to leach from stainless steel cookware, especially in mildly acidic conditions at boiling temperatures.[21]

Natural food sources of nickel include cocoa, nuts, soybean, and oatmeal. Oysters and salmon may accumulate high levels when fished from water with increased concentrations of nickel. Nickel may be present in higher concentrations in certain vegetables such as peas, beans, cabbage, spinach, and lettuce. Certain plants and bacteria have been found to carry nickel-containing enzymes. Nickel, however, has not been shown to be an essential nutrient in humans.[17] Nickel deficiency has been induced in rats, chicks, cows, and goats. Decreasing growth has been noted in these animals as has abnormal morphology and oxidative metabolisms in the liver. Nickel may act as a bioligand cofactor facilitating the gastrointestinal absorption of ferric irons.[22]

### Biological Fate
After nickel enters the body, soluble ions of nickel may be absorbed directly while insoluble compounds may be phagocytosed. Nickel bisulfide ($Ni_3S_2$) and nickel oxide (NiO) are relatively insoluble; however, they play an important role in carcinogenesis when phagocytosed

by cells lining the respiratory tract. Soluble nickel compounds may be absorbed through the gastrointestinal tract from water and food, however, a large percentage of this nickel will be excreted in feces. Soluble nickel that enters the bloodstream may accumulate in the kidneys and be excreted in the urine.[17,18] Nickel may be dermally absorbed by direct contact. Nickel sensitization frequently follows ear piercing when a nickel-containing pin is placed in the wound channel until epithelialization occurs.[23]

### Clinical Effects

Workers in nickel refinery and processing industries exposed by inhalation have a higher incidence of respiratory cancers of the lung, larynx, and nasopharyngeal passages.[24] Occupational nickel carbonyl inhalation in workers has been described as causing adrenal, hepatic, and renal damage leading to death. Inhaled nickel sulfate has been known to cause asthma.[25] Occupational exposure is associated with a higher incidence of spontaneous abortions, congenital structural malformations,[26] and chromosomal aberrations.[27]

The most common adverse health effect in children from nickel is the development of allergies. Nickel is one of the most common causes of contact dermatitis from jewelry, white gold, wrist watches, metal clothing fasteners, and dental prostheses. A nickel allergy may be induced by ear piercing. Nickel dermatitis has been described in infants.[28]

A 2-year-old child who accidentally ingested nickel sulfate ($NiSO_4$) crystals (570 mg of nickel per kilogram) died from cardiac arrest 8 hours after exposure.[17]

### Diagnosis

A urine sample from an acute exposure with a concentration of 5 µg/dL is considered at the upper limits of normal. Acute poisoning is diagnosed at higher levels.

## Treatment

Acute toxicity may be treated with chelating agents especially diethyl-dithiocarbamate (DDC). Disulphiram, which is metabolized to DDC, also may be effective. Penicillamine also has been used in treating acute toxic effects of nickel compounds.[1]

## Regulations

The EPA has designated nickel and its compounds as toxic pollutants. The EPA health advisories for children's water intake are 1.0 mg/L (1-day intake), 1.0 mg/L (10-day intake), and 0.5 mg/L (longer term).

The World Health Organization has classified nickel compounds as group I carcinogens (human carcinogens) and metallic nickel as group IIB carcinogens (possible human carcinogens).[17]

The European Union in 1996 announced a directive to restrict the use of nickel to reduce the prevalence of nickel allergy. The directive prohibits the use of nickel in jewelry, especially earrings, for pierced ears, wristwatches, and clothing that may be in direct contact with the skin for prolonged periods.[29]

## Prevention of Exposure

Because of the high incidence of nickel dermatitis and implications in sensitization to nickel, it would be prudent to warn the public of its widespread use in jewelry and clothes fasteners and alert people with sensitivity to avoid direct prolonged contact on the skin. Avoidance of nickel-containing stainless steel cookware by nickel-sensitive individuals would likewise be prudent in reducing sensitization of atopic individuals.

## Frequently Asked Question

Q  *Should I worry about the nickel in coins, cookware, jewelry, and clothes fasteners? Are these potential sources of carcinogenicity for my child?*

A  Metallic nickel has not been shown to produce cancer in children. Contact with metallic nickel can cause allergic dermatitis generally if the metal is in contact with the skin for prolonged periods. Workers in nickel refineries who inhaled large quantities of nickel salts were found to have a higher risk of cancers of the nasopharynx and lungs. Children are generally not exposed to these sorts of levels from ambient nickel sources.

## References

1. Barceloux DG. Chromium. *J Toxicol Clin Toxicol.* 1999;37:173–194
2. Pellerin C, Booker SM. Reflections on hexavalent chromium: health hazards of an industrial heavyweight. *Environ Health Perspect.* 2000;108:A402–A407
3. Geller RJ. Chromium. In: Sullivan JB, Krieger GR, eds. *Hazardous Materials Toxicology—Clinical Principles of Environmental Health.* Baltimore, MD: Williams & Wilkins; 1992:891–895
4. Agency for Toxic Substances and Disease Registry. *Toxicological Profile for Chromium.* Washington, DC: US Department of Health and Human Services, Public Health Service; 2001
5. Barceloux DG. Manganese. *J Toxicol Clin Toxicol.* 1999;37:293–307
6. Agency for Toxic Substances and Disease Registry. *Toxicological Profile for Manganese.* Washington, DC: US Department of Health and Human Services, Public Health Service; 2000
7. Aschner M. Manganese: brain transport and emerging research needs. *Environ Health Perspect.* 2000;108(suppl 3):429–432
8. Goodman D. How safe is soy infant formula? *Mercola.com Newsletter.* 2001. Available at: http://www.mercola.com/2001/jun/13/soy_formula.htm
9. Pal PK, Samii A, Calne DB. Manganese neurotoxicity: a review of clinical features, imaging and pathology. *Neurotoxicology.* 1999;20:227–238
10. Davis JM. Methylcyclopentadienyl manganese tricarbonyl: health risk uncertainties and research directions. *Environ Health Perspect.* 1998;106(suppl 1):191–201

11. McKinsey K. Running on MMT? *Sci Am.* June 1998

12. McMillan DE. A brief history of the neurobehavioral toxicity of manganese: some unanswered questions. *Neurotoxicology.* 1999;20:499–507

13. Gilmore DA, Bronstein AC. Manganese and magnesium. In: Sullivan JB, Krieger GR, eds. *Hazardous Materials Toxicology—Clinical Principles of Environmental Health.* Baltimore, MD: Williams & Wilkins; 1992:896–902

14. Verity MA. Manganese neurotoxicity: a mechanistic hypothesis. *Neurotoxicology.* 1999;20:489–497

15. Zhang G, Liu D, He P. Effects of manganese on learning abilities in school children. *Zhonghua Yu Fang Yi Xue Za Zhi.* 1995;29:156–158

16. Lauwerys R, Roels H, Genet P, Toussaint G, Bouckaert A, De Cooman S. Fertility of male workers exposed to mercury vapor or to manganese dust: a questionnaire study. *Am J Ind Med.* 1985;7:171–176

17. Agency for Toxic Substances and Disease Registry. *Toxicological Profile for Nickel (update).* Washington, DC: US Department of Health and Human Services, Public Health Service; 1997

18. Snow ET, Costa M. Nickel toxicity and carcinogenesis. In: Rom WN, ed. *Environmental and Occupational Medicine.* 3rd ed. Philadelphia, PA: Lippincott-Raven Publishers; 1998:1057–1062

19. Landsberger S, Jervis RE, Kajrys G, Monaro S. Characterization of trace elemental pollutants in urban snow using proton induced x-ray emission and instrumental neutron activation analysis. *Intern J Environ Anal Chem.* 1983;16:95–130

20. Bennett BG. 1984. Environmental nickel pathways in man. In: Sunderman FW Jr, ed. *Nickel in the Human Environment. Proceedings of a Joint Symposium.* Lyon, France: International Agency for Research on Cancer; March 8–11, 1983:487–495. IARC scientific publication no. 53

21. Kuligowski J, Halperin KM. Stainless steel cookware as a significant source of nickel, chromium, and iron. *Arch Environ Contam Toxicol.* 1992;23:211–215

22. Nielsen FH, Shuler TR, McLeod TG, Zimmerman TJ. Nickel influences iron metabolism through physiologic, pharmacologic and toxicologic mechanisms in the rat. *J Nutr.* 1984;114:1280–1288

23. Larsson-Stymne B, Widstrom L. Ear piercing—cause of nickel allergy in schoolgirls? *Contact Dermatitis.* 1985;13:289–293

24. Goldberg M, Goldberg P, Leclerc A, et al. Epidemiology of respiratory cancers related to nickel mining and refining in New Caledonia (1978–1984). *Int J Cancer.* 1987;40:300–304

25. McConnell LH, Fink JN, Schleuter DP, Schmidt MG Jr. Asthma caused by nickel sensitivity. *Ann Intern Med.* 1973;78:888–890

26. Chashschin VP, Artunina GP, Norseth T. Congenital defects, abortion and other health effects in nickel refinery workers. *Sci Total Environ.* 1994;148:287–291

27. Elias Z, Mur JM, Pierre F, et al. Chromosome aberrations in peripheral blood lymphocytes of welders and characterization of their exposure by biological samples analysis. *J Occup Med.* 1989;31:477–483

28. Ho VC, Johnston MM. Nickel dermatitis in infants. *Contact Dermatitis.* 1986;15:270–273

29. Delescluse J, Dinet Y. Nickel allergy in Europe: the new European legislation. *Dermatology.* 1994;189(suppl 2):56–57

# 22
# Nitrates and Nitrites in Water

Nitrogen, an essential nutrient, is absorbed and incorporated by plants from nitrate or ammonium in soil. The use of nitrogen fertilizer for improved crop yields has generally increased in the United States and globally since the 1950s, peaking in the United States around 1990.[1] Nitrate contamination of water supplies is a serious environmental consequence of modern agricultural activity and increasing urbanization. Nitrate levels in shallow groundwater and some surface waters have increased due to use of nitrogen fertilizers, intensive livestock operations that produce large amounts of animal waste, substandard private septic systems, and municipal wastewater treatment discharges.[2] A recent US Geological Survey National Water Quality Assessment Program report documents elevated nitrate levels in 4 of 33 major aquifers sampled in rural and urban areas.[3] Poorly constructed shallow wells in rural areas are at greatest risk of nitrate contamination. In general, nitrite is not as prevalent in water supplies as nitrate because nitrite is rapidly converted to nitrate, depending on aerobic and bacterial conditions.[4]

High nitrate levels in water can potentially have adverse effects on ecology and public health. Nitrate and other nutrients have been linked to blue-green algal blooms, which can produce toxic bacteria that can negatively impact wildlife and humans.[5,6] Methemoglobinemia in infants may be caused by ingestion of water contaminated with nitrate.[7]

## Nitrate in US Water Supplies
The trend for US water supplies has been a general increase in nitrate levels. The US Environmental Protection Agency (EPA) drinking water standard (maximum contaminant level [MCL]) for public water supplies is 10 mg/L (10 ppm) for nitrate-nitrogen ($NO_3$-N) and 1 mg/L

(1 ppm) for nitrite.[8] The MCLs were set in response to concerns about methemoglobinemia in infants.[9] An EPA nationwide survey of drinking water wells from 1988 to 1990 reported that approximately 1.2% of community water wells and 2.4% of private wells exceeded the nitrate MCL.[10] It was estimated that about 1.5 million people, including 22 500 infants served by private wells, and another 3 million people, including 43 500 infants served by public community wells, were exposed to drinking water nitrate above the MCL.[11] The 1994 Midwest Well Water Survey collected water samples from 5500 domestic wells located in 9 states. Of those samples, 13.4% exceeded the nitrate MCL, with Kansas (24.6%) and Iowa (20.6%) having the highest proportion of samples with nitrate greater than 10 ppm.[12] Proximity to heavy agricultural activity may exacerbate the situation. A North Carolina study (1998) sampled 1600 wells in 15 counties where intensive livestock facilities were located. Of the wells tested, 10.2% had nitrate greater than 10 ppm.[13] In 2002 the Des Moines (IA) Water Works reported 15 to 17 ppm nitrate levels in the Raccoon River (a heavily agricultural watershed), the source of drinking water for more than 300 000 residents of the Des Moines metropolitan area.[14]

**Route and Sources of Exposure**

Ingestion is the route of exposure. Drinking water is the main source of nitrate in infants.[15] In breastfed infants, there is little or no evidence for increased risk of methemoglobinemia from maternal ingestion of nitrate-contaminated water.[16] It is uncertain whether transplacental transfer of nitrates occurs or whether breast milk transfers nitrates to infants.

**Clinical Effects**

Nitrate is rapidly absorbed from the proximal small intestine, and approximately 70% of ingested nitrate is found in urine within 24 hours.[17] Ordinarily, most ingested nitrate is metabolized and excreted unless conditions favor reduction to nitrite. Methemoglobinemia is the primary adverse effect in young infants exposed to nitrate-contaminated drinking water.[18] About 2000 cases of acquired methemoglobinemia were reported in North America and Europe between 1945 to 1971.[19] Recent US data are not easily accessible because only 9 environmental public health surveillance systems monitor for methemoglobinemia. In parts of Central and Eastern Europe, infant methemoglobinemia is a persistent public health problem (see Chapter 40).

While nitrate does not cause methemoglobinemia, it can be converted to nitrite by gut flora. In turn, nitrite converts ferrous (Fe$^{+2}$) iron in hemoglobin to ferric (Fe$^{+3}$) iron resulting in methemoglobin, which is incapable of carrying oxygen. Infants younger than 4 months who are fed formula reconstituted with well water containing nitrate are at the greatest risk for methemoglobinemia. The gastric pH of infants is higher than that in older children and adults, with resultant proliferation of intestinal bacteria that reduce ingested nitrate to more reactive nitrite.[7] Fetal hemoglobin (hemoglobin F), the predominant form in infants up to 3 months of age, is more readily oxidized to methemoglobin by nitrite than is adult hemoglobin (hemoglobin A). The system responsible for reduction of induced methemoglobin to normal ferrous hemoglobin has only about half the activity in infants as in adults.[20]

Methemoglobinemia generally presents with few clinical signs other than cyanosis. Methemoglobin is dark brown and results in obvious cyanosis at levels as low as 3%. Symptoms are generally minimal until methemoglobin levels exceed 20%. Usually cyanosis is manifest well before other symptoms appear unless exposure is intense. The mucous membranes of infants with methemoglobinemia-induced cyanosis tend to have a brownish (rather than blue) cast. The brown discoloration increases with the level of methemoglobin as does irritability, tachypnea, and altered mental status (and complaints of headache in older children). In the absence of respiratory symptoms, history of cardiovascular disease, abnormal pulse, or abnormal oximetry, a diagnosis of methemoglobinemia should be considered in a child who becomes acutely cyanotic and unresponsive to oxygen administration.

## Treatment of Methemoglobinemia

Health professionals who suspect that a child has methemoglobinemia are advised to consult with the local poison control center or a toxicologist to help guide management. An asymptomatic child with cyanosis who has a methemoglobin level of less than 20% usually requires no treatment other than identifying and eliminating the source of exposure. More information on diagnosis and treatment can be found elsewhere.[21,22]

## Prevention of Methemoglobinemia

Clinical treatment alone for methemoglobinemia is not sufficient. It is critical to identify and eliminate the sources of exposure. Assessment of potential nitrate exposure includes questions about family residence, occupation, drinking water, foods ingested, and use of topical medications or folk remedies. Prenatal and newborn care for patients with private wells should include a recommendation for testing well water for nitrate contamination. Water with elevated nitrate levels should not be ingested by infants or used in the preparation of infant formula. Boiling water prior to mixing formula, although a good measure for prevention of microbial contamination, is not a safe practice with nitrate-contaminated water because it will increase nitrate concentration. Boiling water for 1 minute is generally sufficient to kill microorganisms without overconcentrating nitrate. Alternative sources of water include deeper wells, public water supplies, or bottled water free of nitrate. Effective in-home systems for nitrate removal include ion exchange resins and reverse osmosis, which are available but expensive. Water testing for nitrate can be obtained from any reference or public health laboratory using approved EPA laboratory methods.

## Chronic Effects

Epidemiologic studies have reported increased risks for non-cancer health outcomes associated with exposure to elevated levels of nitrate in drinking water, including hyperthyroidism[23] and insulin-dependent diabetes.[24] Maternal transfer of nitrate and nitrite is suggested by a number of studies on reproductive outcomes tentatively linked to high nitrate levels in water supplies.[25-27] Anecdotal reports of spontaneous abortions in Indiana (1991–1993) describe a case study where 3 women experienced a total of 6 spontaneous abortions; the women resided in proximity to each other and consumed drinking water from private wells containing high levels of nitrate (19–26 ppm $NO_3$-N).[28]

Cancer risk from exposure to nitrate in drinking water also has been of interest to epidemiologists. Ingested nitrate can be reduced endogenously to nitrite through bacterial reactions in the saliva, and nitrite can be further reduced to N-nitroso compounds via reaction with amines and amides in the stomach, intestine, and bladder.[29,30] N-nitroso compounds are some of the strongest known carcinogens,[29] can act systemically,[30] and have been found to induce cancer in a variety of organs in more than 40 animal species including higher primates.[31] Most of the epidemiologic data on nitrate in drinking water and cancer risk are from ecologic studies looking at gastric cancer, for which the data are mixed.[32] Elevated risk of cancer of the esophagus, nasopharynx, bladder, prostate, and non-Hodgkin lymphoma also have been reported.[32,33] Case-control studies have reported mixed results for nitrate in drinking water and gastric cancer,[34-36] null results for brain cancer[37] and bladder cancer,[38] and a positive association for non-Hodgkin lymphoma.[39] Cohort studies have reported no association between nitrate in drinking water and gastric cancer,[40] positive associations for bladder and ovarian cancer,[41] and inverse associations for uterine and rectal cancer.[41]

## Frequently Asked Questions

Q *Do commercial treatment systems sufficiently protect against nitrate contamination?*

A Water softeners and charcoal filters do not significantly reduce nitrate concentrations. Reverse osmosis and ion exchange resins do remove nitrate, but are expensive.

Q *Is low-grade nitrate contamination a risk for cancer?*

A Published studies of exposure to nitrate in drinking water and cancer risk show conflicting results.

Q *Are the current MCLs sufficiently strict to protect the population?*

A Most of the population is protected from methemoglobinemia or other potential adverse effects of nitrate at current MCLs.[42] The EPA's drinking water standards for nitrate (10 ppm) and nitrite (1 ppm) are designed to protect the health even of persons who are considered most susceptible. These standards, however, only apply to public water supplies.

Q *Should I have my well water tested? How often?*

A Individuals with private wells should have them tested quarterly for at least 1 year to determine whether episodic elevations of nitrate or bacterial coliforms occur. If those levels are all acceptable, yearly follow-up is recommended.

## References

1. Brown LR, Renner M, Flavin C. *Vital Signs 1997: The Environmental Trends That Are Shaping Our Future.* New York, NY: WW Norton & Co; 1997
2. Nolan BT, Ruddy BC, Hitt KJ, Helsel DR. A national look at nitrate contamination of groundwater. *Water Conditioning and Purification.* 1998;40:76–79
3. US Geological Survey. *The Quality of Our Nation's Waters: Nutrients and Pesticides.* Reston, VA: US Department of the Interior, US Geological Survey; 1999. US Geological Survey Circular 1225
4. Mackerness CW, Keevil CW. Origin and significance of nitrite in water. In: Hill M, ed. *Nitrates and Nitrites in Food and Water.* Chichester, England: Ellis Horwood; 1991:77–92

5. Burgess C. A wave of momentum for toxic algae study. *Environ Health Perspect.* 2001;109:A160–A161

6. Carmichael WW, Azevedo SM, An JS, et al. Human fatalities from cyanobacteria: chemical and biological evidence for cyanotoxins. *Environ Health Perspect.* 2001;109:663–668

7. McKnight GM, Duncan CW, Leifert C, Golden MH. Dietary nitrate in man: friend or foe? *Br J Nutr.* 1999;81:349–358

8. US Environmental Protection Agency. National Primary Drinking Water Regulations: Final Rule, 40. CFR Parts 141, 142, and 143. *Fed Regist.* 1991;3526–3597

9. National Research Council. *Drinking Water and Health.* Washington, DC: National Academy of Sciences; 1977

10. Office of Drinking Water. *National Pesticide Survey: Project Summary.* Washington, DC: US Environmental Protection Agency; 1990

11. US Environmental Protection Agency. *Another Look: National Pesticide Survey: Phase II Report.* Washington, DC: US Environmental Protection Agency; 1992

12. National Center for Environmental Health. *A Survey of the Quality of Water Drawn From Domestic Wells in Nine Midwest States.* Atlanta, GA: Centers for Disease Control and Prevention; 1995. Available at: http://www.cdc.gov/nceh/emergency/wellwater/WellResults.htm

13. North Carolina Division of Public Health. *Contamination of Private Drinking Well Water by Nitrates.* Raleigh, NC: North Carolina Division of Public Health; 1998. Available at: http://www.epi.state.nc.us/epi/mera/ilocontamination.html

14. Beeman P. Nitrate levels surge in Des Moines. *Des Moines Register.* May 17, 2002

15. Litovitz TL, Holm KC, Clancy C, Schmitz BF, Clark LR, Oderda GM. 1992 annual report of the American Association of Poison Control Centers Toxic Exposure Surveillance System. *Am J Emerg Med.* 1993;11:494–555

16. Hartman PE. Nitrates and nitrites: ingestion, pharmacodynamics and toxicology. *Chem Mutagens.* 1982;7:211–294

17. Gangolli SD, van den Brandt PA, Feron VJ, et al. Nitrate, nitrite and N-nitroso compounds. *Eur J Pharmacol.* 1994;292:1–38

18. Committee on Toxicology, National Research Council. *Nitrate and Nitrite in Drinking Water.* Washington, DC: National Academies Press; 1995

19. Reynolds KA. The prevalence of nitrate contamination in the United States. *Water Conditioning and Purification.* 2002;44(1)

20. Smith RP. Toxic responses of the blood. In: Amdur MO, Doull J, Klaassen CD, eds. *Casarett and Doull's Toxicology, The Basic Science of Poisons.* 4th ed. New York, NY: Pergamon Press; 1991:257–281

21. Wright RO, Lewander WJ, Woolf AD. Methemoglobinemia: etiology, pharmacology, and clinical management. *Ann Emerg Med.* 1999;34:646–656

22. Rehman HU. Methemoglobinemia. *West J Med.* 2001;175:193–196

23. Seffner W. Natural water contents and endemic goiter—a review. *Zentralbl Hyg Umweltmed.* 1995;196:381–398

24. Kostraba JN, Gay EC, Rewers M, Hamman RF. Nitrate levels in community drinking waters and risk of IDDM. An ecological analysis. *Diabetes Care.* 1992;15:1505–1508

25. Arbuckle TE, Sherman GJ, Corey PN, Waters D, Lo B. Water nitrates and CNS birth defects: a population-based case-control study. *Arch Environ Health.* 1988;43:162–167

26. Scragg RK, Dorsch MM, McMichael AJ, Baghurst PA. Birth defects and household water supply. Epidemiological studies in the Mount Gambier region of South Australia. *Med J Aust.* 1982;2:577–579

27. Croen LA, Todoroff K, Shaw GM. Maternal exposure to nitrate from drinking water and diet and risk of neural tube defects. *Am J Epidemiol.* 2001;153:325–331

28. Spontaneous abortions possibly related to ingestion of nitrate-contaminated well water—LaGrange County, Indiana, 1991–1994. *MMWR Morb Mortal Wkly Rep.* 1996;45:569–572

29. Walker R. Nitrates, nitrites and N-nitroso compounds: a review of the occurrence in food and diet and the toxicological implications. *Food Addit Contam.* 1990;7:717–768

30. Bruning-Fann CS, Kaneene JB. The effects of nitrate, nitrite and N-nitroso compounds on human health: a review. *Vet Hum Toxicol.* 1993;35:521–538

31. Tricker AR, Preussmann R. Carcinogenic N-nitrosamines in the diet: occurrence, formation, mechanisms and carcinogenic potential. *Mutat Res.* 1991;259:277–289

32. Cantor KP. Drinking water and cancer. *Cancer Causes Control.* 1997;8:292–308

33. Eichholzer M, Gutzwiller F. Dietary nitrates, nitrites, and N-nitroso compounds and cancer risk: a review of the epidemiologic evidence. *Nutr Rev.* 1998;56:95–105

34. Cuello C, Correa P, Haenzel W, et al. Gastric cancer in Columbia. I. Cancer risk and suspect environmental agents. *J Natl Cancer Inst.* 1976;57:1015–1020

35. Rademacher JJ, Young TB, Kanarek MS. Gastric cancer mortality and nitrate levels in Wisconsin drinking water. *Arch Environ Health.* 1992;47:292–294

36. Yang CY, Cheng MF, Tsai SS, Hsieh YL. Calcium, magnesium, and nitrate in drinking water and gastric cancer mortality. *Jpn J Cancer Res.* 1998;89:124–130

37. Steindorf K, Schlehofer B, Becher H, Hornig K, Wahrendorf J. Nitrate in drinking water. A case-control study on primary brain tumors with an embedded drinking water survey in Germany. *Int J Epidemiol.* 1994;23:451–457

38. Ward MH, Cantor KP, Lynch C, Merkle SK. Nitrate in public water supplies and risk of bladder cancer in Iowa, USA. *Epidemiology.* 2001;12 (suppl)S88

39. Ward MH, Mark SD, Cantor KP, Weisenburger DD, Correa-Villasenor A, Zahm SH. Drinking water nitrate and the risk of non-Hodgkin's lymphoma. *Epidemiology.* 1996;7:465–471

40. van Loon AJ, Botterweck AA, Goldbohm RA, Brants HA, van Klaveren JD, van den Brandt PA. Intake of nitrate and nitrite and the risk of gastric cancer: a prospective cohort study. *Br J Cancer.* 1998;78:129–135

41. Weyer PJ, Cerhan JR, Kross BC, et al. Municipal drinking water nitrate level and cancer risk in older women: the Iowa Women's Health Study. *Epidemiology.* 2001;12:327–338

42. Centers for Disease Control and Prevention. Monitoring environmental disease—United States, 1997. *MMWR Morb Mortal Wkly Rep.* 1998;47:522–525

# 23
# Noise

Noise is undesirable sound. Sound is vibration in a medium, usually air, and has frequency (pitch), intensity (loudness), periodicity, and duration. The frequency of sound is measured in cycles per second and is expressed in hertz (Hz) (1 Hz = 60 cycles per second). People respond to frequencies ranging from 20 to 20 000 Hz, but are most sensitive to the sounds in the range of 500 to 3000 Hz, the band of frequencies that includes human speech.

The loudness of sound is measured in terms of pascals (Pa) or decibels (dB). The range of sound limits in human hearing is 0.00002 (the weakest sound that a keen human adult ear can detect under quiet conditions) to 200 Pa (the pressure causing pain in the adult ear). The decibel is a method of compressing this range by expressing the ratio of one sound energy level to another. The unit most commonly used is dB SPL, indicating that the ratio of sound pressure levels is being used. Human speech is approximately 50 dB SPL.

The perceived loudness of sound varies with the frequency. For example, to match the perceived loudness of a 1000-Hz 40-dB SPL tone requires more than 80 dB SPL at 50 Hz and more than 60 dB SPL at 10 000 Hz. This 40-dB SPL equivalency curve is used to determine the measure of sound intensity, referred to as the decibel weighted by the A scale (dBA). Periodicity refers to either continuous sound or impulse sound. Duration is the total length of time of exposure to sound. A recent review of sound characteristics and the development of hearing is available.[1]

Few studies have been done to estimate children's exposure to noise. From available data it is likely that children are routinely exposed to more noise than the 24-hour equivalent noise exposures (Leq24) of 70 dbA recommended as an upper limit by the US

Environmental Protection Agency (EPA) in 1974.[2] A longitudinal study of hearing in suburban and rural Ohio children aged 6 to 18 years found that Leq24 varied from 77 to 84 dB, and exposures were higher in boys than girls.[3]

## Routes of Exposure

Sound waves enter the ear through the external auditory canal and vibrate the eardrum. This vibration in turn travels through the 3 ossicles of the middle ear (the malleus, incus, and stapes), where the stapes vibrates through the oval window, vibrating the fluid of the inner ear, the cochlea. Within the cochlea, the basilar membrane covers the organ of Corti, which is composed of hair cells. Each hair cell responds to a specific frequency of the vibration and converts this signal to a nerve impulse. The impulses, transmitted by auditory nerve, are interpreted as sound or noise by the brain. Loss of hearing originating in the external auditory canal, eardrum, ossicles, or middle ear is called conductive hearing loss and is usually treatable. Loss of hearing originating in the hair cells or sites within the central nervous system is called sensorineural hearing loss and is usually irreversible.

Although sound vibration also may be transmitted to the body directly through the skin, it is not discussed here.

## Clinical Effects

Noise affects hearing and results in several adverse physiological and psychological effects.[4]

Susceptibility to noise-induced hearing loss is highly variable; while some individuals are able to tolerate high noise levels for prolonged periods, other people in the same conditions may lose some hearing.[5] Trauma to the hair cells of the cochlea results in hearing loss. Prolonged exposure to sounds louder than 85 dBA is potentially injurious.[6] Continuous exposure to hazardous levels of noise tends to have its maximum effect in the high-frequency regions of the cochlea. Noise-induced hearing loss usually is most severe around 4000 Hz, with downward extension toward speech frequencies with prolonged exposure. This pattern of loss of frequency perception is true regardless of the frequency of the noise exposure. Impulse noise is more harmful than continuous noise because it bypasses the body's natural protective reaction to noise, the dampening of the ossicles mediated by the facial nerve.[7]

Exposure to loud noise may result in a temporary decrease in the sensitivity of hearing and tinnitus. This condition, called temporary noise-induced threshold shift (NITS), lasts for several hours depending on the degree of exposure, and may become permanent depending on the severity and duration of noise exposure. The prevalence of NITS in one or both ears among children 6 to 19 years of age was recently found to be 12.5% (or 5.2 million children affected).[8] Most children with NITS had an early phase of NITS in only one ear and involving only a single frequency. However, among children with NITS, 4.9% had moderate to profound NITS. Noise-induced threshold shift may be reversible; however, continued excessive noise exposure could lead to progression of NITS to include other frequencies and to increase severity and irreversibility.

The consequences of these measured NITS may be enormous if they progress to a persistent minimal sensorineural hearing loss. In school-aged children, minimal sensorineural hearing loss has been associated with poor school performance and social and emotional dysfunction.[9]

Little evidence is available to suggest that the organs of hearing are more sensitive to noise-induced hearing loss in children than in adults. Children are at increased risk of increased exposure to noise related to their behaviors. Older children play with firecrackers and cap pistols, which can produce noise levels of 134 dBA[10] (see Table 23.1), and teenagers attend loud concerts. Infants cannot remove themselves from noxious noise.

**Table 23.1**
**Average Peak Sound Levels for Selected Toys***

| Toy | Peak Noise Level dBA |
|---|---|
| Music box | 79 |
| Toy mobile phone | 85 |
| Robot soldier | 94 |
| Pull turtle | 95 |
| Musical telephone | 89 |
| Sit-on fire truck | 87 |
| Vacuum cleaner | 83 |
| Laser pistol | 87 |
| Police machine gun | 110 |
| Cap gun fired with caps | 134 |
| Cap gun fired without caps | 114 |
| 007 cap pistol with caps | 127 |
| 007 cap pistol without caps | 118 |

*From the National Institute of Public Health Denmark.[10]

Evidence is available that suggests that exposure to excessive noise during pregnancy may result in high-frequency hearing loss in newborns and may be associated with prematurity and intrauterine growth retardation.[11] Incorporation of individualized environmental care (including reduction of noise) to the management of premature infants decreases time on the ventilator and in oxygen.[12,13]

### *Physiological Effects of Noise*

Noise causes a stress response. For people, the hypothalamic-pituitary-adrenal axis is sensitive to noise as low as 65 dBA, resulting in a 53% increase in plasma 17-OH-corticosteroid levels.[14] Increased excretion of adrenaline and noradrenaline has been demonstrated in humans exposed to noise at 90 dBA for 30 minutes.[15]

Noise contributes to sleep deprivation.[16,17] Noise levels at 40 to 45 dBA result in a 10% to 20% increase in awakening or electroencephalogram (EEG) arousal changes. Noise levels at 50 dBA result in a 25% probability of arousal features on the EEG.[18]

Noise has undesirable cardiovascular effects. Exposure to noise levels greater than 70 dBA causes increases in vasoconstriction, heart rate, and blood pressure.

### Psychological Effects of Noise

Exposure to moderate levels of noise can cause psychological stress.[19] Annoyance, including feelings of bother, interference with activity, and symptoms such as headache, tiredness, and irritability, are common psychological reactions to noise. The degree of annoyance is related to the nature of the sound and individual tolerance. Intense noise can cause personality changes and a reduced ability to cope. Sudden, unexpected noise can cause a startle reaction, which may provoke physiological stress responses.

Work performance can be affected by noise. At low levels it can improve the performance of simple tasks. However, noise may impair intellectual function and performance of complex tasks.

A stress response consisting of acute terror and panic has been described in children in Labrador, Canada, and Germany on exposure to sonic booms.[20] Biochemical evidence of the stress response was found in elevated urinary cortisol levels. Hypertension accompanied a 30-minute exposure to 100 dBA in 60 children aged 11 to 16 years.

### Diagnosis

The typical finding in noise-induced hearing loss is a dip in hearing threshold around 4000 Hz on an audiogram. Physicians in facilities that are unable to provide pure tone audiograms should refer their patients for evaluation. Audiologic evaluation, including pure tone audiometry, should be performed to determine noise-induced hearing loss in children who have no evidence of acute or serous otitis media but have a history of

- In utero exposure to excessive noise by maternal occupation or recreation
- Excessive environmental noise exposure, such as prolonged exposure to cap pistols or "boom boxes"

- Poor school performance
- Short attention span
- Complaining of ringing in the ears, a feeling of fullness in the ears, muffling of hearing, or difficulty in understanding speech
- Speech delay

The American Academy of Pediatrics currently recommends hearing screening for all newborns and at 4, 5, 10, 12, and 18 years of age.[11,21,22]

## Treatment of Clinical Symptoms

There is no known treatment for noise-induced hearing loss.

## Prevention of Exposure

Questions addressed to parents and their children about noise exposure should be part of routine health supervision visits. Reduce noise exposure. Encourage parents and children to

- Avoid loud noises, especially loud impulse noise, whenever possible.
- Avoid toys that make loud noise, especially cap pistols. (There currently is no regulation on the amount of noise toys can make.)
- Avoid the use of firecrackers.
- Reduce the volume on televisions, computers, and radios.
- Turn off televisions, computers, and radios when not in use.
- Use headphones with caution. The volume level of the radio should be low enough so that normal conversation can still be heard.
- Use earplugs if attending a loud event.
- Create a "stimulus haven," the quietest room in the house for play and interactions.[23]

See Table 23.2 for common exposures to noise.

**Table 23.2**
**Decibel Ranges and Effects of Common Sounds**

| Example | Sound Pressure (dBA) | Effect From Exposure |
|---|---|---|
| Breathing | 0–10 | Threshold of hearing |
| Whisper, rustling leaves | 20 | Very quiet |
| Quiet rural area at night | 30 | |
| Library, soft background music | 40 | |
| Quiet suburb (daytime), conversation in living room | 50 | Quiet |
| Conversation in restaurant or average office, background music, chirping bird | 60 | Intrusive |
| Freeway traffic at 15 m, vacuum cleaner, noisy office or party, TV audio | 70 | Annoying |
| Garbage disposal, clothes washer, average factory, freight train at 15 m, food blender, dishwasher, arcade games | 80 | Possible hearing damage |
| Busy urban street, diesel truck | 90 | Hearing damage (8-hour exposure), speech interference |
| Jet takeoff (305 m away), subway, outboard motor, power lawn mower, motorcycle at 8 m, farm tractor, printing plant, jack hammer, garbage truck | 100 | |
| Steel mill, riveting, automobile horn at 1 m, boom box stereo held close to ear | 110 | |
| Thunderclap, textile loom, live rock music, jet takeoff (161 m away), siren, chain saw, stereo in cars | 120 | Human pain threshold |
| Armored personnel carrier, jet takeoff (100 m away), earphones at loud level | 130 | |
| Aircraft carrier deck | 140 | |
| Jet takeoff (25 m), toy cap pistol, firecracker | 150 | Eardrum rupture |

When noise reduction is not possible, hearing protectors need to be worn, such as during occupational exposures, use of power lawn mowers, recreational exposures such as loud concerts, and other situational noise exposures. There are 2 types of hearing protectors—earplugs or earmuffs. Earplugs should fit properly; a slight tug required to remove them indicates correct fit. They are available in most drug stores. Earplugs should be checked while chewing because jaw motion may loosen them. Earmuffs are the most effective type of ear protector and are available at most hardware stores. They have cups lined with sound-absorbing material that are held against the head with a spring band or oil-filled ring that provides a tight seal.

Unfortunately, environmental noise often cannot be controlled, which makes noise reduction or hearing protection difficult. Government regulations are needed to protect parents and children from these noises. The standard for the workplace is no more than 8 hours of exposure to 90 dBA, 4 hours at 95 dBA, and 2 hours at 100 dBA, with no exposure allowed to continuous noise above 115 dBA or impulse noise above 140 dBA. In nonoccupational settings, environmental noise is expressed as a day-night average sound level (DNL). For the protection of public health, the EPA proposed a DNL of 55 dB during waking hours and 45 dB during sleeping hours in neighborhoods, and 45 dB in daytime and 35 dB at night in hospitals. In 1972 Congress passed the Noise Control Act, giving the EPA a mandate to regulate environmental noise. The act placed the EPA in charge of all federal noise activities and ordered other agencies to help develop noise-reduction plans. The EPA's Office of Noise Abatement and Control supported research on noise; established noise standards for new trucks and motorcycles; proposed regulations for tractors, buses, lawn mowers, and jackhammers; started a program to rate the sound levels of consumer products; and developed a "buy quiet" program to encourage federal and state agencies to purchase quiet products. This office was closed in 1982, and no effort is being made to enforce the noise regulations that have been established.

## Frequently Asked Questions

Q  *We live near an airport and the jets fly directly over our house as they take off and land. Will this be harmful to my newborn baby?*

A  If the noise is causing discomfort to the parents' ears, it may be causing pain to the infant. The infant should be observed for sleep disturbances and response to the noise. The Federal Aviation Administration program on Airport Noise Compatibility Planning may be contacted for assessment of noise and possible mitigation. The local state programs listing participating airports can be found at http://www.faa.gov.

Q  *Are there unique hazards to the use of headphones?*

A  There are several reports of hearing loss secondary to the use of headphones. Children and teenagers should be educated about the potential danger of loud music, whether heard in concert halls or through headphones.

## Resource

US Environmental Protection Agency, Office of Air and Radiation, Internet: http://www.epa.gov/oar

## References
1.  Philbin MK, Graven SN, Robertson A. The influence of auditory experience on the fetus, newborn, and preterm infant: report of the sound study group of the national resource center: the physical and developmental environment of the high risk infant. *J Perinatol.* 2000;20(suppl):S1–S142
2.  DeJoy DM. Environmental noise and children: a review of recent findings. *J Aud Res.* 1983;23:181–194
3.  Roche AF, Chumleawc RM, Siervogel RM. *Longitudinal Study of Human Hearing, Its Relationship to Noise and Other Factors. III. Results From the First 5 Years.* Washington, DC: US Environmental Protection Agency/ Aerospace Medical Research Lab; 1982. Report No. AFAMRL-TR-82-68

4. Swift D, Molon T. Disorders of the ear and hearing. In: Brooks S, ed. *Environmental Medicine*. St Louis, MO: Mosby; 1995:250–262

5. Henderson D, Hamernik RP. Biologic bases of noise-induced hearing loss. *Occup Med*. 1995;10:513–534

6. Thompson DA. Ergonomics and the prevention of occupational injuries. In: LaDou J, ed. *Occupational Medicine*. Norwalk, CT: Appleton and Lange; 1990:54

7. Jackler RK, Schindler DN. Occupational hearing loss. In: LaDou J, ed. *Occupational Medicine*. Norwalk, CT: Appleton and Lange; 1990:95–105

8. Niskar AS, Kieszak SM, Holmes AE, Esteban E, Rubin C, Brody DJ. Estimated prevalence of noise-induced hearing threshold shifts among children 6–19 years of age: the Third National Health and Nutrition Examination Survey, 1988–1994, United States. *Pediatrics*. 2001;108:40–43

9. Bess FH, Dodd-Murphy J, Parker RA. Children with minimal sensorineural hearing loss: prevalence, educational performance, and functional status. *Ear Hear*. 1998;19:339–354

10. National Institute of Public Health Denmark. *Health Effects of Noise on Children and Perception of the Risk of Noise*. Bistrup ML, ed. Copenhagen, Denmark: National Institute of Public Health Denmark; 2001:29

11. American Academy of Pediatrics Committee on Environmental Health. Noise: a hazard for the fetus and newborn. *Pediatrics*. 1997;100:724–727

12. Als H, Lawhon G, Brown E, et al. Individualized behavioral and environmental care for the very low birth weight preterm infant at high risk for bronchopulmonary dysplasia: neonatal intensive care unit and developmental outcome. *Pediatrics*. 1986;78:1123–1132

13. Buehler DM, Als H, Duffy FH, McAnulty GB, Liederman J. Effectiveness of individualized developmental care for low-risk preterm infants: behavioral and electrophysiologic evidence. *Pediatrics*. 1995;96:923–932

14. Henkin RI, Knigge KM. Effect of sound on hypothalamic pituitary-adrenal axis. *Am J Physiol*. 1963;204:701–704

15. Frankenhaeuser M, Lundberg U. Immediate and delayed effects of noise on performance and arousal. *Biol Psychol*. 1974;2:127–133

16. Falk SA, Woods NF. Hospital noise—levels and potential health hazards. *N Engl J Med*. 1973;289:774–781

17. Hilton BA. Quantity and quality of patients' sleep and sleep disturbing factors in a respiratory intensive care unit. *J Adv Nurs*. 1976;1:453–468

18. Thiessen GJ. Disturbance of sleep by noise. *J Acoust Soc Am*. 1978;64:216–222

19. Kam PC, Kam AC, Thompson JF. Noise pollution in the anaesthetic and intensive care environment. *Anaesthesia.* 1994;49:982–986
20. Rosenberg J. Jets over Labrador and Quebec: noise effects on human health. *Can Med Assoc J.* 1991;144:869–875
21. American Academy of Pediatrics Committee on Psychosocial Aspects of Child and Family Health. *Guidelines for Health Supervision III.* Elk Grove Village, IL: American Academy of Pediatrics; 1997
22. American Academy of Pediatrics Joint Committee on Infant Hearing. Joint Committee on Infant Hearing 1990 position statement. *AAP News.* April 1991;7:6, 14
23. Wachs TD. Nature of relations between the physical and social microenvironment of the two-year-old child. *Early Dev Parenting.* 1993;2:81–87

# 24
# Pesticides

Pesticides are ubiquitous in the environment. More than 900 chemicals are registered in the United States as pesticides, including insecticides, herbicides, fungicides, rodenticides, fumigants, and insect repellents. The mechanism by which they kill pests often is similar to that which harms or kills human beings. Use of pesticides in the United States doubled from the 1960s to the 1980s to more than 1 billion pounds per year. In a 1996 survey by the US Environmental Protection Agency (EPA), 74% of households were reported to be using 1 or more pesticides in the home or immediate environment.[1]

Pesticides have numerous beneficial effects. When used appropriately for control of insects and rodents, pesticides can assist in the prevention of the spread of disease. Pesticides can have a positive impact on crop yields. These compounds, however, also can be toxic to adults and children. Because pesticides are present in food, medications, homes, schools, and parks, children frequently may be exposed. Children at increased risk of pesticide exposure include those whose parents are farmers or farmworkers, pesticide applicators or landscapers, or children who live adjacent to agricultural areas.[2,3] Children and teenagers may work or play near their parents in the fields, where they may be exposed to pesticides. People who work with pesticides may use these agricultural-strength chemicals at home.[3] Inappropriate applications may cause illness and death.

In response to growing concern about children's exposure to pesticides via food, Congress passed the Food Quality Protection Act (FQPA) of 1996 (PL 104-170).[4] This law is unique in that it explicitly requires that the EPA ensure a "reasonable certainty that no harm will result in infants and children" from exposure to pesticides and that the effects of chemicals that have the same mechanism of action be considered cumulatively. Additional information regarding chronic exposure to small amounts of pesticides is included in Chapter 14.

---

**Food Quality Protection Act (FQPA) of 1996**

Actions generated by the FQPA, modifying the Federal Insecticide, Fungicide and Rodenticide Act and the Federal Food, Drug, and Cosmetic Act:

- Established a single health-based standard for all pesticides in food.
- Benefits, in general, cannot override the health-based standard.
- Prenatal and postnatal effects are to be considered.
- In the absence of data confirming the safety to infants and children, because of their special sensitivities and exposures, an additional uncertainty factor of up to 10 times can be added to the safety values.
- Aggregate risk, the sum of all exposures to the chemical, must be considered in establishing safe levels.
- Cumulative risk, the sum of all exposures to chemicals with similar mechanisms of action, must be considered in establishing safe levels.
- Endocrine disruptors are to be included in the evaluation of safety.
- All existing pesticide registrations are to be reviewed by 2006.
- Expedited review is possible for safer pesticides.
- Risks are to be determined for 1 year and lifetime exposure.

---

This chapter focuses on acute and chronic effects of pesticides and prevention measures.

## Insecticides

The major classes of insecticides are organophosphates, carbamates, pyrethrum and synthetic pyrethroids, organochlorines, and boric acid and borates.

- **Organophosphates.** Organophosphate pesticides account for about one half of the insecticides used in the United States and are responsible for most acute pesticide poisonings. Organophosphates are used on food and are available for insect control in the home and garden, and in institutions such as schools. (Currently organophosphate pesticides are under scrutiny by the EPA under provisions of the FQPA.) The requirements that exposure from all routes be viewed cumulatively and that children's health be directly addressed have resulted in many chemical uses being restricted or eliminated in this category.
- **N-Methyl Carbamates.** N-methyl carbamates are similar to organophosphates. The most toxic carbamate is aldicarb. Carbaryl, bendiocarb, and propoxur are more commonly found in household use and are moderately toxic.
- **Pyrethrum and Synthetic Pyrethroids.** Pyrethrum, an extract of dried chrysanthemum flowers, refers to a composite of 6 insecticidal ingredients known as pyrethrins. Natural pyrethrins are used mainly for indoor bug bombs and aerosols due to their instability in light and heat. Anti-lice shampoos such as A200 and Rid contain pyrethrins. Pyrethroids, synthetic chemicals based on the structure and biological activity of pyrethrum, are modified to increase their stability. The pyrethroids are classified as Type I or Type II (or cyano-pyrethroids); Type II pyrethroids generally are more toxic than the Type I pyrethroids. Pyrethroids are used in agriculture and gardening for control of structural pests (eg, termites) and against lice and scabies (as permethrin, eg, Elimite). Pyrethrum and pyrethroids rapidly penetrate insects and paralyze them.
- **Organochlorines.** Halogenated hydrocarbons were developed in the 1940s for use as insecticides, fungicides, and herbicides. Organochlorines are lipid soluble, have low molecular weight, and persist in the environment. Dichlorodiphenyltrichloroethane (DDT), chlordane, and other organochlorines were enormously successful due to their efficacy and low acute toxicity. Production

of DDT and most other organochlorine compounds was banned in the United States in the 1970s because of concern about their persistence, bioaccumulation in the food chain, possible long-term carcinogenicity, and increasing resistance of the targeted pests. Organochlorines continue to be used in developing countries, including those exporting food to the United States. Lindane (Kwell) continues to be prescribed for lice and scabies, although safer preparations are available. Lindane poses a serious risk of poisoning if accidentally ingested or misused topically. Lindane is to be used only in patients who have failed to respond to adequate doses of other approved agents. As of January 2002, the state of California no longer allowed the sale of prescriptions containing lindane for human use.[5] This action was prompted by recognition that treatment for head lice adds significantly to water pollution. Many of these compounds are known to affect the endocrine system (see Chapter 12).

- **Boric Acid and Borates.** Boric acid commonly is available as a pellet or powder for household insect control. Boric acid and borates generally are considered to be among the less toxic chemicals used for insect control and increasingly are used instead of organophosphate pesticides in settings where children may be present. Though less toxic, this class of compounds was used extensively in the 1950s and 1960s with reports of significant toxicity, especially when ingested.[6,7] Poison control centers increasingly are receiving reports of ingestions of boric acid pellets or powders by children younger than 6 years.[8]

## Other Pesticides

### Herbicides
Herbicides kill unwanted plants in agriculture, in homes, on lawns, in gardens, in parks, on school grounds, and along roadways where children walk, play, and ride bicycles. Herbicides are used by about 14 million households annually.

- **Glyphosate (Roundup, Rodeo).** Glyphosate is a broad-spectrum herbicide used to kill unwanted plants in agriculture and landscapes.
- **Bipyridyls.** The bipyridyls paraquat and diquat are nonselective plant-killing agents preferred in agriculture because they become inactive on contact with soil. These are widely used by municipal and industrial entities.
- **Chlorophenoxy Herbicides.** These include 2,4-dichlorophenoxy-acetic acid (2,4-D or Weedone, Weed-be-gone). The mixture of 2,4-D and the now-banned chlorophenoxy herbicide 2,4,5-trichlorophenoxyacetic acid, known as Agent Orange, was used heavily in South Vietnam and Cambodia for defoliation by the US Armed Forces. The mixture was contaminated with 2,3,7,8-tetrachlorodibenzo-p-dioxin, which is a known human carcinogen and developmental toxicant.

### *Fungicides*

Fungicides include substituted benzenes, thiocarbamates, ethylene bis-dithiocarbamates, copper, organotin, cadmium compounds, elemental sulfur, and miscellaneous compounds such as captan, benomyl, and ipriodine.[9] Organomercury compounds have been banned in the United States due to their extreme toxicity. Fungicides are used to protect grains and perishable produce from mold. These chemicals also are used as seed treatments, on ornamental plants, and in soil. Some fungicides are available in stores for use on garden plants. Fungicides most commonly are applied as a wettable powder or in granular form, and are generally poorly absorbed in these forms via dermal or respiratory routes.

### *Wood Preservatives*

Wood preservatives include pentachlorophenol and copper chromium arsenate (CCA). These preservatives were banned from materials other than wood by the EPA in 1987. Pentachlorophenol is used as a wood preservative for utility poles, cross arms, and fence posts and is a known carcinogen. Copper chromium arsenate is a pesticide used in pressure-treated wood, a product that commonly is used to construct decks, porches, and playground equipment (see Chapter 8).

### Rodenticides

Rodenticides commonly used in US homes are anticoagulants or cholecalciferol. Anticoagulants interfere with the activation of vitamin K-dependent factors (II, VII, IX, X). Examples include warfarins, the 10-fold more potent indanediones, and superwarfarins (eg, brodifacoum), approximately 100 times more potent than the warfarins. Yellow phosphorus, strychnine, and arsenic rodenticides no longer are registered but may be in use from existing stored supplies.

### Insect Repellents

N,N-diethyl-m-toluamide (also known as N,N-diethyl-3-methyl-benzamide)—DEET—is the active ingredient in many insect repellent products. DEET is used to repel insects such as mosquitoes that may transmit viral encephalitis (eg, West Nile Virus) or malaria, and ticks that may carry Lyme disease. Marketed in the United States since 1956 and used by about one third of the US population each year, DEET is available in many commercial products as an aerosol, liquid, lotion, or stick and in impregnated materials such as wristbands. Commercial products registered for direct application to human skin contain from 4% to 99.9% DEET. Concentrations above 30% provide no increase in protection.

Products containing citronella, sold as insect repellents, are not as effective as DEET and therefore not recommended when concern exists about arthropod-borne disease. Permethrin (Permanone, Duranon) is marketed as a spray for tents and clothing, but not for direct application to the skin.[10]

### Sources of Exposure

Children in the United States are almost universally exposed to some degree to pesticides; home and garden pesticide use may result in increased levels of exposure in urban and rural settings.[11]

Prenatal and early childhood exposures may be especially signifi-cant because of the susceptibility of developing organ systems as well as behavioral, physiological, and dietary characteristics of children.[12] Metabolites of organophosphate pesticides were shown to be present in the meconium of all of the 20 newborns tested in a study in New York City.[13] This is indicative of the ubiquitous exposure to these chemicals even in utero.

## Routes of Exposure

Children may be exposed to pesticides through inhalation, ingestion, and dermal absorbtion.

### Inhalation

Pesticides applied as dusts, mists, sprays, or gases may reach the mucous membranes, or the alveoli, where they are absorbed into the bloodstream. Where suburban neighborhoods are interspersed with agricultural lands, chemicals from aerial spraying may drift into residential areas.

Inhalation of the non-insecticide group of pesticides is relatively minor because their volatility is low and, with the exception of the chlorophenoxy herbicides, they are rarely distributed by aerial spray-ing. Fungicides may be inhaled during the process of application, but once applied, they are subject to limited inhalation.

### Ingestion

Ingestion of pesticides may result in acute poisoning. Pesticides stored in food containers (eg, soft drink bottles) pose a special hazard for children. An EPA survey reported that nearly half of US households with a child younger than 5 years had a pesticide stored within the reach of children.[14]

The major problem with ingestion of pesticides is from foods that have been treated with them, especially those grown in home gardens. Infants and children may be exposed through their diets to trace amounts of pesticides applied to food crops (see Chapter 14). People also may be exposed to low levels of organochlorines by eating crops grown in contaminated soil and eating fish from contaminated waters. Pesticides are found in some water supplies: a 1999 EPA survey found that 10.7% of community water system wells contained one or more pesticides that were not removed by standard water treatment technologies (see Chapter 27).[15]

In addition, young children consume measurable amounts of soil, and children with pica can consume up to 100 g/day of soil that may contain persistent organic pesticides as well as heavy metals such as arsenic.

Wood treated with CCA is a potential source of childhood exposure to arsenic. Arsenic is leached from the wood with aging and can accumulate on the wood surface of the soil under playground equipment and decks made with treated wood. Young children are at particular risk of exposure from hand-to-mouth activity.

Accidental ingestion may occur with any of these compounds, especially with the rodenticides. Whether by ingestion or inhalation,

**Table 24.1**
**Number of Calls to Poison Control Centers About Pediatric Pesticide Poisonings, 1999\***

| Pesticide | <6 Years | 6–19 Years |
|---|---|---|
| Anticoagulant rodenticides | 15 892 | 605 |
| Pyrethrins (with or without piperonyl butoxide) | 5422 | 2252 |
| Insect repellents | 4446 | 1092 |
| Organophosphates | 4056 | 1152 |
| Borates/boric acid | 2445 | 158 |
| Veterinary insecticide | 2119 | 614 |
| Carbamates | 1686 | 437 |
| Organochlorines | 1026 | 437 |
| Other/unknown | 6015 | 938 |

\*From Litovitz TL, Klein-Schwartz W, White S.[8]

children frequently have serious exposures to pesticides as seen in calls to poison control centers (see Table 24.1).

## Dermal Absorption

Many pesticides are readily absorbed through the skin. The potential for dermal exposures in children is high because of their relatively large body surface area and extensive contact with lawns, gardens, and floors by crawling and playing on the ground. Lindane (Kwell, for topical scabies and lice treatment) and DEET are absorbed through the skin. Herbicides, the bipyridyls, and fungicides can all create dermal exposures but they generally result in skin irritation and rarely in systemic effects.

## Systems Affected and Clinical Effects

### Parental and Prenatal Exposures

Effects that have been associated with parental or prenatal pesticide exposures include intrauterine growth retardation and prematurity,[16] birth defects,[17] fetal death,[18] and spontaneous abortion.[19] More research is needed to further clarify whether these associations are causal.

## Acute Effects

### Organophosphates

Organophosphates phosphorylate the active site of the enzyme acetylcholinesterase (AChE) at the nerve ending, irreversibly inhibiting this enzyme. The signs and symptoms of acute organophosphate poisoning result from the accumulation of acetylcholine at cholinergic receptors (muscarinic effects), as well as at voluntary muscle (including the diaphragm) and autonomic ganglia (nicotinic effects). Accumulation of acetylcholine in the brain causes sensory and behavioral disturbances, impaired coordination, depressed cognition, and coma (see Table 24.2).

Organophosphates are rapidly distributed throughout the body after inhalation or ingestion. Symptoms usually develop within 4 hours of exposure, but may be delayed up to 12 hours with dermal exposure. Initial symptoms may include headache, dizziness, miosis, nausea, abdominal pain, and diarrhea; anxiety and restlessness may be prominent. With progressive worsening, muscle twitching, weakness, bradycardia, hypersecretion (sweating, salivation, rhinorrhea, bronchorrhea), and profuse diarrhea may develop. Central nervous system (CNS) effects include headache, blurred vision, anxiety, confusion, emotional lability, ataxia, toxic psychosis, vertigo, convulsions, and coma. Cranial nerve palsies have been noted.[20]

More severe intoxications result in sympathetic and nicotinic manifestations with muscle weakness and fasciculations including twitching (particularly in eyelids), tachycardia, muscle cramps, hypertension, and sweating. Finally, paralysis of respiratory and skeletal muscles and convulsions may develop.[9,21] Children are more likely than adults to have CNS signs such as coma and seizures.[21,22]

### N-Methyl Carbamates

Carbamates act similarly to organophosphates in binding AChE, but the bonds are more readily reversible. The clinical symptoms produced are not easily differentiated from those of organophosphate poisoning. While AChE may be low in organophosphate poisoning, it usually is normal in carbamate poisoning.[20] Carbamates may be highly toxic, although the effects of exposure are more short-lived, with some cases abating within 6 to 8 hours.

### Pyrethrum and Synthetic Pyrethroids

Pyrethrum and synthetic pyrethroids are absorbed from the gastrointestinal and respiratory tracts but only very slightly through the skin. Because pyrethrins are metabolized very rapidly by the liver, and most metabolites are promptly excreted by the kidneys, they have low toxicity when ingested.[20] Most problematic are allergic reactions, which

**Table 24.2**
**Acute Effects of Common Pesticide Classes\***

| Pesticide Category | Chemical Examples | Mechanism of Effects, Acute Symptoms | Diagnosis and Treatment |
|---|---|---|---|
| Organophosphates | Chlorpyrifos, diazinon, methyl parathion, azinphos-methyl, naled, malathion, acephate | Irreversible acetylcholinesterase inhibition; nausea, vomiting, hypersecretion, bronchoconstriction, headache | Cholinesterase levels; supportive care, atropine, pralidoxime |
| N-methyl carbamates | Carbaryl, aldicarb | Reversible acetylcholinesterase inhibition; nausea, vomiting, hypersecretion, bronchoconstriction, headache | Cholinesterase levels; supportive care, atropine |
| Pyrethrins | Pyrethrum | Allergic reactions, anaphylaxis, tremor; ataxia at high doses | No diagnostic test; treat allergic reactions with antihistamines, or steroids, as needed |
| Pyrethroids | | | |
| Type I | Allenthrin, permethrin, tetramethrin | Tremors, ataxia, irritability, and enhanced startle response | No diagnostic test; decontamination, supportive care, symptomatic treatment |
| Type II | Deltamethrin, cypermethrin, and fenvalerate | Choreoathetosis, salivation, and seizures | Note: skin contact may cause highly unpleasant, temporary paresthesias, best treated with vitamin E oil preparations |
| Organochlorines | Lindane, endosulfan, dicofol | GABA blockade; uncoordination, tremors, sensory disturbances, dizziness, seizures | Detectable in blood; decontamination, supportive care, cholestyramine to clear enterohepatic recirculation |

**Table 24.2**
**Acute Effects of Common Pesticide Classes\*, *continued***

| Pesticide Category | Chemical Examples | Mechanism of Effects, Acute Symptoms | Diagnosis and Treatment |
|---|---|---|---|
| Chlorophenoxy compounds | 2,4-Dichloro-phenoxyacetic acid (2,4-D) | Acidosis, neuropathy, myopathy; nausea and vomiting, myalgia, headache, myotonia, fever | Detectable in urine; decontamination, forced alkaline diuresis |
| Bipyridyl compounds | Paraquat, diquat | Free radical formation; pulmonary edema, acute tubular necrosis, hepatocellular toxicity | Urine dithionite test (colorimetric); decontamination, do NOT administer oxygen, aggressive hydration, hemoperfusion |
| Anticoagulant rodenticides | Warfarin, brodifacoum, diphencoumarin, diphacinone, pindone | Vitamin K antagonism; hemorrhage | Elevated PT; vitamin K administration |

\*From Reigart JR, Roberts JR.[20]

have occurred in the form of contact dermatitis, anaphylaxis, or asthma.[9] Paresthesias (described as stinging, burning, or itching) may occur when liquid or volatile compounds contact the skin; these rarely last more than 24 hours.[20] Absorption of extraordinarily high doses rarely may cause incoordination, dizziness, headaches, nausea, and diarrhea. A fatal asthma attack in a child attributed to shampooing her dog with an animal shampoo containing pyrethrin has been described.[23]

The active ingredient usually is formulated (mixed with carriers, solvents, or synergists) with "inert ingredients" that may be toxic. For example, xylene (an inert ingredient in some pyrethroid formulations) is a CNS depressant and reproductive toxicant. Synergists (chemicals that inhibit the detoxification process) such as piperonyl butoxide and sulfoxide are of low toxicity. Organophosphates and carbamates often are combined with pyrethroids and may have significant toxicity.

### Organochlorines

The toxic action of organochlorines is primarily on the nervous system. By interfering with the flux of cations across nerve cell membranes, organochlorines produce abnormal nerve function and irritability, which may result in seizures. Disturbances of sensation, coordination, and mental function are characteristic. Lindane poisoning presents with nausea, vomiting, and CNS stimulation or generalized seizures.

### Boric Acid and Borates

Boric dust is irritating to the skin, upper airways, and lower respiratory tract. Ingestion of borates can result in severe gastroenteritis, headache, lethargy, and an intensely erythematous skin rash similar in appearance to a staphylococcal scalded skin syndrome.[24] Metabolic acidosis can occur, leading to shock in severe cases.

## Herbicides

### Glyphosate

At usual exposure levels, glyphosate has a low level of acute toxicity. Ingestions of three quarters of a cup or more (usually as an attempted suicide) have been fatal.[25,26] Symptoms include abdominal pain, vomiting, pulmonary edema, kidney damage, and renal failure. More commonly, lower levels cause skin and eye irritation. The surfactant polyethoxylated tallowamine, added to improve product application, is more toxic than the active ingredient glyphosate. The 2 mixed together (Roundup) may show a synergistic increase in toxicity.

### Bipyridyls (Paraquat and Diquat)

Acute bipyridyl toxicity is thought to involve the production of free radical oxygen and, secondarily, interference with nicotinamide adenine dinucleotide phosphate and nicotinamide adenine dinucleotide phosphate (reduced form). Paraquat and diquat are corrosive to the tissues they contact directly. Initially, local effects of paraquat result in caustic burns to the skin or mucosa. This is followed by a period of multisystem injury with damage to the liver, kidney, myocardium, and skeletal muscle. Two to 14 days following exposure, progressive pulmonary failure occurs due to irreversible alveolar fibrosis. Diquat is less damaging to the skin and does not concentrate in the lungs. Intense nausea, vomiting, and diarrhea may be followed by hypertension, dehydration, renal failure, and shock. Death has occurred after ingestion of as little as 10 mL of a 20% concentration of paraquat in an adult and is common in ingestions exceeding 40 mg/kg. Sufficient amounts of paraquat may be absorbed dermally to produce systemic toxicity and death.

### Chlorophenoxy Herbicides

Chlorophenoxy herbicides primarily are irritants, causing cough, nausea, and emesis. Few cases of large ingestions have been reported. Symptoms include coma, myosis, fever, hypertension, muscle rigidity, and tachycardia. Pulmonary edema, respiratory failure, and rhabdomyolysis may occur.[20,27,28]

### Fungicides

Because a large variety of compounds are used in fungicides, the systems affected and clinical effects vary with each compound. Fungicides rarely are associated with acute poisonings in children due to their low toxicity, poor absorption, and use patterns. However, many of these chemicals are serious respiratory and skin irritants, some are associated with allergic sensitization, and some are linked to chronic effects such as endocrine disruption.[29] Common responses to acute fungicide exposure include rashes, mucous membrane irritation, and respiratory symptoms.

## Rodenticides

### Anticoagulants

Anticoagulants may produce bleeding and are the number one cause of pesticide-related calls to poison control centers among children younger than 6 years. However, data reported by the American Association of Poison Control Centers show no fatalities after anticoagulant ingestion.[30,31]

## Cholecalciferol

Cholecalciferol produces persistent hypercalcemia that induces vaso-constriction resulting in renal dysfunction and a reduced glomerular filtration rate and renal plasma flow. Typically, 2 or 3 days pass between ingestion and the onset of clinical manifestations of hypercalcemia. Calcium levels of 11.5 to 12 mg/dL may produce anorexia, muscle weakness (due to decreased neuromuscular activity), apathy, nausea, vomiting, constipation, and headache. Levels greater than 13 mg/dL may produce bone pain, ectopic calcification, polyuria, hypertension, renal failure, nephrocalcinosis, and cardiac dysrhythmias. Moderately severe hypercalcemia may interrupt bone growth for 6 months.

## Insect Repellents

### DEET

Occasionally, people who use DEET experience adverse reactions, generally consisting of temporary irritation to the skin and eyes. A portion of dermally applied DEET is absorbed systemically.[32] In 1961 a case of encephalitis linked to DEET was reported.[33] Since that time additional reports of adverse reactions included rashes, fevers, seizures, and death (mostly in children).[34,35] The relationship between exposure to DEET and reported neurologic symptoms is of concern. Most of the cases of toxicity involved the use of DEET concentration from 10% to 50% and were related to overdose and misuse. Clinicians evaluating children with unexplained encephalopathy or seizures should consider the possibility of exposure to DEET.[10,36,37] The EPA has established a program to investigate adverse events following DEET use. Physicians should report serious adverse reactions to DEET, including anaphylaxis or seizures, to EPA, 6A2 Processing Desk, 7502C,

1200 Pennsylvania Ave, Washington, DC 20460-0001, or e-mail
spurling.normal@epa.gov.

## Subclinical Effects

A statistical simulation by a committee of the National Academy
of Sciences suggested that for some pesticides, the reference dose (the
dose of a non-cancer toxicant at which no health effects are likely)
may be exceeded by thousands of children daily. Some children may
display mild symptoms of inattention and gastrointestinal, or flulike,
symptoms related to dietary pesticides.[38] Multiple exposures from a
variety of sources (ie, food, yard, school) may be cumulative.[39]

## Chronic Systemic Effects

Many organochlorine pesticides are linked to chronic health effects
such as developmental abnormalities in animals, cancer, and
endocrine disruption.[20,40,41]

## Chronic Neurotoxic Effects

Chronic neurobehavioral or neurologic effects have been reported
in a small proportion of organophosphate poisonings. Symptoms
reported to persist for months or years include headaches, visual
difficulties, problems with memory and concentration, confusion,
unusual fatigue, irritability, and depression.[42] In serious poisonings
with some organophosphates, there have been reports of organophos-
phate-induced delayed polyneuropathy associated with paralysis in the
legs, sensory disturbances, and weaknesses.[43] In one well-documented
case, an infant with hypertonia was diagnosed and treated for cerebral
palsy prior to the discovery that she was suffering from chronic poisonings by an organophosphate pesticide. Her house had been sprayed
by uncertified applicators prior to her birth and continued to have
excessive levels of chemical 9 months later.[44]

There is some evidence of delayed or chronic neurotoxicity associated with pesticide exposure during CNS development. Although
there is plasticity inherent in the development of the nervous system

in the infant and child, toxic exposures during the brain growth spurt may exert subtle, permanent effects on the structure and function of the brain. Some investigators have put forward the hypothesis that exposure to neurotoxicants during early life may result in abnormal behavioral traits such as hyperactivity, decreased attention span, and neurocognitive deficits.[39]

Areas of the brain most commonly affected by pesticides include the limbic system, hippocampus, basal ganglia, and cerebellum.[45] Adult workers acutely or chronically exposed to organophosphate pesticides may develop chronic neurologic abnormalities.[46] Cognitive symptoms in these populations include impairment of memory and psychomotor speed, and affective symptoms including anxiety, irritability, and depression.[47] Visuospatial deficits also have been linked to organophosphate exposure.[48] Standardized neuropsychiatric testing batteries have confirmed these deficits in exposed groups compared with unexposed controls. N-methyl carbamate pesticides have been implicated in similar health effects.[47]

Animal studies have demonstrated periods of vulnerability to neurotoxicants during early life. Single, relatively modest doses of organophosphate, pyrethroid, or organochlorine pesticides during the brain growth spurt in rodents lead to permanent changes in muscarinic receptor levels in the brain and behavioral changes into adulthood.[49,50] These findings are supported by recent evidence that acetylcholinesterase may play a direct role in axonal outgrowth and neuronal differentiation.[51] The widely used organophosphate pesticides chlorpyrifos and diazinon are suspected neuroteratogens and now have been banned by the EPA for general use. These chemicals inhibit deoxyribonucleic acid synthesis in neuronal and glial cells.[52] One observational study in children from a region in Mexico with intensive pesticide use found a variety of developmental delays compared with otherwise similar children living in a region where fewer pesticides were used. The children were similar in growth and physical development. However, significant delays were noted among the exposed children in physical stamina, gross and fine hand-eye coordination, short-term memory, and ability to draw a person.[53]

## Carcinogenic Effects

Several organophosphates are probable (ie, dichlorvos or possible (ie, malathion, tetrachlorvinphos) human carcinogens.[54] Epidemiologic studies have found associations between certain childhood cancers (eg, all brain cancers, non-Hodgkin lymphoma, and leukemia) and pesticide exposure.[55–57] A review of 17 case-control studies and one cohort study supported a possible role for pesticides in childhood leukemia. Most, but not all, of the studies reported elevated risks among children whose parents were occupationally exposed to pesticides or who used pesticides in the home or garden.[58] Several studies have linked home use of pesticides with childhood brain tumors.[59] Particular behaviors associated with increased odds of brain tumors included using sprays or foggers to dispense flea or tick treatments, flea collars, home pesticide bombs, fumigation for termites, pest strips, and lindane shampoo.[39] Several epidemiologic studies in agricultural workers have linked chronic exposures to chlorophenoxy herbicides with non-Hodgkin lymphoma and with sperm abnormalities in males.[41,60,61]

## Diagnostic Methods

The history of exposure is of particular importance. In a review of 190 acute pesticide poisonings, laboratory tests were not often found to be diagnostically helpful.[62] In addition, symptoms of pesticide exposure are likely to be nonspecific. In the case of organophosphate or N-methyl carbamate poisoning, measurement of plasma pseudo-cholinesterase or red blood cell acetylcholinesterase levels are generally rapidly available and may be helpful in confirming a diagnosis. However, due to population variability, these tests are neither sensitive nor specific and must be considered as one piece of the clinical context.

Urine metabolites of some pesticides (organophosphates, chloro-phenoxy herbicides) are measurable, but these tests generally are not available, and there is little information about population reference ranges. These tests should only be ordered in unusual circumstances. Organochlorine pesticides and their metabolites are measurable in blood. Population surveys have shown widespread low-level residues in the general population. Testing for these chemicals should be reserved for unusual circumstances and the results interpreted with caution. There are no existing methods for detecting some pesticides, such as the pyrethroids, in human samples. The mainstay for the diagnosis of pesticide poisoning is maintenance of a high index of suspicion and a careful exposure history.

## Treatment

When a poisoning has occurred, the label of the chemical should be obtained whenever possible. Many pesticides have confusingly similar names. Many active ingredients are sold using the same trade names. Therefore, it is important to ascertain the exact ingredients for any product of concern. The EPA-mandated label contains concise information on specific treatment guidelines, symptoms, and signs and a toll-free telephone number for manufacturer assistance. In an agricultural exposure, the country cooperative extension service agent can provide invaluable knowledge of the local crops, chemical usage patterns, and modes of application.

Regional poison control centers can help with patient evaluation and management and have a medical toxicologist available for consultation. The National Pesticide Telecommunications Network can help answer questions about pesticide identification, toxicology, acute and chronic symptoms, and treatment (see Resources).

Serious poisonings should be managed with guidance from a medical toxicologist and/or a regional poison control center. Immediate decontamination is important. If there is an ingestion, gastric decontamination usually is indicated. If the exposure is dermal, clothing should be removed and the patient should be washed with soap and water. Caregivers should avoid exposure to the chemical. Grossly contaminated patients may need to be decontaminated outside with rescuers using chemical protective gear. Care should be taken to identify other children or adults who may have had similar exposure and need evaluation and treatment. Eliminating a source of contamination may prevent future exposures.[28]

### Insecticides

## Organophosphates

The patient should be decontaminated. Patients who are asymptomatic or only have minor symptoms should be closely observed. Individuals with muscarinic signs and symptoms of organophosphate poisoning are treated with atropine—very large doses may be required to reverse muscarinic symptoms. The most common life-threatening problem is respiratory arrest from bronchorrhea and diaphragmatic paralysis. The most reliable end point of adequate atropinization is control of bronchorrhea (drying of the secretions and clear lungs). Tachycardia before administration of atropine is not a contraindication to administration because early in the acute poisoning, stimulation of autonomic ganglionic nicotinic receptors can activate the sympathetic pathway resulting in transient tachycardia. Eventually stimulation of cardiac muscarinic receptors predominates, resulting in bradycardia.

Pralidoxime (2-PAM, Protopam) breaks the bond in the AChE-phosphate complex and should be used as an antidote for most clinically significant organophosphate poisonings. Pralidoxime affects nicotinic and muscarinic effects of organophosphates. The bond in the AChE-phosphate complex takes up to 24 hours to become an irreversible bond that pralidoxime cannot break. Thus it is important to administer pralidoxime early to prevent irreversible bonding and to preserve diaphragmatic function and prevent intubation. The neuromuscular junction is a nicotinic receptor and is unresponsive to atropine. A blood sample for cholinesterase activity should be obtained prior to administering pralidoxime, and it quickly reactivates the enzyme.[63] The decision to use pralidoxime should not await blood test results, but is based on the clinical picture of the patient.

## N-Methyl Carbamates

Treatment with atropine for carbamate poisoning is the same as for organophosphates. Pralidoxime therapy generally is unnecessary, and in some cases severe reactions and sudden death have occurred with its use.[64] In mixed poisonings involving organophosphates and carbamates or unidentified agents, cautious use of pralidoxime should be considered.

## Pyrethrum and Synthetic Pyrethroids

Generally, ingestion represents little risk. In extremely large ingestions, intubation and lavage may be advised. Dermal paresthesias should be treated with topical application of vitamin E oil preparations.

## Organochlorines

There is no specific antidote for poisoning from organochlorines. Treatment is symptomatic, with use of anticonvulsants for seizures and general supportive measures. Epinephrine is not advised for poisoning from organochlorines because of increased myocardial susceptibility to catecholamines and life-threatening dysrhythmias.

## Boric Acid and Borates

Skin, eye, and gastrointestinal decontamination are the principal treatments. Aggressive hydration, treatment of metabolic acidosis, and oxygenation can be critical to supportive care.

## *Herbicides*

### Glyphosate

There is no specific antidote for glyphosate poisoning. Treatment is supportive.

## Bipyridyl Herbicides (Paraquat and Diquat)

Hemoperfusion has been shown to be ineffective in reducing mortality. In paraquat poisoning, supplemental oxygen may increase lung damage and should be avoided if possible. Renal status should be closely monitored, particularly with diquat because dialysis may be required.

## Chlorophenoxy Herbicides

There is no specific antidote for poisoning from chlorophenoxy herbicides. The patient should be monitored for seizures and signs of multiple organ dysfunction (eg, gastrointestinal irritation or liver, kidney, and muscle damage). Alkalinization of the urine may enhance clearance.

## *Fungicides*

Treatment for fungicide poisoning is guided by the specific compound ingested. Generally decontamination and supportive care are the mainstays of treatment.

## *Rodenticides*

## Anticoagulants

Consulting with a poison control center can assist in determining the significance of the ingestion. In general, for one-time minor ingestions of warfarin-related or superwarfarin-related rodenticides in children younger than 6 years, no hospital visits, decontamination, or prothrombin time determinations are needed. The child should be observed at home, and a physician should be notified if bleeding or bruising occurs. More severe poisonings require monitoring of prothrombin time at 24 and 48 hours following ingestion. Phytonadione or Aquamephyton are appropriate agents for treatment of poisoning with the warfarins or superwarfarins. In several cases of poisoning with superwarfarins, treatment may need to continue for as long as 3 to 4 months.

## *Insect Repellents*

DEET

Treatment for poisoning from DEET is supportive. There is no specific antidote.

### Prevention: Reduction of Pesticide-Related Risks

With the exception of poison baits, as little as 1% of pesticides applied indoors reach the targeted pest. The rest may contaminate surfaces and air in the treated building. Outdoor pesticides may fall on non-targeted organisms, plants, animals, and outdoor furniture and play areas. In addition, material from the outdoor environment can be tracked indoors and add to exposure from dust, floors, and carpets.[65] They may contaminate groundwater, rivers, or wells.

Biomagnification of long-lasting compounds may result in exposure to animals (including humans) at the top of the food chain at concentrations tens of thousands of times greater than those at the bottom of the food chain.

Exposure assessment and counseling about safe practices should be a part of the health maintenance visit, especially for the children of farmworkers, pesticide applicators, and others who work with pesticides. The following safety precautions to safeguard the family's health should be stressed.

**Encourage Families to Avoid the Following Unsafe Pesticide Practices***

- Do not enter a field that has been posted with a sign indicating pesticide treatment. Treated fields should not be entered by anyone until pesticide dust has settled, plants are dry from spray, or the worker is wearing protective clothing.
- Do not use water in drainage ditches or any irrigation system for drinking, washing food or clothing, swimming, or fishing.
- Do not carry lunch or drinks into a treated field.
- Do not put pesticides in unmarked containers or food or drink jars.
- Never take pesticide containers home for use around the house. They are unsafe.
- Do not burn pesticide bags for fuel; they can give off poisonous fumes.
- Do not use pesticides from work around the house.

**Encourage Families to Use Safe Pesticide Practices**

- Wash work clothes separately from other laundry.
- Wash work clothes with detergent and hot water before wearing them again.
- Wash hands and arms after putting clothing into washing machine.
- Change clothing and wash with soap and water before picking up or playing with your children.
- Store pesticides in an area safe from children.
- Cover children's skin if they are with you at work.
- Keep the children and their toys and playthings indoors when there is nearby aerial spraying or spraying that may drift near the house.
- Children and teenagers should avoid work that involves mixing or spraying pesticides.

*Adapted from INFO Letter: Environmental and Occupational Health Briefs.[66]

## Integrated Pest Management

Integrated pest management is an increasingly useful approach to minimizing pesticide use while providing long-term pest control. It integrates chemical and nonchemical methods to provide the least toxic alternative for pest control. Integrated pest management uses regular monitoring to determine if and when treatments are needed. Management tactics include physical (eg, barriers, caulking), mechanical (eg, vacuuming up white flies), cultural (eg, choosing plants well suited to the site), biological (eg, using predators, pathogens such as *Bacillus thuringiensis,* and naturally occurring bacteria that kill insects), and educational (eg, cleaning up roach- and ant-attracting foods in the kitchen). Treatments are not made based on a predetermined schedule, but rather when monitoring indicates that the pest will cause unacceptable economic, medical, or aesthetic damage. Treatments are chosen and timed to be most effective and least hazardous to nontargeted organisms and the general environment.

Integrated pest management programs have been successfully adopted by personal homes, school systems, cities and counties (for parks and roadways), lawns, gardens, and farms across the United States and often have resulted in substantial cost savings. The national Parent Teacher Association passed a resolution to work toward pesticide-free schools.[67,68]

## Frequently Asked Questions

Q   *I am having pest problems in my lawn and garden. Should I get regular preventive applications by a professional service?*

A   Regular lawn treatment exposes people to pesticides unnecessarily. It also may kill insects that are beneficial in controlling the pest population, thereby requiring the use of more chemicals. If a professional lawn service is used, its personnel should (1) regularly monitor the lawn for pests and treat the lawn only when pests exist, (2) offer alternatives to the standard treatment, (3) give advance warning (including neighbors) before applying any pesticides (this allows time to cover outdoor furniture and remove toys and pet food dishes), (4) be trained and certified, (5) give advance notification of the types of chemicals to be used and information on their effects on health, and (6) avoid applications under adverse weather conditions (eg, high winds).

---

**Simple Steps That May Reduce the Need for Pesticides**

1. Grow plant varieties that grow well in the area. A county extension agent or nursery personnel may have advice.
2. Time the watering and fertilizing of the plants according to their needs.
3. Follow recommendations given for mowing grass and pruning plants.
4. Decide what degree of damage from weeds, insects, and diseases can be tolerated, and do not take control measures unless that degree is reached.
5. Consider nonchemical options first when controls are needed. For example, determine whether weeds can be removed by hoeing or pulling.

---

Q  *Is an insect repellent containing DEET safe for use on my children?*

A  Products containing DEET are the most effective mosquito repellents currently available.[69] DEET is also an effective repellent for a variety of other insect pests, including ticks. DEET should be used in areas where there is concern about illness from insect bites. It also can be used when insects are likely to be a nuisance, such as at barbecues or at the beach. While it generally is used without any problems, there have been rare reports of side effects. Usually these problems have occurred with inappropriate use. No definitive studies exist in the scientific literature about what concentration of DEET is safe for children.

The concentration of DEET in products may range from less than 10% to more than 30%. The efficacy of DEET plateaus at a concentration of 30%, the maximum concentration currently recommended for infants and children. The major difference in the efficacy of products relates to their duration of action. Products with concentrations around 10% are effective for periods of approximately 2 hours. As the concentration of DEET increases, the duration of activity increases; for example, a concentration of about 24% has recently been shown to provide an average of 5 hours of protection.

The safety of DEET does not seem to relate to differences in these concentrations. Thus products with a concentration of 30% appear to be as safe as products with a concentration of 10% when used according to the directions on the product labels. A prudent approach would be to select the lowest concentration effective for the amount of time spent outdoors. It is generally agreed that DEET should not be applied more than once a day.

There are no specific data on the skin absorption of DEET as a function of age. However, data on skin absorption of similar substances suggest that absorption through the skin would not differ after an infant has reached a month or 2 of age.[36] It is therefore recommended that DEET not be used for children younger than 2 months.

DEET should not be used in a product that combines the repellent with a sunscreen. Sunscreens are often applied repeatedly because they can be washed off. DEET is not water soluble and will last up to 8 hours. Repeated application may increase the potential toxic effects of DEET.

Q  *How do citronella and Skin So Soft compare to DEET as insect repellents?*

A  Citronella and Skin So Soft have mild repellent properties. DEET is significantly more effective. Therefore, when repellent is being used to prevent insect-borne infection (eg, Lyme disease or arthropod-borne encephalitis), DEET should be used.[69]

| Precautions When Using DEET |
|---|
| 1. Read and carefully follow all directions before using the product. Young children should not apply DEET to themselves. |
| 2. Wear long sleeves and pants when possible and apply repellent to clothing—a long-sleeved shirt with snug collar and cuffs is best. The shirt should be tucked in at the waist. Socks should be tucked over pants, hiking shoes, or boots. |
| 3. Apply DEET sparingly on exposed skin. Do not use DEET underneath clothing. |
| 4. Do not use DEET on the hands of young children. Avoid the eye and mouth areas. |
| 5. Do not apply DEET over cuts, wounds, or irritated skin. |
| 6. Wash treated skin with soap and water on returning indoors. Wash treated clothing. |
| 7. Avoid using sprays in enclosed areas. Do not use DEET near food. |
| 8. Wash the exposed area if an allergic reaction is suspected. |

Q  *We have rodents in and around our home. How can we safely get rid of them?*

A  Most pesticides for controlling rats (rodenticides) available for home use today are the anticoagulants warfarin or superwarfarin (coumarins) or indanediones. They kill the rodents by causing internal bleeding. These anticoagulants also can cause bleeding in children if ingested and therefore must be used carefully. Each year, more than 10 000 children are exposed to these products, making anticoagulant baits one of the most common pesticide ingestions in children younger than 6 years. Fortunately, the amounts usually eaten by young children rarely cause serious injury. Poisoning can be avoided by following the product label and using common sense. Contact your physician or poison control center or the emergency department of the nearest hospital immediately if it is suspected that a child may have ingested a product containing anticoagulants. Alternatives to rodenticides include careful sealing of cracks and crevices, cleaning up brush and debris from outdoor areas where rats may hide, and careful sanitation to leave no food scraps for rodents to eat. Mechanical traps can be effective for controlling a minor rodent problem. These can include snap traps or glue traps. The latter are less likely to cause injuries to small children who might come into contact with the traps.

---

**Measures That May Reduce the Danger of Exposure**

1. Place all rodenticides out of the reach of children and nontarget animals or in tamper-proof bait boxes. Outdoors, place bait inside the entrance of a burrow and then collapse the entrance over the bait.
2. Securely lock or fasten shut the lids of all bait boxes.
3. Place bait in the baffle-protected feeding chamber, never in the runway of the box.
4. Always use sanitation measures in conjunction with pesticides to limit rodent access to food and hiding places. Work with neighbors to secure the neighborhood. If baiting alone is used without sanitation measures, the rodent population will rebound each time the baiting stops. Measures include using rat-proof garbage cans and food storage precautions (including keeping food in the refrigerator), and frequently raking up garden waste (including fallen fruit).

---

| Measures That May Reduce the Danger of Exposure, *continued* |
| --- |
| 5. Modify the habitat by rat-proofing buildings and changing landscaping to eliminate hiding places. |
| 6. Continue to monitor periodically to ensure that rats are not recolonizing. |

Q  *What is the best way to treat my roach problem?*

A  Hygiene measures are key. Cockroaches are found where there is water and food. Eating should be discouraged in areas other than the kitchen. All foodstuffs should be stored in closed containers. Water sources should be eliminated by caulking cracks around faucets and pipe fittings. Cracks and crevices where cockroaches can enter the home should be sealed.

A prudent approach is to minimize exposure to sprays whenever possible. Individual bait stations are recommended. If possible, baiting should be done outside the home as well. Boric acid, formulated for use as a pesticide, is comparatively less toxic than cholinesterase inhibitors and pyrethroids, and may be used in cracks and crevices in areas inaccessible to children.

If these measures are not successful, the family should consult a professional exterminator. If professional extermination is to be done, be certain that this is a licensed firm and find out what insecticide will be used and its possible toxic effects. Before use of any insecticide in the home, all food, dishes, cooking utensils, children's toys, and clothing should be removed or protected from contamination. After application of the insecticide, young children and pregnant women should stay out of the area for as long as possible. The room should be aired well by cross ventilation for 4 to 8 hours before people and pets return. Crawling babies should not be allowed in the area until it has been well vacuumed or mopped and the resident can be certain that the pesticide was not applied in an area where the infant can reach. For example, if the pesticide is applied to the wall, a crawling infant could hold onto the wall or wipe his hands and sustain a significant exposure.

Families should avoid using over-the-counter bug sprays and bug bombs. *The Cockroach Control Manual,* an excellent resource, is available from the University of Nebraska. It includes complete information on an integrative pest management approach including "least toxic methods." It is available for purchase or free download at http://pested.unl.edu/cocktoc.htm.

## Resources

Extoxnet, Internet: http://ace.ace.orst.edu/info/extoxnet, a cooperative effort among the University of California at Davis, Oregon State University, Michigan State University, and Cornell University that provides updated pesticide information in understandable terms. It includes toxicology briefs and information on carcinogenicity, testing, and exposure assessment.

National Center for Environmental Assessment Publications and Information, phone: 513-489-8190, offers free fact sheets on lawn care, pesticide labels, and pesticide safety

National Pesticide Information Center, phone for health professionals: 800-858-7377, phone for general public: 800-858-7378, Internet: http://npic.orst.edu/index.html

Pesticide Educational Center, phone: 415-665-4722

Texas Agricultural Extension Service, Internet: http://www-aes.tamu.edu/doug/med/pgpp.htm, Physician's Guide to Pesticide Poisoning

Toxnet, Internet: http://toxnet.nlm.nih.gov/, a cluster of databases on toxicology, hazardous chemicals, and related areas

University of Nebraska Cooperative Extension, Signs and Symptoms of Pesticide Poisoning. Internet: http://www.ianr.unl.edu/pubs/ pesticides/ec2505.htm

US Environmental Protection Agency, Internet: http://www.epa.gov/
- *Recognition and Management of Pesticide Poisonings.* 5th ed, available at: http://www.epa.gov/oppfead1/safety/healthcare/ handbook/handbook.htm (available in English and Spanish)
- EPA online resources in case of suspected pesticide poisoning: http://www.epa.gov/oppfead1/safety/incaseof.htm http://www.epa.gov/oppfead1/safety/resource.htm
- EPA Office of Pesticide Programs, Communication Services Branch, National Pesticide Hotline: 800-535-PEST, general information phone: 703-305-5017, Internet: http://www.epa.gov/pesticides (general information)
- EPA pamphlets
  - *Citizen's Guide to Pest Control and Pesticide Safety*
  - *Pest Control in the School Environment*
  - *Healthy Lawn, Healthy Environment*

## References

1. Aspelin AL, Grube AH. *Pesticide Industry Sales and Usage: 1996 and 1997 Market Estimates.* Research Triangle Park, NC: US Environmental Protection Agency, Office of Pesticide Programs; 1999. Available at: http://www.epa.gov/oppbead1/pestsales/97pestsales/table_of_ contents1997.html
2. Lu C, Fenske RA, Simcox NJ, Kalman D. Pesticide exposure of children in an agricultural community: evidence of household proximity to farmland and take home exposure pathways. *Environ Res.* 2000;84:290–302
3. Fenske RA, Kissel JC, Lu C, et al. Biologically based pesticide dose estimates for children in an agricultural community. *Environ Health Perspect.* 2000;108:515–520
4. Food Quality Protection Act of 1996. Pub L No 104-170, 110 Stat 1489
5. California Health and Safety Code. State of California Assembly Bill 2318, §111246(2000)

6. Goldbloom RB, Goldbloom A. Boric acid poisoning: report of four cases and a review of 109 cases from the world literature. *J Pediatr.* 1953;43:631–643

7. Wong LC, Heimbach MD, Truscott DR, Duncan BD. Boric acid poisoning: report of 11 cases. *Can Med Assoc J.* 1964;90:1018–1023

8. Litovitz TL, Klein-Schwartz W, White S, et al. 1999 annual report of the American Association of Poison Control Centers Toxic Exposure Surveillance System. *Am J Emerg Med.* 2000;18:517–574

9. Ellenhorn MJ, Schonwald S, Ordog G, Wasserberger J. Pesticides. In: *Ellenhorn's Medical Toxicology: Diagnosis and Treatment of Human Poisoning.* 2nd ed. Baltimore, MD: Williams and Wilkins; 1997:1614–1663

10. Brown M, Hebert AA. Insect repellents: an overview. *J Am Acad Dermatol.* 1997;36:243–249

11. Lu C, Knutson DE, Fisker-Andersen J, Fenske RA. Biological monitoring survey of organophosphorus pesticide exposure among pre-school children in the Seattle metropolitan area. *Environ Health Perspect.* 2001;109:299–303

12. Faustman EM, Silbernagel SM, Fenske RA, Burbacher TM, Ponce RA. Mechanisms underlying children's susceptibility to environmental toxicants. *Environ Health Perspect.* 2000;108(suppl 1):13–21

13. Whyatt RM, Barr DB. Measurement of organophosphate metabolites in postpartum meconium as a potential biomarker of prenatal exposure: a validation study. *Environ Health Perspect.* 2001;109:417–420

14. Whitmore RW, Kelly JE, Reading PL. *National Home and Garden Pesticide Survey: Final Report, Volume 1.* Research Triangle Park, NC: Research Triangle Institute; 1992. Publication RTI/5100/17-01F

15. US Environmental Protection Agency, Office of Water. *A Review of Contaminant Occurrence in Public Water Systems.* Washington, DC: US Environmental Protection Agency; 1999. EPA Publication 816-R-99-006

16. Longnecker MP, Klebanoff MA, Zhou H, Brock JW. Association between maternal serum concentration of the DDT metabolite DDE and preterm and small-for-gestational-age babies at birth. *Lancet.* 2001;358:110–114

17. Garry VF, Schreinemachers D, Harkins ME, Griffith J. Pesticide appliers, biocides, and birth defects in rural Minnesota. *Environ Health Perspect.* 1996;104:394–399

18. Bell EM, Hertz-Picciotto I, Beaumont JJ. A case-control study of pesticides and fetal death due to congenital anomalies. *Epidemiology.* 2001;12:148–156

19. Arbuckle TE, Lin Z, Mery LS. An exploratory analysis of the effect of pesticide exposure on the risk of spontaneous abortion in an Ontario farm population. *Environ Health Perspect.* 2001;109:851–857

20. Reigart JR, Roberts JR. *Recognition and Management of Pesticide Poisonings.* 5th ed. Washington, DC: US Environmental Protection Agency; 1999

21. Zwiener RJ, Ginsburg CM. Organophosphate and carbamate poisoning in infants and children. *Pediatrics.* 1988;81:121–126

22. Sofer S, Tal A, Shahak E. Carbamate and organophosphate poisoning in early childhood. *Pediatr Emerg Care.* 1989;5:222–225

23. Wagner SL. Fatal asthma in a child after use of an animal shampoo containing pyrethrin. *West J Med.* 2000;173:86–87

24. Tangermann RH, Etzel RA, Mortimer L, Penner GD, Paschal DG. An outbreak of a food-related illness resembling boric acid poisoning. *Arch Environ Contam Toxicol.* 1992;23:142–144

25. Menkes DB, Temple WA, Edwards IR. Intentional self-poisoning with glyphosate-containing herbicides. *Hum Exp Toxicol.* 1991;10:103–107

26. Talbot AR, Shiaw MH, Huang JS, et al. Acute poisoning with a glyphosate-surfactant herbicide (Roundup): a review of 93 cases. *Hum Exp Toxicol.* 1991;10:1–8

27. O'Malley M. Clinical evaluation of pesticide exposure and poisonings. *Lancet.* 1997;349:1161–1166

28. American Academy of Pediatrics Committee on Injury and Poison Prevention. Rodgers GC Jr, ed. *Handbook of Common Poisonings in Children.* 3rd ed. Elk Grove Village, IL: American Academy of Pediatrics; 1994

29. Kelce WR, Monosson E, Gamcsik MP, Laws SC, Gray LE Jr. Environmental hormone disruptors: evidence that vinclozolin developmental toxicity is mediated by antiandrogenic metabolites. *Toxicol Appl Pharmacol.* 1994;126:276–285

30. Litovitz T, Manoguerra A. Comparison of pediatric poisoning hazards: an analysis of 3.8 million exposure incidents. A report from the American Association of Poison Control Centers. *Pediatrics.* 1992;89:999–1006

31. Litovitz TL, Klein-Schwartz W, Dyer KS, Shannon M, Lee S, Powers M. 1997 annual report of the American Association of Poison Control Centers Toxic Exposure Surveillance System. *Am J Emerg Med.* 1998;16:443–497

32. Selim S, Hartnagel RE Jr, Osimitz TG, Gabriel KL, Schoenig GP. Absorption, metabolism, and excretion of N,N-diethyl-m-toluamide following dermal application to human volunteers. *Fundam Appl Toxicol.* 1995;25:95–100

33. Gryboski J, Weinstein D, Ordway N. Toxic encephalopathy apparently related to the use of an insect repellent. *N Engl J Med.* 1961;264:289–291

34. Centers for Disease Control and Prevention. Seizures temporally associated with use of DEET insect repellent—New York and Connecticut. *MMWR Morb Mortal Wkly Rep.* 1989;38:678–680

35. Veltri JC, Osimitz TG, Bradford DC, Page BC. Retrospective analysis of calls to poison control centers resulting from exposure to the insect repellent N,N-diethyl-m-toluamide (DEET) from 1985–1989. *J Toxicol Clin Toxicol.* 1994;32:1–16

36. Osimitz TG, Murphy JV. Neurological effects associated with use of the insect repellent N,N-diethyl-m-toluamide (DEET). *J Toxicol Clin Toxicol.* 1997;35:435–441

37. Garrettson L. DEET: caution for children still needed [commentary]. *J Toxicol Clin Toxicol.* 1997;35:443–445

38. National Research Council. *Pesticides in the Diets of Infants and Children.* Washington, DC: National Academies Press; 1993

39. Schettler T, Stein J, Reich F, Valenti M. *In Harm's Way: Toxic Threats to Child Development.* Cambridge, MA: Greater Boston Physicians for Social Responsibility; 2000

40. Vonier PM, Crain DA, McLachlan JA, Guillette LJ Jr, Arnold SF. Interaction of environmental chemicals with the estrogen and progesterone receptors from the oviduct of the American alligator. *Environ Health Perspect.* 1996;104:1318–1322

41. Lerda D, Rizzi R. Study of reproductive function in persons occupationally exposed to 2,4-dichlorophenoxyacetic acid (2,4-D). *Mutat Res.* 1991;262:47–50

42. Steenland K, Jenkins B, Ames RG, O'Malley M, Chrislip D, Russo J. Chronic neurological sequelae to organophosphate pesticide poisoning. *Am J Public Health.* 1994;84:731–736

43. Savage EP, Keefe TJ, Mounce LM, Heaton RK, Lewis JA, Burcar PJ. Chronic neurological sequelae of acute organophosphate pesticide poisoning. *Arch Environ Health.* 1988;43:38–45

44. Wagner SL, Orwick DL. Chronic organophosphate exposure associated with transient hypertonia in an infant. *Pediatrics.* 1994;94:94–97

45. Keifer MC, Mahurin RK. Chronic neurologic effects of pesticide overexposure. *Occup Med.* 1997;12:291–304

46. Steenland K, Dick RB, Howell RJ, et al. Neurologic function among termiticide applicators exposed to chlorpyrifos. *Environ Health Perspect.* 2000;108:293–300

47. Jamal GA. Neurological syndromes of organophosphorus compounds. *Adverse Drug React Toxicol Rev.* 1997;16:133–170

48. Fiedler N, Kipen H, Kelly-McNeil K, Fenske R. Long-term use of organophosphates and neuropsychological performance. *Am J Ind Med.* 1997;32:487–496

49. Ahlbom J, Fredriksson A, Eriksson P. Exposure to an organophosphate (DFP) during a defined period in neonatal life induces permanent changes in brain muscarinic receptors and behaviour in adult mice. *Brain Res.* 1995;677:13–19

50. Ahlbom J, Fredriksson A, Eriksson P. Neonatal exposure to a type-I pyrethroid (bioallethrin) induces dose-response changes in brain muscarinic receptors and behaviour in neonatal and adult mice. *Brain Res.* 1994;645:318–324

51. Brimijoin S, Koenigsberger C. Cholinesterases in neural development: new findings and toxicologic implications. *Environ Health Perspect.* 1999;107(suppl 1):59–64

52. Qiao D, Seidler FJ, Slotkin TA. Developmental neurotoxicity of chlorpyrifos modeled in vitro: comparative effects of metabolites and other cholinesterase inhibitors on DNA synthesis in PC12 and C6 cells. *Environ Health Perspect.* 2001;109:909–913

53. Guillette EA, Meza MM, Aquilar MG, Soto AD, Garcia IE. An anthropological approach to the evaluation of preschool children exposed to pesticides in Mexico. *Environ Health Perspect.* 1998;106:347–353

54. US Environmental Protection Agency, Office of Pesticide Programs. List of chemicals evaluated for carcinogenic potential. Washington, DC: US Environmental Protection Agency; 2000. Available at: http://www.epa.gov/pesticides/carlist

55. Kristensen P, Andersen A, Irgens LM, Bye AS, Sundheim L. Cancer in offspring of parents engaged in agricultural activities in Norway: incidence and risk factors in the farm environment. *Int J Cancer.* 1996;65:39–50

56. Alexander FE, Patheal SL, Biondi A, et al. Transplacental chemical exposure and risk of infant leukemia with MLL gene fusion. *Cancer Res.* 2001;61:2542–2546

57. Buckley JD, Meadows AT, Kadin ME, LeBeau MM, Siegel S, Robinson LL. Pesticide exposures in children with non-Hodgkin lymphoma. *Cancer.* 2000;89:2315–2321

58. Zahm SH, Ward MH. Pesticides and childhood cancer. *Environ Health Perspect.* 1998;106(suppl 3):893–908

59. Davis JR, Brownson RC, Garcia R, Bentz BJ, Turner A. Family pesticide use and childhood brain cancer. *Arch Environ Contam Toxicol.* 1993;24:87–92

60. Fontana A, Picoco C, Masala G, Prastaro C, Vineisx P. Incidence rates of lymphomas and environmental measurements of phenoxy herbicides: ecological analysis and case-control study. *Arch Environ Health.* 1998;53:384–387

61. Zahm SH. Mortality study of pesticide applicators and other employees of a lawn care service company. *J Occup Environ Med.* 1997;39:1055–1067

62. Lessenger JE, Estock MD, Younglove T. An analysis of 190 cases of suspected pesticide illness. *J Am Board Fam Pract.* 1995;8:278–282

63. Cholinesterase-inhibiting pesticide toxicity. In: Wagner S, ed. *Case Studies in Environmental Medicine.* Atlanta, GA: Agency for Toxic Substances and Disease Registry; 1993

64. Kurtz PH. Pralidoxime in the treatment of carbamate intoxication. *Am J Emerg Med.* 1990;8:68–70

65. Nishioka MG, Lewis RG, Brinkman MC, Burkholder HM, Hines CE, Menkedick JR. Distribution of 2,4-D in air and on surfaces inside residences after lawn applications: comparing exposure estimates from various media for young children. *Environ Health Perspect.* 2001;109:1185–1191

66. INFO Letter: Environmental and Occupational Health Briefs. Vol. 9, No. 4. Piscataway, NJ: Environmental and Health Risk Communications Division; 1996

67. Child Proofing our Communities Campaign. *Poisoned Schools: Invisible Threats, Visible Actions.* Falls Church, VA: Center for Health, Environment, and Justice; 2001

68. Rose RI. Pesticides and public health: integrated methods of mosquito management. *Emerg Infect Dis.* 2001;7:17–23

69. Fradin MS, Day JF. Comparative efficacy of insect repellents against mosquito bites. *N Engl J Med.* 2002;347:13–18

# 25
# Polychlorinated Biphenyls, Dibenzofurans, and Dibenzodioxins

Polychlorinated biphenyls (PCBs) are compounds with 2 linked phenyl rings and variable degrees of chlorination. They are clear, nonvolatile, hydrophobic oils that resist metabolism and persist in the environment. About 1.5 million metric tons were produced starting in the 1930s. They were banned in the United States and northern Europe in the late 1970s. Much of what was made is still somewhere in the environment. The PCBs were used primarily in the electrical industry as insulators and dielectrics, especially for applications in which a fire hazard was present, such as in heavy transformers. During the 1960s, analytical chemists interested in dichlorodiphenyl-trichloroethane (DDT) residues in the tissues of pelagic birds began identifying background peaks in their chromatograms as PCBs. Since then, numerous studies throughout the world have shown detectable levels of PCBs in human tissue and human milk; except for DDT and its analogues, PCBs are the most dispersed of the halogenated hydrocarbon pollutant chemicals.[1]

Polychlorinated dibenzofurans (PCDFs) are partially oxidized PCBs. They were not made intentionally but appear as contaminants in PCBs that have undergone high temperature applications or have been in fires or explosions. Polychlorinated dibenzodioxins (PCDDs), commonly referred to as dioxins, also are contaminants. These compounds were formed during the manufacture of hexachlorophene, pentachlorophenol, and the phenoxyacid herbicides 2,4,5 trichloro-phenoxyacetic acid (a component of Agent Orange) and silvex, under what would now be considered poorly controlled conditions. They also are formed, albeit at very low yield, during paper bleaching and waste incineration. One dioxin congener, 2,3,7,8-tetrachlorodibenzo-p-dioxin (TCDD), may be the most toxic synthetic chemical known.[2]

## Routes and Sources of Exposure

Children may be exposed through ingestion, inhalation, and dermal exposure. Dermal exposure poses less risk because PCBs are incompletely absorbed through the skin. The source of exposure for most people to all of these compounds is contaminated food. Because the chemicals are not well metabolized or excreted, even very small daily doses accumulate to measurable amounts over years. The most concentrated source is sport fish from contaminated waters because the residues bioconcentrate and fish usually is the food at the highest trophic level consumed by humans. Bioconcentration also increases exposure for the Arctic Inuit who eat blubber of sea mammals, themselves fish eaters.[3] In certain areas of the Arctic, dietary intakes of PCBs exceed established national and international guidelines.[4] In areas where PCB contamination has been a problem, state and local health departments have issued advisories that recommend limiting the consumption of contaminated fish. The major dietary source for young children is human milk, from which they absorb and store these chemicals (see Chapter 3).

Predictable occupational exposure to these compounds is now rare and would be most likely for those involved in the cleanup of hazardous waste sites or repair work for electrical utilities. Heavy electrical equipment produced decades ago still is in service, and transformers may leak or become damaged during fires or explosions, thus exposing workers and the environment to PCBs or PCDFs. Substantial quantities of PCBs still are present in older industrial facilities other than electric utilities, such as railroads. Modern herbicides are not contaminated with PCDDs, and while there is exposure from waste incineration and paper bleaching, the amounts are very small.

## Systems Affected and Clinical Effects

Exposure to commonly encountered levels of PCBs is associated with lower developmental/IQ test scores, including lower psychomotor scores from the newborn period through 2 years of age,[5] defects in short-term memory in 7-month-olds[6] and 4-year-olds,[7] and lowered IQs in 42-month-olds[8,9] and 11-year-olds.[10] Prenatal exposure to PCBs from the mother's body burden, rather than exposure through human milk, seems to account for most, but not all,[9] of the findings. There also may be subclinical effects on thyroid function in the newborn.[11] The results of studies on birth weight and low-dose exposure have been inconsistent. See Table 25.1 for a list of reported signs and symptoms by age at occurrence.

Two mass poisonings have occurred in Asia in which cooking oil was inadvertently mixed with PCBs that were heat-degraded, and thus heavily contaminated with PCDFs. In 1968 an epidemic of acne among residents of Kyusha province in Japan was traced to the use of such cooking oil. About 2000 people were eventually given the diagnosis of *Yusho* (oil disease).[12] Among 13 women who were pregnant around the time of exposure, one of the children was stillborn and was deeply and diffusely pigmented (a "cola-colored" baby). Some of the live-born children were small, hyperbilirubinemic, and pigmented and had conjunctival swelling with dilatation of the sebaceous glands of the eyelid. Follow-up of the children up to 9 years later showed apathy, lethargy, and soft neurologic signs. The growth deficit apparent at birth resolved by about 4 years of age. An extraordinarily similar outbreak occurred in Taiwan in 1979.[13] In Taiwan, 117 children who were born during or after the food contamination in 1979 and thus exposed to their mothers' body burden of PCBs and PCDFs were examined in 1985[14] and have been followed since. They have a variety of ectodermal defects, such as excess pigmentation, carious teeth, poor nail formation, and short stature. They have persistent behavioral abnormalities[15] and cognitive impairment, on the average about 5 to 8 IQ

**Table 25.1**
**Reported Signs and Symptoms by Age at Occurrence From PCBs, PCDFs, PCDDs, and TCDD\***

| Prenatal Exposure to Low Levels of PCBs | |
|---|---|
| • Newborns | Decrease in birth weight |
| • Infants | Motor delay detectable from age newborn to 2 years |
| • 7-month-olds | Defects in visual recognition memory |
| • 42-month-olds | Lower IQ (may be some contribution from postnatal exposure) |
| • 4-year-olds | Defects in short-term memory |
| • 11-year-olds | Delays in cognitive development |
| **Prenatal Exposure to High Levels of PCBs/PCDFs (Asian Poisonings)** | |
| • Newborns | Low birth weight, conjunctivitis, natal teeth, pigmentation |
| • Infant through school age | Delays on all cognitive domains tested; behavior disorder; growth retardation; abnormal development of hair, nails, and teeth; pigmentation; increased risk of bronchitis |
| • Puberty | Small penis size but normal development in boys; growth delay but normal development in girls |
| **Direct Ingestion of High Doses of PCBs/PCDFs** | |
| • Any age | Chloracne, keratoses, and pigmentation; mixed peripheral neuropathy; gastritis |
| **Dermal Exposure to High Levels of TCDD** | |
| • Children | Probably higher absorbed dose for a given exposure than adults, chloracne, liver function test abnormalities |

\*PCBs, polychlorinated biphenyls; PCDFs, polychlorinated dibenzofurans; PCDDs, polychlorinated dibenzodioxins; TCDD, 2,3,7,8-tetrachlorobenzo-p-dioxin.

points. Furthermore, the delay is as severe in children born up to 6 years after exposure as it is in those born in 1979.[16]

A chemical plant explosion released kilogram quantities of TCDD in Seveso, Italy, in 1975. The highest recorded serum levels of TCDD in humans occurred in children in the most heavily exposed areas in this incident.[17] Children in the area near the explosion had chloracne, most pronounced on areas unprotected by clothing,[18] and some had abnormal liver function tests.[19] In Vietnam, spraying with Agent

Orange during the Vietnam War has left a legacy of TCDD contamination still detectable in breast milk.[20] There are anecdotal reports of toxicity in the children, but no systematic study has been reported. The offspring of male Vietnam veterans, who may have had exposure from Agent Orange, show no clear excess of malformations[21]; no data are available on the offspring of female veterans.

Studies assessing the carcinogenic potential of PCBs in animals and humans have shown inconsistent results.[22]

## Diagnostic Methods

Although many laboratories can measure PCBs, there are no agreed-on methods, quality assurance programs, or reference values available, and no laboratory is licensed to measure these chemicals for diagnostic or therapeutic use. Thus any measurement would have to be regarded as research and would be interpretable only within a research project. The PCDFs and PCDDs are much more difficult to measure, and no clinical interpretation is available if the measurement is done. Because any of these compounds can appear in human milk, it occasionally seems useful to measure them in a clinical setting. However, any reasonably sensitive method will detect PCBs in most samples of human milk. Thus far all expert bodies that have considered this topic recommend breastfeeding and do not recommend testing of milk. More information is included in Chapter 3.

## Treatment

No regimen is known to lower body burden of these compounds. In Asia, treatments that have been tried include cholestyramine, sauna bathing, and fasting, none of which work. Breastfeeding does lower the levels, by about 20% for each 6 months of lactation. Theoretically, this would increase the risk to the child, but so far the morbidity attributable to exposure to these compounds has come from prenatal exposure to maternal body burden rather than from exposure through breast milk (see Chapter 3).

## Regulation

Polychlorinated biphenyls are banned from new production throughout the world. Any waste substance, commonly waste oils, with more than 50 ppm of PCBs must be handled as a hazardous substance and disposed of as hazardous waste. Polychlorinated biphenyls are unavoidable contaminants of foods, and so have "temporary tolerances," which are levels that, if found in a food in commerce, result in a requirement from the US Food and Drug Administration that the food be removed from the market. For infant and junior foods, the tolerance is 1.5 ppm fat basis for PCBs; for fish, it is 5 ppm fat basis. There are no tolerances for PCDFs or PCDDs.

The Food and Agriculture Organization and the World Health Organization (WHO) publish "allowable daily intakes." For PCBs, the allowable daily intake is 6 µg/kg per day, which is about the median for a fully breastfed 5-kg infant. There are no allowable daily intakes for PCDDs or PCDFs. There is a "tolerable daily intake" (reflecting greater uncertainty in the data) of 4 pg/kg per day of toxic equivalents of TCDD. Note that, although intake by breastfed children might commonly exceed this level, the WHO explicitly advised there to be no change in the organization's policy to recommend breastfeeding despite the presence of the pollutant chemicals.[23]

The concept of "toxic equivalency" arises out of the dilemma faced by those who regulate these compounds. Exposure to a single compound of this class is unusual; rather, most human exposure is to mixtures of dozens or more of these compounds. Many PCBs, PCDFs, and dioxins other than TCDD have a spectrum of toxic effects similar to that of TCDD, but the doses at which they produce those effects vary over orders of magnitude, with TCDD being the most potent. Much if not all of the toxicity of TCDD is thought to begin when it binds to the aryl hydrocarbon hydroxylase (Ah) receptor. There are assays available that measure receptor binding, thus a given compound can be compared to TCDD in terms of its abilities to bind to the receptor. The ratio of receptor binding can be used as a conversion factor to estimate the toxicity of a compound relative to TCDD; multiplying the amount of the compound times its conversion factor yields a "toxic equivalent" (TEQ) amount of TCDD. The conversion factors are thus called "toxic equivalency factors." They can be calculated for any compound that binds to the Ah receptor. The TEQ for a mixture can be estimated by adding the TEQs for the individual compounds present. The 1998 revision of the tolerable daily intake for TCDD was the first time that it was expressed in TEQs, rather than as an amount of TCDD per se. This makes biological sense because the typical diet contains more TEQs from compounds other than TCDD, especially PCBs, than from TCDD itself, thus it makes little sense to consider only part of a mixture of compounds with similar toxicity. On the other hand, there are other forms of toxicity that some of these compounds possess, such as neurotoxicity, that are not related to Ah receptor binding, and thus will not be captured by the TEQ approach. Nonetheless, using TEQs to think about the problem of mixtures of compounds with relatively similar toxicity seems like a step in the right direction, recognizing that the toxicology of mixtures in general is not well understood and a great deal of work will be necessary before it is understood. There is a good discussion of the use of toxic equivalency in the documents supporting the 1998 tolerable daily intake recommendation for TCDD.[22]

## Alternatives

Polychlorinated biphenyls have been replaced mostly by mineral oils. Polychlorinated dibenzodioxins and PCDFs were never made deliberately, and no product is now contaminated at the levels seen during the 1960s.

## Frequently Asked Questions

Q *Should I be concerned about dioxins in coffee filters, diapers, tampons, etc?*

A Paper products usually are bleached by using chlorine bleaches. The reaction between the chlorine and the lignins in the wood fiber produces many complex chlorinated organic compounds, among them TCDD. The amounts are minuscule, and avoiding products that have been bleached using chlorine is unlikely to produce a discernable health benefit. Unbleached products, or products bleached using oxygen, are sometimes available and can be substituted. They should be free of such residues.

Q *How do I know whether fish or other foods have PCBs or dioxins in them?*

A The food supply has trace amounts of all of these compounds. Commercial foods are regulated, and so should not have more than minimal amounts. Among unregulated foods, the most likely source of higher exposure is sport fish. States in which these compounds have been a problem, such as those around the Great Lakes, have advisories concerning the consumption of noncommercial fish, and these should be available from the state health department.

Q *If PCBs were banned in the 1970s and are no longer produced, why are they still a problem?*

A Polychlorinated biphenyls and compounds like them were used and dispersed at a time when their persistence seemed to be desirable and the consequences of that persistence unappreciated. Polychlorinated biphenyls and DDT break down either very slowly or not at all in the environment. Parts of the Great Lakes and the Hudson River still have sludge heavily contaminated by PCBs that were probably made in the 1960s. Compounds with this degree of persistence are no longer used for applications that allow such pollution to occur, but the amounts in the environment when the ban occurred were sufficient to produce contaminated sediment for subsequent decades, with no clear end in sight.

## Resource

US Environmental Protection Agency (EPA), Internet: http://www.epa.gov/OST/fish. This Web address lists EPA guidelines for states for the development of fish advisories for PCBs and other persistent contaminants.

## References

1. World Health Organization. *Polychlorinated Biphenyls and Terphenyls.* 2nd ed. Environmental Health Criteria, 140. Geneva, Switzerland: World Health Organization; 1993

2. Dioxin's lethality compared to other poisons. *Chemical and Engineering News.* June 6, 1983;45

3. Dewailly E, Nantel A, Weber JP, Meyer F. High levels of PCBs in breast milk of Inuit women from arctic Quebec. *Bull Environ Contam Toxicol.* 1989;43:641–646

4. Hansen JC, Reiersen LO, Wilson S. Arctic Monitoring and Assessment Programme (AMAP): strategy and results with focus on the human health assessment under the second phase of AMAP, 1998–2003. *Int J Circumpolar Health.* 2002;61:300–318

5. Rogan WJ, Gladen BC. PCBs, DDE, and child development at 18 and 24 months. *Ann Epidemiol.* 1991;1:407–413

6. Jacobson SW, Fein GG, Jacobson JL, Schwartz PM, Dowler JK. The effect of intrauterine PCB exposure on visual recognition memory. *Child Dev.* 1985;56:853–860

7. Jacobson JL, Jacobson SW, Humphrey HE. Effects of in utero exposure to polychlorinated biphenyls and related contaminants on cognitive functioning in young children. *J Pediatr.* 1990;116:38–45

8. Patandin S, Lanting CI, Mulder PG, Boersma ER, Sauer PJ, Weisglas-Kuperus N. Effects of environmental exposure to polychlorinated biphenyls and dioxins on cognitive abilities in Dutch children at 42 months of age. *J Pediatr.* 1999;134:33–41

9. Walkowiak J, Wiener JA, Fastabend A, et al. Environmental exposure to polychlorinated biphenyls and quality of the home environment: effects on psychodevelopment in early childhood. *Lancet.* 2001;358:1602–1607

10. Jacobson JL, Jacobson SW. Intellectual impairment in children exposed to polychlorinated biphenyls in utero. *N Engl J Med.* 1996;335:783–789

11. Brouwer A, Longnecker MP, Birnbaum LS, et al. Characterization of potential endocrine-related health effects at low-dose levels of exposure to PCBs. *Environ Health Perspect.* 1999;107(suppl 4):639–649

12. Kuratsune M. Yusho, with reference to Yu-Cheng. In: Kimbrough RD, Jensen AA, eds. *Halogenated Biphenyls, Terphenyls, Naphthalenes, Dibenzodioxins, and Related Products, Topics in Environmental Health.* 2nd rev ed. Amsterdam, The Netherlands: Elsevier, 1989:381–400

13. Hsu ST, Ma CI, Hsu SK, Wu SS, Hsu NH, Yeh CC. Discovery and epidemiology of PCB poisoning in Taiwan. *Am J Ind Med.* 1984;5:71–79

14. Rogan WJ, Gladen BC, Hung KL, et al. Congenital poisoning by polychlorinated biphenyls and their contaminants in Taiwan. *Science.* 1988;241:334–346

15. Chen YC, Yu ML, Rogan WJ, Gladen BC, Hsu CC. A 6-year follow-up of behavior and activity disorders in the Taiwan Yu-Cheng children. *Am J Public Health.* 1994;84:415–421

16. Chen YC, Guo YL, Hsu CC, Rogan WJ. Cognitive development of Yu-Cheng ("oil disease") children prenatally exposed to heat-degraded PCBs. *JAMA.* 1992;268:3213–3218

17. Mocarelli P, Needham LL, Moracchi A, et al. Serum concentrations of 2,3,7,8-tetrachlorodibenzo-p-dioxin and test results from selected residents of Seveso, Italy. *J Toxicol Environ Health.* 1991;32:357–366

18. Caramaschi F, del Corno G, Favaretti C, Giambelluca SE, Montesarchio E, Fara GM. Chloracne following environmental contamination by TCDD in Seveso, Italy. *Int J Epidemiol.* 1981;10:135–143

19. Mocarelli P, Marocchi A, Brambilla P, Gerthoux P, Young DS, Mantel N. Clinical laboratory manifestations of exposure to dioxin in children. A six-year study of the effects of an environmental disaster near Seveso, Italy. *JAMA.* 1986;256:2687–2695

20. Schecter A, Dai LC, Thuy LT, et al. Agent Orange and the Vietnamese: the persistence of elevated dioxin levels in human tissues. *Am J Public Health.* 1995;85:516–522

21. Erickson JD, Mulinare J, McClain PW, et al. Vietnam veterans' risks for fathering babies with birth defects. *JAMA.* 1984;252:903–912

22. Cogliano VJ. Assessing the cancer risk from environmental PCBs. *Environ Health Perspect.* 1998;106:317–323

23. Consultation on assessment of the health risk of dioxins; re-evaluation of the tolerable daily intake (TDI): executive summary. *Food Addit Contam.* 2000;17:223–240

# 26
# Ultraviolet Light

The sun is responsible for life on earth because of its essential role in photosynthesis. The infrared portion of the sun provides warmth to humans. Sunlight drives biological rhythms and promotes feelings of well-being. Humans need sunlight for the production of vitamin D in the absence of supplementation. In addition to beneficial effects, exposure to the ultraviolet (UV) component of the sunlight spectrum results in adverse effects on human health.

Sunlight is divided into visible light, ranging from 400 nm (violet) to 700 nm (red); infrared, or greater than 700 nm, also called heat; and UV radiation (UVR), or less than 400 nm. Ultraviolet radiation is divided into UV-A (320–400 nm), also called black (invisible) light; UV-B (290–320 nm), which is more skin-penetrating; and UV-C (<290 nm). Ultraviolet-C is completely absorbed by stratospheric ozone; no UV-C reaches the earth's surface. Most UV-B is absorbed by stratospheric ozone, but no UV-A is absorbed.[1] Ultraviolet-B is more intense during summer than during winter, at midday compared with early morning or late afternoon, in places closer to the equator than in temperate zones, and at high altitudes. Sand, snow, concrete, and water can reflect up to 85% of sunlight, resulting in greater exposure.[2]

Ultraviolet-B constitutes less than 0.5% of sunlight but is responsible for most of the acute and chronic sun damage to normal skin. Exposure to UVR during childhood can result in substantial morbidity and even mortality later in life.

## Route of Exposure

Individuals are exposed to UVR through direct contact to the skin and eyes while they are outdoors in the sunlight or when they are exposed to artificial sources of UVR emitted by sunlamps and sunbeds.

## Systems Affected

The skin, eyes, and immune system are affected.

## Clinical Effects

### Erythema and Sunburn

Erythema and sunburn are acute reactions to excessive amounts of UVR. Exposure to UVR causes vasodilatation and an increase in the volume of blood in the dermis, resulting in erythema. The minimal erythemal dose depends on factors such as skin type and thickness, the amount of melanin in the epidermis and the capacity of the epidermis to produce melanin after sun exposure, and the intensity of the radiation. Six sun-reactive skin classifications have been developed (see Table 26.1).

The ability of UVR to produce erythema depends on the radiation wavelength expressed as the erythema action spectrum; for erythema and sunburn the action spectrum is mainly in the UV-B range.[3]

### Tanning

Tanning is a protective response to sun exposure.[4] Immediate pigment darkening is the result of oxidation of existing melanin after exposure to visible light and UV-A. Immediate pigment darkening becomes visible within several minutes and usually fades within 1 to 2 hours. Delayed tanning occurs when new melanin is formed as a result of

**Table 26.1**
**Classification of Sun-Reactive Skin Types**

| Skin Type | History of Sunburning or Tanning |
|---|---|
| I | Always burns easily, never tans |
| II | Always burns easily, tans minimally |
| III | Burns moderately, tans gradually and uniformly (light brown) |
| IV | Burns minimally, always tans well (moderate brown) |
| V | Rarely burns, tans profusely (dark brown) |
| VI | Never burns, deeply pigmented (black) |

UV-B exposure. Delayed tanning becomes apparent 2 to 3 days after exposure, peaks at 7 to 10 days, and may persist for weeks or months.

### Non-melanoma Skin Cancer

Non-melanoma skin cancer (NMSC) includes basal cell carcinoma (BCC) and squamous cell carcinoma (SCC). In the US adult population, NMSC is by far the most common malignant neoplasm, accounting for more than 40% of all cancers with more than 1 million cases every year. The exact number of cases of NMSC in the United States is not precisely known because physicians are not required to report these to cancer registries. Non-melanoma skin cancer is rarely fatal unless left untreated; nevertheless, the American Cancer Society (ACS) estimated that 2200 people die of NMSC per year.[5]

In general, NMSC occurs in maximally sun-exposed areas of fair-skinned persons and is uncommon in blacks; cumulative sun exposure over long periods is considered to be important in pathogenesis. Biological evidence implicates sunlight exposure in the pathogenesis of skin cancer: SCC developed in mouse skin chronically exposed to UVR.[6]

Non-melanoma skin cancer is extremely rare in children in the absence of predisposing conditions.[7]

### Cutaneous Malignant Melanoma

Exposure to large amounts of sunlight that is episodic and relatively infrequent is important in the pathogenesis of cutaneous malignant melanoma (referred to hereafter as melanoma). Although much less common than NMSC, melanoma is a serious public health issue. The incidence rates of melanoma in the United States have risen more rapidly than any other cancer, with the exception of lung cancer incidence in women. The lifetime risk of melanoma was 1 in 1500 in 1930, 1 in 250 in 1980, 1 in 120 in 1987, 1 in 75 in 2000, and estimated at 1 in 71 in 2001.[8] Melanoma accounts for about 4% of skin cancer cases, but causes about 79% of skin cancer deaths. The ACS estimates that about 54 200 melanomas will be diagnosed in 2003 and that about 7600 people are expected to die of the disease.[9] Although melanoma is potentially curable if detected in the early stages, melanoma that has metastasized has a grave prognosis. Thus efforts have been directed toward prevention and early detection.

The reason for the increase in the incidence of melanoma is complex and incompletely understood but is felt to be related to the population's increased exposure to the sun over the last 50 years. During that time, the protective stratospheric ozone layer was depleted due to the widespread use of chlorofluorocarbons, resulting in more intense UVR reaching the earth's surfaces. Changes in fashion norms, more leisure time, and more time spent outdoors have resulted in more skin exposure. Other factors, yet to be determined, are most likely involved.

Increasing age is a risk factor for melanoma, with most melanomas occurring in people older than 50 years. Melanoma occurs in young adults but is rare in children. Family history also increases risk: a person's risk of developing melanoma increases if there are one or more first-degree relatives (mother, father, brother, or sister) with melanoma.

Epidemiologic evidence supports the role of sunlight in the pathogenesis of most, but not all, cases of melanoma.

1. Latitude: There is an inverse relationship between latitude and the incidence and mortality rates of melanoma in whites, with higher rates found closer to the equator (where the amount of sunlight is greater).[10]
2. Race and pigmentation: According to the National Cancer Institute, melanoma occurs predominantly in whites with an incidence approximately 20 times greater for white men and women than for blacks,[11] and the mortality rate among whites is 5 times greater than for blacks.[12] There is, in general, an inverse relationship between incidence and the skin pigmentation of people in various countries in the world. Melanin decreases the transmission of

UVR. This may protect melanocytes from sunlight-induced changes that lead to their malignant transformation.[4]

3. Childhood exposure: Episodic high exposures sufficient to cause sunburn, particularly during childhood and adolescence, increase the risk of melanoma.[13-15] Blistering sunburns at ages 15 to 20 years (but not after age 30 years) were significantly associated with increased risk (relative risk of 2.2 for more than 5 sunburns vs none).[16] Migration studies indicate that high exposure to sunlight during childhood sets the stage for high rates of melanoma in adulthood.[17]

Approximately 25% of lifetime sun exposure occurs before the age of 18 years.[18] In childhood and adolescence, melanocytes may be more sensitive to the sun, resulting in alteration of their deoxyribonucleic acid (DNA), possibly leading to the formation of unstable moles that may become malignant. Sunlight exposure and blistering sunburns during youth may be more intense than later in life because of child and adolescent behavior patterns. Passing through critical stages of carcinogenesis early in life may increase the chance of completing the remaining stages. One of these stages may involve the formation of nevi (moles), particularly dysplastic nevi.

4. Nevi: Acute sun exposure is implicated in the development of nevi in children. The number of nevi increases with age,[19] nevi occur with more frequency on sun-exposed areas, and the number of nevi on exposed areas increases with the total cumulative sun exposure during childhood and adolescence.[20] Children with light skin who tend to burn rather than tan have more nevi at all ages, and children who have more severe sunburns have more nevi.[19]

There is a relationship between the number and type of melanocytic nevi and the development of melanoma. Dysplastic melanocytic nevi, which may represent a reaction to solar injury, are considered precursor lesions that increase risk.[21] The presence of congenital nevi greater than 1.5 cm in diameter also increases risk.[22]

The familial dysplastic nevus syndrome is a disorder with the following features: (1) a distinctive appearance of abnormal melanocytic nevi, (2) unique histologic features of the nevi, (3) autosomal dominant pattern of inheritance, and (4) hypermutability of fibroblasts and lymphoblasts. Fibroblasts and lymphoblasts from patients with this syndrome are abnormally sensitive to UV damage, and persons with this syndrome are at markedly higher risk for the development of melanoma.[21]

Biological evidence also suggests that sunlight exposure is important in the pathogenesis of melanoma. Studies in opossums suggest that portions of the UV-A spectrum may play a role in the pathogenesis of melanoma.[23] Melanoma has been induced in human foreskins grafted onto immunologically tolerant animals exposed to UVR.[24] Melanomas frequently are found in people with xeroderma pigmentosum (XP) and related disorders in which there is a genetically determined defect in the repair of DNA damaged by UVR and a high risk of NMSC.[25]

Cellular studies provide additional evidence. Ultraviolet-B exposure damages DNA, resulting in UV-induced lesions, primarily cyclobutane pyrimidine dimmers and pyrimidine (6-4) pyrimidone photoproducts.[4] The incomplete repair of DNA damage results in mutations.[4] Ultraviolet-A causes oxidative damage to DNA that is potentially mutagenic.[4]

Exposure to sunbeds and sunlamps, which produce primarily UV-A, also is associated with increased risk of developing melanoma.[26]

### *Phototoxicity and Photoallergy*

Chemical photosensitivity refers to an adverse cutaneous reaction that occurs when certain chemicals or drugs are applied topically or taken systemically at the same time that a person is exposed to UV or visible radiation. Phototoxicity is a form of chemical photosensitivity that does not depend on an immunologic response because the reaction can occur on the person's first exposure to the offending agent. Most phototoxic agents are activated in the UV-A range (320–400 nm). Photoallergy is an acquired altered reactivity of the skin that is dependent on antigen-antibody or cell-mediated hypersensitivity.[27] Phyto-photodermatitis is a skin eruption resulting from the interaction of sunlight and photosensitizing compounds. The most common phototoxic compounds are the furocoumarins (psoralens) contained in a wide variety of plants such as limes, lemons, and celery.

Persons who take medications or use topical agents that are sensitizing should avoid all sun exposure, if possible, and completely avoid all UV-A from artificial sources. The consequences of exposure can be uncomfortable, serious, or life threatening.[27] Sensitizing medications include sulfonamides, tretinoin, tetracyclines, and thiazides.

### Skin Aging

Long-term exposure to sunlight without protection starting in childhood causes wrinkles and varying degrees of skin thickening and thinning. The cumulative effects of excessive unprotected sun exposure weaken the skin's elasticity, leading to sagging cheeks, deeper facial wrinkles, and skin discoloration later in life.[28]

### Effects on the Eye

In adults, more than 90% of UVR is absorbed by the anterior structure of the eye. Ultraviolet radiation can contribute to the development of age-related cataracts, pterygium, photodermatitis, and cancer of the skin around the eye.[29] Cataract formation seems to be positively correlated with decreasing latitude and increasing UV-B and total sunlight exposure.[27] Gazing directly into the sun (as can occur during an eclipse) can result in focal burns to the retina (solar retinopathy).[30]

Melanoma of the uveal tract, the most common primary intra-ocular malignant neoplasm in adults, is associated with a tendency to sunburn and with intense exposure to UVR.[31]

## *Effects on the Immune System*

Exposure to UVR contributes to immunosuppression, increasingly recognized as important in the development of skin cancer.[32] In mice, contact hypersensitivity and delayed-type hypersensitivity can be suppressed by exposure to UVR. In humans, exposure to UVR doses achieved at midday in the summer sun causes suppression of contact hypersensitivity similar to that demonstrated in mice.[33] People exposed to immunosuppressive agents develop large numbers of squamous cell carcinomas.[34,35] Immunosuppression is thought to play an important role in the growth of skin cancer, progression of certain infections, and vaccine response.

## Treatment of Clinical Syndromes

Pediatricians will rarely encounter patients with NMSC or melanoma. Patients at high risk, including children with XP and related disorders and those with a large number of nevi and a family history of melanoma, should be treated in collaboration with a dermatologist. Sunburns should be treated with cool compresses and analgesics. Instruction about preventing future sunburns should be given at the time of the burn.

## Prevention of Exposure

Although other major risk factors (eg, precursor lesions, age, race, previous melanoma, and family history) also are associated with melanoma, solar radiation is the only risk factor that is avoidable.

Pediatricians have an important role in education beginning in infancy, and later when developmental stages result in new patterns of sun exposure (eg, when the child begins to walk, before starting school, and before entering adolescence).[36] Preteens and teens may need special reinforcement because they often are susceptible to societal notions of beauty and health. Teen counseling should include warnings about using sunbeds and sunlamps, which increase the risk of developing skin cancer.[37]

All parents and children should receive advice about sun protection. Not all children sunburn easily, but people of all skin types can experience skin cancer, skin aging, and sun-related damage to the immune system. Children who should receive special attention include those with XP, who must avoid all UVR, and those with familial dysplastic nevus syndrome, with excessive numbers of nevi, or with 2 or more family members with melanoma. Children showing signs of excessive sun exposure (eg, freckles) also should receive special instruction.

### Avoiding Exposure

Infants younger than 6 months should be kept out of direct sunlight. They should be dressed in cool, comfortable clothing and wear hats with brims. Children's activities should be planned to avoid peak-intensity midday sun (10 am–4 pm).

Seeking shade is somewhat useful but people can still sunburn because light is scattered and reflected. A fair-skinned person sitting under a tree can burn in less than an hour. Shade provides relief from heat, possibly providing a false sense of security about UV protection. Clouds decrease UV intensity but not to the same extent that they decrease heat intensity, which also may result in overexposure.[3]

### Clothes

Clothes offer the simplest and often most practical means of sun protection. One study showed that wearing clothing decreases the development of nevi.[38] Protective factors in clothing include style, weave, and chemical enhancement. Clothes that cover more of the body provide more protection; sun-protective styles cover to the neck, elbows, and knees. A tighter weave lets in less sunlight than a looser weave.[39] Treating fabrics with chemical absorbers or washing them with optical brighteners increases UV protectiveness.

In 1996 Australia and New Zealand established standards for the UV protectiveness of clothing. The United States developed standards in 2001. The UV protection factor (UPF) measures a fabric's ability to block UVR from passing through the fabric and reaching the skin. The UPF is classified from 15 to 50+; 15 to 24 is rated as "Good"; 25 to 39, "Very Good"; and 40 to 50+, "Excellent" UV protection. The UPF of fabrics can be altered by shrinking, stretching, and wetness. Shrinking increases the UPF; stretching decreases the UPF. If cotton fabrics get wet, the UPF decreases. Sun-protective clothing and fabrics are not regulated by the US Food and Drug Administration (FDA) or any other government agency, but the Federal Trade Commission monitors sun-protective claims.

### Window Glass

Window glass blocks virtually all UV-B and at least half of all UV-A energy.

### Sunscreens

Sunscreen is the method of sun protection most commonly used.[40,41] Sunscreens reduce the intensity of UVR affecting the epidermis, thus preventing erythema and sunburn. Opaque sunscreens, including zinc oxide and titanium dioxide, do not selectively absorb UVR, but reflect and scatter all light. They are useful for patients with photosensitivity and other disorders who require protection from full-spectrum UVR, but may be cosmetically unacceptable.[2] Chemical sunscreens absorb UV rays, decreasing the intensity of UVR affecting the epidermis.

The sun protection factor (SPF) is a grading system developed to quantify the degree of protection from erythema provided by using a sunscreen; the higher the SPF, the greater the protection. Sun protection factor pertains only to UV-B. For example, a person who would normally experience a sunburn in 10 minutes can be protected up to about 150 minutes (10 x 15) with an SPF-15 sunscreen. Sunscreens with an SPF of 15 or more theoretically filter more than 92% of the UV-B responsible for erythema; sunscreens with an SPF of 30 filter out about 97% of the UV-B. In actual use, the SPF often is substantially lower than expected because the amount used is less than half the recommended amount.[2,42] An SPF of 15 should be adequate in most cases.

The regular use of a broad-spectrum sunscreen preparation can prevent solar (actinic) keratoses, which are precursor lesions of SCC.[43,44] One randomized clinical trial showed that sunscreen also decreases the risk of developing SCC.[45] In contrast, sunscreen users have been found to have a higher risk of melanoma and BCC and more nevi.[38] These observations have led to concern that people who use sunscreens spend more time in the sun.[46] The American College of Preventive Medicine and others have questioned the use of sunscreen in preventing cancer.[47] The ACS and the American Academy of Dermatology continue to recommend sunscreen use as part of a program of sun avoidance.[48]

Sunscreens should be used when a child might sunburn. Although there are no data showing that sunscreens prevent melanoma, there is no benefit in burning and it should be avoided.

The issue of whether sunscreen is safe for infants younger than 6 months is controversial. There are concerns that human skin in infants younger than 6 months may have different absorptive characteristics and that biological systems that metabolize and excrete drugs may not be fully developed.[49] The Australian Cancer Society concluded that there is no evidence to suggest that using sunscreen on small areas of a baby's skin is associated with any long-term effects. They recommend that sunscreen be used when physical protection, such as clothing, hats, and shade, is not adequate.[50] On the basis of available evidence, it is reasonable to tell parents what is known about the safety of sunscreens in infants younger than 6 months and to emphasize the importance of avoiding high-risk exposure. In situations where the infant's skin is not protected adequately by clothing, it may be reasonable to apply sunscreen to small areas, such as the face and the backs of the hands.[51]

Preparations that contain a combination of sunscreen with the insecticide N-N-diethyl-m-toluamide (DEET) should not be used because they may result in overexposure to DEET (see Chapter 24).

### The Ultraviolet Index

The UV index was developed in 1994 by the National Weather Service in consultation with the EPA and the Centers for Disease Control and Prevention. The UV index predicts the intensity of UV light for the following day based on the sun's position, cloud movements, altitude, ozone data, and other factors. It is conservatively calculated based on effects on skin types that burn easily. Higher numbers predict more intense UV light during midday of the following day (see Table 26.2). The index is available online for thousands of cities at http://www.weather.com. It also is printed in the weather section of many daily newspapers and reported through weather reports of local radio, television, and weather stations.[52]

### Eye Protection

Wearing a hat with a brim can reduce UV-B exposure to the eyes by 50%. Sunglasses should be worn whenever the child may be in the sun long enough to get a sunburn or tan. Sunglasses should be chosen to block at least 99% of UV-B and UV-A rays.[53]

**Table 26.2**
**Exposure Levels Predicted by the Ultraviolet Index***

| Index Value | Exposure Level | Time in the Sun Needed for Burn |
| --- | --- | --- |
| 0–2 | Minimal | 1 h |
| 3–4 | Low | 30–60 min |
| 5–6 | Moderate | 20–30 min |
| 7–9 | High | 13–20 min |
| 10–15 | Very high | <13 min |

*These ultraviolet effects are on unprotected skin type II, which always burns easily and tans minimally.

### Changes in Knowledge and Attitudes

Pediatricians alone cannot change social concepts in which a suntan is equated with health and beauty. School programs and public education campaigns must address this issue. Australia, which has the world's highest incidence of melanoma, has mounted a long sun-safety campaign urging citizens to "Slip, Slop, Slap": slip on a shirt, slop on some sunscreen, slap on a hat. The effects of these measures indicate that there has been a shift in knowledge and attitudes about sun exposure accompanied by behavior change.[54] The incidence of melanoma and NMSC is leveling off in young people and is dropping in some instances.[54,55]

### Frequently Asked Questions

Q *Why is a baby at special risk from sunburn?*

A A baby's skin is thinner than an adult's and burns more easily. Even dark-skinned babies may be sunburned. Babies cannot tell you if they are too hot or beginning to burn and cannot get out of the sun without an adult's help. Babies also need an adult to dress them properly and to apply sunscreen.

Q *What can I do to protect my child?*

A Babies younger than 6 months should be kept out of direct sunlight because of the risk of heat stroke. They should be moved under a tree, umbrella, or stroller canopy, although on reflective surfaces an umbrella or canopy may reduce UVR exposure by only 50%.

Q *What factors in clothing can offer protection against sunburn?*

A Some fabrics have a UPF rating showing how much sun protection they offer. Even if a fabric doesn't have a UPF rating, it may offer excellent sun protection. Some fabrics, such as polyester crepe, bleached cotton, and viscose, are quite transparent to UVR and should be avoided in the sun. Other fibers, such as unbleached cotton, can absorb UVR. High-luster polyesters and even thin, satiny silk can be highly protective because they reflect radiation. Weave also is important; in general, the tighter the weave or knit, the higher the protection offered. To assess protection, parents can hold the material up to a window or lamp and see how much light gets through. Darker clothes also generally offer more protection. Virtually all garments lose about a third of their sun-protective ability when wet.

Q  *How should I apply sunscreen to my baby?*

A  The sunscreen needs to be applied to the parts of the baby's skin that will be exposed to the sun. It also should be applied around the eyes, avoiding the eyelids. If he or she cries or complains that the sunscreen burns the eyes, the parent should try a different brand or try a sunscreen stick or a preparation made with titanium dioxide or zinc oxide. If a rash develops, the pediatrician can make another suggestion.

When choosing a sunscreen, parents should look for the words "broad-spectrum" on the label—it means that the sunscreen will screen out the UV-B and UV-A rays. An SPF of 15 should be adequate in most cases.

Parents should apply sunscreen liberally and rub it in well before going outdoors, making sure to cover all exposed areas, especially the child's face, nose, ears, feet, and hands, and even the backs of the knees. Sunscreen should be used even on cloudy days, because the sun's rays can penetrate through the clouds. Zinc oxide can be used as extra protection on the nose, cheeks, tops of the ears, and the shoulders. Zinc oxide should not be blended into the skin.

It is important to remember that using sunscreen is only one part of a total program of sun protection. Sunscreens should be used to prevent burning and not as a reason to stay in the sun longer.

Q *Why are some sunscreens labeled "PABA-free"?*

A Para-aminobenzoic acid (PABA) is an ingredient used in many sunscreens. Some people have a rash or a burning sensation when using preparations containing PABA, and some PABA preparations can cause a yellow discoloration on clothing. Other chemicals used in sunscreen preparations also can cause allergic or phototoxic reactions.[56,57]

Q *Does adhering to sun-safe practices such as covering up and using sunscreen put a breastfeeding baby at risk for rickets by blocking skin conversion of vitamin D precursors into vitamin D?*

A Breast milk is the optimal nutrition for infants but does not contain sufficient vitamin D to meet infants' requirements. Vitamin D needs can be met by exposure to direct sunlight. Because we recommend that infants should be protected from sun exposure with clothing, hats, and sunscreen, the American Academy of Pediatrics recently recommended that all breastfed infants (as well as infants receiving less than 500 mL/d of infant formula) receive supplementation with vitamin D.[58]

Q *Are tanning salons safe? How about self-tanning products?*

A People who use sunlamps or go to tanning salons are exposed primarily to UV-A. The tan that occurs represents a protective response to the harmful rays of the sun. Skin damage occurs whether a tan comes from the sun itself or from artificial light from a tanning salon. Although our culture often equates a suntan with health and beauty, that image contributes to skin damage and cancer. Tanning salons are not safe.

"Sunless" or "self-tanning" products use a chemical, dihydroxyacetone, which when applied to the skin darkens it without exposure to UVR. Some self-tanning products contain sunscreen, but others do not, so consumers should read the labels carefully because they may not be protected when they go outside into the sun. Tanning oils or baby oil may make skin look shiny and soft, but they provide no protection from the sun.

Q  *How do I choose sunglasses for my child?*

A  There are no government regulations on the amount of UVR that sunglasses must block. Sunglasses are regulated as medical devices by the FDA and may be labeled as UV protected if they meet certain standards. Parents should look for a label that states that the lenses block at least 99% of UV-A and 99% of UV-B rays.

Protection is provided by a chemical coating applied to the lenses. Lens color has nothing to do with UV protection. Ski goggles and contact lenses with UV protection also are recommended.

It is never too early for a child, even an infant, to wear sunglasses. Larger lenses, well fitted and close to the surface of the eye, provide the best protection.

## Resources

American Academy of Pediatrics (AAP), Internet: http://www.aap.org. The AAP provides a patient education brochure titled *Fun in the Sun.*

American Cancer Society, Internet: http://www.cancer.org

American Sun Protection Association, Internet: http://www.americansun.org

Centers for Disease Control and Prevention Choose Your Cover Campaign, Internet: http://www.cdc.gov/ChooseYourCover

National Council on Skin Cancer Prevention, Internet: http://www.skincancerprevention.org. The council comprises 25 organizations (including the AAP) whose staffs have experience, expertise, and knowledge in the area of disease prevention and education.

National Skin Cancer Foundation, Internet: http://www.skincancer.org. The foundation is dedicated to nationwide public and professional education programs aimed at increasing public awareness, sun protection and sun safety, skin self-examination, children's education, melanoma understanding, and continuing medical education.

US Environmental Protection Agency SunWise Program, Internet: http://www.epa.gov/sunwise1/publications.html

World Health Organization (WHO), Internet: http://www.who.int/en. "Solar Radiation and Human Health: Too Much Sun Is Dangerous" (Fact Sheet 227) is available on the WHO Web site at http://www.who.int/inf-fs/en/fact227.html.

## References

1. Sparling B. *Basic Chemistry of Ozone Depletion*. Moffet Field, CA: NASA Advanced Supercomputing. Available at: http://www.nas.nasa.gov/About/Education/Ozone/chemistry.html
2. Gilchrest BA. Actinic injury. *Annu Rev Med*. 1990;41:199–210
3. Diffey BL. Ultraviolet radiation and human health. *Clin Dermatol*. 1998;16:83–89
4. Gilchrest BA, Eller MS, Geller AC, Yaar M. The pathogenesis of melanoma induced by ultraviolet radiation. *N Engl J Med*. 1999;340:1341–1348
5. American Cancer Society. *What Are the Key Statistics for Non-Melanoma Skin Cancer?* Available at: http//www.cancer.org/docroot/CRI/content/ CRI_2_4_1X_What_are_the_key_statistics_for_skin_cancer_ 51.asp?sitearea=
6. deGruijl FR, Forbes PD. UV-induced skin cancer in a hairless mouse model. *Bioessays*. 1995;17:651–660
7. Sasson M, Mallory SB. Malignant primary skin tumors in children. *Curr Opin Pediatr*. 1996;8:372–377
8. Kim T. Melanoma risk 1 in 71 today, still climbing. *Skin Allergy News*. March 2001:44
9. American Cancer Society. *How Many People Get Melanoma Skin Cancer?* Available at: http://www.cancer.org/docroot/CRI/content/CRI_2_2_1X_ How_many_people_get_melanoma_skin_cancer_50.asp?sitearea=

10. Kopf AW, Kripke ML, Stern RS. Sun and malignant melanoma. *J Am Acad Dermatol.* 1984;11:674–684

11. National Cancer Institute. *Surveillance, Epidemiology and End Results. Incidence, Melanoma of the Skin.* Available at: http://seer.cancer.gov/faststats/html/inc_melan.html

12. National Cancer Institute. *Surveillance, Epidemiology and End Results. Mortality, Melanoma of the Skin.* Available at: http://seer.cancer.gov/faststats/html/mor_melan.html

13. Marks R. Prevention and control of melanoma: a public health approach. *CA Cancer J Clin.* 1996;46:199–216

14. Lew RA, Sober AJ, Cook N, Marvell R, Fitzpatrick TB. Sun exposure habits in patients with cutaneous melanoma: a case control study. *J Dermatol Surg Oncol.* 1983;9:981–986

15. Cress RD, Holly EA, Ahn DK. Cutaneous melanoma in women. V. Characteristics of those who tan and those who burn when exposed to summer sun. *Epidemiology.* 1995;6:538–543

16. Weinstock MA, Colditz GA, Willett WC, et al. Nonfamilial cutaneous melanoma incidence in women associated with sun exposure before 20 years of age. *Pediatrics.* 1989;84:199–204

17. Khlat M, Vail A, Parkin M, Green A. Mortality from melanoma in migrants to Australia: variation by age at arrival and duration of stay. *Am J Epidemiol.* 1992;135:1103–1113

18. Godar DE, Urbach F, Gasparro FP, van der Leun JC. UV doses of young adults. *Photochem Photobiol.* 2003;77:453–457

19. Gallagher RP, McLean DI, Yang CP, et al. Suntan, sunburn, and pigmentation factors and the frequency of acquired melanocytic nevi in children. Similarities to melanoma: the Vancouver Mole Study. *Arch Dermatol.* 1990;126:770–776

20. Holman CD, Armstrong BK. Pigmentary traits, ethnic origin, benign nevi, and family history as risk factors for cutaneous malignant melanoma. *J Natl Cancer Inst.* 1984;72:257–266

21. Clark WH Jr. The dysplastic nevus syndrome. *Arch Dermatol.* 1988;124:1207–1210

22. Kopf AW, Bart RS, Hennessey P. Congenital nevocytic nevi and malignant melanomas. *J Am Acad Dermatol.* 1979;1:123–130

23. Ley RD. Ultraviolet radiation A-induced precursors of cutaneous melanoma in Monodelphis domestica. *Cancer Res.* 1997;57:3682–3684

24. Atillasoy ES, Seykora JT, Soballe PW, et al. UVB induces atypical melanocytic lesions and melanoma in human skin. *Am J Pathol.* 1998;152:1179–1186

25. Taylor AM, McConville CM, Byrd PJ. Cancer and DNA processing disorders. *Br Med Bull.* 1994;50:708–717

26. Westdahl J, Olsson H, Masback A, et al. Use of sunbeds or sunlamps and malignant melanoma in southern Sweden. *Am J Epidemiol.* 1994;140:691–699

27. Council on Scientific Affairs, American Medical Association. Harmful effects of ultraviolet radiation. *JAMA.* 1989;262:380–384

28. Gilmore GD. Sunscreens: a review of the skin cancer protection value and educational opportunities. *J Sch Health.* 1989;59:210–213

29. National Society to Prevent Blindness, American Optometric Association, American Academy of Ophthalmology. *Statement on Ocular Ultraviolet Radiation Hazards in Sunlight.* St Louis, MO: American Optometric Association; 1993

30. Wong SC, Eke T, Ziakas NG. Eclipse burns: a prospective study of solar retinopathy following the 1999 solar eclipse. *Lancet.* 2001;357:199–200

31. Holly EA, Ashton DA, Char DH, Kristiansen JJ, Ahn DK. Uveal melanoma in relation to ultraviolet light exposure and host factors. *Cancer Res.* 1990;50:5773–5777

32. Ullrich SE. Photoimmune suppression and photocarcinogenesis. *Front Biosci.* 2002;7:d684–d703

33. Selgrade MK, Repacholi MH, Koren HS. Ultraviolet radiation-induced immune modulation: potential consequences for infectious, allergic, and autoimmune disease. *Environ Health Perspect.* 1997;105:332–334

34. DiGiovanna JJ. Posttransplantation skin cancer: scope of the problem, management, and role for systemic retinoid chemoprevention. *Transplant Proc.* 1998;30:2771–2775

35. Bouwes-Bavinck JN, Robertson I, Wainwright RW, Green A. Excessive numbers of skin cancers and pre-malignant skin lesions in an Australian heart transplant recipient. *Br Heart J.* 1995;74:468–470

36. Williams ML, Sagebiel RW. Sunburns, melanoma, and the pediatrician. *Pediatrics.* 1989;84:381–382

37. Karagas MR, Stannard VA, Mott LA, Slattery MJ, Spencer SK, Weinstock MA. Use of tanning devices and risk of basal cell and squamous cell skin cancers. *J Natl Cancer Inst.* 2002;94:224–226

38. Autier P, Dore JF, Cattaruzza MS, et al. Sunscreen use, wearing clothes, and number of nevi in 6- to 7-year-old European children. European Organization for Research and Treatment of Cancer Melanoma Cooperative Group. *J Natl Cancer Inst.* 1998;90:1873–1880

39. Welsh C, Diffey B. The protection against solar actinic radiation afforded by common clothing fabrics. *Clin Exp Dermatol.* 1981;6:577–582

40. Robinson JK, Rigel DS, Amonette RA. Trends in sun exposure knowledge, attitudes, and behaviors: 1986 to 1996. *J Am Acad Dermatol.* 1997;37:179–186

41. Robinson JK, Rigel DS, Amonette RA. Summertime sun protection used by adults for their children. *J Am Acad Dermatol.* 2000;42:746–753

42. Sunscreens: are they safe and effective? *Med Lett Drugs Ther.* 1999;41:43–44

43. Thompson SC, Jolley D, Marks R. Reduction of solar keratoses by regular sunscreen use. *N Engl J Med.* 1993;329:1147–1151

44. Naylor MF, Boyd A, Smith DW, Cameron GS, Hubbard D, Nelder KH. High sun protection factor sunscreens in the suppression of actinic neoplasia. *Arch Dermatol.* 1995;131:170–175

45. Green A, Williams G, Neale R, et al. Daily sunscreen application and betacarotene supplementation in prevention of basal-cell and squamous-cell carcinomas of the skin: a randomised controlled trial. *Lancet.* 1999;354:723–729

46. Autier P, Dore JF, Negrier S, et al. Sunscreen use and duration of sun exposure: a double-blind, randomized trial. *J Natl Cancer Inst.* 1999;91:1304–1309

47. Hill L, Ferrini RL. Skin cancer prevention and screening: summary of the American College of Preventive Medicine's practice policy statements. *CA Cancer J Clin.* 1998;48:232–235

48. McDonald CJ. American Cancer Society perspective on the American College of Preventive Medicine's policy statements on skin cancer prevention and screening. *CA Cancer J Clin.* 1998;48:229–231

49. Sunscreen drug products for over-the-counter human use: tentative final monograph. *Fed Regist.* May 12, 1993;58:28194

50. Australian Cancer Society. *Policy statement: babies and sunscreen.* Sydney, Australia: Australia Cancer Society; 1998

51. American Academy of Pediatrics Committee on Environmental Health. Ultraviolet light: a hazard to children. *Pediatrics.* 1999;104:328–333

52. US Environmental Protection Agency. *The Federal Experimental Ultraviolet Index: What You Need to Know.* Washington, DC: US Environmental Protection Agency; 1994. EPA Publication 430-F-94-016

53. Wagner RS. Why children must wear sunglasses. *Contemp Pediatr.* 1995;12:27–37

54. Marks R. Two decades of the public health approach to skin cancer control in Australia: why, how and where are we now? *Australas J Dermatol.* 1999;40:1–5

55. Giles GG, Armstrong BK, Burton RC, Staples MP, Thursfield VJ. Has mortality from melanoma stopped rising in Australia? Analysis of trends between 1931 and 1994. *BMJ.* 1996;312:1121–1125

56. Trevisi P, Vincenzi C, Chieregato C, Guerra L, Tosti A. Sunscreen sensitization: a three-year study. *Dermatology.* 1994;189:55–57

57. Cook N, Freeman S. Report of 19 cases of photoallergic contact dermatitis to sunscreens seen at the Skin and Cancer Foundation. *Australas J Dermatol.* 2001;42:257–259

58. Garner LM, Greer FR; American Academy of Pediatrics Section on Breastfeeding, Committee on Nutrition. Prevention of rickets and vitamin D deficiency: new guidelines for vitamin D intake. *Pediatrics.* 2003;111:908–910

# 27
# Water Pollutants

Safety of water is of primary importance to child health. Water is used for drinking, cooking, and preparation of infant formulas for children who are not breastfed. Water is an important medium for irrigating crops and for growing food for fish; pollutants in water can thus enter the food supply. Water is important for bathing and swimming; contaminated water can result in exposures to children who may swallow or have skin contact with pollutants.

Although 70% of the earth is covered by water, only 3% of the earth's water is fresh. Of that 3%, two thirds is frozen in glaciers and ice caps, leaving only 1% available for human use. Freshwater is classified as either groundwater, such as underground aquifers (0.7%), or surface water, such as lakes and rivers (0.3%), but less than half of the liquid freshwater in the world is readily accessible.[1] Water pollution results from sources of contamination termed either point or nonpoint. Point sources of pollution include municipal wastewater treatment plant discharges and industrial wastewater discharges into surface waters. Nonpoint sources of pollution are more difficult to identify and control and include agricultural runoff, urban runoff, soil contamination, and atmospheric deposition. Pollutants contaminate surface waters or soils directly and seep into underground aquifers to contaminate groundwater as well. In the United States, approximately half of drinking water comes from groundwater, with the other half coming from either surface water or mixed surface water and groundwater sources.[2] Preserving an adequate supply of quality freshwater is essential to public health and ecological integrity but is threatened by increasing population pressure and industrial and agricultural production, which can result in pollution.

Water pollutants can be categorized as biological agents, chemicals, or radionuclides (see Table 27.1). Hundreds of biological agents and thousands of chemical agents can be found in water. For many water pollutants, little is known of their long-term health effects. Federal regulations were not required until passage of the Safe Drinking Water Act of 1974; they exist for only a small percentage of the contaminants that have been identified in water. Federal standards apply to community water supplies serving 25 or more customers. Some states have standards for smaller suppliers, but private wells are not regulated. Modern water treatment facilities have made the drinking water in the United States among the safest in the world, eliminating most

**Table 27.1**
**Examples of Some Water Pollutants, Common Sources, and Systems Affected**

| Pollutant Category (Specific Examples) | Common Sources | Systems Affected |
|---|---|---|
| **Biological Agents** | | |
| **Bacteria** | | |
| *Campylobacter* species | Feces: human, animal | Gastrointestinal |
| *Escherichia coli* | Feces: human, animal | Gastrointestinal |
| *Salmonella* species | Feces: human, animal | Gastrointestinal |
| *Shigella coli* | Feces: human | Gastrointestinal |
| *Vibrio* species | Feces: human, animal | Gastrointestinal |
| **Viruses** | | |
| Calicivirus | Feces: human | Gastrointestinal |
| Enterovirus | Feces: human | Gastrointestinal, neurologic |
| Hepatitis A virus | Feces: human | Gastrointestinal (liver) |
| Rotavirus | Feces: human | Gastrointestinal |
| **Parasites** | | |
| *Balantidium coli* | Feces: human, animal | Gastrointestinal |
| *Cryptosporidium parvum* | Feces: human, animal | Gastrointestinal |
| *Entamoeba histolytica* | Feces: human | Gastrointestinal |
| *Giardia lamblia* | Feces: human, animal | Gastrointestinal |
| **Natural Toxins** | | |
| Microcystins | Cyanobacteria | Gastrointestinal, neurologic |
| *Pfiesteria* toxins | *Pfiesteria piscicida* | Neurologic, dermatologic |

| Pollutant Category (Specific Examples) | Common Sources | Systems Affected |
| --- | --- | --- |
| **Chemicals** | | |
| **Inorganic** | | |
| Arsenic | Ores, smelting, pesticides | Lung, kidney, and skin cancer; cardiovascular |
| Chromium | Ores, steel and pulp mills | Cancer (chromium VI) |
| Lead | Pipes, solder, soil | Neurologic |
| Mercury (inorganic) | Waste incineration, burning coal, mercury use, volcanoes | Kidney damage |
| Nitrates | Nitrogen fertilizer, leaching from septic tanks, sewage; erosion of natural deposits | Methemoglobinemia in infants |
| **Organic** | | |
| Benzene, other organics | Leaking gasoline storage tanks | Leukemia |
| Pesticides | Agricultural use, urban runoff | Multiple |
| Polychlorinated biphenyls | Transformers, industry | Multiple |
| Trichloroethylene | Degreasing, dry cleaning | Cancer |
| **Disinfectants and Disinfection By-products** | | |
| Chloramines | Water chlorination | Eye/nose irritation; stomach discomfort, anemia |
| Chlorine | Water chlorination | Eye/nose irritation; stomach discomfort |
| Chlorine dioxide | Water chlorination | Anemia; infants and young children; nervous system effects |

Table 27.1
Examples of Some Water Pollutants, Common Sources, and Systems Affected,
*continued*

| Pollutant Category (Specific Examples) | Common Sources | Systems Affected |
|---|---|---|
| **Disinfectants and Disinfection By-products** | | |
| Haloacetic acid | By-product of drinking water disinfection | Increased risk of cancer |
| Trihalomethanes | By-product of drinking water disinfection | Liver, kidney, or central nervous system problems; increased risk of cancer |
| **Radionuclides** | | |
| Radon | Natural uranium | Lung cancer |

waterborne bacterial illnesses. Nonetheless about 30 waterborne disease outbreaks are reported each year in the United States and doubtless many others occur that are not recognized and/or reported.[3]

The discussion in this chapter will be limited to a few representative examples of each of the categories of water pollutants. While biological contamination of drinking water represents the largest threat to human health worldwide, it will not be extensively discussed in this chapter. See the 2003 *Red Book*® for information about infectious diarrheal diseases.[4] Details on specific pollutants can be found in other chapters in this book.

## Routes and Sources of Exposure

Children drink more water per kilogram of body weight than do adults. Drinking water is consumed in a number of forms: as water, as an addition to reconstituted infant formula, in juice and other drinks, and in cooking. To the extent that children consume breast milk or drinks from outside the home (eg, fresh milk and juice, premixed formulas, and sodas) they have less consumption of tap water.

Household water supplies can result in inhalation exposures. If volatile substances (eg, organic solvents) or gases (eg, radon gas) are present, these will enter the home during showering, bathing, and other activities. It has been estimated that 50% of the total exposure to volatile organic compounds in drinking water is via this inhalation route.

Water can cause exposure via other sources. When contaminated water is used for the irrigation of foods, the foods may become contaminated (see Chapter 14). Fish and shellfish harvested from polluted fresh and marine waters also are important sources of exposure to water pollutants; in many cases pollutants are concentrated by shellfish and fish.[5] Contaminated bathing water can result in exposures via ingestion or dermal contact as well. Young children particularly are at risk because they swallow more water when bathing than do older children and adults.

The fetus also may be exposed to pollutants when a pregnant woman ingests water in which water pollutants have bioaccumulated. Methylmercury and polychlorinated biphenyls (PCBs) in fish have been particularly important in this regard because they accumulate in the body and are not readily excreted. These toxicants may be found in the body years after exposure.

## Contaminants in Water

### Biological Agents

**Microorganisms.** Drinking and bathing water may contain numerous pathogens, which have the ability to survive in the water for variable periods. Some of these agents are listed in Table 27.1. Certain of these agents (eg, certain parasites) form small cysts, which pass through standard filters and are quite resistant to water disinfectants.[4] Waterborne illness usually results in mild gastroenteritis with diarrhea. Even when water systems are in compliance with federal and local regulations, sporadic and epidemic illnesses occur.[6] This is of particular concern for infants and immunocompromised persons exposed to pathogens such as *Cryptosporidium* despite state-of-the-art water treatment. In the United States, it is rare to have serious dysentery or enteric fever due to *Vibrio cholerae* and *Salmonella typhi* except in areas where water quality is compromised. Contaminated bathing waters frequently are associated with viral upper respiratory and gastrointestinal infections. Syndromes associated with illnesses from various pathogens are described in the 2003 *Red Book*.[4]

**Natural Toxins.** Natural toxins may produce acute or chronic illnesses and a variety of clinical syndromes. Water from ponds and lakes, as well as municipal and recreational waters, under certain conditions may contain cyanobacteria (blue-green algae), including *Microcystis aeruginosa.* These bacteria produce cyanotoxins such as microcystins, some of which are hepatotoxic and neurotoxic compounds.[7] Microcystins produced by cyanobacteria have been linked to liver failure and death in patients who underwent hemodialysis at a dialysis center supplied by untreated water from a lake with massive growth of blue-green algae.[8]

Water from the rivers flowing into the Chesapeake Bay on the eastern shore of the United States periodically may be contaminated with *Pfiesteria piscicida* and other dinoflagellates that can produce neurotoxins.[9] The rate of contamination by cyanobacteria and *Pfiesteria* is unknown but thought to be infrequent. Chronic, daily exposure to waterways containing toxin-producing *Pfiesteria* dinoflagellates has been associated with learning and memory difficulties in a small sample of adults in Maryland.[9]

### *Chemical Contaminants*

Water and sediments in water are the ultimate sinks for many chemicals produced and used by humans. There are more than 15 000 chemicals produced at more than 10 000 pounds per year in the United States, and thousands of new chemicals are introduced into use each year. Few of these chemicals have been tested. Even among the 2800 chemicals used at more than a million pounds per year, more than half have not been tested for toxic effects on humans.[10]

Thousands of synthetic organic chemicals are used in agricultural and industrial processes. According to the US Geological Survey, many of these chemicals, as well as antibiotics and other pharmaceuticals (including estrogens), pesticides, and certain industrial chemicals, frequently are found in the waters of the United States, particularly downstream from factories and cities.[11]

## Inorganic Chemicals

**Arsenic.** Arsenic, a ubiquitous metal, can be found in the environment in organic and inorganic states and in valence states of 0, 3, and 5. Human activities, such as smelting, coal burning, wood preservation, pesticide distribution, and other industrial processes, produce at least 3 times more arsenic than natural processes.[12] The toxicity of arsenic to humans depends on the form, with organic being less toxic than inorganic and pentavalent being less toxic than trivalent. Except in electronics, industrial uses of arsenicals are decreasing. Drinking water and food represent the major sources of arsenic for humans. Clinical effects of arsenic are discussed in Chapter 8. Arsenic is a known human carcinogen[12]; however, its natural occurrence in drinking water and the expense of removal have caused the US Environmental Protection Agency (EPA) to set a standard that is much higher than the usual level for protection against a carcinogen.

**Chromium.** Chromium in drinking water is regulated to protect against exposure to one of the valence states of chromium, chromium VI (hexavalent chromium), which is a carcinogen.

**Lead.** Drinking water represents a potential route of exposure to lead. In the past 2 decades, expanded regulations and monitoring of drinking water have made most large municipal water supplies safe from exposure to lead. Nevertheless, some homes in the United States have lead levels in water above acceptable levels. Chicago, Boston, and other cities historically used 100% lead piping to connect water mains to homes. Millions of these lead connectors still exist. In addition, lead solder, used to connect copper pipes, was widely used until the late 1980s. Drinking water, particularly that which is soft (ie, low in calcium or magnesium), or below a neutral pH, causes lead to leach from lead connector pipes or soldered joints. Clinical effects of lead exposure are discussed in Chapter 19. Lead in drinking water is controlled by limiting the corrosiveness of the water (ie, the ability of the water to leach lead from these materials) and eliminated by removing lead pipes or pipes with lead solder.

**Methylmercury.** Mercury in fish originates from natural sources and from combustion sources that release mercury into the air, such as coal-fired power plants used for generating electrical energy and municipal waste incinerators that burn garbage.[13] Atmospheric mercury ultimately is deposited into lakes and rivers by dustfall, rain, and snow. In the aquatic environment, mercury is converted by sediment bacteria into methylmercury, which becomes concentrated in the muscle tissues of fish by direct absorption from the water and by biomagnification up through the aquatic food chain. Clinical effects of mercury exposure are discussed in Chapter 20. Although mercury is regulated as a drinking water contaminant, the most important source of exposure is through consumption of methylmercury-contaminated fish.[14]

### Organic Chemicals

**Components of Gasoline.** Gasoline has been stored in underground tanks that have over the years developed leakages, causing toxic chemicals to rapidly move into groundwater and eventually into drinking water supplies. Probably the most toxic component of gasoline is benzene. Along with other gasoline constituents (some of which also are very toxic), it enters the water when gasoline is spilled, or when gasoline tanks leak into the ground, and from other industrial sources. Thousands of other compounds in gasoline are of unknown toxicity. Another toxic compound in gasoline is methyl tertiary butyl ether

(MTBE). The 1990 Clean Air Act required MTBE or ethanol as components of gasoline formulations in areas exceeding the carbon monoxide standard, purportedly to reduce smog in warm weather and to reduce carbon monoxide as a product of combustion in cold weather. This latter use has been discontinued, and the EPA no longer requires MTBE for smog control. Methyl tertiary butyl ether has a strong odor in air and water, and the EPA regulates it for this characteristic. There are conflicting data about carcinogenicity. California regulates MTBE as a carcinogen; the federal government (the EPA and the National Toxicology Program) do not classify it as a carcinogen. Benzene is known to cause leukemia in humans[15] and aplastic anemia at high doses (see Chapter 15).

**Nitrates.** Nitrates enter the water supply from urban and agricultural runoff of nitrogen fertilizers. They also may be produced by bacterial action on animal waste runoff. Nitrates themselves are not toxic to humans, but can be converted to more reactive and toxic nitrites by gut bacteria. Nitrates in drinking water above the EPA level of 10 mg/L may cause fatal methemoglobinemia in infants (see Chapter 22).

**Pesticides.** Pesticides may not be removed by conventional drinking water treatment. As detection technologies have improved, increasingly low concentrations of common insecticides, herbicides, and fungicides have been documented in drinking water.[16]

Some of the older pesticides were designed to be persistent in the environment for years, and can be found distributed worldwide in water and soil. Newer pesticides degrade more quickly, but still contaminate water. Concentrations in water often correlate with growing seasons in agricultural areas and rainy seasons in more urban settings.

Chemical contamination of groundwater in municipal and private wells has been found in the past 2 decades. Private wells may become contaminated with agricultural pesticides. During the late 1970s and early 1980s, aldicarb, a carbamate pesticide, was found in private wells in New York, California, Maine, and Florida. In Wisconsin, where aldicarb was used to treat potatoes about 300 private wells were found to be contaminated.[17] Environmental analyses revealed that the water-soluble pesticide leached through the sandy soils often favored for growing potatoes and other crops.

While high-level, acute poisoning is well understood for most pesticides (see Chapter 24), low-level, chronic, and mixed exposures are poorly studied, particularly in infants and children. Consequently, great uncertainty exists about the significance of contamination of drinking water with pesticides.

**Polychlorinated Biphenyls and Dioxins.** Polychlorinated biphenyls were intentionally manufactured as industrial insulating fluids. Dioxins and furans (collectively termed "dioxins") are formed inadvertently via manufacture of other chemicals (eg, PCBs, paper pulp bleaching, and incineration). Polychlorinated biphenyls and dioxins have very low solubility in water and are not found in drinking water. They are a problem because they readily bioaccumulate in the fat of wildlife, are very resistant to biological degradation, and remain in the environment for decades. The sediments of many lakes and rivers are contaminated with PCBs and/or dioxins. Contaminated sediments, a nonpoint source, are still the major source of PCBs and dioxins found in fish and wildlife (see Chapter 14). Dioxins and PCBs are associated with risks of cancer and developmental toxicity.[15,18]

**Trichloroethylene.** In 1986 an association was found between childhood leukemia and drinking water supplied from 2 municipal wells in Woburn, MA.[19] The 2 wells were contaminated with the animal carcinogens trichloroethylene, tetrachloroethylene, and chloroform.[15] Childhood leukemia rates in Woburn reported between 1964 and 1983 were twice the national rates. Some chemical disposal pits, used for several decades, were suspected as the source of these chlorinated products. Although the 2 affected wells were shut down immediately on discovery of the contamination, exposure to these carcinogens is believed to have occurred for many years. Despite years of study, it is not yet known whether the association between trichloroethylene and childhood leukemia is causal.

**Disinfectants and Disinfection By-products.** In the 1970s chlorination of waters having high natural organic content (eg, humic and tannic acids) was found to cause the formation of chloroform and other chlorinated compounds called trihalomethanes (THMs). Some residual levels of the disinfectants chlorine and chlorine dioxide are found in tap water. Epidemiologic studies show a correlation between THM-containing drinking water and increases in the rates of rectal and bladder cancer.[20] As a result of extensive testing of the water supplies in the United States, cancer risk analysis of the chemicals found, and suggestive epidemiologic studies in 1981, the EPA issued a maximum contaminant level for THM in water. One chlorination by-product, bromodichloromethane, has recently been associated with a higher risk of fetal loss in 2 epidemiologic studies and one animal study. It also seems to have sperm toxicity.[21–24] This is an emerging issue, and research is ongoing.

### Radionuclides

#### Radon
Radon gas is a product of the radioactive decay of uranium. It enters the water supply naturally and becomes aerosolized during use of tap water. Radon further breaks down into radon "daughters" or "progeny." Radon in water is important because during showering, radon may be inhaled. Lung cancer in adults has been linked to inhalation of radon progeny.[25] An association of radon with gastrointestinal cancer has been suggested in a few epidemiologic studies (see Chapter 17). More evidence is being collected to better assess these risks.

## Prevention of Exposure

The public health successes of the 20th century in eliminating epidemic cholera and typhoid fever are dramatic evidence of the importance of prevention in managing drinking and recreational water supplies. Historically, water and waste management were local responsibilities. During the environmental movement in the 1970s, Congress enacted laws that unified standards, resulting in the development of high-quality drinking and recreational waters.

### Public Water Supplies

The EPA and state agencies require that municipal or commercial water suppliers serving more than 25 people meet all standards developed under the Safe Drinking Water Act of 1974 and its amendments (see Table 27.2). The Water Pollution Control Act (1972) and the Resource Conservation and Recovery Act (1976) require industrial, commercial, and municipal facilities to meet requirements to prevent contamination of surface and groundwaters.

In 1987 increased findings of water supplies contaminated with industrial chemicals led the EPA to promulgate drinking water standards for 8 volatile organic compounds, including those most often found in contaminated wells. The EPA and state environmental agencies also require municipal water supplies to meet specific standards for pesticides that have been found in groundwater and surface water.[26] Restrictions have been placed on the use of pesticides, which may leach into waters. Drinking water also must meet a standard for disinfectants and disinfectant by-products (see Table 27.2). The benefits of disinfection of drinking water in reducing waterborne diseases far outweigh the risks from traces of disinfection by-products in drinking water.

### Private Wells

Private wells are not federally regulated. The EPA estimates that 42 million people in the United States get drinking water from private wells. Contamination of well water can occur if the well is shallow,

**Table 27.2**
**Selected National Primary Drinking Water Regulations 2002***

| Contaminant | Type of Standard[†] | Standard |
|---|---|---|
| **Microbiologic Contaminants** | | |
| *Cryptosporidium* | TT | 99% removal/inactivation |
| *Giardia lamblia* | TT | 99.9% removal/inactivation |
| Heterotrophic plate count (HPC)[‡] | TT | ≤500 bacterial colonies/mL |
| Total coliforms (including fecal coliforms and *Escherichia coli*) | MCL | <5.0% of samples/month allowed to contain fecal coliforms and *Escherichia coli* |
| Turbidity[§] | TT | Can never exceed 1 unit; <0.3 unit in 95% of daily samples (per month) |
| Viruses (enteric) | TT | 99.99% removal/inactivation |
| **Inorganic Chemicals** | | **Standard (mg/L = ppm)** |
| Arsenic | MCL | 0.010 (as of 1/23/06) |
| Barium | MCL | 2 |
| Beryllium | MCL | 0.004 |
| Cadmium | MCL | 0.005 |
| Chromium (total) | MCL | 0.1 |
| Fluoride | MCL | 4.0 |
| Lead | TT | If >10% of tap water samples exceed 0.015 water must be treated to control corrosiveness |
| Mercury (inorganic) | MCL | 0.002 |
| Nitrate (as N) | MCL | 10 |
| Selenium | MCL | 0.05 |
| **Organic Chemicals** | | |
| Alachlor | MCL | 0.002 |
| Atrazine | MCL | 0.003 |
| Benzene | MCL | 0.005 |
| Benzo(a)pyrene | MCL | 0.0002 |
| Carbofuran | MCL | 0.04 |
| Carbon tetrachloride | MCL | 0.005 |

**Table 27.2**
**Selected National Primary Drinking Water Regulations 2002\*, *continued***

| Contaminant | Type of Standard† | Standard (mg/L = ppm) |
|---|---|---|
| **Organic Chemicals, *continued*** | | |
| Chlordane | MCL | 0.002 |
| 2,4-D | MCL | 0.07 |
| 1,2-Dibromo-3-chloropropane (DBCP) | MCL | 0.0002 |
| p-Dichlorobenzene | MCL | 0.075 |
| 1,2-Dichloroethane | MCL | 0.005 |
| 1,1-Dichloroethylene | MCL | 0.007 |
| Dichloromethane | MCL | 0.005 |
| 1,2-Dichloropropane | MCL | 0.005 |
| Di(2-ethylhexyl) phthalate | MCL | 0.006 |
| Dioxin (2,3,7,8-TCDD) | MCL | 0.00000003 |
| Endrin | MCL | 0.002 |
| Ethelyne dibromide | MCL | 0.00005 |
| Glyphosate | MCL | 0.7 |
| Heptachlor | MCL | 0.0004 |
| Hexachlorobenzene | MCL | 0.001 |
| Lindane | MCL | 0.0002 |
| Methoxychlor | MCL | 0.04 |
| Polychlorinated biphenyls | MCL | 0.0005 |
| Pentachlorophenol | MCL | 0.001 |
| Tetrachloroethylene | MCL | 0.005 |
| 2,4,5-T, Silvex | MCL | 0.05 |
| 1,1,1-Trichloroethane | MCL | 0.2 |
| 1,1,2-Trichloroethane | MCL | 0.005 |
| Trichloroethylene | MCL | 0.005 |
| Vinyl chloride | MCL | 0.002 |
| Xylenes (total) | MCL | 10 |

| Contaminant | Type of Standard[†] | Standard |
|---|---|---|
| **Disinfectants/Disinfectant By-products** | | |
| Bromate | MCL | 0.01 |
| Chloramines (as $Cl_2$) | MRDL | 4.0 |
| Chlorine (as $Cl_2$) | MRDL | 4.0 |
| Chlorine dioxide (as $ClO_2$) | MRDL | 0.8 |
| Chlorite | MCL | 1.0 |
| Haloacetic acid | MCL | 0.06 |
| Trihalomethanes | MCL | 0.08 |
| **Radionuclides** | | |
| Alpha particles | MCL | 15 pCi/L[‖] |
| Beta particles and photon emitters | MCL | 4 mrem/y[¶] |
| Radium-226 and radium-228 | MCL | 5 pCi/L |
| Uranium | MCL | 30 µg/L (as of 12/08/03) |

* From US Environmental Protection Agency.[26]

† MCL, maximum contaminant level; TT, treatment technique; MRDL, maximum residual disinfectant level.

‡ Heterotrophic plate count (HPC): HPC has no health effects but is an analytic method used to measure the variety of bacteria common in water. The lower the concentration of bacteria in water, the better maintained is the water system.

§ Turbidity: A measure of water cloudiness used to determine water quality and filtration effectiveness. Higher turbidity levels are often associated with higher levels of disease-producing organisms.

‖ pCi/L, picocurie per liter.

¶ mrem/y, millirem per year.

in porous soil, old, poorly maintained, near a leaky septic tank, or downhill from agricultural fields or intensive livestock operations. Each state has different testing procedures, sometimes requiring testing only at transfer of land ownership. Testing of private wells is the responsibility of individual homeowners, but in some states may be performed at no cost by the health department if recommended by a health care provider. In rural areas, physicians can ask patients if their wells have been tested by local or county health departments within the last year for coliforms and nitrates. Guidance for testing and water treatment for owners of private wells is available from the State of Wisconsin at http://www.dnr.state.wi.us/org/water/dwg/prih2o.htm.

In agricultural areas, higher than normal levels of nitrates or coliform bacteria may indicate the presence of pesticides. If so, parents can contact state health and environmental agencies to determine if their well water should be tested for specific pesticides. State agencies may conduct the testing without cost or may recommend private laboratories. Extensive pesticide testing should not be encouraged due to the cost and the rarity of pesticide contamination.

### Home Treatment Systems
Home water filtration and treatment systems that remove lead, chlorine by-products, traces of organic compounds, and bacteria are increasingly popular. These systems, which may attach to the end of a water faucet, generally provide limited health benefits. Most drinking water sources keep contaminants below EPA standards and state criteria. In addition, small, end-of-the-faucet filtration systems are not always highly effective in removing trace substances. If not properly maintained, filters using activated carbon can provide media for the growth of bacteria. Unless the carbon filter is frequently replaced, the first morning draw of tap water can have unacceptable levels of bacteria. In spite of potential drawbacks, some home water systems can be effective in removing lead and other toxic substances. These systems, however, do not remove fluoride.

Home drinking treatment systems or filters are not encouraged unless a chemical problem has been identified. Even then, it is more effective, on a communitywide basis, to have the municipal or commercial water source personnel correct the problem as required by law than to have homeowners assume the responsibility. However, if families prefer to treat water, it is important to ensure that the treatment system removes the pollutants of concern and that the system is maintained so that it functions well and does not become contaminated.

### Contaminants in Fish

Physicians living in active fishing areas with advisories related to PCBs or mercury should ask women and children if their consumption of fish is in accordance with state-issued fish advisories. Freshwater fish generally have higher levels of contaminants than saltwater fish.[27–31] Saltwater fish, generally low in contaminants, are the main fish purchased in the marketplace. However, a few saltwater fish may have higher levels of contaminants than freshwater fish. They include swordfish, shark, king mackerel, tilefish, and tuna, which are long-lived, predatory fish capable of bioaccumulating methylmercury.

---

To reduce hazards from fish consumption, inform parents to
- Eat pan fish rather than predator fish (shark, swordfish, tuna).
- Eat small game fish rather than large ones.
- Eat fewer fatty fish (mackerel, carp, catfish, lake trout), which accumulate higher levels of chemical toxicants.
- Trim skin and fatty areas where contaminants such as PCBs and dichlorodiphenyltrichloroethane (DDT) accumulate. (Note: Trimming fatty areas will have no effect on consumption of methylmercury, which accumulates in fish muscle.)
- Advise women of childbearing age, pregnant women, nursing mothers, and young children to follow fish advisories.
- Know state fish advisories obtained from state health, environmental, and conservation departments.

---

**Current Federal Fish Advisories**

Health scientists in the Great Lakes states, the Agency for Toxic Substances and Disease Registry (ATSDR), and the EPA have recommended limiting PCB intake to protect the developing fetus from neurologic effects. This has resulted in fish advisories in the Great Lakes region. These advisories also may protect the general public from adverse immune system effects and theoretical cancer risks of ingesting PCBs. For example, fish advisories for Lake Michigan recommend that individuals not eat more than one meal per month of salmon (with an average of 0.7 ppm PCBs), for a maximum of 12 meals per year. Women and children are advised to wait a month before eating another meal of Lake Michigan salmon or any other fish from a restricted category to prevent PCBs from building up in the body. Instructions also are provided to help reduce PCB exposures by cleaning (eg, fat removal) and cooking methods.[27–31]

Guidelines for maximum exposure to mercury have been established by the EPA at 0.1 µg/kg per day,[13] by the US Food and Drug Administration (FDA) at 0.4 µg/kg per day,[32] and by the ATSDR at 0.3 µg/kg per day.[33] The FDA and most states advise that pregnant women, young children, and women of childbearing age should not eat fish with mercury levels greater than 0.5 ppm. Most state health agencies advise limiting intake of freshwater fish having greater than 0.2 ppm of mercury, and the FDA advises that people at higher risk eat no more than 12 oz of fish a week, on average. Other states simply recommend that women and children not eat any large predator fish that tend to concentrate mercury.

**Frequently Asked Questions**

Q  *Should I buy bottled water?*

A  Unless there are known contamination problems of the drinking water, families should not be encouraged to buy bottled water. Bottled water is not required to meet any higher standards than tap water, and can cost 500 to 1000 times as much.

Q *Should I boil my baby's water or use a home water treatment system?*

A If on a public water supply that meets standards, parents should not boil their infant's drinking water or use a home water treatment system unless the drinking water is contaminated. Drinking water should be boiled only when the water supplier or health or environmental agency issues such instructions. The Centers for Disease Control and Prevention and the EPA state that people with special health needs (eg, those who are immunocompromised) may wish to boil or treat their drinking water. Boiling tap water for 1 minute inactivates or destroys biological agents, but boiling water longer than 1 minute may concentrate contaminants. Point-of-use filters also may be considered but only if they are clearly labeled to remove particles 1 μm or less in diameter. Unless carefully evaluated and well maintained, home water treatment systems often are ineffective and may even contribute to exposure to waterborne bacteria.

Q *Is it true that federal and state regulations ensure the safety of drinking water?*

A In most cases, regulations provide very safe water. Nonetheless, almost 10% of the population drinks water that does not meet the regulations. Violations are higher where water supply systems serve fewer than 1000 people. Some standards (eg, for *Cryptosporidium*) only apply to systems that serve more than 10 000 people. The new lower standard of the allowable level of arsenic in water is phasing in slowly over the next 2 years. Information on drinking water quality and violations can be obtained from the water supplier or state health and environmental agencies. Even water in compliance with all standards may contain harmful contamination. Consumers are given annual written statements of any violations by their public water supply in consumer confidence reports. Many public water suppliers maintain Web sites with current surveillance information.

Q *Should I get my water tested?*

A Under most circumstances, it is not necessary to have drinking water tested. If the local water supply fails to meet a standard, pressure should be exerted on politicians to correct the problem, rather than have people test their own water. As a precaution, people who use private wells less than 50 ft (15 m) deep and have septic systems should have them tested yearly for coliforms (see Table 27.2). In agricultural areas, quarterly testing of private wells for 1 year is recommended followed by yearly nitrate testing if results of quarterly tests are normal.

Q *Do the benefits of eating fish outweigh the risks from PCBs, mercury, and other contaminants?*

A Fish provide a diet high in protein and low in saturated fats. The consumption of fish may reduce the risk of coronary disease. State and federal health agencies recommend that people who frequently consume freshwater fish follow fish advisories. This permits the consumer to reap the potential benefits of fish consumption and minimize risks due to the intake of PCBs and mercury.

**Resources**

Agency for Toxic Substances and Disease Registry, Information Center, Internet: http://www.atsdr.cdc.gov

Local and State Health Departments

US Environmental Protection Agency regional offices are listed in the local telephone book; EPA Safe Drinking Water Hotline, 800/426-4791, Internet: http://www.epa.gov/ost/fish

US Fish and Wildlife Service, Department of the Interior, Internet: http://www.fws.gov

## References

1. Okum DA. Water quality management. In: Last JM, Wallace RB, eds. *Public Health and Preventive Medicine.* 13th ed. Norwalk, CT: Appleton & Lange; 1992:619–648

2. Ruttenber AJ. Water: pollution and availability. In: Blumenthal DS, Ruttenber AJ, eds. *Introduction to Environmental Health.* 2nd ed. New York, NY: Springer Publishing Co, Inc; 1995:221–254

3. Craun GF. The epidemiology of waterborne disease: the importance of drinking water disinfection. In: Talbott EO, Craun GF, eds. *Introduction to Environmental Epidemiology.* Boca Raton, FL: Lewis Publishers; 1995:123–150

4. American Academy of Pediatrics Committee on Infectious Diseases. Pickering LK, ed. *Red Book®: 2003 Report of the Committee on Infectious Diseases.* 26th ed. Elk Grove Village, IL: American Academy of Pediatrics; 2003

5. Bowen EL, Hu H. Food contamination due to environmental pollution. In: Chivian E, McCally H, Hu H, Haines A, eds. *Critical Condition: Human Health and the Environment.* Cambridge, MA: MIT Press; 1993

6. Payment P, Richardson L, Siemiatycki J, Dewar R, Edwardes M, Franco E. A randomized trial to evaluate the risk of gastrointestinal disease due to consumption of drinking water meeting current microbiological standards. *Am J Public Health.* 1991;81:703–708

7. Codd GA, Ward CJ, Bell SG. Cyanobacterial toxins: occurrence, modes of action, health effects and exposure routes. *Arch Toxicol Suppl.* 1997; 19:399–410

8. Pouria S, de Andrade A, Barbosa J, et al. Fatal microcystin intoxication in haemodialysis unit in Caruaru, Brazil. *Lancet.* 1998;352:21–26

9. Grattan LM, Oldach D, Perl TM, et al. Learning and memory difficulties after environmental exposure to waterways containing toxic-producing *Pfiesteria* or *Pfiesteria*-like dinoflagellates. *Lancet.* 1998;352:532–539

10. Goldman LR. Chemicals and children's environment: what we don't know about risks. *Environ Health Perspect.* 1998;106(suppl 3):875–880

11. Kolpin DW, Furlong ET, Meyer MT, et al. Pharmaceuticals, hormones, and other organic wastewater contaminants in US streams, 1999–2000: a national reconnaissance. *Environ Sci Technol.* 2002;36:1202–1211

12. National Academy of Sciences. *Arsenic in Drinking Water.* Washington, DC: National Academies Press; 1999:330

13. Goldman LR, Shannon MW, American Academy of Pediatrics Committee on Environmental Health. Technical report: mercury in the environment: implications for pediatricians. *Pediatrics.* 2001;108:197–205

14. Harada Y. Congenital (or fetal) Minamata disease. In: Study Group of Minamata Disease, ed. *Minamata Disease.* Japan: Kumamoto University, 1968:93–117

15. National Toxicology Program. *9th Report on Carcinogens (Revised).* Washington, DC: Public Health Services, US Department of Health and Human Services; 2001

16. US Geological Survey National Water Quality Assessment Program. NAWQA Pesticide National Synthesis Program. Available at: http://ca.water.usgs.gov/pnsp/

17. Mirkin IR, Anderson HA, Hanrahan L, Hong R, Golubjatnikov R, Belluck D. Changes in T-lymphocyte distribution associated with ingestion of aldicarb-contaminated drinking water: a follow-up study. *Environ Res.* 1990;51:35–50

18. Jacobson JL, Jacobson SW. Intellectual impairment in children exposed to polychlorinated biphenyls in utero. *N Engl J Med.* 1996;335:783–789

19. National Research Council. *Environmental Epidemiology: Public Health and Hazardous Wastes.* Washington, DC: National Academies Press; 1991:1

20. Morris RD, Audet AM, Angelillo IF, Chalmers TC, Mosteller F. Chlorination, chlorination by-products, and cancer: a meta-analysis. *Am J Public Health.* 1992;82:955–963

21. Klinefelter GR, Suarez JD, Roberts NL, DeAngelo AB. Preliminary screening for the potential of drinking water disinfection byproducts to alter male reproduction. *Reprod Toxicol.* 1995;9:571–578

22. Waller K, Swan SH, DeLorenze G, Hopkins B. Trihalomethanes in drinking water and spontaneous abortion. *Epidemiology.* 1998;9:134–140

23. Bielmeier SR, Best DS, Guidici DL, Narotsky MG. Pregnancy loss in the rat caused by bromodichloromethane. *Toxicol Sci.* 2001;59:309–315

24. King WD, Dodds L, Allen AC. Relation between stillbirth and specific chlorination by-products in public water supplies. *Environ Health Perspect.* 2000;108:883–886

25. Bean JA, Isacson P, Hahne RM, Kohler J. Drinking water and cancer incidence in Iowa. II. Radioactivity in drinking water. *Am J Epidemiol.* 1982;116:924–932

26. US Environmental Protection Agency, Office of Ground Water & Drinking Water. List of Drinking Water Contaminants and MCL. Available at: http://www.epa.gov/safewater/mcl.htm

27. US Environmental Protection Agency, Office of Water. *Drinking Water Regulations and Health: What You Need to Know.* Washington, DC: Environmental Protection Agency; 1999. EPA Publication 816-K-99-001

28. Anderson HA. *Protocol for a Uniform Great Lakes Sport Fish Advisory.* Madison, WI: Wisconsin Department of Health and Family Services; 1993

29. Minnesota Department of Public Health. *Fish and Your Health: Environmental Exposure to PCBs.* June 1993

30. Minnesota Department of Public Health. *An Expectant Mother's Guide.* August 1994

31. Minnesota Department of Public Health. *Mercury in the Environment.* May 1996

32. Tollefson L, Cordle F. Methylmercury in fish: a review of residue levels, fish consumption and regulatory action in the United States. *Environ Health Perspect.* 1986;68:203–208

33. Agency for Toxic Substances and Disease Registry. *Toxicological Profile for Mercury.* Atlanta, GA: US Public Health Service; 1999

# 28
# Child Care Settings

Every day 13 million preschoolers—including 6 million infants and toddlers, regardless of their mother's work status—are in some form of non-parental care.[1] This accounts for nearly 60% of all children younger than age 6 years. Typical child care arrangements for young children when parents work are child care centers (29%), family child care homes (15%), parents (24%), relatives (25%), and in-home caregivers other than the parent or relative (5%).[1] Children enter care as early as 6 weeks of age and can be in care for as many as 40 hours per week until they reach school age.[2] Millions of school-aged children are in after-school and summer activities, and nearly 7 million children are home alone after school each week while their parents work.[2]

Child care settings are located in single-family homes or buildings specifically designed for child care or within office buildings, schools, churches, malls, health clubs, and other sites. The American Public Health Association and American Academy of Pediatrics (AAP) recommend that these child care settings be designed or modified to meet current standards published in *Caring for Our Children: National Health and Safety Performance Standards—Guidelines for Out-of-Home Child Care Programs.*[3] These standards, which apply to all aspects of child care settings, including environmental health aspects, should be met regardless of the setting or whether the care provided is full time or part time.[2]

States establish and enforce child care licensing regulations that include health and safety requirements. The scope and intensity of state enforcement activities differ among the provider types within states as well as among states overall. For example, most states do not regulate some types of providers such as relatives or in-home nannies and au pairs.[4] Child care centers typically have more health and safety regulations and oversight compared with family child care homes, hourly drop-off care, and preschool programs (particularly if they operate part time). One study suggests compliance with regulations depends on agreement of child care providers with the rationale for the regulations as well as the quality and frequency of inspection.[2] The licensing and enforcement activities most commonly considered to be critical are background checks, monitoring visits, sanctions, training for licensing staff, and caseload of licensing staff.[4]

The occurrence of environmental hazards in child care varies widely and is influenced by

- Type of setting
- Licensing requirements
- Location and age of the structure
- Past use of the land or structure
- Current use of other parts of the structure
- Behaviors and practices of adults in the setting
- Prevalence of hazards in the community

Hazards in a child care setting can adversely affect a group of children. On the other hand, children may benefit when hazards are reduced or controlled. For example, children exposed to environmental tobacco smoke (ETS), radon, or lead paint at home may reduce their total daily exposure by spending time in child care.

### Environmental Hazards in Child Care Settings

Environmental hazards in child care settings are expected to be similar to those found in other environments (see Table 28.1). Of the few studies that document environmental hazards in child care, indoor air quality, ETS, lead, and pesticides are noted to be of concern (see chapters 6, 13, 19, and 24).

**Table 28.1**
**Environmental Hazards in Child Care Settings**

| Environmental Hazard | Indoor Sources | Outdoor Sources |
|---|---|---|
| **Poor air quality** | | |
| Carbon monoxide (CO) | • CO from malfunctioning or improperly vented fuel-burning appliances such as stoves, furnaces, fireplaces, clothes dryers, water heaters, and space heaters<br>• Poorly maintained home heating system such as dirty furnace filter or a blocked flue | • Playground located near high-traffic area or near the exhaust outlet of a building<br>• Auto, truck, or bus exhaust from attached garages, nearby roads, or idling parking areas |
| Environmental tobacco smoke | • Smoking in the child care area<br>• A multiple-use building with a smoking area that is not properly ventilated and exhausted to the outside | • Fresh air intake (eg, doorway) located near an outside smoking area or an exhaust outlet that emits tobacco smoke in an area where children play |
| Molds and other biological pollutants | • Plumbing leaks, roof leaks, and flooding provide the moisture for molds and other biological pollutants | • Water from river or sewer overflows |
| Volatile organic compounds (VOCs) | • VOCs from building materials and furnishings (eg, formaldehyde), paints, cleaning supplies, and coverings on floors | |

**Table 28.1**
**Environmental Hazards in Child Care Settings,** *continued*

| Environmental Hazard | Indoor Sources | Outdoor Sources |
|---|---|---|
| **Other chemical hazards** | | |
| Lead and other heavy metals | • Leaded dust or paint chips, particularly on floors, windowsills, and window wells, and during renovation of pre-1978 structures<br>• Leaded paint on furniture or toys, leaded ceramic dishware, plumbing, remedies, and other sources<br>• Arts and crafts supplies, paints, acidic foods or beverages placed in galvanized containers | • Leaded soil or leaded paint on the building's exterior, fences, sheds, or playground equipment<br>• Improperly contained materials from renovations in the vicinity of the setting<br>• Soil contamination at the site from prior industrial use or geological mineral deposits<br>• Toxic clays and play structures or contents of storage areas accessible to children |
| Pesticides such as lawn and garden chemicals, herbicides, insecticides, rodenticides, sanitizers, and disinfectants | • Improper storage, labeling, handling, or use of pesticides in any child care area, particularly in the following high-risk areas: diaper changing, food preparation and storage, carpeted areas, laundry, maintenance and custodial supply rooms, rooms where children eat and play, as well as other areas prone to infestation of pests<br>• Infested food preparation and storage areas, bedding, laundry rooms, and spaces under sinks due to preventable problems such as poor sanitation, water leaks, and unprotected openings to the outside | • Improper storage, labeling, handling, or use of chemical products in any area accessible to children, particularly unsecured storage sheds<br>• Infested playgrounds and storage sheds, space under sheds, debris, and clutter or dense foliage near the foundation |

| Environmental Hazard | Indoor Sources | Outdoor Sources |
|---|---|---|
| **Other hazards** | | |
| Other household drugs or chemicals such as medications, cosmetics, chemical products, pool chemicals, and petroleum products for outdoor maintenance equipment | • Improper storage, labeling, handling, or use of medications or chemicals in any child care area | • Improper storage, labeling, handling, or use of chemical products in any area accessible to children, particularly unsecured storage sheds |
| **Physical hazards** | | |
| Asbestos | • Friable, non-intact asbestos in exposed insulation, ceilings, floors, or duct work<br>• Renovation without appropriate asbestos containment | • Disasters (eg, collapse of the World Trade Center towers) |
| Noise | • Room design or materials that amplify sounds | • Adjacent roadways, airports, or industrial sources of sound |
| Radon | • Cracks and openings in foundations allow this naturally occurring radioactive gas to leak through the ground into buildings | |
| Ultraviolet radiation | | • Excessive sun exposure because of inadequate shade on the playground, nonrestricted time and duration of outdoor play, and inadequate use of sun-protective clothing and sunscreen |

## Environmental Tobacco Smoke

Licensed child care centers are more likely to have smoke-free policies and enforce these policies compared with family child care homes. In a 1993 national survey of US licensed child care centers, 55% of the centers reported being smoke-free indoors and outdoors.[4] In the remaining 45% of child care centers, smoking was not totally prohibited in the building. Children may be exposed when employees are allowed to smoke when children are not present, or when they smoke in another part of the building that shares a common ventilation system with the center.[4]

While the prevalence of smoking among adults in family child care homes is largely unknown, one study suggests that ETS is an important hazard in this setting. Exposure to caregiver smoking was low for children cared for in child care centers (<1%), but high for children cared for in other homes (26%) or in their own homes (26%).[4] This is in contrast with the rate of smoking among mothers who cared for their own children at home (17%). Infants whose mothers smoked were more likely to have a caregiver who smoked. During an infant's first 3 years, approximately one fifth of those with nonsmoking mothers were in a care setting with a caregiver who smoked.

## Indoor Air Quality

Children spend 80% to 90% of their time indoors (home, child care, school, after-school care, etc) and indoor air quality is an important health concern (see Chapter 6) stimulating federal initiatives such as *Indoor Air Quality: Tools for Schools*[5] and *Home\*A\*Syst/Farm\*A\*Syst.*[6] Pollutants that contribute to poor indoor air quality include ETS, molds and other biological products, combustion by-products, and volatile organic compounds (VOCs). Only one indoor air quality in child care study[7] was located, and it investigated carbon dioxide ($CO_2$) levels in 91 child care centers in Quebec, Canada. Ninety percent had $CO_2$ levels that exceeded the office building standard.[7] Increased $CO_2$ levels were associated with the number of children in a given area.

A high $CO_2$ level (>1000 ppm) can be used as a rough indicator of the effectiveness of ventilation and can serve as a marker for other indoor air pollutants.[7]

## Lead

There are few studies of lead hazards in child care. The prevalence of lead in family child care homes is probably similar to the prevalence among homes in the community. A survey of schools, preschools, and child care centers conducted in Washington state found that 62% of 75 facilities built before 1979 contained leaded paint, and 31% contained elevated leaded soil or dust.[4]

Lead exposure is probably underestimated by routine surveillance systems. When lead paint is identified in the home of a child who has been poisoned by lead, sources of lead in the home are identified. Sources of lead away from the home (such as child care settings) are more likely to be overlooked. Two studies of children attending child care centers with high environmental lead levels (in paint, dust, or soil)[8,9] found only one child who had a confirmed blood lead level exceeding 10 µg/dL (12 µg/dL).[9] These results, however, cannot be generalized to all child care settings. In both studies, the average age of the participants was about 5 years, and in one study, the rate of participation was low.[8] Children in these 2 studies may have been protected from lead exposure by continual supervision, high frequency of hand washing (averaging once per hour), and standard cleaning practices, including daily wet mopping of floors. Therefore, there are no data showing that child care settings are a significant source of environmental lead. The risk of exposure may be higher with younger children, poor hygiene and maintenance practices, or when housing renovations occur without appropriate testing and containment measures.

Federal regulations address the problem of lead only in the child's home. Federal funding for remediation of lead hazards can be applied to homes, but not to child care settings.

## Pesticides and Other Toxic Household Products

Children are highly vulnerable to pesticides (see Chapter 24). While no studies specifically address pesticides in child care settings, it is probably similar to home, school, and other settings in the community. Communities where children are at increased risk of pesticide exposure include agricultural areas as well as urban and other settings where pesticides are used extensively in schools, homes, and child care centers for control of cockroaches, rats, and other pests. The use of pesticides in child care settings is common because young children in child care spill food that attracts pests, and many of the buildings used for child care are old and poorly maintained for control of pests by other means. Children can be exposed to pesticides in child care through a variety of sources such as

- Pesticide residues from indoor or outdoor pesticide use (may be found in the indoor air, surfaces, household dust, and soil/drift)
- Pets
- Residues on food
- Playground structures made of wood treated with wood-preserving pesticides such as copper chromium arsenate
- Lawn and garden products
- Insect repellents

The incidence of poisoning by pesticides and other household products (such as medications [incorrect administration of or exposure to], arts and crafts materials, toxic plants, and petroleum products) was higher when children were in their own homes.[10] Children in child care centers may be protected somewhat because they usually are supervised by an adult, the facility and equipment are designed for children, and licensing procedures and public health inspections help to eliminate hazards. However, the potential for poisonings is real. In Colorado, health inspectors visiting child care settings 2 weeks after licensing inspections found toxic chemicals accessible to children in

68% of the settings.[11]  Some products such as pesticides may be used
as directed but still are not safe to use in child care settings.[12]

**Characteristics of Child Care That May Exacerbate Hazards**

Several child care characteristics impact its environmental quality.
First, low salaries (the average salary of a child care worker is $14,820
per year)[13] and lack of benefits generate high staff turnover among
child care providers. Because approximately one third of child care
staff leave their centers each year, child care service operators need to
continually educate new employees.[14] In addition, 31 states require no
training in early childhood care and education, intensifying the need
for voluntary continuing education.[9] Second, child care businesses
usually operate with a low profit margin. The largest portion of a
family child care home or child care center budget is dedicated to staff
salaries. Tuition funded by public assistance often is at low, fixed dollar
amounts. These financial conditions result in limited funds for preventive measures such as pest control by a professional and appropriate lead hazard abatement remodeling or renovation. It is important
to note when considering measures to reduce or eliminate environmental hazards that it is difficult for child care programs to temporarily close. Third, when a child care center is located within a larger
facility, such as a church or office building, hazards may arise due
to practices that occur in other parts of the facility.

**Measures to Prevent or Control Environmental Hazards in a
Child Care Setting**

*Caring for Our Children: The National Health and Safety Performance
Standards—Guidelines for Out-of-Home Child Care Programs* identifies
numerous prevention and control measures.[3] Some of these are discussed here, but the standards should be consulted for details on the
features of the facility and the operational activities that reduce environmental risks.

## *Primary Prevention*

### Site Selection

An environmental audit, from a child and adult perspective, should be conducted prior to selecting a child care site and before new construction begins or an existing building is renovated. The environmental audit should at least include assessments of (1) historical land use to determine the potential for soil contamination with toxic or hazardous waste such as old gasoline storage; (2) molds, lead, and asbestos in older buildings; (3) potential sources of infestation, noise, air pollution, and toxic exposures; (4) location of the playground in relation to stagnant water, roadways, industrial emissions, and building exhaust outlets; and (5) access to a safe drinking water supply (public or private), a public sewer or approved septic tank system, and other utilities such as electricity. While geological factors may suggest potential radon exposure, there are no reliable methods of testing for radon prior to construction.

### Architectural Design and Building Materials

Modern homes and buildings are more tightly sealed, and mechanical cooling and heating systems are common in all climate zones. Thousands of new materials used as goods, finishes, and furnishings have increased sources of indoor pollution.[15] Indoor air quality from an architectural design and building materials perspective depends on (1) the absence of pollutants (source management—includes removal, substitution, and encapsulation), (2) the power of ventilation systems to supply fresh air indoors, (3) the ability of local exhausts and air cleaning through filtration to remove pollutants, and (4) controlling exposure to pollutants such as cleaning products through the principles of time of use and location of use.[16] Prevention and control measures include frequent air exchanges and sufficient ventilation (especially bathrooms, diapering areas, and kitchens) of air to the outside; some windows that open, preferably offering cross ventilation;

and properly placed fresh-air intakes, which prevent exhaust from automobiles and the building systems from reaching hazardous levels inside. Electrostatic air cleaners and high-efficiency filtration systems can be used. Pesticide use can be reduced by sealing openings and using screens on the doors and windows. Less toxic building materials, paints, cleaners, and other products that contain pollutants can be selected to minimize levels of toxic substances.[15]

## Child Care Regulation and Monitoring

Before construction or remodeling is started, consultation with an environmental health specialist (such as those located in local health departments) to review construction or remodeling plans is essential to prevent environmental hazards. State or local health departments may need to develop additional environmental health regulations that specifically address child care facilities. Child care settings should be monitored by trained licensors who visit during construction or remodeling, inspect them prior to opening and routinely during operation, and investigate complaints. All parts of the child care setting, not only the food service area, must be inspected to identify potential environmental hazards so preventive actions can be implemented. Table 28.2 provides key environmental health questions to include in a routine health and safety inspection of a child care facility. Refer to *Caring for Our Children: National Health and Safety Performance Standards—Guidelines for Out-of-Home Child Care Programs* for a comprehensive listing of standards and rationale.[3]

## Education

Continued education of child care providers was shown to be a strong predictor of few safety hazards in child care centers in a study of child care centers in Sweden.[17] Through Healthy Child Care America, a national campaign initiated in 1995 by the US Department of Health and Human Services' Maternal and Child Health Bureau and Child Care Bureau and coordinated by the AAP, many states now have a

**Table 28.2**
**Some Key Questions to Assess Potential Environmental Hazards in a Child Care Setting**

| | |
|---|---|
| • | Is the child care setting smoke-free? Is there a smoke-free child care policy? |
| • | Does the facility appear clean, in good repair, and without water-marked areas or areas of peeling and chipping paint? |
| • | Is there any evidence of water damage or mold in the facility? Have flooding or plumbing problems occurred? Are there musty odors? |
| • | Are the rooms adequately ventilated? |
| • | Has the child care center or home been tested for radon? |
| • | Are fuel-burning furnaces, stoves, or other equipment in use? |
| • | Are medications and chemical products properly labeled and stored in areas inaccessible to children and in a manner so as not to contaminate food? Are staff members trained in the safe use of chemical products and administration of medications? |
| • | Are arts and crafts supplies free of hazardous substances and labeled in compliance with the American Society for Testing and Materials? |
| • | Are the kitchen and bathroom areas operated in compliance with health department regulations? |
| • | Are hand-washing policies followed and monitored? Are soap and clean towels always available? |
| • | Are indoor and outdoor storage closets and sheds locked so their contents are inaccessible to children? All maintenance, lawn care and other hazardous equipment, and chemical products (such as gasoline, paints, pesticides, and cleaning products) must be inaccessible to children. |
| • | If the building was constructed before 1978, has the building been assessed for lead paint, dust, and soil hazards, as well as asbestos hazards? Homes and other buildings built before 1978 may contain lead, and those built before 1950 have the most lead. If remodeling or renovation work is under way, have lead and asbestos hazards been assessed, and have children been protected from the release of these potentially hazardous toxicants? |
| • | Is there standing water? |
| • | Is integrated pest management used? |
| • | Are there adequate shady areas for play outside? |

child care health consultation system established to respond to child care providers' health and safety educational needs. Often this state child care health consultation system includes personnel from local health departments with expertise in environmental hazards, communicable diseases, injury control, nutrition, sanitation, and safety. Health professionals who provide child care consultation can assist child care providers to identify environmental hazards, understand the associated health risks, and implement preventive actions. Many times, child care providers seek consultation directly from their community's pediatricians, nurse practitioners, nurses, and other health professionals in pediatric offices. More information for these pediatric health care providers can be obtained in the resource *The Pediatrician's Role in Promoting Health and Safety in Child Care* (available through the AAP at http://www.aap.org). It includes specific strategies such as advocacy, training and consultation, and policy making.

To prevent environmental health hazards, all employees, including maintenance personnel, need to be included in continuing education. For example, janitorial and custodial staff should be regularly monitored to ensure the safest practices. The Occupational Safety and Health Administration requires that Material Safety Data Sheets (MSDS) be kept on file to explain health hazards, proper use and storage procedures, and emergency procedures in case of toxic chemical exposure. Staff also may use MSDS to choose nontoxic chemicals.

Child care providers may not have knowledge about, or experience or supervisory support in, administering medications. To avoid having child care providers administer medications to children, pediatricians may consider prescribing formulations that require fewer dosages or altering the time of administration. When medications must be given while a child is in child care, specific written instructions should be either on the bottle or on a separate piece of paper. Instructions are especially important for medications that are used on an as-needed basis. Instructions are needed for prescription and nonprescription medications and topical preparations such as sunscreen.

## Child Care Program Policies and Procedures

Child care providers are well positioned to respond quickly and appropriately to environmental hazards. By developing child care policies, safe practices can become part of everyday practice. For example, (1) smoking should be prohibited (even among non-caregivers in a family child care home) while children are present and in areas where children may be exposed to ETS—even better, at any time in areas that children will use; (2) plumbing leaks, roof leaks, and flooding should be cleaned up within 24 hours and wet areas cleansed with detergent and water to prevent growth of molds and other biological pollutants; (3) emergency preparedness plans should include procedures for responding to hazardous material incidents and chemical/biological/radiologic threats; and (4) staff should receive education in administration of medications and use of chemicals.

### Secondary Prevention

Some hazardous situations in child care settings may be avoided by educating child care providers and others working in child care settings to recognize and appropriately control hazards (eg, by properly storing or using chemicals). Other hazards may require more costly and complex measures. For example, when extensive mold is found, interim control measures may be needed before full remediation is possible. Remediation procedures should meet applicable standards and regulations. If conditions are potentially hazardous, the center may need to be shut down. When the facility has limited financial resources, environmental health regulators play an important role in ensuring that the health of children is not jeopardized. This may require community collaboration to offset the burden of cost.

### Disease in a Child Attending Out-of-Home Child Care

When a child's illness or symptoms may have an environmental etiology, parents, health care personnel, and public health investigators should evaluate potential exposures in the child's home environment and out-of-home settings.

## Frequently Asked Questions

Q *How can I make my child care facility safe for children with asthma?*

A The 2 most important steps that a child care facility can take to prevent asthma attacks in children are to prohibit smoking and to keep the facility free of molds and other biological pollutants. Of the 13 million children 5 years and younger enrolled in child care in the United States, an estimated 1.4 million have asthma (about 1 child in every 11).[18] Child care programs need to have specific information (provided by the parent or guardian and the child's physician) on file for each child with asthma. The information should explain the child's triggers, medications and how to use them, symptoms that indicate when their asthma is worsening or getting out of control, and what to do in an asthma emergency. The Asthma and Allergy Foundation of America, New England Chapter, has an Asthma-Friendly Child Care Checklist (revised summer 2001), available in English, Spanish, Haitian Creole, and Portuguese, that has useful ideas for making child care environments safe for children with asthma and allergies. It can be ordered through their Web site (http://www.asthmaandallergies.org) or by calling 877-2-ASTHMA. The National Heart, Lung, and Blood Institute also has a similar but shorter checklist—*How Asthma-Friendly Is Your Child-Care Setting?*—available in English and Spanish, which includes an extensive list of resources for child care providers (http://www.nhlbi.nih.gov/health/public/lung/asthma/child_ca.htm).

Q *Are sandboxes and sand safe for children?*

A Sandboxes are safe if constructed and filled with appropriate materials and properly maintained. Sandbox frames are sometimes made with inexpensive railroad ties, which may cause splinters and may be saturated with creosote, a carcinogen. Nontoxic landscaping timbers or non-wood containers are preferred.

In 1986 concern was first expressed that some types of commercially available play sand contained tremolite, a fibrous substance found in some crushed limestone and crushed marble (see Chapter 9). It was hypothesized that the long-term effects of exposure to tremolite would be identical to those of asbestos. Despite these concerns, the US Consumer Product Safety Commission (CPSC) denied a petition prohibiting marketing of play sand containing significant levels of tremolite. The CPSC currently has no standards or labeling requirements regarding the source or content of sand.

Directors of child care facilities and parents may have difficulty determining what sand is safe. They should attempt to buy only natural river, beach, or silica-based materials. They should avoid products that are made from crushed limestone or crushed marble, or those that are obviously dusty. When there is doubt, parents may send a sample of sand to a laboratory for determination of asbestos content. Information about reliable laboratories can be obtained from the US Environmental Protection Agency Regional Asbestos Coordinators (see Resources, Chapter 9).

Once installed, the sandbox should be covered to prevent contamination with animal feces and parasites. Sand should be raked regularly to remove debris and dry it out. A sand rake does a better job than a garden rake.

Q *Which chemical disinfectants and sanitizers are safe to use in child care settings?*

A While chemical disinfectants and sanitizers are essential to control communicable diseases in the child care setting, they are potentially hazardous to children, particularly if the products are in concentrated form. Products must be stored in their original labeled containers and in places inaccessible to children. Diluted disinfectants and sanitizers in spray bottles must be labeled and stored safely out of the reach of children. Solutions should not be sprayed when children are close by to avoid inhalation and exposure of their skin and eyes.

Before using any chemical, read the product label carefully and the manufacturer's MSDS. Consult with public health personnel if you have questions. It is important to read and follow label instructions. Factors to consider when selecting a chemical disinfectant are: Is it inactivated by organic matter? Is it affected by hard water? Does it leave a residue? Is it corrosive by nature? Is it a skin, eye, or respiratory irritant? Is it toxic (by skin absorption, ingestion, or inhalation)? What is its effective shelf life after dilution? Household bleach (chlorine as sodium hypochlorite) is active against most microorganisms, including bacterial spores, and can be used as a disinfectant or sanitizer depending on its concentration. See Table 28.3 for instructions on diluting bleach with water. Bleach is available at various strengths. Household or laundry bleach is a solution of 5.25%, or 52 500 ppm, of sodium hypochlorite. The ultra form is only slightly more concentrated and should be diluted and used in the same fashion as ordinary strength household bleach. Higher strength industrial bleach solutions are not appropriate to use in child care settings.

Household bleach is effective, economical, convenient, and readily available at grocery stores. It can be corrosive to some metal, rubber, and plastic materials. Bleach solutions gradually lose their strength, so fresh solutions must be prepared daily and stock solutions replaced every few months. In child care settings, a bleach solution is typically applied using spray bottles. Spray bottles should be labeled with the name of the solution and the dilution. Contact time is important. What is typically observed in a child care setting is "spray and wipe." Bleach solution should be left on for at least 2

**Table 28.3**
**Diluting Bleach**

| Type of Object or Surface | Amount of Household Bleach to Add to Water | Concentration (ppm) |
|---|---|---|
| To disinfect environmental surfaces, such as door knobs, counter tops, changing areas, and toilet areas | 1/4 cup in 1 gallon of water<br>1 tablespoon in 1 quart of water | 500–800 |
| To sanitize mouth and food contact surfaces, such as crib railings, mouthing toys, dishes, utensils, and high chair trays | 1 tablespoon in 1 gallon of water | 100 |

minutes before being wiped off. It can be allowed to dry because it leaves no residue.

Household bleach can be used to sanitize dishes and eating utensils. The concentration of chlorine used in the process is much less than that used for disinfecting other objects. One rationale for sanitizing (as opposed to disinfecting) dishes and eating utensils is that these objects are typically contaminated by only one person and are washed and rinsed thoroughly before being treated with the sanitizing agent. Other objects typically are contaminated by more than one person, and less thoroughly washed, resulting in a potentially greater microbial load and diversity of microorganisms. Bleach (the sanitizer/disinfectant) and ammonia (the cleaner) should never be mixed.

Q *Is it important to clean first before disinfecting or sanitizing?*

A Soiled objects or surfaces will block the effects of a disinfectant or sanitizer. First, clean objects and surfaces with detergent and water, and then rinse them. Then sanitize or disinfect as necessary to reduce the level of harmful pathogens.

Q *What is the difference between sanitizing and disinfecting?*

A Sanitizing is designed to greatly reduce the number of pathogens to a level that is unlikely to cause disease and is the process used after visible dirt is removed from a surface. Sanitizing refers to the application of heat or a chemical, such as household bleach, to clean surfaces that is sufficient to yield a 99.9% reduction in representative (but not all) disease-causing microorganisms of public health importance. An example of cumulative heat treatment is found in the operation of some household dishwashers. Household dishwashers that effectively sanitize dishes and utensils using hot water may be used to clean and sanitize the outer surfaces of plastic toys. However, dishwashers that use a heating element to dry dishes should be used with caution to avoid melting soft plastic toys. Some dishwashers may permit the heating element used for drying to be deactivated while retaining the sanitizing process. Child care staff can consult the manufacturer's user's guide. Mouth and food contact surfaces (eg, crib railings, mouthing toys, dishes, high chair trays) should be sanitized.

Disinfecting is more rigorous than sanitizing. It refers to the application of cumulative heat or a chemical that results in elimination of almost all microorganisms from inanimate surfaces. Pathogens of public health importance and nearly all other microorganisms are eliminated, but not to the degree achieved by sterilization. Environmental surfaces such as changing tables and counter tops should be disinfected. Refer to *Caring for Our Children: National Health and Safety Performance Standards—Guidelines for Out-of-Home Child Care Programs* for more details.[3]

Q *Is it beneficial to use cleaners that contain disinfectants?*

A Proper disinfection or sanitizing of a surface requires that the surface be cleaned (using soap or detergent and a water rinse) prior to disinfecting or sanitizing.[19] By separating out the cleaning and disinfecting processes you will reduce the amount of disinfectant chemicals used. Remember that not all items and surfaces require sanitizing or disinfecting. Guidelines for cleaning, sanitizing, and disinfecting can be found in *Caring for Our Children: National Health and Safety Performance Standards—Guidelines for Out-of-Home Child Care Programs.*[3]

Q *What are alternative or less toxic homemade cleaning products and are they safe?*

A Alternative or less toxic cleaners are cleaners made from ingredients such as baking soda, liquid soap, and vinegar. For example, an all-purpose floor cleaner might consist of 2 tablespoons of liquid soap or detergent and 1 gallon of hot water. Many of the ingredients are inexpensive, so you may save money over time. They also may require more "elbow grease"; you may have to scrub harder. While the ingredients in homemade cleaners (eg, baking soda for scrubbing, vinegar for cutting grease) are safer, all are not nontoxic. Treat them as you would any other cleaner, with caution.

Q *Should I place my child in child care if a "no smoking" policy is not in place?*

A No. Children should not be exposed to ETS, and smoke-free policies should be written or stated, enforced, and monitored by the director of the center and parents. Children also can be exposed to ETS if persons other than employees are allowed to smoke when children are present, or when the facility has shared ventilation or air spaces that allow ETS to drift (see Chapter 13).

Q *I know that there are health concerns related to carpeting. What precautions should I take?*

A The ideal floor is warm to the touch, skid-proof, easily cleanable, moisture resistant, nontoxic, and does not generate static electricity.[16] This can best be achieved by using hard flooring materials. Carpets are an easy gathering place for biological pollutants such as molds and dust mites, as well as lead dust and pesticide residues. Instead of wall-to-wall carpeting, consider using area rugs (that are secured to avoid slipping) on hard surfaces; these tend to be easier to clean than installed carpeting. Carpets, pads, and adhesives emit VOCs (also called off-gassing). For children, the elderly, and people with lung conditions, allergies, and allergic-type sensitivities, fairly low amounts of VOCs may have health effects such as headaches; nausea; irritation to eyes, nose, and throat; and difficulty breathing. If installing new carpet, look for low–VOC-emitting carpets and nontoxic adhesives and pads. Ask the carpet store or installer to air out the carpet for at least 24 to 48 hours in the store or warehouse. During installation, make sure the room is well ventilated. After the carpet is installed continue to ventilate and wait at least 72 hours before using the room. Other preventive measures include: vacuum daily using a good filtering vacuum cleaner; leave shoes worn out-of-doors at the entry way; choose carpet that cleans easily; do not saturate the carpet when wet-cleaning, and ensure the carpet is dry within 24 hours; and use low- or no-solvent cleaning products. Thoroughly clean and dry water-damaged carpets within 24 hours or consider removal and replacement. Be aware that some carpet comes already treated with antimicrobial products. When possible avoid the use of pesticides on carpeting.[20]

Q *Are air cleaners that generate ozone safe and effective to use in my child care program?*

A No. Ozone generators that are sold as air cleaners intentionally produce the gas ozone. Manufacturers and vendors of ozone devices often use terms such as "energized oxygen" or "pure air" to suggest that ozone is a healthy kind of oxygen.[21] Ozone is a toxic gas. For more information, see the EPA indoor air quality publications at http://www.epa.gov/iaq/pubs/ozonegen.html.

Q *Should pets be allowed in child care settings?*

A Many child care providers who care for children in their homes have pets, and many centers include pets as part of their educational program. However, when bringing a pet into the child care setting, you need to follow guidelines to protect the health and safety of the children. The health and safety risks include allergies, injuries (eg, dog and cat bites), and infections (eg, salmonellosis caused by common bacteria carried by such animals as chickens, iguanas, and turtles). While no pet is perfect, there are some that are more suitable to a child care setting than others. The health department can give you guidance on regulations for pets in the child care setting. Specific guidelines can be found in *Caring for Our Children: National Health and Safety Performance Standards— Guidelines for Out-of-Home Child Care Programs*[3]. Iowa State University Extension also has a very concise, clear, and user-friendly handout, *Child Care and Pets* (March 1999), which can be found at http://www.extension.iastate.edu/Publications/PM1783.pdf.

Q *I just got a call from my neighbor, and she would like to donate her home playground equipment to my child care program. I have a copy of the CPSC's Handbook for Public Playground Safety (http://www.cpsc.gov/cpscpub/pubs/playpubs.html), and her playground equipment doesn't seem to meet their guidelines but I'm not sure. What should I do?*

A Playground equipment is the leading source of childhood injury. Many deaths and injuries occur on home playgrounds.[22] Since 1981 the CPSC has worked to strengthen playground safety guidelines and standards. If you are uncertain if the playground equipment meets CPSC guidelines, get professional advice. Contact your local parks and recreation office or the National Recreation and Park Association (http://www.nrpa.org), and they will be able to connect you with a certified playground inspector in the area. This person can determine the safety of the equipment as well as provide you with advice as to what type of equipment would best suit the ages of the children in your care and your physical space, and the type and amount of shock-absorbing surfacing needed around play equipment.

## Resources

American Academy of Pediatrics and American Public Health Association. *Caring for Our Children: National Health and Safety Performance Standards—Guidelines for Out-of-Home Child Care Programs,* 2nd Edition. It is available in electronic format at the National Resource Center for Health and Safety in Child Care's Web site at http://nrc.uchsc.edu and in hard copy through the American Academy of Pediatrics and the American Public Health Association. Child care regulations for every state are posted on the federally funded National Resource Center for Health and Safety in Child Care's Web site at http://nrc.uchsc.edu. This site also has a search engine for accessing specific child care topics by state.

Healthy Child Care America Campaign. American Academy of Pediatrics, Internet: http://www.aap.org/advocacy/hcca/network.htm. This includes a list of state contacts and resource materials and links.

## References

1. Children's Defense Fund. *Overview of Child Care, Early Education, and School-Age Care.* Washington, DC: Children's Defense Fund; 1999. Available at: http://www.childrensdefense.org/childcare/99_overview.pdf
2. Children's Defense Fund. *Child Care Basics.* Washington, DC: Children's Defense Fund; 2001. Available at: www.childrensdefense.org/cc_facts.htm
3. American Public Health Association, American Academy of Pediatrics. *Caring for Our Children: National Health and Safety Performance Standards—Guidelines for Out-of-Home Child Care Programs.* 2nd ed. Washington, DC: American Public Health Association, and Elk Grove Village, IL: American Academy of Pediatrics; 2002
4. General Accounting Office. *Child Care: State Efforts to Enforce Safety and Health Requirements.* Washington, DC: General Accounting Office; 2000. Available at: http://www.gao.gov/new.items/he00028.pdf
5. US Environmental Protection Agency, Indoor Environments Division. *Indoor Air Quality: Tools for Schools.* IAQ Coordinator's Guide. Available at: http://www.epa.gov/iaq/schools/tools4s2.html
6. Home*A*Syst. *Help Yourself to a Healthy Home: Protect Your Children's Health.* Available at: http://www.uwex.edu/homeasyst/text.html

7. Daneault S, Beausoleil M, Messing K. Air quality during the winter in Quebec day-care centers. *Am J Public Health.* 1992;82:432–434

8. Washington State Department of Health. *Environmental Lead Survey in Public and Private Schools, Preschools and Day Care Centers.* Olympia, WA: Washington State Department of Health; 1995:1–20

9. Weismann DN, Dusdieker LB, Cherryholmes KL, Hausler W Jr, Dungy CI. Elevated environmental lead levels in a day care setting. *Arch Pediatr Adolesc Med.* 1995;149:878–881

10. Gunn WJ, Pinsky PF, Sacks JJ, Schonberger LB. Injuries and poisoning in out-of-home child care and home care. *Am J Dis Child.* 1991;145:779–781

11. Aronson SS. Role of the pediatrician in setting and using standards for child care. *Pediatrics.* 1993;91:239–243

12. Fenske RA, Black KG, Elkner KP, et al. Potential exposure and health risks of infants following indoor residential pesticide applications. *Am J Public Health.* 1990;80:689–693

13. Shulman K. *The High Cost of Child Care Puts Quality Care Out of Reach for Many Families.* Washington, DC: Children's Defense Fund; 2000. Available at: http://www.childrensdefense.org/pdf/highcost.pdf

14. Bank H, Behr A, Schulman K. *State Developments in Child Care, Early Education, and School-Age Care.* Washington, DC: Children's Defense Fund; 2000:57. Available at: http://www.childrensdefense.org/pdf/2000_state_dev.pdf

15. Olds AR. *Child Care Design Guide.* New York, NY: McGraw-Hill; 2001

16. US Environmental Protection Agency. *IAQ Design Tools for Schools.* Washington, DC: US Environmental Protection Agency; 2001. Available at: http://www.epa.gov/iaq/schooldesign

17. Sellstrom E, Bremberg S. Education of staff—a key factor for a safe environment in day care. *Acta Paediatr.* 2000;89:601–607

18. Asthma and Allergy Foundation of America, New England Chapter. *For Child Care Providers.* Available at: http://www.asthmaandallergies.org/childcare.html

19. Healthy Child Care Pennsylvania. *Preventing Spread of Infectious Disease in Child Care.* Pennsylvania Chapter, American Academy of Pediatrics; 2001

20. Vermont Department of Health. *An Air Quality Fact Sheet on Carpet.* Burlington, VT: Vermont Department of Health. Available at: http://www.state.vt.us/health/_hp/airquality/carpet/carpet.htm

21. US Environmental Protection Agency. *Ozone Generators that are Sold as Air Cleaners: An Assessment of Effectiveness and Health Consequences.* Washington, DC: US Environmental Protection Agency. Available at: http://www.epa.gov/iaq/pubs/ozonegen.html

22. US Consumer Product Safety Commission. *Home Playground Equipment-Related Deaths and Injuries.* Washington, DC: US Consumer Product Safety Commission; 2001. Available at: http://www.cpsc.gov/library/playground.pdf

# 29
# Preconceptional and Prenatal Exposures

Environmental exposures associated with poor health outcomes may occur in the womb. In addition, some data suggest that harmful exposures also may occur to the ova and sperm prior to life in the womb. Parents may not be aware of the associations of preconceptional and prenatal exposures with the health of their children.

Occupational and environmental risks to the fetus are becoming increasingly important as more women enter the workforce. In 2001 46.6% of the US workforce was women (approximately 62.9 million female workers).[1] Sixty-four percent of working women are of reproductive age.[2] It is estimated that 52% of pregnant women work.[3] (This is an estimated number because no US Department of Labor or Bureau of Labor Statistics figures exist to quantify the percent of working women who give birth each year or the birth rate among employed women). The number of births in 2000 was 4.1 million. Assuming that multiple births are negligible, approximately 2.1 million infants were born to working mothers.

Concern with preconceptional and prenatal exposures is based on the knowledge that there are critical periods during development when the fetus is much more vulnerable to exposures than at other times. A well-known example is the exposure to thalidomide and limb reduction defects. In addition, thalidomide causes autism in infants exposed during gestational days 20 to 24, a window of only 5 days.[4,5] Differing vulnerability to ionizing radiation and microcephaly also are well known (a period of extreme vulnerability to ionizing radiation exists from gestational age 10 to 17 weeks).[6] These windows have not been clearly defined for most exposures.

This chapter describes preconceptional and prenatal exposures and the spectrum of adverse outcomes known to be associated with parental occupational and environmental exposures.

## Nonconcurrent Exposures

Environmental exposures that result in an affected newborn may occur before conception. Exposures to the ova or sperm before conception (preconceptional exposures) may lead to the development of an abnormal fetus, or a woman's exposure may result in a delayed exposure to the developing fetus by the ongoing elimination of the chemical from the mother's body (secondary fetal exposure). Because the initial exposure is prior to conception, these exposures are nonconcurrent with the pregnancy. For some chemicals, such as the organohalogens, the fetus can be affected by nonconcurrent and concurrent maternal exposures.

### *Preconceptional Exposures*

Exposures to the Ovum
The ovum from which the fetus is derived develops during the early fetal life of the mother and arrests in the prophase of the cell cycle until ovulation, which may occur up to 50 years later. The notion of the vulnerability of the oocyte to environmental exposures is supported by the rising incidence of nondisjunctional events, such as Trisomy 21, with increasing maternal age, and therefore with prolonged environmental exposure. Environmental exposures to the oocyte have been measured in samples of human follicular fluid (and in seminal plasma).[7]

The easiest outcome to measure is loss of fertility. Loss of ova from such exposures may reduce fertility as reported in women born to mothers who smoke.[8,9] Few outcome studies on environmental exposures have been reported, however, due to the lengthy period from exposure to outcome in such transgenerational studies. The population of women who took diethylstilbestrol (DES) during pregnancy is an exception because the exposure was well documented.[10,11] Several reports on transgenerational effects from DES exposure (effects in individuals whose grandmothers took DES during pregnancy [ie, DES grandchildren]) have been made. These include increased incidence of hypospadias in grandsons (prevalence ratio of 21.3, 95% confidence interval [CI], 6.5–70.1)[12] and prematurity of DES grandsons and grandaughters.[11,12]

## Exposures to the Sperm

In contrast to effects on ova, effects on sperm can be measured relatively easily in the next generation, so there is more evidence in the literature to suggest that paternal occupational exposures before conception may constitute a risk to the fetus. The sperm itself represents a vulnerable stage to the effects of mutagens; in its final form the sperm has no deoxyribonucleic acid repair mechanisms. Cancer is not usually thought to be a result of in utero exposures. New data, however, suggest that the preconceptional sperm may be a vulnerable target for carcinogenesis. The risk of cancer in the offspring and paternal occupation has been extensively studied. One recent study reported increased risk of central nervous system (CNS) tumors with paternal occupational exposure to pesticides (relative risk [RR] 2.36; 95% CI, 1.27–4.39) and work as a painter (RR 2.18; 95% CI, 1.26–3.78),[13] and leukemia with paternal woodwork (RR 2.18; 95% CI, 1.26–3.78). In 1998 48 published studies representing more than 1000 specific occupational/ cancer combinations were reviewed.[14] Important findings were that (1) occupations and exposures of fathers were investigated much more frequently than those of mothers, and (2) the studies have limitations related to the quality of the exposure assessment, small numbers of exposed cases, multiple comparisons, and possible bias toward the reporting of positive results. Despite these limitations, evidence was found for associations of childhood leukemia with paternal exposure to solvents, paints, and employment in motor vehicle–related occupations.

The studies on the association of birth defects with paternal occupation also have been recently reviewed and found to have many of the same limitations as the studies of paternal occupation and cancer.[15] However, birth defects were repeatedly reported to be associated with several common paternal occupations (janitors, painters, printers, firefighters, those in occupations exposed to solvents; and in occupations related to agriculture). Additional evidence that paternal exposures may result in fetal abnormalities comes from observations that certain fetal birth defects are associated with older fathers. These abnormalities include ventricular septal defects, atrial septal defects, and situs inversus.[16] The strongest association between advanced paternal age and birth defects is for achondroplasia.[17]

## Secondary Fetal Exposure: Maternal Body Burden

Nonconcurrent fetal exposure may result from ongoing excretion or mobilization of chemicals stored in the mother's body. Adipose tissue and skeletal tissue are known storage sites for various chemicals. Polychlorinated biphenyls (PCBs) are stored in adipose tissue. Following a Taiwanese poisoning episode with PCBs, children born up to 6 years after maternal exposure had similar developmental abnormalities (developmental delays, mildly disordered behavior, and increased activity levels) as those found in children born within 1 year of maternal exposure.[18,19] The developmental delay persisted in these children at all times measured. Thus these children had significant adverse effects from maternal exposure to PCBs that occurred up to 6 years before their birth.

The major repository for lead is bone, where the turnover rate is approximately 25 to 30 years. Chronic lead exposure results in significant accumulation of lead in the skeleton. During pregnancy, calcium turnover is greatly increased,[20] which may increase mobilization of lead stores from bone. Demonstration of significant fetal exposure because of an elevated maternal body burden of lead comes from 2 case reports of children with congenital lead poisoning delivered to women inadequately treated for childhood plumbism.[21,22]

## Concurrent Maternal Exposures

Exposures to the mother concurrent with pregnancy can come from many sources. Five common sources include maternal occupation, "paraoccupation," air, water, and diet. A recent article lists Internet resources for estimating the risk of exposures to pregnant women.[23]

## Maternal Occupation

Several maternal occupations have been shown to increase the risk of a poor outcome of pregnancy. The strongest associations between workplace exposures and poor reproductive outcome (eg, spontaneous abortion, miscarriage, and birth defects) have been found for lead, mercury, organic solvents, ethylene oxide, and ionizing radiation.[24] A summary of multiple chemical reagents and their potential as possible teratogens is available[24] (see Table 29.1).

Recent concerns have focused on maternal exposure to solvents and birth defects, primarily due to the large number of women involved in computer chip manufacture and the working conditions in such plants. A large multicenter case-control study showed an odds ratio of 1.44 (95% CI, 1.10–1.90) for congenital malformations and glycol ether exposure.[25] In another study, 32 infants born to women exposed occupationally to organic solvents were compared with 28 control infants on their performance of color vision and visual acuity.[26] Solvent-exposed children had significantly higher error scores on red-green and blue-yellow color discrimination, as well as poorer visual acuity compared with the unexposed group. Clinical red-green color vision loss was found in 3 of the 32 in the exposed group compared with none in the unexposed group.

## Paraoccupation

Other important sources of maternal exposure may occur through paraoccupational routes. These exposures occur when the father or others bring or track home occupational chemicals, the home itself is in an occupational setting, or industrial chemicals are purposely brought home for home use.

## Air

Air is an important source of exposure to the pregnant woman and fetus. For example, exposure of the mother to environmental tobacco

Table 29.1
Agents Associated With Adverse Female Reproductive Capacity or Developmental
Effects in Human and Animal Studies*†

| Agent | Human Outcomes | Strength of Association in Humans‡ | Animal Outcomes | Strength of Association in Animals‡ |
|---|---|---|---|---|
| Anesthetic gases¶ | Reduced fertility, spontaneous abortion | 1,3 | Birth defects | 1,3 |
| Arsenic | Spontaneous abortion, low birth weight | 1 | Birth defects, fetal loss | 2 |
| Benzo(a)pyrene | None | NA§ | Birth defects | 1 |
| Cadmium | None | NA | Fetal loss, birth defects | 2 |
| Carbon disulfide | Menstrual disorders, spontaneous abortion | 1 | Birth defects | 1 |
| Carbon monoxide | Low birth weight, fetal death (high doses) | 1 | Birth defects, neonatal mortality | 2 |
| Chlordecone | None | NA | Fetal loss | 2,3 |
| Chloroform | None | NA | Fetal loss | 1 |
| Chloroprene | None | NA | Birth defects | 2,3 |
| Ethylene glycol ethers | Spontaneous abortion | 1 | Birth defects | 2 |
| Ethylene oxide | Spontaneous abortion | 1 | Fetal loss | 1 |
| Formamides | None | NA | Fetal loss, birth defects | 2 |
| Inorganic mercury¶ | Menstrual disorders, spontaneous abortion | 1 | Fetal loss, birth defects | 1 |
| Lead¶ | Spontaneous abortion, prematurity, neurologic dysfunction in child | 2 | Birth defects, fetal loss | 2 |
| Organic mercury | Central nervous system (CNS) malformation, cerebral palsy | 2 | Birth defects, fetal loss | 2 |
| Physical stress | Prematurity | 2 | None | NA |
| Polybrominated biphenyls | None | NA | Fetal loss | 2 |

| Agent | Human Outcomes | Strength of Association in Humans[‡] | Animal Outcomes | Strength of Association in Animals[‡] |
|---|---|---|---|---|
| Polychlorinated biphenyls (PCBs) | Neonatal PCB syndrome (low birth weight, hyper-pigmentation, eye abnormalities) | 2 | Low birth weight, fetal loss | 2 |
| Radiation, ionizing | Menstrual disorders, CNS defects, skeletal & eye abnormalities, mental retardation, childhood cancer | 2 | Fetal loss, birth defects | 2 |
| Selenium | Spontaneous abortion | 3 | Low birth weight, birth defects | 2 |
| Tellurium | None | NA | Birth defects | 2 |
| 2,4-Dichloro-phenoxyacetic acid (2,4-D) | Skeletal defects | 4 | Birth defects | 1 |
| 2,4,5-Trichloro-phenoxyacetic acid (2,4,5-T) | Skeletal defects | 4 | Birth defects | 1 |
| Video display terminals | Spontaneous abortion | 4 | Birth defects | 1 |
| Vinyl chloride[¶] | CNS defects | 1 | Birth defects | 1,4 |
| Xylene | Menstrual disorders, fetal loss | 1 | Fetal loss, birth defects | 1 |

*From Welch LS.[24]

[†] Major studies of the reproductive health effects of exposure to dioxin are currently in progress.

[‡] 1, limited data; 2, strong positive data; 3, limited negative data; 4, strong negative data.

[§] Not applicable because no adverse outcomes were observed.

[¶] Symbol used to designate agents that may have male-mediated effects.

smoke (ETS) has been linked to decreased birth weight,[27] increased risk of sudden infant death syndrome,[28] and predisposition to persistent pulmonary hypertension.[29]

## Water

Because the embryo and fetus develop through multiple short critical periods, the quality of water consumed by a pregnant woman is a daily concern; a yearly average of contaminants is not sufficient to protect the developing fetus. Public and well water supplies can vary greatly over the course of a year. A recent review of the relationship of drinking water contaminants to adverse pregnancy outcomes illustrates the risk from exposure to by-products of chlorinated water disinfectants.[30] These studies show a moderate association between trihalomethane exposure and small for gestational age, neural tube defects, and spontaneous abortions.[30] Excess neural tube defects, oral clefts, cardiac defects, and choanal atresia were found in studies evaluating trichloroethylene-contaminated drinking water.

## Diet

Diet may be an important vehicle for exposure. In Minamata Bay, Japan, methylmercury from an acetaldehyde-producing plant contaminated the food chain in the 1950s.[31] Pregnant women from a fishing village on the same bay gave birth to severely neurologically damaged infants, whereas the women had only mild transient paresthesias or no symptoms at all. The safe limit of organic and inorganic mercury ingestion for a pregnant woman is the subject of much discussion and ongoing research.[32]

## Pathways of Fetal Exposure

### Placenta-Dependent Pathways

Two possible routes of fetal exposure to environmental hazards are placenta-dependent pathways and placenta-independent pathways. For a placenta-dependent chemical to reach the fetus, it must first enter the mother's bloodstream and then cross the placenta in significant amounts. Not all environmental toxicants meet these criteria. Three properties that enable chemicals to cross the placenta are low molecular weight, fat solubility, and resemblance to nutrients that are specifically transported. Information about an individual chemical's ability to cross the placenta may be found through a literature search using PubMed, or by reviewing its Material Safety Data Sheet.

An example of a low molecular weight compound is carbon monoxide (CO). Carbon monoxide is an asphyxiant because it displaces oxygen from hemoglobin, forming carboxyhemoglobin (COHb). If enough COHb accumulates in the circulation, cellular metabolism is impaired by the inhibition of oxygen transport, delivery, and use. Fetal COHb accumulates more slowly than maternal COHb but increases to a steady state approximately 10% greater than in the maternal circulation. Thus nonfatal CO poisoning of the mother may prove fatal to the fetus.

Examples of fat-soluble chemicals that readily cross the placenta are ethanol and polycyclic hydrocarbons. (Benzo[a]pyrene, a carcinogen present in ETS, is a member of this class of compounds.) Ethanol causes fetal alcohol syndrome. In pregnant ewes, intravenous infusion of ethanol results in identical maternal and fetal blood alcohol levels.[33] Polychlorinated biphenyls have been measured in equal concentrations in fetal and maternal blood.[34]

Calcium is a nutrient that is actively transported across the placenta to provide the fetus with 100 to 140 mg/kg of calcium per day during the third trimester. It is thought that lead is transported by the calcium transporter. The fetal blood lead concentration is equivalent to the maternal blood lead concentration. Recent animal studies have demonstrated that calcium supplementation may reduce the transfer of lead from prepregnancy maternal exposures to the fetus.[35]

### Placenta-Independent Pathways

Placenta-independent hazards to the fetus include ionizing radiation, heat, noise, and possibly electromagnetic fields. Ionizing radiation is a well-characterized teratogen (see Chapter 17). Much of our knowledge about the effects of radiation comes from studies of the survivors of the atomic bombs in Hiroshima and Nagasaki.[36]

Heat may directly penetrate to the fetus, and exposure to heat in the first trimester has been associated with neural tube defects.[37] Noise has a waveform, which may be transmitted to the fetus. Noise has been associated with certain birth defects, prematurity, and low birth weight.[38]

Not all forms of radiation are hazardous to the fetus. Neither radon nor ultraviolet light reach the fetus.

## Spectrum of Outcomes

Because of the complexity of development and of developmental processes from the fertilized egg to the newborn infant, sites of action of chemicals and radiation are numerous. An intrauterine exposure to radiation or chemicals may result in a broad array of phenotypic effects that often are not thought of as teratogenic effects. Table 29.2 lists some of the phenotypes that may be seen.

The environment has been strongly linked to birth defects. In a study of 371 933 women, the relative risk of a child's being born with a birth defect similar to the birth defect affecting the preceding sibling was investigated.[39] The relative risk of a similar birth defect was 11.6 (95% CI, 9.3–14.0) and dropped by more than 50% when the mother changed her living environment between the 2 pregnancies.

**Table 29.2**
**Spectrum of Phenotypic Effects**

| |
|---|
| • Infertility |
| • Spontaneous abortion/miscarriage |
| • Preterm birth |
| • Intrauterine growth retardation |
| • Microcephaly |
| • Major and minor malformations |
| • Deformations |
| • Metabolic dysfunction |
| • Cognitive dysfunction |
| • Behavioral dysfunction |
| • Pulmonary dysfunction |
| • Hearing loss |
| • Endocrine dysfunction |
| • Effects on vision |
| • Cancer |

Developmental neurotoxicity deserves special mention. The development of the CNS requires expression of unique proteins in specific cell populations during specific critical windows of time. There is concern that injury to these populations may result in neurodevelopmental disorders such as mental retardation, autism, dyslexia, and attention-deficit/hyperactivity disorder. It is estimated that 3% to 8% of the 4 million children born each year in the United States are affected by a neurodevelopmental disability.[40] Some are caused by genetic aberrations (Down syndrome, Fragile X syndrome), some by perinatal anoxia or meningitis, and some by exposure to drugs (eg, alcohol, cocaine). However, for most of the neurodevelopmental disabilities, the cause is unknown. Environmental chemicals, such as lead, tobacco, PCBs, and mercury, are known developmental neurotoxicants. Of the chemicals produced in or imported into the United States at more than 1 million pounds a year, fewer than 10% have been tested to determine whether they have the potential to cause developmental damage.[41] As of 1998, of all chemicals regulated by the US Environmental Protection Agency, only 12 have had any developmental neurotoxicity testing.[42] Thus it remains a possibility that neurodevelopmental disabilities arising in the newborn period are linked to in utero chemical exposures.

## Prevention of Exposure

Each pregnant woman should be asked an occupational and environmental exposure history. It is not enough to know the woman's occupation. The clinician must ascertain the nature of her work, the nature of her partner's work, their hobbies and home activities, and the characteristics of their residence and neighborhood.[43] Additional areas of inquiry include the composition of their diet and use of tobacco, alcohol, or other recreational drugs. The clinician should inquire about medicines (prescribed, over-the-counter, or natural/alternative/herbal) used during the pregnancy.

Pediatric environmental health continues to evolve, elucidating sources of potential harm. What can one do now with the limited information available? First, women who work have a right to know about the chemicals with which they work, and they have a right to be protected from harmful exposures. Material Safety Data Sheets are available to any employee who requests them. These sheets supply information about potential reproductive hazards. Personal protective gear should be available, and increased monitoring of potential exposures instituted. In certain instances, temporary job shifting may prevent potential exposure.

## Frequently Asked Question

Q  *What can I do to prevent birth defects?*

A  If you are a woman of childbearing age, take a folic acid supplement every day. Ingesting 0.4 mg (400 µg) of folic acid per day will prevent certain kinds of birth defects, particularly defects of the nervous system. Because many pregnancies are not planned and women may not know they are pregnant until the first trimester is well under way, folic acid should be taken by all women of childbearing age. Folic acid is available as part of many multivitamin supplements. Do not smoke and try not to be around others who smoke. If you work with chemicals, become as informed as possible about the possible risks those chemicals could pose to your unborn child.

## Resource

Agency for Toxic Substances and Disease Registry, Internet: http://www.atsdr.cdc.gov. A discussion of the pros and cons of MSDS, as well as a link to the MSDS, can be found at http://www.atsdr.cdc.gov/HEC/CSEM/exphistory/identifying_agents.html#Material

# References

1. US Department of Labor, Bureau of Labor Statistics. *20 Leading Occupations of Employed Women: 2001 Annual Averages.* Washington, DC: US Department of Labor; 2001. Available at: http://www.dol.gov/wb/wb_pubs/20lead2001.htm
2. US Department of Labor, Bureau of Labor Statistics. http://www.bls.gov
3. Waldfogel J. Family leave coverage in the 1990s. *Monthly Labor Review.* 1999;October:13–20
4. Miller MT, Stromland K. Thalidomide embryopathy: a sight into autism? *Teratology.* 1993;47:387–388
5. London E, Etzel RA. The environment as an etiologic factor in autism: a new direction for research. *Environ Health Perspect.* 2000;108(suppl 3): 401–404
6. Yamazaki JN, Schull WJ. Perinatal loss and neurological abnormalities among children of the atomic bomb. Nagasaki and Hiroshima revisited, 1949 to 1989. *JAMA.* 1990;264:605–609
7. Younglai EV, Foster WG, Hughes EG, Trim K, Jarrell JF. Levels of environmental contaminants in human follicular fluid, serum, and seminal plasma of couples undergoing in vitro fertilization. *Arch Environ Contam Toxicol.* 2002;43:121–126
8. Weinberg CR, Wilcox AJ, Baird DD. Reduced fecundability in women with prenatal exposure to cigarette smoking. *Am J Epidemiol.* 1989;129:1072–1078
9. Munafo M, Murphy M, Whiteman D, Hey K. Does cigarette smoking increase time to conception? *J Biosoc Sci.* 2002;34:65–73
10. Herbst AL, Hubby MM, Azizi F, Makaii MM. Reproductive and gynecologic surgical experience in diethylstilbestrol-exposed daughters. *Am J Obstet Gynecol.* 1981;141:1019–1028
11. Herbst AL, Hubby MM, Blough RR, Azizi F. A comparison of pregnancy experience in DES-exposed and DES-unexposed daughters. *J Reprod Med.* 1980;24:62–69
12. Klip H, Verloop J, van Gool JD, Koster ME, Burger CW, van Leeuwen FE. Hypospadias in sons of women exposed to diethystilbestrol in utero: a cohort study. *Lancet.* 2002;359:1102–1107
13. Feychting M, Plato N, Nise G, Ahlbom A. Paternal occupational exposures and childhood cancer. *Environ Health Perspect.* 2001;109:193–196
14. Colt JS, Blair A. Parental occupational exposures and risk of childhood cancer. *Environ Health Perspect.* 1998;106(suppl 3):909–925

15. Chia SE, Shi LM. A review of recent epidemiological studies on paternal occupations and birth defects. *Occup Environ Med.* 2002;59:149–155

16. Lian ZH, Zack MM, Erickson JD. Paternal age and the occurrence of birth defects. *Am J Hum Genet.* 1986;39:648–660

17. Rousseau F, Bonaventure J, Legeai-Mallet L, et al. Mutations in the gene encoding fibroblast growth factor receptor-3 in achondroplasia. *Nature.* 1994;371:252–254

18. Chen YC, Guo YL, Hsu CC, Rogan WJ. Cognitive development of Yu-Cheng ("oil disease") children prenatally exposed to heat-degraded PCBs. *JAMA.* 1992;268:3213–3218

19. Chen YC, Yu ML, Rogan WJ, Gladen BC, Hsu CC. A 6-year follow-up of behavior and activity disorders in the Taiwan Yu-Cheng children. *Am J Public Health.* 1994;84:415–421

20. Bezerra FF, Laboissiere FP, King JC, Donangelo CM. Pregnancy and lactation affect markers of calcium and bone metabolism differently in adolescent and adult women with low calcium intakes. *J Nutr.* 2002;132:2183–2187

21. Shannon MW, Graef JW. Lead intoxication in infancy. *Pediatrics.* 1992;89:87–90

22. Thompson GN, Robertson EF, Fitzgerald S. Lead mobilization during pregnancy. *Med J Aust.* 1985;143:131

23. Polifka JE, Faustman EM. Developmental toxicity: web resources for evaluating risk in humans. *Toxicology.* 2002;173:35–65

24. Welch LS. Reproductive and developmental hazards. In: *Case Studies in Environmental Medicine: Taking an Exposure History.* Atlanta, GA: Agency for Toxic Substances and Disease Registry; 2000. ATSDR Publication ATSDR-HE-CS-2001-002. Available at: http://www.atsdr.cdc.gov/HEC/CSEM/exphistory/index.html

25. Cordier S, Bergeret A, Goujard J, et al. Congenital malformation and maternal occupational exposure to glycol ethers. Occupational Exposure and Congenital Malformations Working Group. *Epidemiology.* 1997;8:355–363

26. Till C, Westall CA, Rovet JF, Koren G. Effects of maternal occupational exposure to organic solvents on offspring visual functioning: a prospective controlled study. *Teratology.* 2001;64:134–141

27. Haddow JE, Knight GL, Palomaki GE, McCarthy JE. Second-trimester serum cotinine levels in nonsmokers in relation to birth weight. *Am J Obstet Gynecol.* 1988;159:481–484

28. Nicholl JP, O'Cathain A. Epidemiology of babies dying at different ages from the sudden infant death syndrome. *J Epidemiol Community Health.* 1989;43:133–139

29. Bearer C, Emerson RK, O'Riordan MA, Roitman E, Shakleton C. Maternal tobacco smoke exposure and persistent pulmonary hypertension of the newborn. *Environ Health Perspect.* 1997;105:202–206

30. Bove F, Shim Y, Zeitz P. Drinking water contaminants and adverse pregnancy outcomes: a review. *Environ Health Perspect.* 2002;110 (suppl 1):61–74

31. Harada M. Methyl mercury poisoning due to environmental contamination ("Minamata disease"). In: Oehme FW, ed. *Toxicity of Heavy Metals in the Environment.* New York, NY: Marcel Dekker; 1978:261

32. Goldman LR, Shannon MW, American Academy of Pediatrics Committee on Environmental Health. Technical report: mercury in the environment: implications for pediatricians. *Pediatrics.* 2001;108:197–205

33. Clarke DW, Smith GN, Patrick J, Richardson B, Brien JF. Activity of alcohol dehydrogenase and aldehyde dehydrogenase in maternal liver, fetal liver and placenta of the near-term pregnant ewe. *Dev Pharmacol Ther.* 1989;12:35–41

34. Bush B, Snow J, Koblintz R. Polychlorobyphenyl (PCB) congeners, p,p′-DDE, and hexachlorobenzene in maternal and fetal cord blood from mothers in upstate New York. *Arch Environ Contam Toxicol.* 1984;13:517–527

35. Han S, Pfizenmaier DH, Garcia E, et al. Effects of lead exposure before pregnancy and dietary calcium during pregnancy on fetal development and lead accumulation. *Environ Health Perspect.* 2000;108:527–531

36. Blot WJ. Growth and development following prenatal and childhood exposure to atom radiation. *J Radiat Res (Tokyo).* 1975;16(suppl):82–88

37. Milunsky A, Ulcickas M, Rothman KJ, Willett W, Jick SS, Jick H. Maternal heat exposure and neural tube defects. *JAMA.* 1992;268:882–885

38. American Academy of Pediatrics Committee on Environmental Health. Noise: a hazard for the fetus and newborn. *Pediatrics.* 1997;100:724–727

39. Lie RT, Wilcox AJ, Skajaerven R. A population-based study of the risk of recurrence of birth defects. *N Engl J Med.* 1994; 331:1–4

40. Weiss B, Landrigan PJ. The developing brain and the environment: an introduction. *Environ Health Perspect.* 2000;108(suppl 3):373–374

41. Goldman LR, Koduru S. Chemicals in the environment and developmental toxicity to children: a public health and policy perspective. *Environ Health Perspect.* 2000;108(suppl 3):443–448

42. Makris S, Raffaele K, Sette W, Seed J. *A Retrospective Analysis of Twelve Developmental Neurotoxicity Studies.* Washington, DC: US Environmental Protection Agency Office of Prevention, Pesticides, and Toxic Substances. Available at: www.epa.gov/scipoly/sap/1998/december/neuro.pdf

43. Agency for Toxic Substances and Disease Registry. *Case Studies in Environmental Medicine: Taking an Exposure History.* Atlanta, GA: Agency for Toxic Substances and Disease Registry; 2000. ATSDR Publication ATSDR-CS-2001-0002. Available at: http://www.atsdr.cdc.gov/HEC/CSEM/exphistory/index.html

# 30
# Schools

Because school-aged children may spend 35 to 50 hours per week in and around school facilities while in transit on buses, during school, recess, and in after-school programs, pediatricians need to be alert to considering and assessing problems arising from those settings.[1] Even younger children spend time in school buildings in kindergarten, pre-school, and child care programs. Exacerbation of respiratory symptoms; academic difficulties in achievement, attention, and focus; and behavioral problems that have no other specific etiology may be linked to the school environment, especially if such problems are of relatively sudden onset. A pediatrician may need to serve as diagnostician and advocate for the child. In addition to the history and physical examination, a careful environmental assessment of the school may be needed. If the school environment is a possible source of the problem, evaluation of the school needs to be done by someone with expertise in this area. Subsequently, the pediatrician, in collaboration with other concerned individuals, may need to assume an advocacy role to promote correction of environmental exposures in the school setting. This chapter discusses the following problems in the school setting: indoor air quality, biological agents, radon, asbestos, pesticides, lead, noise, and the outdoor environment. Additional information can be found in the chapters on each specific topic.

## Indoor Air Quality

Table 30.1 presents selected sources of indoor air pollutants in schools.[2]

Many school buildings are old and poorly maintained. The average US school is 42 years old.[3] A recent incident in New York City illustrated the extreme of problems caused by indoor air pollution in a

Table 30.1
Typical Sources of Indoor Air Pollutants*

| Outside Sources | Building Equipment | Components/ Furnishings | Other Indoor Sources |
|---|---|---|---|
| **Polluted Outdoor Air** <br>• Pollen, dust, fungal spores <br>• Industrial emissions <br>• Vehicle emissions <br><br>**Nearby Sources** <br>• Loading docks <br>• Odors from dumpsters <br>• Unsanitary debris or building exhausts near outdoor air intakes <br><br>**Underground Sources** <br>• Radon <br>• Pesticides <br>• Leakage from underground storage tanks | **HVAC† Equipment** <br>• Microbiological growth in drip pans, ductwork, coils, and humidifiers <br>• Improper venting of combustion products <br>• Dust or debris in ductwork <br><br>**Non-HVAC Equipment** <br>• Emissions from office equipment (volatile organic compounds, ozone) <br>• Emissions from shops, labs, cleaning processes | **Components** <br>• Microbiological growth on soiled or water-damaged materials <br>• Dry traps that allow the passage of sewer gas <br>• Materials containing volatile organic compounds, inorganic compounds, or damaged asbestos <br>• Materials that produce particles (dust) <br><br>**Furnishings** <br>• Emissions from new furnishings and floorings <br>• Microbiological growth on or in soiled water-damaged furnishings | • Science laboratories <br>• Vocational arts areas <br>• Copy/print areas <br>• Food prep areas <br>• Smoking lounges <br>• Cleaning materials <br>• Emissions from trash <br>• Pesticides <br>• Volatile organic compounds from paint, chalk, and adhesives <br>• Occupants with communicable diseases <br>• Dry-erase markers and similar pens <br>• Insects and other pests <br>• Personal care products |

*Adapted from US Environmental Protection Agency.[2]
†HVAC, heating, ventilating, and air conditioning.

building heated by a coal-fired furnace. In February 1998, 75 children and several adults became ill when carbon monoxide and other fumes escaped from the furnace. The cause was attributed to human error and improper functioning of a fan used to force air into the furnace.[4]

Many problems with indoor air quality in schools are common to all large buildings. There are, however, other pollutants unique to schools including those released into the air from art and craft supplies, chemistry and biology laboratories, and wood and metal shops.

A report by the US Government Accounting Office noted that more than half the schools surveyed had at least one environmental pollutant that could affect air quality.[5] The indoor air may directly influence a child's learning by affecting alertness, attentiveness, and absenteeism and indirectly by affecting the performance and productivity of teachers. Indoor air pollutants can originate within the building or be drawn in from outdoors and may consist of particles, fibers, mists, molds, bacteria, and gases. Levels of air pollutants can vary within the school building or even within a single classroom. Levels can vary with time; pollutants may increase acutely on the day floor stripping is done, or may increase continuously from growth of molds on damp walls and ceilings or heating, ventilating, and air-conditioning (HVAC) systems.

Attributing a child's symptoms to indoor air problems in a particular building can be difficult. Multiple pollutants may be involved. Common signs and symptoms, and clues to indoor air quality problems are shown in Table 30.2.

The US Environmental Protection Agency (EPA) provides extensive resources for evaluating the school environment and procedures that can be used for remediation (see Resources).

### Sick Building Syndrome and Building-Related Illness

*Sick building syndrome* (SBS) is a term first used during the 1970s.[6] It is used to describe situations in which building occupants experience acute health and comfort effects that seem to be linked to time spent in a building, but no specific illness or cause can be identified. The complaints may be localized in a particular room or zone, or may be widespread throughout the building. In contrast, the term *building-related illness* (BRI) is used when symptoms of diagnosable illness are

**Table 30.2**
**Poor Indoor Air Quality**

| **Common Signs and Symptoms** |
| --- |
| • Headache |
| • Fatigue |
| • Shortness of breath |
| • Nasal congestion |
| • Cough and sneezing |
| • Eye, nose, throat, and skin irritation |
| • Nausea and syncope |
| • Nosebleeds |
| **Clues Suggesting Indoor Air Quality Problems** |
| • There is a stuffy or musty odor when entering the building or room in the morning. |
| • Symptoms are widespread in a class or within the school. |
| • Symptoms disappear or diminish with sufficient time out of the school building (weekends). |
| • Onset is sudden after some change at the school (painting, remodeling, pesticide use). |
| • Affected persons have symptoms indoors but not outdoors. |

identified and can be attributed directly to airborne building contaminants. Symptoms of SBS and BRI may abate when the people are not in the building. Poor design, maintenance, and operation of the structure's ventilation systems have been identified as causes of SBS, as have biological contaminants and indoor and outdoor chemical contaminants.[2] Another theory suggests that very low levels of specific pollutants may be present and may act synergistically, or in combination, to cause health problems.

## Remedial Actions for Sick Building Syndrome

In the absence of readily identifiable problems, appropriate people (eg, school or school district personnel, building investigation specialists, industrial hygienists, and state and local government environmental health specialists) should investigate the school, paying particular attention to the design, operation, and maintenance of the HVAC systems, and correct contributing conditions. Investigation of the HVAC systems can be a complex problem and requires a specialist in this area because airflow, humidity, and temperature need to vary with use, occupancy levels, and type of potential pollutants.

Relative humidity in schools should be between 30% and 50% and airflow between 15 and 20 cubic ft/min per person. Carbon dioxide levels, which depend on occupancy, should be less than 1000 ppm when a room has been occupied for 4 to 6 hours.[2] Rules of thumb for indoor air in schools have been published.[7]

### Biological Agents

Biological air pollutants are found to some degree in every school and home and may generate toxic or allergic reactions if excessive exposure occurs. Sources include outdoor air, human occupants who shed viruses and bacteria, animal dander brought in on children's clothing, insects and other arthropods that shed allergens, and damp indoor surfaces and water reservoirs (eg, humidifiers) where bacteria and molds can grow. Molds may produce mycotoxins, fungal metabolites with toxic effects ranging from short-term irritation to immunosuppression, and cancer.[8,9] Most information related to diseases caused by mycotoxins concerns ingestion of contaminated food.[10] However, mycotoxins are contained on some mold spores that can enter the body through the respiratory tract.[11] One reported case of neurotoxic symptoms was related to airborne mycotoxin exposure in a heavily contaminated environment.[12]

Exposure to dust mites may be a problem; clutter, carpets, stuffed furniture, and stuffed toys are common sources. High relative humidity encourages dust mite multiplication and allows bacteria and mold growth. Damp surfaces and high humidity may result from flooding; continually damp carpet; inadequate exhaust of bathrooms; kitchen-generated moisture; appliances such as humidifiers, dehumidifiers, and air conditioners; and drip pans under cooling coils (as in refrigerators).

---

**Biological Agents
Diagnostic Clues**

---

Is the relative humidity in the classroom/school consistently higher than 50%?

Are humidifiers or other water-spray systems used? How often are they cleaned? Are they cleaned according to manufacturers' directions?

Have flooding or leaks occurred?

Is there evidence of mold growth (visible growth or musty odors)?

Are organic materials handled in the school?

Is carpet installed on damp or unventilated concrete floors?

Are there pets in the school?

Is there evidence of cockroaches or rodents?

Are bacterial odors present (fishy or locker-room smells)?

Is adequate outdoor air provided (sufficient number of air changes per hour)?

---

## Remedial Action for Biological Contaminants

- Provide adequate fresh air ventilation (15–20 cu ft/min per person).[7]
- Be sure there is no standing water in air conditioners. Maintain HVAC systems, humidifiers, and dehumidifiers according to manufacturers' instructions.
- Repair leaks and seepage. Thoroughly clean and dry water-damaged carpets and building materials within 24 hours of damage, or remove and replace them.
- Keep relative humidity at 30% to 50%. Use exhaust fans in bathrooms, pools, showers, and kitchens.
- Vacuum carpets regularly. While it is important to keep an area as dust-free as possible, cleaning activities often resuspend fine particles. Sensitive persons should avoid such exposure and have others perform the vacuuming, or use a commercially available high-efficiency particulate air (HEPA)-filtered vacuum.[13]

### *Volatile Organic Compounds*

Volatile organic compounds (VOCs) include a wide range of chemicals emitted as gases at room temperature.[14,15] These include a variety of solvents and other compounds released from such diverse sources as paint, adhesives, new building materials, office copiers, permanent markers, arts and crafts materials, science room materials, cleaning products, air fresheners, and carbonless paper. Concentrations of many VOCs are consistently higher indoors than outdoors.

Many of these items carry precautionary labels specifying risks and procedures for safe use; some do not.

| **Volatile Organic Compounds**<br>**Diagnostic Clues** |
| --- |
| Has the child used or been in the room with art, craft, or photographic materials, or do fumes from print shops or auto welding share the same ventilation system?<br>Are chemical cleaners used extensively or stored in the school?<br>Is remodeling underway or has it recently been done?<br>Has the child recently used or been exposed to paints or solvents? |

## Remedial Action for Volatile Organic Compounds

• Increase ventilation when using products that emit VOCs, and meet or exceed any label precautions. Do not store opened containers of unused paints and similar materials in the school.

• If formaldehyde is the potential cause of the problem, identify, and, if possible, remove the source. If removal is not possible, reduce exposure by using sealants on cabinets, paneling, and other furnishings. To be effective, any such coating must cover all surfaces and edges and remain intact.[16]

## Prevention of Indoor Air Quality Problems

Prevention provides the greatest overall health benefit. Pediatricians can enlist the cooperation of teachers, administrators, and parents in taking preventive actions. A practical yet flexible plan can be found in the *Indoor Air Quality Tools for Schools* kit (see Resources), designed with the understanding that schools have few monetary and human resources available to address this issue. The following are a variety of methods that can be used to control concentrations of indoor air pollutants, and may cost very little or nothing at all.

1. Educate the school and staff about the sources and effects of pollutants under their control.
2. Manage the source, which includes removal of offending substances, substitution, airing out, and sealing off materials where practical. The best source management is prevention, such as eliminating smoking within and around the school.
3. Maintain optimal operation of the HVAC systems, with special attention to rooms or areas that are major sources of pollutants.
4. Control exposure, which includes knowledge of time of use and location of use. An example of time of use would be to strip and wax floors after school dismissal on Friday. Location of use involves moving the contaminating source as far as possible from occupants.

## Radon

The EPA measured radon levels in a randomly selected sample of 927 public schools during the 1990 to 1991 school year. Short-term screening measurements were made by placing radon detectors in all frequently occupied, ground-contact schoolrooms for 7 days.

Survey results showed that 2.7% of the schoolrooms had short-term radon measurements above the EPA action level of 4 pCi/L of air.[17] Since then the EPA has estimated that 19.3% of US schools have at least one room with levels at or above 4 pCi/L and has recommended remedial action when any measurements exceed these levels.[18] Although testing is not required, it is highly recommended. Testing the school for radon is the only way to determine whether the school has a radon problem (see Chapter 17).

## Asbestos

Asbestos was used extensively in schools until the 1970s. In 1980 the EPA estimated that more than 8500 schools contained deteriorating asbestos and more than 3 million students and 250 000 teachers and other adults were at risk of exposure in schools.[19]

To prevent asbestos exposure in schools, the EPA, in compliance with the Asbestos Hazard Emergency Response Act of 1986, developed a systematic strategy for dealing with asbestos in schools and other buildings.

The asbestos hazard legislation mandates that every room and every surface of every school—public, private, and parochial—must be systematically inspected for the presence of asbestos every 3 years by a trained and certified inspector. Monitoring of levels of asbestos in air in schools is of little value because release typically is episodic and usually is missed in sampling. If asbestos is found by visual inspection, 3 options exist for dealing with it: removal, containment, or watchful waiting.

Removal (termed *abatement*) has been found necessary only in approximately 10% of school buildings. It is mandatory when deteriorating asbestos is readily accessible to children or when renovation of asbestos-containing surfaces or equipment is about to occur. It is essential that abatement be done by properly trained and certified workers in a properly sealed situation.

Containment of asbestos behind drywall, drop ceilings, or other enclosures has proven a useful approach for dealing with asbestos in schools. It has been the strategy most commonly followed. Use of this strategy requires that careful records be kept on the location of enveloped asbestos.

Watchful waiting (termed *operations and maintenance*) means that nothing is done immediately with asbestos in place, but that its presence, location, and condition are carefully recorded. This approach is permissible when no potential for immediate contact between children and asbestos exists. If renovations are planned or deterioration occurs, the decision must be revisited, and containment or abatement may be required. Any school district that chooses to follow the operations and maintenance option is required by law to reinspect every 3 years and to maintain detailed records of the location and condition of any asbestos. These inspection records must be available to the public.

## Pesticides

Schools are susceptible to pest problems because they are large, may be in poor repair, have multiple entrances and exits, prepare and serve food, serve large numbers of children, and are heavily stocked with books and other supplies and equipment that provide habitats for pests. Some school buildings are aging, multilevel, and under severe budgetary constraints, making maintenance and physical plant improvements difficult. Often pest problems are approached in a unimodal fashion involving spraying of pesticides inside and outside the school building. Children may be exposed to high levels of pesticides from "routine" spraying.

Herbicides often are used on school grounds to control weed growth. The most commonly used chemical is glyphosphate, which has a low level of toxicity. However, abdominal pain and vomiting may occur, and skin and eye irritation is common. The presumed inert ingredient, polyethoxylated tallowamine, which is used to improve application, may be more toxic than the herbicide itself.[20]

Integrated pest management (IPM) is a cost-effective and environmentally sensitive approach to pest management that uses knowledge of pest life cycles and their interactions with the environment in addition to the judicious use of pesticides. An IPM program has been shown to reduce pest problems while decreasing the use of pesticides by using substitutes for chemical treatments and, when chemicals are used, timing treatments to maximize pest destruction based on life cycle characteristics. A hallmark of a successful IPM program is that it is less expensive, less toxic, and more effective than the practice of routine scheduled pesticide spraying. The EPA has developed an approach to IPM for schools that offers step-by-step guidance to local school officials for development, implementation, and evaluation.[21] Because the health effects of pesticide exposure on children are of concern, though not well studied, an approach that reduces their exposure to these chemicals is desirable (see Chapter 24). It is now recommended that schools use an IPM methodology, post notices of pesticide use, and notify parents of such use. Several states currently have statutes requiring these actions.[22]

## Lead

Schools built before the 1970s are likely to contain leaded materials on walls, woodwork, stairwells, and window casings and sills. Other sources include deteriorating paint, lead pipes, lead-lined water coolers, water fixtures, and lead-containing art supplies. Outside the buildings, playground soil may be contaminated, with higher concentrations found closest to the school walls where paint has flaked off and accumulated, or near major thoroughfares, under bridges, and in inner-city playgrounds. Children may be exposed to lead if the school is near a point source, such as a smelter or battery manufacturing plant (see Chapter 19).

In contrast to data available on US housing, to our knowledge no studies have comprehensively and systematically assessed the presence of lead in schools and preschools nationwide. There are no comprehensive federal laws pertaining to lead exposure in schools, though schools are indirectly affected by many existing federal regulations. High concentrations of lead can accumulate in water overnight, on weekends, and over school holidays. Schools are not required to meet the 1991 EPA action level of 15 ppb because the EPA only regulates public water systems, not end users. Some school systems may have their own wells. Schools should meet or exceed relevant federal and state laws, and they are encouraged to test drinking water at the tap and to meet a recommended lead level of 15 ppb or less. The Lead Contamination Control Act of 1988 banned the sale of water coolers that were not lead-free and required manufacturers to repair, replace, or recall existing lead-containing water coolers.

## Art Supplies

The Labeling of Hazardous Art Materials Act of 1988 requires labeling of art materials that contain substances such as lead, chromium, mercury, and a variety of solvents where exposure constitutes a health hazard (see Chapter 33).

## Noise

Noise levels greater than 60 dBA can not only be intrusive and annoying, but can also interfere with cognitive activities. Children with attention-deficit/hyperactivity disorder may be especially affected because they may have difficulty focusing on important information rather than on background noise[23] (see Chapter 23).

## Outdoor Environments

Preschool- and school-aged children spend part of every school day in the outdoor environment of the school. In addition there are many sport activities carried out in the school play area after school and on weekends. Environmental hazards include outdoor pollution, contaminated soil, play equipment, and ultraviolet light.

Many urban schools are built on land of low value, such as previous industrial sites, and in high-traffic areas. Such sites may increase the hazards that children face in their outdoor activities.

## Contaminated Soil

Schools may be located on or near "brownfields" (land used for industrial purposes, polluted, abandoned, and later designated for development). The soil may be contaminated with heavy metals and their derivatives, polychlorinated biphenyls, dioxins, and leakage from old underground storage tanks and off-gassing of solvents such as methane and trichlorethylene. Corrective measures are designed to meet residential soil standards, but such standards are determined for adults but not for children.[24] Checking state standards is necessary to ascertain the level required. Primary prevention is ideal when new school siting considers these problems. Remediation measures for existing schools may include covering the contaminated soil with clean soil; however, disruption of the soil cover may occur from planting of trees or bushes, and children may disrupt this coverage by playing on or digging in the soil.[25] Additionally, soil contaminants, including pesticides and herbicides, can be transported into the school by foot.[26]

## Play Equipment

Wooden play equipment usually is made from pressure-treated wood, which may contain arsenic and chromium or pentachlorphenol (see Chapter 8).

## Ultraviolet Light

Excessive exposure to ultraviolet light can be especially hazardous to children and can result in serious effects in later life, including skin cancers, retinal damage, and immune system disorders.[27] The most dangerous times of day are from about 10 am to 4 pm, which corresponds to recess and lunchtimes. Avoiding exposures during these times, timing outside activities and choosing shady areas whenever possible, wearing clothing and hats, and using sunscreens are indicated. Using coverings over play structures is another possible approach. Guidelines for school programs to prevent skin cancer have been published[28] (see Chapter 26).

## Frequently Asked Questions

Q  *My child's school is hot and dry. What should I do?*

A  The first thing to determine is the relative humidity present in your child's classroom. The building maintenance supervisor should be able to provide that information. An alternative is to determine this yourself with a temperature/humidity device available in most general merchandise stores. The ideal relative humidity for school rooms is between 30% and 50%. If the relative humidity is below or above this range, you can request that the school adjust this by modification of the controls of the HVAC system or opening windows.

Q  *Asbestos has recently been discovered on the ceiling of my child's school. Should my child have a chest x-ray? Will cancer develop in my child?*

A  Asbestos on the ceiling does not by itself constitute a health hazard. Ask the school for a copy of the Asbestos Hazard Emergency Response Act plan, then ask school authorities to determine through visual inspection whether the asbestos is breaking up and whether it is likely liberating fibers into the air. If fibers are being liberated, it is essential that abatement or enclosure is instituted immediately by professionals and that children be evacuated from the affected area until the remedial work is completed and the area cleaned and tested. A chest radiograph is not indicated because asbestos produces no acute changes in the lungs. The risk of lung cancer or of mesothelioma from brief exposure is very unlikely.

If, on the other hand, the asbestos has actively been liberating fibers and this situation has persisted for many weeks or months, it must be promptly remediated, and intensified efforts to prevent children from starting to smoke become a particularly high priority.

Q *Our school board has done asbestos inspections as required by federal law, but it will not let parents see the results. Do parents have a right to see this information?*

A Yes. Federal law requires that this information be made available to parents and pediatricians. First, call the education department and log a written complaint, keeping a copy. If the problem persists, you should call the regional office of the EPA and seek guidance from the regional asbestos coordinator.

Q *How do I know if there is a problem with lead in the school?*

A To find out whether your child's school has lead hazards, contact the local school district or the principal of the school to learn whether inspection or testing has been done. Ask to see a copy of the results. Contact your state or local health department or education department to learn what regulations exist for testing various systems in the schools for lead and what the requirements are for remediating any lead hazards.

Remember that even if there is lead in the paint in your child's school, it does not necessarily pose a hazard if the paint is in good shape and inaccessible to your child. However, a hazard may be present if leaded paint or plaster is loose, peeling, or chipping. If the child attends an old school in poor repair, and if it has paint flakes or chips on carpets or along baseboards, the flakes are presumptively laden with lead and should be treated as a priority repair. The classroom should be closed until cleanup and testing is completed.

## Resources

US Environmental Protection Agency. The *Indoor Air Quality Tools for Schools* kit includes "Indoor Air Pollutants: An Introduction for Health Professionals." For more information on the indoor air quality kit, e-mail iaqinfo@aol.com, phone 800-438-4318, or fax 703-356-5386 or go to http://www.epa.gov/iaq/schools/tools4s2.html. For assistance and guidance in dealing with known or suspected adverse effects of indoor air pollution, contact EPA Indoor Air Quality Information at 866-837-3721.

For more information about mold remediation, see *Mold Remediation in Schools and Commercial Buildings* (EPA 402-K-01-001) March 2001 at http://www.epa.gov/iaq.

## References

1. American Academy of Pediatrics Committee on Environmental Hazards. Asbestos exposure in schools. *Pediatrics.* 1987;79:301–305
2. US Environmental Protection Agency. *Tools for Schools.* Washington, DC: US Environmental Protection Agency; 2002. Available at: http://www.epa.gov/iaq/schools/tools4s2.html
3. US Department of Education. *The Condition of Education 2000.* Washington, DC: National Center for Education Statistics; 2000. Report NCES 2000-062
4. McFadden RD. Students sickened when fumes from coal furnace seep through school. *New York Times.* February 3, 1998:B1
5. US Government Accounting Office. *School Facilities: Conditions of America's Schools.* Washington, DC: US General Accounting Office; 1995. GAO Report #HEHS-95-61
6. Gammage RB, Kaye SV. *Indoor Air and Human Health.* Chelsea, MI: Lewis Publishers, Inc; 1985
7. Etzel RA. Indoor air pollutants in homes and schools. *Pediatr Clin North Am.* 2001;48:1153–1165
8. Etzel RA. Mycotoxins. *JAMA.* 2002;287:425–427
9. Rotter BA, Prelusky DB, Pestka JJ. Toxicology of deoxynivalenol (vomitoxin). *J Toxicol Environ Health.* 1996;48:1–34
10. Bhat RV, Beedu SR, Ramakrishna Y, Munshi KL. Outbreak of trichothecene mycotoxicosis associated with consumption of mould-damaged wheat products in Kashmir Valley, India. *Lancet.* 1989;1:35–37

11. Etzel RA. *Stachybotrys. Curr Opin Pediatr.* 2003;15:103–106
12. Croft WA, Jarvis BB, Yatawara CS. Airborne outbreak of trichothecene toxicosis. *Atmospheric Environ.* 1986;20:549–552
13. Wheeler AE. System selection. *ASHRAE Journal.* 1998;June:12–16
14. Menzies D, Bourbeau J. Building-related illnesses. *N Engl J Med.* 1997;337:1524–1531
15. Gold DR. Indoor air pollution. *Clin Chest Med.* 1992;13:215–229
16. Samet JM, Spengler JD, eds. *Indoor Air Pollution: A Health Perspective.* Baltimore, MD: Johns Hopkins University Press; 1991
17. US Environmental Protection Agency. *National School Radon Survey.* Washington, DC: US Environmental Protection Agency; 1992
18. US Environmental Protection Agency. *Radon Levels in Schools.* Washington, DC: US Environmental Protection Agency; 1993. EPA Publication 402-R-92-014
19. US Environmental Protection Agency. *Support Document for Proposed Rule on Friable Asbestos-Containing Materials in School Buildings: Health Effects and Magnitude of Exposure.* Washington, DC: US Environmental Protection Agency Office of Testing and evaluation, Office of Pesticides and Toxic Substances; 1980. EPA Publication 560/12-80-003
20. Reigart JR, Roberts JR, eds. *Recognition and Management of Pesticide Poisonings.* 5th ed. Washington, DC: US Environmental Protection Agency; 1999. EPA Publication 735-R-98-003. Available at: http://www.epa.gov/oppfead1/safety/healthcare/handbook/handbook.htm
21. US Environmental Protection Agency, Office of Pesticide Programs. *Pest Control in the School Environment: Adopting Integrated Pest Management.* Washington, DC: US Environmental Protection Agency; 1993. EPA Publication 735-F-93-012
22. Owens K, Feldman J. The schooling of state pesticide laws—2002 Update. *Pesticides and You.* 2000;20:16–23
23. Zentall SS. Research on the educational implications of attention deficit hyperactivity disorder. *Except Child.* 1993;60:143–153
24. Center for Health, Environment and Justice. *Poisoned Schools: Invisible Threats, Visible Actions.* Falls Church, VA: Center for Health, Environment and Justice; 2000
25. Calabrese EJ, Stanek EJ, James RC, Roberts SM. Soil ingestion: a concern for acute toxicity in children. *Environ Health Perspect.* 1997;105:1354–1358

26. Nishioka MG, Lewis RG, Brinkman MC, Burkholder HM, Hines CE, Menkedick JR. Distribution of 2,4-D in air and on surfaces inside residences after lawn applications: comparing exposure estimates from various media for young children. *Environ Health Perspect.* 2001;109:1185–1191

27. American Academy of Pediatrics Committee on Environmental Health. Ultraviolet light: a hazard to children. *Pediatrics.* 1999;104:328–333

28. Glanz K, Saraiya M, Wechsler H. Guidelines for school programs to prevent skin cancer. *MMWR Recomm Rep.* 2002;51:1–18

# 31

# Waste Sites

The potential adverse impact of hazardous waste sites on human health may be a source of concern to families and health professionals. The Agency for Toxic Substances and Disease Registry (ATSDR), a component of the US Department of Health and Human Services, estimates that 3 to 4 million American children live within 1 mile of a hazardous waste site.[1] Uncontrolled hazardous waste sites are prevalent throughout the world. Although accurate worldwide data are lacking, the US Environmental Protection Agency (EPA) listed approximately 15 000 sites in the United States in 1996. On the basis of a hazard ranking system, 1371 were listed or proposed for listing on the National Priorities List (NPL).[2,3] Each of the 50 states has at least one NPL site; 5 states (California, Michigan, New Jersey, New York, and Pennsylvania) contain 37% of all the sites and 30% of the children and youth (from birth through 17 years of age) in the United States.[4] Most (65%–70%) uncontrolled hazardous waste sites in the United States are waste storage/treatment facilities (including landfills) or former industrial properties.[5] Many of these properties have been abandoned and most have more than one major chemical contaminant. Less common are waste recycling facilities and mining sites, which may be active, inactive, or abandoned. Some of the substances found in uncontrolled hazardous waste sites are heavy metals such as lead, chromium, and arsenic and organic solvents such as trichloroethylene and benzene.[5] Children living in urban areas may have greater risks of exposure to hazardous waste because of nearby "brownfield" sites. A brownfield is a tract of land that has been developed for industrial purposes, polluted, abandoned, and later designated by municipalities for redevelopment. An additional group of hazardous waste sites is associated with federal government facilities, in particular military facilities and nuclear energy complexes. See Table 31.1 for federal legislation covering waste sites and unintentional releases. The National Research Council has cited 17 482 contaminated sites at 1855 military installations and 3700 sites at 500 nuclear facilities.[6] Some of these sites cover large geographic areas and are contaminated with complex mixtures of wastes.

Certain types of waste sites and chemical contaminants are in preponderance in distinct regions of the country. For example, the New England states have many sites related to old economy industries, such as mills, radium clock factories, and metal plating and tanning facilities; the common contaminants are lead, arsenic, chromium, radium, and mercury. In contrast, several southwestern states have waste sites related to refining and petrochemicals, wood treatment, and mining and smelting; the common contaminants are volatile organic compounds, pentachlorophenol, lead, arsenic, and creosote.[7]

**Table 31.1**
**US Legislation Covering Waste Sites and Unintentional Releases**

| 1980 | The *Comprehensive Environmental Response, Compensation, and Liability Act (CERCLA) of 1980* established ATSDR as an agency of the Public Health Service with mandates to (1) establish a National Exposure and Disease Registry; (2) create an inventory of health information on hazardous substances; (3) create a list of closed and restricted-access sites; (4) provide medical assistance during hazardous substance emergencies; and (5) determine the relationship between hazardous substance exposures and illness. |
|---|---|
| 1984 | The *Resource Conservation and Recovery Act (RCRA),* as amended in 1984, mandated that ATSDR work with the EPA to (1) identify new hazardous waste sites to be regulated; (2) conduct health assessments at RCRA sites at EPA's request; and (3) consider petitions for health assessments by the public or states. |
| 1986 | The *Superfund Amendments and Reauthorization Act (SARA)* of 1986 broadened ATSDR's responsibilities in the areas or public health assessments, establishment and maintenance of toxicologic databases, information dissemination, and medical education. |

When the EPA places a site on the NPL, the Superfund Act (passed in 1980* and amended in 1986†) provides monies for remediation (cleanup) of the site and an array of public health actions in nearby communities. The ATSDR conducts public health assessments to evaluate the potential health hazards faced by communities in proximity to every proposed, listed, or former NPL site and in response to petitions from individuals. In many cases this work is conducted by state health departments under ATSDR sponsorship and review. A site is assigned a hazard category according to the human health hazard it poses on the basis of professional judgment and weight-of-evidence criteria.[5] In the 3-year period from 1993 to 1995, this process indicated a health hazard at 49% of sites and an urgent hazard at 4% of sites.[5] A site-specific epidemiologic investigation or other type of investigation is needed to establish the actual hazard to health. Of the public health assessments conducted at 1371 sites, 60% to 70% have included recommendations that address the need for intervention to interrupt ongoing exposure pathways.[4] These interventions have included provision of alternate drinking water, issuance of fish consumption advisories, posting of warning notices, restriction of site access, and (rarely) relocation of community residents.

*The Comprehensive Environmental Response, Compensation, and Liability Act of 1980.
†The Superfund Amendment and Reauthorization Act of 1986.

## Routes and Sources of Exposure

Routes of exposure are ingestion, inhalation, and through the skin. Children may be exposed through contaminated groundwater, surface water, drinking water, air, surface soil, sediment, or consumable plants or animals.

Children often find waste sites interesting. They may ignore or fail to notice warning signs, find or create openings in fences, or otherwise gain access to restricted places on or near a site.[8] Often there is considerable variation in exposure depending on climate, season, and time of day.

Recognizing that proximity to a waste site may be an important risk factor for children, ATSDR initiated a process of routinely collecting standardized information on populations and demographics at NPL sites. This process uses Geographic Information Systems (GIS) to determine the number of people living within 1 mile of the boundaries of a hazardous waste site. The process ascertains the number of children living within the 1-mile polygon, and alerts site investigators to the children's presence.

## Clinical Effects

The effect that exposure to a hazardous substance(s) has on an infant's or child's health is related to the nature of the pollutant, the dose received, the toxicity of the substance, and the individual's susceptibility.

The overall impact of hazardous waste sites on national health is difficult to assess because of conflicting information from epidemiologic studies and limitations of the methodologies used.[9] Many studies have been interpreted as "negative," meaning that no statistically significant increase in adverse health effects was found. These observations may reflect the true absence of adverse effects or the inability to detect such effects due to inadequacies in study design or sample size. For example, many studies that found little if any excess risks of adverse effects defined their target populations crudely, based on linear distance from a site, instead of documented environmental pathways and routes of exposure. Likewise, studies interpreted as "positive" may reflect a true effect or other types of study design flaws, such as misclassification of exposure or inappropriate choice of comparison groups. Improved study methods, such as those that generate real-time exposure models via computerized GIS, hold greater promise in associating exposure to site contaminants with adverse health effects.

Adverse health effects have been reported in some, but not all, investigations of communities around hazardous waste sites.[9,10] These effects have ranged from nonspecific symptoms such as headache, fatigue, and irritative symptoms, to specific conditions such as low birth weight,[11] congenital heart defects,[12] and a constellation of neurobehavioral deficits.[13] Most investigations have included some children in the study population, but only a few have focused primarily on health effects in infants and children. In these studies, it is difficult to know whether proximity to the waste site or some other factor(s) is responsible for the health outcome. The following are examples of findings considered "positive":

- Children exposed to trichloroethylene in drinking water supplies at 15 different sites in 5 states had increased reporting of speech and hearing impairments.[14]
- Neural tube defects in racial minority newborns were associated with maternal residence in a census tract that had a Superfund site.[15]
- Preterm birth was associated with exposure to $^{131}$I at the Hanford nuclear site in Washington state.[15]
- Gestational exposure to drinking water contaminated with perchlorate was associated with measures of decreased thyroid function in neonates.[16]
- Children exposed to lead from a smelter showed poor neurobehavioral function and peripheral nerve function when tested as young adults 15 to 20 years later.[17]

- Children living near a municipal waste incinerator had a 3-fold increase in risk of lower respiratory tract illnesses.[18]

An array of information resources is available on the health hazards of 275 individual toxic substances. This information is provided in a variety of formats intended for different audiences. The ATSDR Toxicological Profiles, in particular, systematically review the toxicology, pharmacokinetics, epidemiology, exposure, environmental fate, and transport of the substances. Additional information specific to children's health and developmental issues is provided in profiles covering most commonly encountered substances. Individual profiles are available on CD-ROM from CRC Press (Boca Raton, FL), and in hard copy from ATSDR and at http://www.atsdr.cdc.gov/toxpro2.html.

Disruption of community cultures and daily life has been observed following toxic releases. For example, persistently high indoor air levels of mercury vapor forced authorities to relocate residents from their own condominium building.[19] The source of the mercury was residual pools of condensed liquid metal from a factory that had been housed in the same building decades prior to its renovation. Frequently, the awareness of environmental risks and hazards in communities with waste sites has led to increased concern and stress within communities.

## Diagnostic Methods

An exposed infant or child can remain asymptomatic, develop non-specific symptoms, or develop signs and symptoms frequently associated with common medical conditions. Because of this range of outcomes, a history of exposure should be obtained when evaluating the etiology of unexplained symptoms. Standardized approaches to taking an exposure history are available.[20,21]

### Individual Evaluation

As in other aspects of medicine, the history guides laboratory testing. Blood or urine tests may be indicated when a child is symptomatic and there is a recent history of a specific exposure (eg, when a child has climbed over a fence and played in a site known to be contaminated with a specific toxicant). Generally, laboratory tests to document exposure are not recommended in the absence of signs or symptoms.

### Community Studies

In formal epidemiologic studies, laboratory biological tests may be useful to determine if there is an association between exposure and any adverse health effects.

A biomarker of exposure provides a reasonable measure of the internal body level of a substance over a period that depends on the pharmacokinetics of that substance. Testing may be performed on blood (for lead), urine (for metallic mercury, arsenic), breast milk (for polychlorinated biphenyls), or other tissue. Analytical methods and human reference ranges are available for many of the substances found most commonly at hazardous waste sites. In some cases, age-specific reference ranges are available to facilitate interpretation of levels found in infants and children. It may be difficult to interpret the results, however, when reference ranges for children are not available.

Highly sensitive standardized medical test batteries are available for use in epidemiologic studies to evaluate subclinical and clinical organ damage or dysfunction related to noncancer health conditions, such as immune function disorders,[22] kidney dysfunction,[23] lung and respiratory diseases,[24] and neurotoxic disorders.[13] Because of their low specificity, these test batteries are not useful outside the context of a formal study.

### Treatment

Treatment of acute exposure to one or more substances from a hazardous waste site depends on the substance; the route, dose, and duration of exposure; and the presence of any symptoms or ill effects.[25]

A 2-part video titled *ATSDR's Community Challenge* gives emergency medical services personnel and hospital emergency departments the necessary guidance to plan for incidents involving human exposure to hazardous materials. The available videos are

- **Part I:** *Hazardous Materials Response and the Emergency Medical System*
- **Part II:** *Hazardous Materials Response and the Hospital Emergency Department*

## Consultation

Consultation is available on potentially toxic exposures and possible ill effects from such exposures. A North American network of Pediatric Environmental Health Specialty Units has been formed to provide information, receive referrals, and offer training in the diagnosis and treatment of illnesses associated with exposure to toxic substances and other environmental health risks (see Resources).

## Prevention of Exposure

In the United States, the EPA is responsible for cleaning up waste sites under the Superfund Act. Experience at hundreds of communities near waste sites has demonstrated the value and importance of early and extensive community involvement. This is usually not a simple process. However, government agencies have made considerable progress in these areas by forming community assistance panels; awarding assistance grants; and developing valid methods of needs assessment, health risk communication, and community outreach. These methods have enhanced the agencies' abilities to recognize the value of community input, address community needs, and focus attention to those needed areas.[7]

**Prevention of Exposure**
**Engineering Controls**
Destroy contaminants by incineration or by chemical or
biological reactions.
Remove the contaminants to a safer location.
Disrupt the exposure pathway (eg, an alternate water supply or
perimeter fence).
Use dust control and other measures to protect workers and
neighbors during the cleanup process.
Develop engineering solutions to eliminate relatively small,
acute problems (removal actions).
Develop "remedial actions," engineering solutions that involve
complex planning to permanently solve a complicated waste
site problem.

**Administrative Controls**
Temporarily or permanently relocate residents.
Restrict deeds (eg, to prevent future use of the land for residential
or child care purposes).
Enact ordinances to control future land use.
Communicate health advisories (eg, warnings about eating fish or
swimming in certain waters).

**Personal Preventive Actions**
Comply with advisories mentioned previously.
Connect to a safer water supply.
Fence children's play areas to avoid exposure to soil contaminants.

## Frequently Asked Questions

Q *I am confused by the conflicting information I hear about the risks to my children from waste sites. Can you clarify this?*

A The risks depend on the amount, type, and duration of exposure and the types of chemicals involved. However, it is difficult to know the exact details of a child's exposure, so it is difficult to know the risk precisely. In addition, for many chemicals, the effects of exposure in childhood are not well known and only can be estimated from the toxic effects found in experiments with animals.

Q *Did exposure from a waste site cause my child's illness? or One of my children has an illness that is linked to the waste site. Will my other children become ill also?*

A It is difficult to prove that one child's illness was caused by exposure to one particular waste site. Most of the illnesses that can be caused by exposure to toxic chemicals have more than one possible cause. Also, not every child who is so exposed becomes ill. A linkage is more likely if several children (or adults) become ill at about the same time, the same place, or following the same exposure.

Q *Will my child get cancer from exposure to a waste site?*

A Although a number of chemicals found at waste sites are carcinogens (known or predicted to cause cancer), the chances of getting cancer from exposure to a waste site is thought to be small. If the child was exposed to one or more carcinogens, the amount and duration of the exposure are important risk factors. Most experts believe that development of cancer is unlikely unless there has been exposure for many years.

Q *Is my child's learning disability (or attention-deficit disorder) caused by exposure to a waste site?*

A A number of chemicals found at waste sites may affect the nervous system. They include heavy metals (eg, lead and mercury), organic solvents (eg, toluene), and certain types of pesticides (eg, carbamates and organophosphates). The risk to the child depends on how long the child was exposed, the child's age at exposure, the degree of exposure, and the child's susceptibility.

Q *How can I protect my child from future exposure to hazardous waste sites?*

A It is best to avoid areas where soil is contaminated by hazardous waste. Explain to children the meaning and importance of posted warning signs, and strongly advise children to stay out of restricted areas. Do not let children swim in streams or other bodies of water that are known to be contaminated. Such conditions usually are posted, but if there is doubt, the local health department should be contacted. Know the source of your household drinking water and if uncertain about contaminants, have it tested. Children, pregnant women, and others should not eat certain fish caught from contaminated waters. Fishing license brochures available locally list advisories on which fish are safe to eat. If a parent or other caregiver works at a hazardous waste site, soiled work clothes should not be brought into the home. Dust can be a source of exposure for children.

**Resources**

Agency for Toxic Substances and Disease Registry (ATSDR) (educational materials, medical management guidelines for acute toxicity, toxicity information for individual chemicals, Toxicological Profiles publications) phone: 888-42-ATSDR (888-422-8737) or 404-498-0110, Child Health Web site: http://www.atsdr.cdc.gov/child, chemical emergencies and accidental releases, phone: 404-498-0100 *(information available 24 hours a day)*

The ATSDR provides 24-hour technical and scientific support (emergency response hotline, 404-498-0120) for chemical emergencies (including terrorist threats) such as spills, explosions, and transportation accidents throughout the United States. The ATSDR also provides health consultations for people exposed to individual substances or mixtures.

Their 3-volume reference text, *Managing Hazardous Materials Incidents: Medical Management Guidelines for Acute Chemical Exposures,* contains the following information:

- **Volume I:** *Emergency Medical Services: A Planning Guide for the Management of Contaminated Patients*
- **Volume II:** *Hospital Emergency Departments: A Planning Guide for the Management of Contaminated Patients*
- **Volume III:** *Medical Management Guidelines for Acute Chemical Exposures*

In particular, ATSDR has addressed issues related to children with respect to the prehospital (Volume I) and hospital management (Volume II) of children who may be chemically contaminated. Appropriate revisions, including pediatric updates, also are being made to Volume III, which addresses medical management of patients who have been exposed to specific chemicals.

Association of Occupational and Environmental Clinics, phone: 202-347-4976, Internet: www.aoec.org

Chemical poisoning emergencies
Internet: http://www.toxicologyonline.com/poison.asp

Pediatric Environmental Health Specialty Units, Internet: http://www.aoec.org/pesu.htm

Poison control centers, phone: see local telephone directory, Internet: http://www.toxicologyonline.com/poison.asp

**Additional Information**
Superfund Records of Decision, Internet: http://www.epa.gov/superfund/sites/rods/index.htm

US Environmental Protection Agency WasteWise Helpline: 800-372-9473, Internet: http://www.epa.gov/epaoswer/non-hw/reduce/wstewise/; chemical spills, oil spills, threats phone: 800-424-8802, Internet: http://www.epa.gov/oilspill/oilhow.htm

## References

1. Amler RW, Smith L, eds. *Achievements in Children's Environmental Health.* Atlanta, GA: US Department of Health and Human Services, Agency for Toxic Substances and Disease Registry; 2001

2. US Environmental Protection Agency. National Priorities List for hazardous waste sites: proposed rule. *Federal Register.* 1996;61:67678–67682

3. US Environmental Protection Agency. National Priorities List for uncontrolled hazardous waste sites: final rule. *Federal Register.* 1996;61:67655–67677

4. Agency for Toxic Substances and Disease Registry. *Hazardous Substances Release/Health Effects Database (HazDat).* Atlanta, GA: US Department of Health and Human Services, Public Health Service, Agency for Toxic Substances and Disease Registry; 1999

5. Agency for Toxic Substances and Disease Registry. *Report to Congress, 1993, 1994, 1995.* Atlanta, GA: US Department of Health and Human Services, Public Health Service, Agency for Toxic Substances and Disease Registry; 1996

6. National Research Council. *Ranking Hazardous-Waste Sites for Remedial Action.* Washington, DC: National Academies Press; 1994;29,37

7. Amler RW, Falk H. Opportunities and challenges in community environmental health evaluations. *Environ Epidemiol Toxicol.* 2000;2:51–55

8. Agency for Toxic Substances and Disease Registry. *Healthy Children–Toxic Environments: Acting on the Unique Vulnerability of Children Who Dwell Near Hazardous Waste Sites. Report of the Child Health Workgroup, Board of Scientific Counselors.* Atlanta, GA: US Department of Health and Human Services, Public Health Service, Agency for Toxic Substances and Disease Registry; 1997

9. Johnson BL. *Impact of Hazardous Waste on Human Health.* Boca Raton FL: Lewis Publishers; 1999

10. Elliott P, Briggs D, Morris S, et al. Risk of adverse birth outcomes in populations living near landfill sites. *BMJ.* 2001;323:363–368

11. Amler RW. Assessment of reproductive disorders and birth defects in communities near hazardous chemical sites: introduction. *Reprod Toxicol.* 1997;11:221–222

12. Savitz DA, Bornschein RL, Amler RW, et al. Assessment of reproductive disorders and birth defects in communities near hazardous chemical sites. I. Birth defects and developmental disorders. *Reprod Toxicol.* 1997;11:223–230

13. Amler RW, Gibertinin M, eds. *Pediatric Environmental Neurobehavioral Test Battery.* Atlanta, GA: US Department of Health and Human Services, Public Health Service, Agency for Toxic Substances and Disease Registry; 1996

14. Agency for Toxic Substances and Disease Registry. *National Exposure Registry Trichloroethylene (TCE) Subregistry Baseline Technical Report (Revised).* Atlanta, GA: US Department of Health and Human Services, Public Health Service, Agency for Toxic Substances and Disease Registry; 1994

15. Orr M, Bove F, Kaye W, Stone M. Elevated birth defects in racial or ethnic minority children of women living near hazardous waste sites. *Int J Hyg Environ Health.* 2002;205:19–27

16. Brechner RJ, Parkhurst GD, Humble WO, Brown MB, Herman WH. Ammonium perchlorate contamination of Colorado River drinking water is associated with abnormal thyroid function in newborns in Arizona. *J Occup Environ Med.* 2000;42:777–782

17. Agency for Toxic Substances and Disease Registry. *A Cohort Study of Current and Previous Residents of the Silver Valley: Assessment of Lead Exposure and Health Outcomes.* Atlanta, GA: US Department of Health and Human Services, Public Health Service, Agency for Toxic Substances and Disease Registry; 1997

18. Agency for Toxic Substances and Disease Registry. *Study of Effect of Residential Proximity to Waste Incinerators on Lower Respiratory Illness in Children.* Atlanta, GA: US Department of Health and Human Services, Public Health Service, Agency for Toxic Substances and Disease Registry; 1995

19. Centers for Disease Control and Prevention. Mercury exposure among residents of a building formerly used for industrial purposes—New Jersey, 1995. *MMWR Morb Mortal Wkly Rep.* 1996;45:422–424

20. Agency for Toxic Substances and Disease Registry. *Case Studies in Environmental Medicine: Taking an Exposure History.* Atlanta, GA: US Department of Health and Human Services, Public Health Service, Agency for Toxic Substances and Disease Registry; 2000. ATSDR Publication ATSDR-HE-CS-2001-0002. Available at: http://www.atsdr.cdc.gov/HEC/CSEM/exphistory/index.html

21. Agency for Toxic Substances and Disease Registry. *Case Studies in Environmental Medicine: Pediatric Environmental Medicine. Principles of Environmental Medical Evaluation.* Atlanta, GA: US Department of Health and Human Services, Agency for Toxic Substances and Disease Registry; 2003:24

22. Straight JM, Kipen HM, Vogt RF, Amler RW. *Immune Function Test Batteries for Use in Environmental Health Field Studies.* Atlanta, GA: US Department of Health and Human Services, Public Health Service, Agency for Toxic Substances and Disease Registry; 1994

23. Amler RW, Mueller PW, Schultz MG. *Biomarkers of Kidney Function for Environmental Health Field Studies.* Atlanta, GA: US Department of Health and Human Services, Public Health Service, Agency for Toxic Substances and Disease Registry; 1998

24. Metcalf SW, Samet J, Hanrahan J, Schwartz D, Hunninghake G. *A Standardized Test Battery for Lungs and Respiratory Diseases for Use in Environmental Health Field Studies.* Atlanta, GA: US Department of Health and Human Services, Public Health Service, Agency for Toxic Substances and Disease Registry; 1994

25. Agency for Toxic Substances and Disease Registry. *Managing Hazardous Materials Incidents: Medical Management Guidelines for Acute Chemical Exposures.* Atlanta, GA: US Department of Health and Human Services, Public Health Service, Agency for Toxic Substances and Disease Registry; 2001

# 32
# Workplaces

More than 80% of high school students work during some time in the year as part of their normal weekly schedule.[1] Each year, work-related injuries kill about 70 US adolescents and children younger than 18 years. About 70 000 additional teens are injured at work badly enough to seek emergency department care.[2] Their exposures to dangerous machinery and hazardous chemicals seldom are addressed by health care providers. Adult occupational medicine professionals rarely see teens, and pediatricians until recently have not become involved in the occupational health and safety of their adolescent patients. The injury and fatality statistics suggest that children, adolescents, and their families need the input of their primary care providers into the occupational choices they make and the job training they receive. The systems that regulate youth employment need information from pediatricians on occupational injury and illness seen in pediatric practices. Advocacy efforts to improve youth occupational safety and health already in progress at the state and national levels also need pediatric input. Issues of acute toxicity and safety need to be addressed most urgently, but chronic or delayed health effects also need to be considered.

## Background
Currently more than 5 million adolescents younger than 18 years are legally employed in the United States during some combination of after-school, weekend, and summer hours. An additional 1 to 2 million are believed to be employed in violation of wage, hour, or safety regulations.[3] Efforts to improve school-to-work transitions are placing more teenagers into the workplace, and even school-based vocational/technical education that simulates employment conditions may in-

volve hazardous conditions, including chemical exposures. National priorities for volunteer community involvement support increased participation of adolescents in nonpaid activities such as rehabilitation of old housing that may still carry the same risks of exposures as paid employment.[4] The largest number of employed youth are aged 14 years and older. However, children aged 10 years or younger also are working, delivering newspapers or working on farms.

While there are no large-scale studies that describe illness or death resulting from exposures in the workplace among teenagers, large studies do exist that document occupational injuries among working adolescents, suggesting that there also is a problem with teenage exposure to hazardous substances in the workplace. In the past decade, despite laws intended to protect teenaged workers, every year at least 70 children younger than 18 years die from work on the job site.[2,5] The occupational fatality rate for employed youth is greater than the rate of occupational death for adult workers, especially in the 3 highest types of occupational mortality: motor vehicle crashes, homicides, and machinery-related deaths.[6,7] Approximately 3% of youth occupational deaths may be attributable to poisonings rather than injuries, but this number is extremely variable, ranging from 4% of North Carolina medical examiner reports of youth occupational fatalities[8] to 7% of poisoning deaths among New York state adolescent workers' compensation fatality cases.[9] More than 65 000 to 70 000 children and adolescents are injured severely enough to seek care in emergency departments.[2,10] These numbers likely underestimate the true extent of the problem, perhaps because many people assume a child or adolescent's occupation is "student" and never inquire or record further information about employed occupation. Many adolescent occupational injury studies serve as markers for concern about occupational exposures, and this is reinforced by our knowledge about exposure-related fatalities.[6,9–14]

## Regulation of Hours and Hazards in Adolescent Employment

The Fair Labor Standards Act (FLSA) of 1938 remains the major
federal law that regulates work for youth younger than 18 years.[15]
The law has 2 parts—the protection of education through regulation of permitted hours of work in a day and in a week, and the protection of health and safety through prohibition of work on dangerous
machinery or with hazardous chemicals via Hazard Orders. Under the
FLSA, adolescents younger than 18 years are prohibited from working
with hazardous chemicals in nonagricultural jobs.[16] Prohibitions on
chemical work in agriculture extend only to age 16 years, and work by
children and adolescents on their own family farms is unregulated.[17]
(A table listing permitted hours and prohibited occupations can be
found on the National Institute for Occupational Safety and Health
[NIOSH] Web site. See Resources.)

Many states also have laws regulating child labor, and if more stringent than the federal law, state law supersedes. Many businesses, particularly small ones, may not be covered by either federal or state law,
and discerning exactly who, if anyone, has jurisdiction for child labor
in small business or agriculture often is complex. Recent trends toward
increased use of contract workers, especially for newspaper delivery
and janitorial services, are problematic because they leave unclear
who is responsible for education, supervision, health, and safety.

Another major area of legal exemptions is vocational/technical
training. Because such training is assumed to occur with supervision
in a safe environment, restrictions based on safety concerns may be
waived for students in various types of training. No systematic surveillance of exposure resulting in illness or injury has been conducted in
school-based learning sites or on job sites, but studies of shop-related
injuries and of work-related poison control center calls suggest that
there is reason for concern.[18,19] From 1992 to 1996, 1008 Utah children in grades 7 through 12 were reported by school personnel to be
injured in shop class. Of the 7 (all high school students) who were

injured badly enough to require hospital admission, 6 were injured using a table saw and 1 was injured using automotive cleaning fluid. That student sustained second-degree burns of the face and upper extremity.[18] Consultations requested of the Massachusetts Poison Control Center from 1991 to 1996 included 124 cases of occupational exposures to working teens aged 14 to 17 years. Moderate to severe injuries were sustained by 18 of these youth, with almost half being related to caustics or cleaning compounds.[19]

### Work Permits

In approximately half the states, adolescents must obtain a work permit issued by their school before seeking or starting a job. Some states require the signature of a physician, which offers an opportunity to provide anticipatory guidance about safety at work.

### Enforcement of Child Labor Laws

Child labor laws are enforced by the federal and state labor departments. Labor inspectors are responsible for enforcing wage, hour, and safety laws for all workers. Thus most child labor is investigated only when a complaint is made, usually by a parent or occasionally by business personnel. The number of inspectors available to enforce child labor laws is small, and the fines for child labor violations historically have been small. Some states recently have increased fines, particularly for repeated violations. Two continuing widespread hours violation problems include keeping teenagers at work too late on school nights or having them clock out at an appropriate time but continue to work without pay.

The most critical aspect of child labor law violation relates to safety because of the repeated association between fatalities and safety violations. If an employer does not abide by wage and hour laws, it may be reasonable to assume that the employer is not following laws to protect the health and safety of the teenager.[20,21] Exposures of legally employed youth to potentially hazardous materials may occur in job activities that violate the law, jobs not covered by the law because of business size or production, or activities outside their major job title, especially cleaning. Family businesses, especially agriculture, are disproportionately represented among child work injury fatalities, including children younger than 14 years,[22] suggesting that exposures also are important in agriculture and other family businesses.

## Routes of Exposure

### Dermal

Some chemical exposures involve absorption through the skin or through breaks in the skin. Examples include pesticide exposure in lawn care and agriculture[23]; nicotine exposure while harvesting tobacco[24]; and solvent exposure in screen printing shops,[25] leather shops, and auto body shops. It is important to remember that cloth gloves and sneakers do not provide adequate protection, and that if soaked with a chemical, clothing may even worsen exposure if not promptly removed. While generally considered with injury rather than exposures, electrocution and radiation could be considered here. Electrocutions, more than 50% of which involved contact with power lines, were the third leading cause of occupational death among 16- and 17-year-olds from 1980 to 1989.[26]

### Inhalation

Inhalation injuries result from breathing chemical fumes or particles. Adolescents involved in new home construction as part of school programs may have such exposures while using spray foam around windows.[27] Other examples include metal fumes (lead) and isocyanates found in auto body paint and some types of shellac that are pulmonary sensitizers. Environmental tobacco smoke is a hazard for restaurant workers where the restaurant has a smoking section.[28] Inhalation of solvents may occur during cleanup activities in a variety of workplaces,[29] ranging from fast food to shop class, and may have neurotoxic and hepatotoxic effects.

## Ingestion

Lead and other heavy metals may be ingested. Lead hazards have been found in auto body shop environments.[30] Given that attention to hygiene is protective, one of the populations at potential special risk is children functioning at a preschool age (those with mental retardation), among whom oral behaviors are much more common than normal for their age. By preferentially channeling such children into vocational education in the United States, the risk is increased and must be considered in planning for the placement of the student.

## Clinical Effects

There is no surveillance system in place in the United States specifically for monitoring children's occupational exposures. With the exception of noise, for which there are studies of clinical effects and preventive interventions,[31] information on clinical effects is gathered piecemeal. Three major sources of data have been (1) case reports of exposures and acute poisonings from the literature and from within adolescent occupational injury studies (many of the latter are based on workers' compensation reports); (2) adult occupational medicine literature about exposures that may be extrapolated to adolescents working in similar jobs; and (3) concerns about the safety of various exposures based on a combination of our knowledge of chemical toxicology and of adolescent growth, development, physiology, and anatomy. Recent work suggests that poison control centers also may serve as valuable though incomplete adolescent occupational exposure surveillance systems.[19]

## Examples of Exposures and Acute Poisonings

Data from a study of more than 17 000 Washington state workers' compensation awards to adolescent workers (aged 11–17) from 1988 to 1991 included almost 900 (4.9%) awards for toxic exposures.[6] Cases from Massachusetts and Kentucky suggest that acute adolescent occupational exposures are occurring; the most common agents are cleaning solutions, and the most common work site involved is food service.[19,32] As an example of a typical case scenario, a teen working in a fast-food restaurant is hired to work at the counter, but at the end of a shift becomes part of the cleanup crew. Cleaning involves use of various chemicals, sometimes informally mixed. The adolescent usually has had no training in safe handling or use of those chemicals, with potentially life-threatening results. Such cases are significantly undercounted, given the many teens who are exposed but do not die or become sick enough to be reported to a poison control center or workers' compensation system.

Teens employed on farms or with lawn care companies also may be at risk of hazardous exposures. A 1989 survey of 50 migrant farmworkers younger than 18 years in New York state found that 11% had mixed or applied pesticides despite child labor laws that prohibit work with hazardous chemicals.[33] No protective equipment was used other than gloves, and it was unclear whether the gloves were impermeable. More than 15% of the youth surveyed reported having had symptoms consistent with organophosphate poisoning, but few had sought medical care. More than 40% had worked in fields wet with pesticides, violating field reentry times suggested by chemical manufacturers, and 40% had been sprayed with pesticides while at work in the fields directly by crop-dusting planes or indirectly by drifting chemicals from planes or tractors. Similar observations were made among 323 North Carolina 4-H students, 69% of whom were working on the farm of a relative. Use of pesticides or other farm chemicals was reported by 29% of girls and 59% of boys. Sickness related to pesticide or other chemical exposures was reported by 3% of girls and 11% of boys.[34]

## Examples of Exposures With Chronic Effects

### Noise

Wisconsin high school students with active involvement in farm work were found to have more than twice the risk of early noise-induced hearing loss than their peers who did not work on farms.[31,35] There was a clear relationship between amount of noise exposure and degree of hearing loss. Among farming students with greater noise exposure, 74% had evidence of some hearing loss in at least one ear. Only 9% of farming students reported using any hearing protection devices.

### *Repetitive Motion*

While there is little available direct data about adolescents, a study including slightly older female supermarket cashiers was notable for the prevalence of self-reported carpal tunnel symptoms (62.5%) related to use of laser scanners, years worked as a cashier, and number of hours per week worked. This is a concern given the large number of teenaged girls employed as supermarket cashiers, and given that teens may have additional school or leisure computer time adding to the potential for repetitive motion problems.[36]

### Diagnostic Methods

A thorough history (including an occupational history) and physical examination are most important. Patients should be screened for the presence of heavy metals or other specific substances if appropriate (eg, for lead when renovating old houses). When the substance itself cannot be measured, end-organ effects of exposure should be measured (ie, hepatocellular enzymes following solvent exposure). In acute events, it is very important that the substance and its original container(s) be saved for analysis if needed. The case of a 16-year-old Kentucky teenager who died after suffering a witnessed cardiorespiratory arrest while scrubbing a hot grill with a mixture of cleaning solutions will probably never be definitively diagnosed because the contents of the mixture were unknown after being thrown away.

### Treatment of Clinical Symptoms

Treatments range from determining and eliminating the source of low-level chronic exposure to advanced cardiac life support in some acute poisonings. It is critical to have knowledge of proper rescue measures to ensure the safety of the rescuer. Specific suggestions for medical treatment also may be provided by a poison control center.

## Prevention of Exposure

Prevention through a combination of training and engineering controls is important. Knowledge of substances used and potential routes of exposure is needed first. Proper ergonomics are important in preventing repetitive motion disorders. Chronic back problems may be better prevented if the size of the lifting teenager and the size of the load are carefully matched.

A 4-year program to prevent noise-induced hearing loss was effective in getting Wisconsin farm tractor-driving adolescents to wear hearing protection devices. The adolescents received yearly hearing tests showing them the pre-intervention hearing decrement, plus an educational intervention over 4 school years and 3 summers. In this program, modeled after an industrial hearing protection program, students tested noise levels on their own farms, were provided with frequent reminders through school contact and mailings home, received classroom education that included a video of music with hearing frequencies deleted, and were provided with different types of hearing protection (earmuffs and earplugs) with demonstrations on how to use them. Student self-report of planned future hearing protection device use increased from 23% to 81% among the 375 study students, while it increased from 24% to only 43% in a comparison group.[31]

### Office-Based Strategies

As a routine part of preventive care visits, but also other visits such as sports physicals, pediatricians are encouraged to find out which of their patients work, where they are working, what their job duties are, the types of chemicals they use in their work, and whether they have received any training about working safely with that chemical. Because 80% of teenagers work at some point in the year, every teenager needs an occupational history, with a focus on potential hazards (see Table 32.1). Such a history should include work that may be unpaid helping on a family farm or non-farm business, vocational training at school in shop and other classes, and school-related work-study or other on-the-job site placements. Pediatricians also should ask if adolescent patients are volunteers on projects such as summer church housing rehabilitation work, which may have exposures. It is very important to include such a history for teenagers with learning disabilities, developmental delays, or various causes of mental retardation. Knowledge of first aid and the presence of an adult supervisor on site also are important. Although some workplaces are exempt from the FLSA, all workers legally have the right to know about the chemicals with which they work. Discussion of these issues provides an opportunity for physicians to educate teens about safety.

Pediatricians need to know their state child labor laws. Each state Department of Labor provides a 1-page poster summarizing work hours, wages, and occupations permitted for adolescents of different ages. This poster must be posted prominently in every workplace. In some states, the office of the US Department of Labor also can provide information.

Information about exposures can be obtained from industrial hygiene and occupational medicine professionals, union or corporate health and safety employees, and local Committee on Occupational Safety and Health groups. State-based Occupational Safety and Health Administration training sections also may be helpful. Employers are legally responsible for educating workers about chemical exposures and usage.

The adolescent's employment should be considered when diagnosing an illness (eg, chronic fatigue in an adolescent who makes silk screens can be caused by chronic solvent intoxication if he works and/or sleeps in an area with inadequate ventilation). The adolescent's employment also should be considered in the medical management

**Table 32.1**
**Potential Job-Related Exposures**

| |
|---|
| • Blood-borne pathogens in nursing homes/hospitals |
| • Cleaning agents in restaurants, nursing homes, and schools |
| • Pesticides in lawn care work, farm work, and when buildings are sprayed |
| • Isocyanates (pulmonary sensitizers) during auto body repair or roofing with newer forms of roofing materials |
| • Benzene when pumping gas |
| • Lead from radiators in auto body repair and home renovation |
| • Asbestos in auto brake repair, renovation/demolition of old buildings |
| • Solvents in T-shirt screening |
| • Secondhand smoke in waitstaff jobs |
| • Heat in dishwashing and outdoor work in the summer or in hot climates |
| • Cold in areas with cold weather and outdoor jobs, potentially exacerbated by wet conditions contributing to faster heat loss (in gas station work, construction work, ski area work, and whitewater guiding) |
| • Asthma-producing wood dusts in shop and furniture making |
| • Welding fumes and eye exposures |
| • Cosmetology chemicals and dyes |
| • Tetanus and other biological/infectious hazards in farming (hypersensitivity pneumonitis), veterinary clinics |
| • Noise-induced hearing loss in farming and factory work |
| • Nicotine in harvest of tobacco (green tobacco sickness) |

of known illnesses (eg, asthma that may have been previously under control may flare up when working in the smoking section of a restaurant).

Pediatricians can provide guidance in the choice of occupations for adolescents with chronic diseases. Employment opportunities, which may be fewer than those for their peers, are important for their development and future adult employment.

Pediatricians should be familiar with state workers' compensation laws; adolescents may be eligible for compensation for medical expenses and lost wages/lost time due to illnesses from an occupational exposure.

Rules governing which industries and workers are covered and when benefits begin differ from state to state.

Pediatricians need to advocate for age-appropriate rehabilitation and follow-up for those injured on the job. Although agricultural-related injuries often are not covered, workers' compensation should pay for many cases of rehabilitation resulting from occupational injury/exposure.

## Help Parents Make Informed Decisions About the Safety of Their Adolescent at Work

Pediatricians should talk with parents about the potential risks and benefits of work for their adolescent. Many parents are unaware of injury risk or risks associated with chemical exposures and the need for their adolescent to receive training about safely using chemicals. Guidance may help reduce the risks. Parents should be educated about normal patterns of adolescent growth and development and related appropriate expectations. Teenagers who are small for their age, especially those who work on farms, are unable to fit into adult-sized protective equipment, which may result in exposures. Teenagers who are large for their age may be cognitively or emotionally immature and should not be expected to perform physical tasks with the judgment of an experienced adult. While realizing that responsibilities for teenagers should increase within safe limits, parents need support in decisions about safety. Faced with pressure from their children or their children's friends, parents may doubt the wisdom of their decisions. Support for safety is important as families weigh the appropriate limits of teenage independence. Parents also should be encouraged to be role models for safety. Parents who are farmers or farmworkers, for example, can demonstrate and discuss the judicious use, safe handling, safe storage, and safe disposal of chemicals with their adolescent while working together. Parents should be encouraged to discuss exposures to noise and dusts and to share information on protective measures and minimizing exposures.

## Take-Home Exposure

Take-home exposure refers to poisoning of a child from chemicals, fibers, or metal dusts brought home from a work site by a parent. Lead is one of the best known examples: a parent employed in a job with lead exposure such as bridge repair, auto battery repair, or work at a firing range may inadvertently bring home sufficient lead dust on clothing to give a child lead poisoning (see Chapter 19).[37–41] In evaluating a child with known heavy metal poisoning, parental occupations always should be considered. Mercury, pesticides, fiberglass, and asbestos are among other known take-home exposures.

## In-Home Exposures

Work conducted by parents in a home setting may put children living or visiting there at risk for chemical exposures. Kitchen-table assembly of radar detectors, which involves dipping wires in lead, may create a poisoning hazard for children in the household. Backyard work on car batteries has been a cause of pediatric lead poisoning in the children of that home or neighbors' homes.[37]

A new and widespread hazard involves the clandestine home manufacture of methamphetamine.[42] The chemicals involved in the processes (besides being extremely volatile) include carcinogens, reproductive hazards, neurotoxins, and corrosive materials. These are sufficiently toxic that law enforcement personnel have begun to treat such sites as hazardous for their own protection.[42] When they move in to break up an operation, they wear extensive personal protective equipment or seek assistance from a hazardous materials unit. Children removed from such homes may be placed in foster care without thought of related medical needs. These children need medical evaluation for potential exposure to neurotoxic and hepatotoxic solvents and appropriate follow-up.

## Frequently Asked Questions

Q *My teenager has asthma, for which she takes daily medication. She wants to get a part-time job. Can I help direct her to work that won't cause her asthma to flare up?*

A Teenagers need to ask potential employers about the tasks they will be doing and what types of chemicals they may be exposed to during work. A restaurant with a smoking section is not a wise choice for a teen with asthma. This teen might be better advised to seek work in a smoke-free establishment. In any job, parents should be concerned about adult supervision, job training, and safety instruction. It is important for parents to visit the workplace. A job that requires personal protective equipment suggests a possible risk that should be explored. Potential chemical exposures in vocational education, shop class, work-study, and volunteer work also need to be considered.

Q *Are teens more vulnerable to work exposure than adults because their systems (especially immune) aren't yet fully developed?*

A Public awareness of research performed to assess dietary and respiratory exposures among preschoolers (especially to pesticides) sometimes has led to assumptions about higher risks for adolescent workers. There is no definitive science to answer this question at present. However, by adolescence the immune system is essentially fully developed, so it is not likely to be more vulnerable. In advocating for adolescent occupational health and safety, it is important not to incorrectly exaggerate the risks that we do know exist, lest it lessen our credibility about the real risks.

If we know, however, that an exposure is hazardous for adults, we should assume that it is likely to be at least as hazardous for adolescents, and protect them from that exposure.

Q *Should teenagers be allowed to work with harzardous substances?*

A There are a number of concerns when teens work with hazardous chemicals. There may be potential risks of earlier exposure to substances (especially oncogenic ones) associated with disease after a long latency period. In addition, if a substance accumulates over time in the body and the effects are dose-related, teen workers have potential for increased exposure because they started earlier. Furthermore, what we know about the effects of chemotherapy effects on rapidly growing cells creates a theoretical worry that the rapid growth period of adolescence plus exposure to a potential carcinogen may increase cancer risk. Given that adolescence is a time of endocrine changes, it might be a time of increased vulnerability to chemicals that are endocrine disruptors, including a number of pesticides. Male and female adolescents are of child-bearing age, so the acute and latent reproductive hazards to which they are exposed should be of concern.

Q *Can a teenager who is still growing safely do manual labor with heavy equipment?*

A Occupational back injury data plus new knowledge related to overuse injuries among young gymnasts and baseball players suggest that periods of rapid growth may put an individual at increased risk for severe and chronic musculoskeletal injuries, especially if there are too many repetitions of a movement.[43] This has implications for farm work, cashier work, and any work with repetitive motion.

Q *Should I be concerned that my developmentally challenged teenager is taking a shop class?*

A In the United States adolescents with learning and developmental disabilities are preferentially routed into environments with vocational education and manual work, with potentially greater and riskier exposures. Those functioning at a preschool level may have more oral behaviors, placing them at increased risk.

Q  *Are teens less vulnerable to workplace exposure because they're young and healthy? When we were young we worked without all these protections.*

A  Risks of exposures can be small or life-threatening depending on the chemical. Teens/children are just as vulnerable to enclosed space exposures, and will, like adults, die in an oxygen-deprived environment, such as in a tank they are cleaning that was previously full of chemicals. Theoretically, if a chemical becomes less toxic when metabolized, and teens metabolize better/faster than adults, then its chemical effects could potentially be less toxic for a young worker. But if the metabolite is what poisons, they could be at increased risk. Because one is unlikely to know which situation pertains for any given chemical in advance, testing it only can be done with risk of illness or death. Thus prudent protection against exposure is always the best approach.

**Resources**

Child Labor Coalition, Internet: http://www.stopchildlabor.org/index.html. This is a coalition of diverse organizations and individuals (including the American Academy of Pediatrics, consumer groups, medical professionals, universities, unions, and religious organizations) interested in all aspects of international and US child labor. They have organized conferences, meet monthly, and maintain one of the most up-to-date watches in the nation on federal and state child labor law changes.

Committees on Occupational Safety and Health (COSH). Like union health and safety officers, most community-based COSH groups maintain staff capable of answering questions about occupational exposures.

Department of Labor. Contact your state Department of Labor for information on child labor laws, wages, hours of work, safety regulations including Hazard Orders that prohibit specific types of hazardous exposures, and problems with any of those areas. A poster summarizing child labor law often is available. Some states have health and safety/training officers within their labor departments, which can be especially helpful. In some states, you will be told to call the local office of the US Department of Labor.

National Child Labor Committee, phone: 212-840-1801, Internet: http://www.kapow.org/nclc.htm. The committee was founded in 1904 and has historical and legal information. The committee also continues to advocate for the safe employment of adolescents.

National Institute for Occupational Safety and Health (NIOSH), phone: 800-356-4674, Internet: http://www.cdc.gov/niosh/homepage.html. This institute deals with scientific, research, and educational aspects. The Web site contains information on hours and safety regulations, and hazards and how to protect against them, including a sheet for teens themselves. The site links to all other major sites containing information relevant to the health and safety of young workers.

The Division of Safety Research in the Morgantown, WV, NIOSH office, phone: 304-285-5894, has expertise in the scientific, research, and educational aspects; work also is being done in the NIOSH office in Cincinnati, OH, concerning exposures in vocational/technical education settings. In May 1995 NIOSH published "Alert-Request for Assistance in Preventing Deaths and Injuries of Adolescent Workers." This booklet (Department of Health and Human Services Publication No. 95-125, available from NIOSH) has background information and a tear-out page to post in the office or to copy for adolescent patients and their parents or for community work.

NIOSH also funds educational resource centers and academic departments of occupational medicine. These centers educate occupational and environmental medicine physicians and provide continuing education on occupational injury and exposures to many different types of workers.

Occupational Safety and Health Administration (OSHA), phone: 800-321-OSHA (6742), Internet: http://www.osha.gov. This is the federal agency that deals with regulatory and enforcement issues. If a teenager has a question about a specific hazard, the teenager or parent (with permission) can call OSHA for assistance. This can be done anonymously, but sometimes an employee may be identifiable. Pediatricians should consider this route especially when concerned about imminent danger to other adolescents in that workplace. OSHA offices can be found in your local phone directory.

Youthwrk e-mail list. This is a mailing list for professionals and volunteers working with youth to discuss programs and issues relating to their work. Questions are posted, as are information and opinions from the federal, state, university and front-line levels on issues pertaining to health and safety of young workers. To subscribe, go to http://lists.extension.umn.edu/mailman/listinfo/youthwrk.

## References

1. Institute of Medicine, Committee on Health and Safety Implications of Child Labor, National Research Council. *Protecting Youth at Work: Health, Safety and Development of Working Children and Adolescents in the United States.* Washington, DC: National Academies Press; 1998
2. National Institute of Occupational Safety and Health. *Are You A Working Teen? What You Should Know About Safety and Health on the Job.* Washington, DC: US Department of Health and Human Services; 1997. DHHS (NIOSH) Publication 97-132. Available at: http://www.cdc.gov/niosh/adoldoc.htm
3. American Academy of Pediatrics Committee on Environmental Health. The hazards of child labor. *Pediatrics.* 1995;95:311–313
4. American Academy of Pediatrics Committee on Injury and Poison Prevention. Injuries in the workplace. In: Widome MD, ed. *Injury Prevention and Control for Children and Youth.* 3rd ed. Elk Grove Village, IL: American Academy of Pediatrics; 1997:119–134
5. Centers for Disease Control and Prevention. Work-related injuries and illnesses associated with child labor—United States, 1993. *MMWR Morb Mortal Wkly Rep.* 1996;45:464–468

6. Miller M. *Occupational Injuries Among Adolescents in Washington State, 1988–91: A Review of Workers' Compensation Data*. Olympia, WA: Safety and Health Assessment and Research for Prevention, Washington State Department of Labor and Industries; 1995. Technical report #35-1-1995

7. Castillo DN, Malit BD. Occupational injury deaths of 16 and 17 year olds in the US: trends and comparisons with older workers. *Inj Prev.* 1997;3:277–281

8. Loomis DP, Richardson DB, Wolf SH, Runyan CW, Butts JD. Fatal occupational injuries in a southern state. *Am J Epidemiol.*1997;145:1089–1099

9. Bellville R, Pollack SH, Godbold JH, Landrigan PJ. Occupational injuries among working adolescents in New York State. *JAMA.* 1993; 269:2754–2759

10. Brooks DR, Davis LK, Gallagher SS. Work-related injuries among Massachusetts children: a study based on emergency department data. *Am J Ind Med.* 1993;24:313–324

11. Bush D, Baker R. *Young Workers at Risk: Health and Safety Education and the Schools*. Berkeley, CA: Labor Occupational Health Program; 1994

12. Cooper SP, Rothstein MA. Health hazards among working children in Texas. *South Med J.* 1995;88:550–554

13. Banco L, Lapidus G, Braddock M. Work-related injury among Connecticut minors. *Pediatrics.* 1992;89:957–960

14. Parker DL, Carl WR, French LR, Martin FB. Characteristics of adolescent work injuries reported to the Minnesota Department of Labor and Industry. *Am J Public Health.* 1994;84:606–611

15. Fair Labor Standards Act of 1938 29USC 201, CFR 570–580

16. US Department of Labor. *Child Labor Requirements in Nonagricultural Occupations Under the Fair Labor Standards Act*. Washington, DC: Employment Standards Administration, Wage and Hour Division; 1985. Child Labor Bull 101

17. US Department of Labor. *Child Labor Requirements in Agriculture Under the Fair Labor Standards Act*. Washington, DC: Employment Standards Administration, Wage and Hour Division, 1984. Child Labor Bull 102

18. Knight S, Junkins EP Jr, Lightfood AC, Cazier CF, Olson LM. Injuries sustained by students in shop class. *Pediatrics.* 2000;106:10–13

19. Woolf AD, Flynn E. Workplace toxic exposures involving adolescents aged 14 to 19 years: one poison center's experience. *Arch Pediatr Adolesc Med.* 2000;154:234–239

20. Suruda A, Halperin W. Work-related deaths in children. *Am J Ind Med.* 1991;19:739–745

21. Dunn KA, Runyan CW. Deaths at work among children and adolescents. *Am J Dis Child.* 1993;147:1044–1047

22. Derstine B. Youth workers at risk of fatal injuries. Presented at: 122nd Annual Meeting of the American Public Health Association; 1994; Washington, DC

23. Curwin B, Sanderson W, Reynolds S, Hein M, Alavanja M. Pesticide use and practices in an Iowa farm family pesticide exposure study. *J Agric Saf Health.* 2002;8:423–433

24. Gelbach SH, Williams WA, Perry LD, Woodall JS. Green-tobacco sickness. An illness of tobacco harvesters. *JAMA* 1974;229:1880–1883

25. Horstman SW, Browning SR, Szeluga R, Burzycki J, Stebbins A. Solvent exposures in screen printing shops. *J Environ Sci Health Part A Tox Hazard Subst Environ Eng.* 2001;36:1957–1973

26. National Institute of Occupational Safety and Health. *Alert-Request for Assistance in Preventing Deaths and Injuries of Adolescent Workers.* Washington, DC: US Department of Health and Human Services; 1995. DHHS (NIOSH) publication 95-125

27. Hosein HR, Farkas S. Risk associated with the spray application of polyurethane foam. *Am Ind Hyg Assoc J.* 1981;42:663–665

28. Husgafvel-Pursiainen K, Sorsa M, Engstrom K, Einisto P. Passive smoking at work: biochemical and biological measures of exposure to environmental tobacco smoke. *Int Arch Occup Environ Health.* 1987;59:337–345

29. Woolf AD. Health hazards for children at work. *J Toxicol Clin Toxicol.* 2002;40:477–482

30. Enander RT, Gute DM, Cohen HJ, Brown LC, Desmaris AM, Missaghian R. Chemical characterization of sanding dust and methylene chloride usage in auto refinishing: implications for occupational and environmental health. *AIHA J* (Farifax, VA). 2002;63:741–749

31. Knobloch MJ, Broste SK. A hearing conversation program for Wisconsin youth working in agriculture. *J Sch Health.* 1998;68:313–318

32. Pollack SH, Scheurich-Payne SL, Bryant S. The nature of occupational injury among Kentucky adolescents. Presented at: Occupational Injury Symposium; 1996; Sydney, Australia

33. Pollack S, McConnell R, Gallelli M, Schmidt J, Obregon R, Landrigan P. Pesticide exposure and working conditions among migrant farmworker children in western New York State. In: Proceedings of the 118th Annual Meeting of the American Public Health Association; 1990; New York, NY. 317

34. Cohen LR, Runyan CW, Dunn KA, Schulman MD. Work patterns and occupational hazard exposures of North Carolina adolescents in 4-H clubs. *Inj Prev.* 1996;2:274–277

35. Broste SK, Hansen DA, Strand RL, Stueland DT. Hearing loss among high school farm students. *Am J Public Health.* 1989;79:619–622

36. Margolis W, Krause JF. The prevalence of carpal tunnel syndrome symptoms in female supermarket checkers. *J Occup Med.* 1987;29:953–956

37. Gittleman JL, Engelgau MM, Shaw J, Wille KK, Seligman PJ. Lead poisoning among battery reclamation workers in Alabama. *J Occup Med.* 1994;36:526–532

38. Piacitelli GM, Whelan EA, Ewers LM, Sieber WK. Lead contamination in automobiles of lead-exposed bridgeworkers. *Appl Occup Environ Hyg.* 1995;10:849–855

39. Gerson M, Van den Eeden SK, Gahagan P. Take-home lead poisoning in a child from his father's occupational exposure. *Am J Ind Med.* 1996;29:507–508

40. Piacitelli GM, Whelan EA, Sieber WK, Gerwel B. Elevated lead contamination in homes of construction workers. *Am Ind Hyg Assoc J.* 1997;58:447–454

41. Whelan EA, Piacitelli GM, Gerwel B, et al. Elevated blood lead levels in children of construction workers. *Am J Public Health.* 1997;87:1352–1355

42. Willers-Russo LJ. Three fatalities involving phosphine gas, produced as a result of methamphetamine manufacturing. *J Forensic Sci.* 1999;44:647–652

43. Hutchinson MR, Ireland ML. Overuse and throwing injuries in the skeletally immature athlete. *Instr Course Lect.* 2003;52:25–36

# 33
# Arts and Crafts

Children begin to use and enjoy arts and crafts materials when they are young. Arts and crafts materials abound in homes, child care settings, schools, churches, and park and recreation facilities. Many of these materials contain ingredients that are known to be hazardous. Parents, teachers, and adults and teens working with children may not be aware of the potential health hazards associated with these common materials.

Dangerous chemicals found in art materials can be divided into metals, solvents, and dusts or fibers.[1] Lead and other toxic metals such as mercury, cadmium, and cobalt are found in paints, pastels, pigments, inks, glazes, enamels, and solder.[2] Legal bans on lead and other metals in paint do not apply to artists' paints, which are used in painting, drawing, ceramics, silk-screening, making stained glass, and other activities that may be part of art projects involving children or adolescents.[3] Some papier-mâché products contain heavy metals from inks found in magazines. Hazardous organic solvents such as turpentine, kerosene, mineral spirits, xylene, benzene, methyl alcohol, and formaldehyde are used in painting, silk-screening, and shellacking, as well as in cleaning tools and preparation of work surfaces.[4] Rubber cement, spray-on enamels, and spray-on fixatives are common art products that also contain organic solvents.[5] Dusts and fibers containing hazardous materials such as asbestos, silica, talc, lead, cadmium, and mercury are generated during reconstitution of powdered pigments, glazes and clay, and the use of pastels.

Physical art hazards result from exposure to noise, dangerous mechanical and power tools, machinery and materials storage, and waste disposal practices. These hazards are most likely to occur in industrial arts settings and often are regulated under Occupational

Safety and Health Administration (OSHA) and US Environmental Protection Agency (EPA) rules.[6]

## Routes of Exposure

The wide variety of arts and crafts activities and materials used by children and adolescents permits the full spectrum of routes of exposure, which depend on the specific activity, materials used, and age of the child.

Inhalation is a major route of exposure for volatile organic solvents, dusts, and fibers. Exposure can occur during normal use, especially if ventilation is inadequate or necessary personal protective equipment is not available or properly used. Exposure also can occur through inappropriate exploring of new materials by "sniff testing." Finally, intentional inhalation such as glue sniffing can result in high-level exposure through the lungs.

Unintentional ingestion is the route of exposure for many art hazards and may occur when common art materials are improperly stored in unlabeled or empty food containers. Even properly labeled art materials may be ingested by young or developmentally delayed children. Ingestion also may occur through nail biting, thumb sucking, or other hand-to-mouth behaviors common in children.

Dermal absorption may occur from improper handling of hazardous art materials, accidental spills, or contact with cuts or abrasions. Exposure through the conjunctivae may occur from spills, splashes, and eye rubbing.

Physical hazards cause injury in a variety of ways. Noise standards developed to protect adult workers may be exceeded in secondary school industrial arts workshops, exposing children to potential hearing loss. Use of potentially dangerous equipment may result in cuts, crush injuries, fractures, or amputations. Power equipment may cause electrical injury or fires and can release carbon monoxide. Techniques requiring repetitive motion may cause tendonitis, carpal tunnel syndrome, or other injuries. Most of these hazards can be minimized through proper industrial hygiene evaluation, engineering measures, and use of personal protective equipment.

## Systems Affected and Clinical Effects

Relatively little is known about the effects on children of chronic low-level exposures to hazardous art materials. No case reports of illness in children from low-level exposures to arts and crafts hazards have been described in the literature. Extrapolation from adult experience is questionable, but raises the theoretical possibilities that chronic low-level exposures to hazardous art materials in childhood could exacerbate or cause allergies, hypersensitivity and asthma, central and peripheral nerve damage, psychological and behavioral changes, respiratory damage, skin changes, or cancer.

## Diagnostic Methods and Treatment

Diagnosis and treatment are specific to each type of exposure and illness.

## Prevention of Exposure

A variety of preventive measures may greatly reduce exposure to arts and crafts hazards. Toxicity from long-term, low-level childhood exposure has not been documented. Nonetheless, it is prudent to implement measures designed to prevent exposures that in theory may be harmful. Some measures apply to all environments in which children use arts and crafts materials; others apply specifically to institutions.

Careful art material selection can eliminate much of the risk from arts and crafts materials. For children, only materials certified to be safe should be selected (see Table 33.1). Materials should be properly labeled, purchased new or sealed in original containers with full instructions, and used with adult supervision according to manufacturer's instructions. The US Consumer Product Safety Commission (CPSC) considers a child as anyone younger than 13 years or attending grade school or below. As children mature, their ability to follow directions, use precautions, and understand risks will allow for careful

**Table 33.1**
**Recommendations for Selecting Art Materials for Children Younger Than 13 Years**

| |
|---|
| • Read the label and instructions on all arts and craft materials. |
| • Buy only products labeled "Conforms to ASTM D4236" and that bear the AP (Approved Product)/CP (Certified Product)/HL Health Label (Non-Toxic) seals of the Art & Creative Materials Institute. |
| • Do not use materials labeled "Keep out of Reach of Children" or "Not for Use by Children." |
| • Do not use materials marked with the words "Poison," "Danger," "Warning," or "Caution," or that contain hazard warnings on the label. |
| • Do not use donated or found materials unless in the original containers with full labeling. |

use of adult art materials and techniques that require precautions for safe use.

Arts and crafts materials are labeled in a variety of ways. The familiar AP (Approved Product), CP (Certified Product), and HL Health Label (Non-Toxic) seals of the Art & Creative Materials Institute (ACMI) certify that an art material can be used by everyone, even children and impaired adults, without risk of acute or chronic health hazards. This program covers about 80% of all children's art materials and about 95% of all fine art materials sold in the United States.

In 1983 the American Society for Testing and Materials (ASTM) developed a national voluntary standard, ASTM D4236, *Labeling of Art Materials for Chronic Health Hazards.* This standard requires that art materials must be evaluated by a toxicologist and, if labeling is required, conform to stringent labeling requirements that include the identity of hazardous ingredients, risks associated with use, precautions to take to prevent harm, first aid measures, and sources of further information. All products certified by the ACMI have conformed to this standard since its inception. In 1990 the Labeling for Hazardous Art Materials Act went into effect. This act made the "voluntary" ASTM D4236 standard mandatory for all art materials imported or sold in the United States. This act, which is administered by the CPSC, requires that hazardous consumer products, including art materials, have warnings to "keep out of reach of children" (for acute health hazards) or that they "should not be used by children" (for chronic health hazards).

Occasionally art materials available for purchase are improperly labeled. Crayons containing high levels of lead have been labeled "nontoxic." To make sure that an art material has been evaluated by a toxicologist, parents should look for the statement, "conforms to ASTM D4236" covering chronic health hazards and an ACMI seal for acute and chronic health hazards.[7] Good ventilation in rooms used for arts and crafts activities is always important (see Chapter 6).

Proper storage and cleanup also are essential. Materials should only be stored in original, fully labeled containers. Appropriate cleanup at the end of an art session includes closing and storing all containers, cleaning all tools, wiping down all used surfaces, and washing hands thoroughly. Adult art and hobby materials should be similarly labeled and stored out of the reach of children. Half of all artists work in home studios, many of which are in living areas where children also live and may be exposed.

Close supervision of all children during arts and crafts activities can prevent injuries and poisonings, ensure proper use of materials, and allow for the observation of adverse reactions. Eating or drinking should not occur while using art materials. Cuts and abrasions should be covered if they are likely to come in contact with materials being used.

Central ordering at the district or state level in public schools and other large institutions can facilitate the selection of safe art materials. Prevention begins with selection of the safest materials.

Emergency protocols should be in place in case of an injury, poisoning, or allergic reaction. The local poison control center number should be prominently posted. Adequate flushing facilities should be provided in case of spills or eye splashes. Material Safety Data Sheets

(MSDS) should be available on site for all hazardous materials that may be used in high school industrial arts classes. Adult supervisors should have proper first aid and emergency response skills and training.

Art safety education for all supervising adults and teens is desirable. Art activities are common in church schools, child care settings, preschools, elementary and secondary schools, hospitals, chronic care institutions, therapeutic facilities, and at art festivals. Whenever possible, teachers, group leaders, and responsible adults and teens should be trained in art safety. Art teachers should be thoroughly trained in safety for all techniques they use in the classroom. Children with special vulnerabilities should be identified and appropriate measures taken to protect their health. These could include children with asthma and allergies who might be hypersensitive to normally tolerated exposures. Children with physical, psychological, or learning disabilities may need special assistance in the use of some equipment or in understanding instructions and following safety techniques.[8]

Industrial arts programs should follow OSHA, EPA, and state guidelines for ventilation, physical plant, fire safety systems, and personal protective equipment. These programs for older children and young adults should have a formal health and safety component.

## Frequently Asked Question

Q *Are water-based art supplies always safe?*

A Some water-based, cold-water dyes are sensitizers. Long-term health effects have not been thoroughly studied. In general, water-based supplies are preferable because they avoid the need for organic solvents. Accidental ingestion of even small amounts of organic solvents can be fatal.

## Resources

American Association of Poison Control Centers, Internet: http://www.aapcc.org. Poison control centers are the best resources for medical response to acute exposures. This Web site has listings for state, regional, and Canadian centers including addresses, emergency telephone numbers, fax numbers, and e-mail addresses.

American Industrial Hygiene Association, phone: 703-849-8888, fax: 703-207-3561, e-mail: infonet@aiha.org, Internet: http://www.aiha.org. This organization gives guidance to institutions designing and managing industrial arts facilities and programs.

Art & Creative Materials Institute (ACMI), phone: 781-293-4100, fax: 781-294-0808, Internet: http://www.acminet.org. The ACMI, an organization of art and craft manufacturers, develops standards for the safety and quality of art materials; manages a certification program to ensure the safety of children's art and craft materials and the accuracy of labels of adult art materials that are potentially hazardous; develops and distributes information on the safe use of art and craft materials; provides lists of certified products (those that are safe for children and adult art materials that may have a hazard potential) to individuals, CPSC, state health agencies, and school authorities; and provides consultations for concerned individuals. The ACMI can put you in touch with toxicologists to answer questions about health concerns.

Public Interest Research Group (PIRG), phone: 202-546-9707, fax: 202-546-2461, e-mail: uspirg@pirg.org, Internet: http://www. pirg.org. Several state PIRGs have conducted surveys of art hazards in schools. Similar methodology was employed by all. Reports may be obtained from individual state groups.

US Consumer Product Safety Commission (CPSC), phone: 800-638-2772, Internet: http://www.cpsc.gov. The CPSC is responsible for developing and managing regulations to support the Labeling for Hazardous Art Materials Act and the Federal Hazardous Substances Act. They instigate actions on mislabeled products and/or misbranded hazardous substances (products whose labels do not conform to these acts), which may involve confiscations, product recalls, or other legal actions. The CPSC's Web site contains general product safety information and recent press releases. To report a dangerous product or product-related injury or illness, call CPSC's hotline at 800-638-2772 or e-mail info@cpsc.gov.

US Environmental Protection Agency, phone: 202-272-0167, Internet: http://www.epa.gov or http://www.epa.gov/epahome/postal.htm.

## References

1. Amdur MO, Doull J, Klaassen CD, eds. *Casarett and Doull's Toxicology: The Basic Science of Poisons.* 4th ed. New York, NY: McGraw Hill; 1991
2. Babin A, Peltz PA, Rossol M. *Children's Art Supplies Can Be Toxic.* New York, NY: Center for Safety in the Arts; 1992
3. McCann MF. Occupational and environmental hazards in art. *Environ Res.* 1992;59:139–144
4. Lesser SH, Weiss SJ. Art hazards. *Am J Emerg Med.* 1995;13:451–458
5. McCann M. *Artist Beware.* New York, NY: Lyons and Burford Publishers; 1992
6. McCann M. *School Safety Procedures for Art and Industrial Art Programs.* New York, NY: Center for Safety in the Arts, 1994
7. Lu PC. A health hazard assessment in school arts and crafts. *J Environ Pathol Toxicol Oncol.* 1992;11:12–17
8. Rossol M. The first art hazards course. *J Environ Pathol Toxicol Oncol.* 1992;11:28–32

# 34
# Asthma

Asthma is a chronic respiratory disease characterized by bronchial hyperresponsiveness, intermittent reversible airway obstruction, and airway inflammation.[1] This chapter primarily focuses on environmental triggers in children with asthma but will briefly review factors that influence the development of asthma.

Genetic and environmental factors contribute to the development of asthma, and early life exposures may play an important role. It is likely that recent changes in children's environments have contributed to the increasing prevalence of asthma. Recent studies suggest that the neonatal immune system tends to favor an allergic (IgE promoting) response to certain environmental allergens (eg, dust mite). This response is mediated in part through infant T helper cells that tend to release a series of cytokines that promote the development of an "allergic (IgE promoting)" B cell response to certain environmental allergens. The T cell cytokine profile that favors an IgE response is termed a Th2 response. In contrast, as the immune system matures, naive T cells tend to release a different mix of cytokines in response to environmental allergens that favor an IgG promoting (Th1) response. It is postulated that exposures to environmental stimuli during early childhood could either further enhance the Th2 response or shift the balance toward the Th1 response depending on the stimuli and/or genetic predisposition.[1,2] Proposed hypotheses on environmental factors that may favor the Th2 response include improved hygiene, changes in diet, changes in intestinal flora due to increased use of antibiotics, increased exposure to allergens due to changes in housing and lifestyle, obesity and reduced physical activity, and changes in the prenatal environment.[3] The "hygiene hypothesis" postulates that early childhood infections (which promote a Th1 response) are becoming less frequent, favoring a persistent Th2 im-balance.[1,4] Observations that the presence of an older sibling and early child care attendance are associated with a reduced incidence of asthma support this hypothesis. The development of a Th2 (IgE) response to common environmental contaminants in the air (eg, house-dust mites, cockroach antigens, and cat allergens) is strongly correlated with the development of childhood asthma.[2,5] The relationship between early life exposures and allergic sensitization is not completely understood. As an example of the complexity, exposure to high levels of cat allergen during infancy may protect children developing asthma, except if the mother has a history of asthma.[6,7] Once sensitized to aeroallergens, optimal management of asthma includes control of exposures to environmental triggers.[3]

Major indoor triggers of asthma include environmental tobacco smoke (ETS), respiratory irritants such as volatile organic compounds (VOCs) and fragrances, animal and insect allergens (such as dander and cockroach antigen), and molds (Table 34.1). Although most agents that exacerbate asthma in children are inhaled, asthma may be exacerbated in some atopic individuals who touch (eg, latex) or ingest certain products (eg, peanuts).

Outdoor air pollution also has been associated with asthma exacerbations.[8]

## Indoor Environmental Precipitants

### Environmental Tobacco Smoke

Forty-three percent of children in the United States live with at least one smoking parent.[9] Children whose mothers smoke have more wheezing symptoms and a higher incidence of lower respiratory tract illnesses compared with those with mothers who do not smoke.[10] The greatest effect seems to be related to maternal smoking during pregnancy and/or early infancy,[11] perhaps due to inflammatory stimuli on lung parenchyma during a period of rapid lung development and prolonged close exposure to the mother. Exposure to ETS is associated

**Table 34.1**
**Common Indoor and Outdoor Agents Precipitating Asthma**

| Agent | Major Sources |
|---|---|
| **Indoor** | |
| Environmental tobacco smoke | Cigarettes, cigars, other tobacco products |
| Wood smoke | Fireplaces and wood-burning stoves |
| Molds | Floods, roof leaks, plumbing leaks, wet basements, air-conditioning units |
| Nitrogen oxides | Space heaters, gas-fueled cooking stoves |
| Odors or fragrances | Sprays, deodorizers, cosmetics, household cleaning products, pesticides |
| Volatile organic compounds | Building and insulation materials, cleaning agents, solvents, pesticides, sealants, adhesives, combustion products, molds |
| **Allergens** | |
| Dust mites | Bedding (pillows, mattress, box springs, bed linens), carpets, soft upholstered furniture, draperies, stuffed toys |
| Animal allergens (dander, saliva, urine) | Cats, dogs, rodents |
| Cockroaches | Kitchens, bathrooms (near food and water sources) |
| **Outdoor** | |
| Pollens | Seasonal release from flowering plants |
| Molds | Ubiquitous in soil, increased in wet environments and decaying organic matter (eg, wood chips) |
| Ozone ($O_3$) | Motor vehicle exhaust, power plants |
| Particulate matter | Combustion sources (eg, diesel engines, industry, wood burning) |
| Sulfur dioxide ($SO_2$) | Burning of coal (coal-fired power plants, other industrial sources) |

with an increase in asthma attacks, earlier symptom onset, increased medication use, and a more prolonged recovery from acute attacks.[12,13] Maternal smoking of half a pack or more per day has been associated with an increased risk of developing asthma in children.[11] Acute short-term ETS exposure has been demonstrated to increase bronchial hyperreactivity, requiring as long as 3 weeks to recover baseline pulmonary function following exposure.[14,15]

### *Other Indoor Irritants*

In the home, other common sources of air pollutants that may act as respiratory irritants include gas stoves and woodstoves, space heaters (gas or kerosene) and fireplaces, and furnishings and construction materials that release organic gases and vapors.[16] Epidemiologic evidence for the role of these indoor air pollutants in exacerbating asthma is limited but suggestive of associations between exposures to these pollutants and asthma exacerbations.[16,17]

Gas stoves or ovens can generate high levels of nitrogen dioxide indoors, especially when there is inadequate ventilation or the gas stove is used as an ancillary heat source. Poorly ventilated fireplaces can produce substantial levels of wood smoke indoors.

Volatile organic compounds and fragrances may induce acute asthma episodes in sensitive individuals.[18] The mechanism of action is unknown, but presumed to be nonspecific irritation. Formaldehyde is emitted from many consumer products, including new carpets, paper products (eg, tissues, towels, and bags), urea-formaldehyde foam insulation, and glues used in plywood and pressed-board products. Formaldehyde is a known respiratory irritant in the occupational setting and a common air pollutant in the home (see Chapter 6).[16]

### *Allergenic Precipitants*

#### Animal Allergens

Animal allergens are glycoproteins that often induce an IgE response in humans. These allergens usually are found in saliva, sebaceous glands (dog and cat), or sometimes in the urine (rodents). Allergies to cow hair or horsehair and dander also have been reported, primarily through occupational exposures.[16] The spread of allergens in the environment has been studied primarily for cats; however, the route of spread is likely to be similar for domestic furry animals.[16] Cat allergen-containing material dries and adheres to many surfaces (eg, animal fur or hair, bedding, and clothing) and often can be transported to other environments via this route. Once an animal enters the room, small airborne allergen-containing particles (diameter <5 μm) can be detected. These small particles remain suspended in the air for hours. Once the allergen-containing particle is inhaled, it is easily deposited in distal airways. Clinical manifestations of animal allergy range from mild cutaneous urticaria to rhinoconjunctivitis to life-threatening bronchospasm and anaphylaxis. Although symptoms may occur instantly following exposure, it is more common for upper and lower respiratory tract symptoms to develop within 30 minutes. Low-level chronic exposures may not trigger clinically significant symptoms for several days.

**Cats.** The severity of allergic reactions to cats is greater than reactions to other common domestic pets. More than 6 million US residents have allergies to cats, and up to 40% of atopic patients demonstrate skin test sensitivity.[19] The major allergen *Fel d I* is present in high concentration in the saliva and sebaceous and anal glands of cats. The grooming habits of cats result in a large amount of saliva on the fur, and cat allergen can be spread via small airborne particles. Children with cats can transmit cat allergens to schoolrooms and may create an environment that can precipitate asthma in sensitized children.[20] Once a cat is removed from an indoor environment, the allergen may persist for months.

**Dogs.** Dogs are the most common domesticated animal species found in US homes. Five percent to 30% of atopic patients have a positive skin test to the major allergen *Can f I,* although many do not demonstrate clinical symptoms or have positive bronchoprovocation tests.[21] It seems that more variations in clinical sensitivity exist between dog breeds, and breed-specific allergens have been suggested.[22]

Nevertheless, no dog breed is considered nonallergenic. As with cat allergen, the highest concentrations of *Can f I* are found in canine fur and dander.[23]

**Rodents.** Exposure to rodents can occur from their presence as pests or pets in the home. Rat and mouse allergens are produced primarily in urine.[16] Through transfer, the fur and dander often contain high amounts of allergen. The prevalence of mouse allergen can be widespread in inner-city homes.[24] Among inner-city children with asthma, there was an association between mouse allergen in house-dust samples and sensitization to mouse allergen, especially among those asthmatics with atopy to multiple allergens on skin testing. The relationship between mouse allergen exposure and asthma morbidity was less clear.[25]

**Birds.** In the occupational setting, hypersensitivity pneumonitis can be associated with antigens from bird excreta and proteinaceous materials found in dust dispersed from birds; however, it is unclear whether birds cause allergy and asthma.[16] Large quantities of dust mites have been documented in feathers, and dust mite allergen is the likely source of the allergic stimulus from feather-containing items in the home, including pillows, comforters, bedding, and down-filled clothes.[16]

## Cockroaches

The incidence of cockroach hypersensitivity is related to the degree of infestation found in the living environment, although nonresidential exposures (eg, schools) may cause allergy in an individual whose residence is not infested. Cockroach infestations are more common in warm, moist environments with readily accessible food sources. Although the highest allergen levels typically are found in the kitchen, significantly elevated concentrations of roach allergen also are found in bedrooms or television-watching areas, particularly if food is consumed in these places.

Numerous species of cockroaches have been described in the United States, and 3 predominant species have been associated with IgE antibody production. The German roach, *Blattella germanica,* is the source of 2 primary antigens, *Bla g 1* and *Bla g 2;* however, significant cross-reactivity exists between cockroach antigens. Cockroach allergens have been described as principal triggers of allergic rhinitis and asthma. Positive skin tests to cockroach antigens can be found in up to 60% of urban residents with asthma. Although several parts of the cockroach are allergenic, the whole body and feces seem to be more potent. Cockroach allergens may behave like the dust mite antigen; that is, they are carried on large particles that become airborne for short periods during active disturbance. Levels of allergen in places where children spend a significant period may be most important. Inner-city children with asthma, cockroach allergy, and exposure to elevated levels of cockroach allergen in bedroom dust had more days of wheezing, more missed school days, and more emergency department visits and hospitalizations than nonsensitized and/or nonexposed asthmatic children. Hospitalization rates for children who were sensitized and exposed to excessive levels of cockroach allergen were nearly 3 times as high as for those with low exposure and sensitivity.[16,26]

## House-Dust Mites *(Dermatophagoides)*

House-dust mites probably play a major role in inducing the asthmatic phenotype and triggering asthma exacerbations in sensitized children. Mite antigen commonly is found where human dander is found, and the principal allergens—*Der p I* and *Der p II*—are found in the outer membrane of mite fecal particles. Indoor environments that provide optimal growth conditions for *Dermatophagoides* species have a relative humidity greater than 55% and temperatures between 22°C and 26°C, but dust mites can survive laundering at moderate temperatures. Under optimal conditions, mites proliferate on mattress surfaces, carpeting, and upholstered furniture, each of which contains a large amount of human dander, its primary food source. A gram of dust may contain 1000 mites and 250 000 fecal pellets. Pellet diameters range from 10 to 40 μm and therefore are not easily transported into the lower airway passages. Exposure occurs either by proximity of the nasopharyngeal mucosa to mite reservoirs (especially mattresses, pillows, carpets, bed linens, clothes, and soft toys) or to airborne antigen resuspended during housecleaning activities.

## Indoor Mold Allergens

Molds are most prominent in climates with increased ambient humidity, although some can grow in relatively dry areas. Species of common indoor molds (eg, *Aspergillus, Penicillium,* and *Cladosporium*) require sufficient moisture for growth, and places where indoor mold growth is commonly found include household areas with high humidity (eg, basements, crawl spaces, ground floors, bathrooms, and areas with standing water such as air-conditioner condensers) and areas with recent moisture damage. Carpeting, ceilings, and paneled or hollow walls also are common reservoirs.

Dampness and the presence of mold should be suspected when there is visible mold or mildew in the home, a moldy or musty smell, evidence of water condensation on windowsills (excluding immediately after showers or cooking in the kitchen), or the use of a humidifier. Epidemiologic studies have suggested an association between dampness and mold in the homes and asthma symptoms.[16,27,28] Because dampness and visible mold growth could be indicators for dust mite allergen exposure, the relative contribution of fungi versus other allergens (eg, house-dust mite) is not entirely clear. However, several studies have found decreased respiratory symptoms in the presence of dampness after adjusting for levels of dust mite allergen.[29,30]

## Miscellaneous Allergens

**Latex.** Latex may cause an allergic response either by direct contact or by inhalation of latex particles. Symptoms range from cutaneous eruption, sneezing, and bronchospasm to anaphylaxis.[31]

Widespread use of latex gloves and revised processing procedures, making the allergen more potent, may have contributed to the increase in reported cases. Most sensitivities occur in medical personnel, food service workers, or environmental service workers, although household exposures to balloons, gloves, condoms, and certain sporting equipment also may trigger allergic responses. Children with increased exposure to latex (eg, those with urogenital abnormalities, cerebral palsy, and preterm infants) are at increased risk of developing latex allergy. Up to one third of children with spina bifida have been reported to have positive skin tests to latex.[31]

**Food.** Many foods contain allergenic proteins that can trigger asthma or anaphylactic reactions in sensitized individuals. Nuts, fish, shellfish, and milk are the most commonly associated foods. Although oral ingestion typically is needed to elicit symptoms, contact with aerosolized particulates and oils that contain the offending antigens can induce symptoms in highly allergic individuals. In rare individuals, food additives, including sulfites and food coloring (especially tartrazine), also can be highly allergenic.

## Outdoor Environmental Precipitants

### Outdoor Air Pollution

Currently more than 120 million Americans live in areas that fail to meet the 1997 National Ambient Air Quality Standards for at least one of the criteria pollutants. Ozone and particulate matter are of special concern. Levels of these air pollutants are high enough in many parts of the United States to present respiratory hazards to children with asthma (see Chapter 7).

### Ozone

Ambient ozone is formed by the action of sunlight on nitrogen oxides and reactive hydrocarbons (both of which are emitted by motor vehicles and industrial sources) under stable weather conditions. The levels tend to be highest on warm, sunny, windless days and often peak in the mid-afternoon.

During the warm season, ozone concentrations exceed the National Ambient Air Quality Standards in many urban and rural areas of the United States, with highest levels often being reached in suburban regions of major metropolitan areas.

Ozone is a powerful oxidant and respiratory irritant. Increased rates of hospitalization and acute visits for asthma exacerbations have been associated with high ozone days.[32,33] A recent study found an increased incidence of asthma associated with heavy exercise among children living in communities with high levels of ozone air pollution.[34]

### Particulate Matter

Particulate matter is a heterogeneous mixture of airborne particles. In urban areas, motor vehicle exhaust (especially diesel), industry, and wood smoke are important sources of particulate pollution. Particulate pollution has been associated with asthma exacerbations and bronchitis symptoms in children with asthma.

### Sulfur Dioxide

Sulfur dioxide ($SO_2$) is an extreme respiratory irritant and can cause asthma exacerbations. Principal sources of $SO_2$ include coal-fired power plants, paper and pulp mills, refineries, and other industries. Although ambient levels of $SO_2$ are below the national air quality standard in most areas of the United States, $SO_2$ levels can be increased in areas near these sources.

For additional information on health effects of outdoor air pollution, see Chapter 7.

## Outdoor Allergens

Outdoor air contains a variety of allergens, most of which arise from plant pollens and mold (fungal) spores. Seasonal exposures to high concentrations of tree, grass, and ragweed pollens that occur in the spring and late summer can induce respiratory symptoms, such as sneezing, rhinitis, and bronchospasm in sensitized children. Spores from mold, such as *Alternaria* and *Aspergillus,* commonly are found in damp, wooded areas, including the wood chips often used as ground cover in playgrounds. These allergens also can cause acute and recurrent asthma exacerbations.[35] Exposure to outdoor fungal spores has been implicated in fatal exacerbations of asthma.[36,37] Asthma attacks that occur during thunderstorms have also been linked to increased fungal spores in the outdoor air.[38]

## Diagnosis

The diagnosis of asthma is suggested by a clinical history of wheezing and/or cough that is episodic, nocturnal, or exertional and occurs apart from acute respiratory infections.[3] Atopy and a family history of asthma and/or atopy are strong predictors of persistent asthma. Pulmonary function testing in children younger than 5 years is seldom reproducible, and response to a therapeutic trial of bronchodilator and/or anti-inflammatory medications frequently is helpful in confirming the diagnosis. Chest roentgenography may reveal the presence of peribronchial thickening and hyperinflation, which may help determine the chronicity of illness and also help evaluate other diagnostic possibilities such as congenital anomaly or foreign body. Baseline pulmonary function testing may demonstrate a decreased forced expiratory volume in 1 second ($FEV_1$ or forced expiratory flow), and a decreased midexpiratory phase ($FEV_{25-75}$) compared with predicted norms. Prebronchodilator and postbronchodilator spirometry ($>15\%$ $FEV_1$ improvement), methacholine, exercise, or cold air bronchoprovocation ($\geq 20\%$ $FEV_1$ decrease) may help diagnose asthma in the patient with mild symptoms. Daily or diurnal variability in peak flow measurements also may help.

Determination of the degree of atopy may be helpful in diagnosing asthma. Skin prick test responses to inhaled antigens or specific foods may help confirm suspected triggers. The radioallergosorbent test

(RAST) generally is less sensitive than skin prick tests, although it may be more readily available and easily tolerated (but more expensive) when screening a patient for numerous potential sensitivities.

## Treatment Goals

Goals of asthma therapy include preventing chronic and troublesome symptoms, maintaining normal pulmonary function, maintaining normal activity levels, preventing recurrent exacerbations, and minimizing emergency department visits and hospitalizations. Medications are categorized into the following 2 general classes: (1) long-term preventive medications that achieve and maintain control of persistent asthma and (2) quick-relief medications that treat acute symptoms and exacerbations. The "step care" approach to asthma therapy emphasizes initiating higher-level therapy at the onset of treatment to control symptoms, and then "stepping down" the use of quick-relief medications followed by control medications. Preventive medications include inhaled corticosteroids and non-steroid medications, such as leukotriene receptor antagonists, and long-acting beta-adrenergic agonists. Relief medications are largely inhaled rapid-acting adrenergic agonists.[3]

Allergen immunotherapy is available for many allergens and has had some success. Immunotherapy should not take the place of efforts to control exposure to allergens. Guidelines discussing all aspects of asthma treatment, including the potential use of immunotherapy, have been published.[3]

## Control Measures for Allergens and Irritants

Avoiding environmental allergens and irritants is one of the primary goals of good asthma management. Skin testing or in vitro testing and appropriate counseling about appropriate environmental control strategies are recommended for all children with persistent asthma who are exposed to perennial indoor allergens.[3]

Most control measures have been directed at the control of chronic asthma symptoms and the prevention of asthma exacerbations.[39,40] Possible interventions to decrease the risk of developing asthma currently are being investigated.[3] To date food allergen avoidance diets prenatally or postnatally have not been successful in decreasing the incidence of asthma. Randomized controlled trials are ongoing to evaluate the effect on asthma incidence of aggressive dust mite control during pregnancy and early life.[40] Primary prevention of asthma should include efforts to reduce a child's exposure to tobacco smoke, including in utero exposure.

Complete control of many of the environmental allergens is difficult, and multiple intervention strategies are recommended. Several expert reviews outline priorities for allergen avoidance.[3,16,40,41] Recommendations follow the basic principles of control of sources. Recommendations for aggressive and continual attention to multiple reservoirs are especially relevant for children who require multiple medications to control their symptoms. Barriers to implementation of indoor environmental control strategies for low-income children with asthma recently have been evaluated.[42]

### Environmental Tobacco Smoke and Other Indoor Irritants

Smoking has been banned in many public places. Pediatricians should counsel parents on smoking cessation and eliminate sources of smoke in the child's environment (see Chapter 13). There is no evidence that ventilation and air-cleaning methods will effectively decrease ETS exposures to children.[16]

For indoor combustion appliances (eg, gas or kerosene space heaters, gas stoves, and wood-burning fireplaces or woodstoves), adequate ventilation is imperative. Gas or kerosene space heaters, which are often used in cold climates where they may be on for prolonged periods,[16] should not be used in unvented spaces because of the risk of carbon monoxide poisoning. Sealant coatings or coverings are sometimes applied over formaldehyde-containing materials to decrease emissions. Furniture, carpets, and building materials emit the highest levels of VOCs during the first months after manufacturing, and adequate ventilation should be supplied during and immediately after installation. Low-emission carpets, adhesives, and building materials are now commercially available but there are no clinical studies comparing asthma exacerbations among children in homes with traditional versus low-emission carpets. Alternative products that contain few or no VOCs or fragrances, such as paint and finishes with low VOCs, low non-aerosol and unscented cleaners, and cosmetics, should be encouraged.

### *Indoor Allergens*

Animal Allergens
The preferred treatment for animal allergy is to avoid animals that provoke reaction. Removal of the animal from the home or keeping the pet outdoors (eg, in the garage) is strongly recommended. If removal of the animal is not possible or acceptable, efforts should be made to control all the sites where pet allergens accumulate as well as the source.[43]

Control of the major cat allergen *Fel d I* is difficult. Even if the cat is removed from the home, it may take more than 3 months to reduce the levels of allergen. Aggressive cleaning (eg, removing carpets and washing walls and furniture) may accelerate the process. Many cat-sensitive patients are exposed to cat allergens outside their home and should receive advice about avoidance in other settings.

If the cat remains in the home, measures should include the restriction of pets to one area of the home and the creation of a safe room in the child's bedroom by not allowing pets into the room and keeping the door closed. Dense filter material may be placed over forced air outlets to trap airborne dander particles. Washing cats may decrease the amount of cat dander and dried saliva in the environment.[3,43]

Other methods include removal of carpeting and heavily contaminated items, use of high-efficiency particulate air (HEPA) filter
vacuums and filters, regular damp mopping, weekly cat bathing, and
washing cat-contaminated items. Experimentally, many of these methods have been found to reduce airborne cat allergen levels temporarily
by about 90%.[43] The HEPA filters are effective for cat allergen only
when used in conjunction with the other measures.[16]

Avoidance of early exposure to pets has been promoted to avoid
sensitization. However, recent studies suggest that in some children,
early contact with cats and dogs may in fact prevent allergy more
effectively than avoidance of these animals.[6,7] Further studies are
needed to resolve this issue.

Dog allergens provoke significant bronchial hyperresponsiveness
in people less often than do cat allergens. The decrease in response
may be due to antigens that vary among breeds and among sources
(dander, hair, saliva, and serum extracts), and because more dogs
reside outside and better tolerate regular bathing. Guidelines recommended for minimizing cat allergen exposure should also be followed
for minimizing dog allergen exposure.

Levels of airborne rodent urinary allergens have been reduced
in most laboratory environments by regulations that mandate rapid
room air exchanges and high-efficiency filters. No intervention
strategies have been studied for populations exposed by infestations
in housing.

## Dust Mites

Eliminating mite exposure reduces symptoms and the degree of
nonspecific bronchial hyperreactivity.[44] Because dust mite allergen
is carried on relatively large particles, exposure is mostly related to
breathing allergen that is resuspended during activity. Encasement
of mattresses, pillows, and box springs in allergen-impermeable covers
is the single most important avoidance measure to reduce mite exposure. Plastic or vinyl covers are an economical choice for box springs

but may be uncomfortable for use on mattresses and pillows. Vapor- or air-permeable covers that prevent the passage of allergens are available but more costly.[40,41]

Clinical intervention trials have shown substantial allergen reduction and improvement in asthma symptoms with dust-mite allergen reduction methods (impervious pillow and mattress covers and weekly hot water washing of bed linens [>130°F (55°C)]). This is higher than the temperature of 120°F recommended by the American Academy of Pediatrics; significant skin burns can be sustained within seconds of exposure to water at this temperature. As an alternative, water temperature could be elevated during linen washing (ideally when the children are at school or asleep) and returned to a lower temperature once laundering is complete. One study suggests that normal laundering (adequate room, moderately warm water, and a variety of commercial laundry detergents) is sufficient to extract most mite and cat allergens from bedding.[45] Further studies are needed to determine whether there are any differences in clinical outcomes after different laundering conditions.

Alternatives to hot water washing that kill mites include drying bedding outside in the sun (dust mites are sensitive to sunlight), drying in a tumble drier at 130°F for at least 20 minutes, and placing soft toys in the freezer.[3,41] Dry cleaning blankets kills mites but is less effective in removing allergens.[41]

Carpeting, a major source of mite antigen and proliferation, should be removed when possible, especially in the bedroom. A single vacuuming may decrease the mite burden by only 35% for a carpeted surface, but by 80% for a solid surface. If possible, upholstered furniture should be replaced with washable vinyl, leather, or wood. Window shades are preferable to curtains or venetian blinds. If curtains are used, they should be made of washable fabric. Blinds should be made of vinyl. Although acaricides (chemicals that kill mites) containing benzyl benzoate or tannic acid may reduce antigen levels on carpeting and upholstery, they must be reapplied every 3 months. Using acaricides is far less effective than removing carpet followed by regular damp mopping of hardwood or vinyl flooring. Therefore, many experts no longer recommend the use of acaricides in routine management of allergen avoidance.[3]

Because dust mite allergen becomes airborne only during disturbances and falls rapidly, and there is little opportunity for air cleaners to have an effect. Vacuum cleaners that incorporate a HEPA filter or double-thickness bag to prevent leakage of allergen may be helpful.[41]

Strategies to control humidity to limit dust mite growth vary according to climate.[16,41] In humid climates (ie, at least 8 months per year with relative outdoor humidity ≥50%), controlling reservoirs for dust mites is key. Successful dehumidification of homes is very difficult in truly humid climates (eg, southeastern United States). Air conditioning to maintain indoor relative humidity below 50% requires tight housing and may be expensive to achieve. In areas of moderate or seasonal humidity, mite growth may be strongly seasonal and growth can be substantially higher in areas of the house that maintain humidity (eg, carpets laid on a concrete slab). During dry seasons, opening windows for an hour per day will ensure removal of humidity from the house.[16] In dry climates (eg, the upper Midwest, the mountain states [altitude ≥5000 feet]), and the southwestern United States, mite growth in homes is minimal unless the house is humidified.

## Cockroaches

Cockroaches may be found wherever water, heat, and organic material are present.[46] It is essential to minimize organic material on open surfaces to reduce infestation. Other measures are storing all foodstuffs in sealed containers, eliminating water sources, eating only in the kitchen, placing trash out daily, caulking all cracks around faucets and pipe fittings, and placing roach gel baits and bait stations in kitchens and bathrooms.[3,47] Boric acid can be used in areas that are not accessible to children. When considering the use of other pesticides, families must balance the risks of cockroaches, severity of asthma, and risks of pesticide use. The use of the least toxic alternatives for pest control should be employed (see Chapter 24). Families should avoid using over-the-counter "bug sprays" because they may cause toxic reactions.

Cockroach allergens are carried on particles similar in size to dust mite allergens. Therefore cockroach allergens may be related to resuspension of settled dust. Concentrations of cockroach allergen are higher in the kitchen but often are found in bedrooms. The same physical barrier and cleaning interventions recommended for dust mite allergen should reduce exposure to cockroach allergen. Research efforts are in progress to determine the optimal methods needed to reduce cockroach allergen in infested homes that will decrease asthma symptoms.

## Molds
Dehumidifiers can be considered for areas with consistently elevated humidity levels, with a target humidity less than 50% relative humidity. Dehumidifiers reduce ambient humidity, but do not significantly reduce growth on surfaces in contact with groundwater. To effectively control further growth on these surfaces, the water source must be eliminated. Eliminating indoor organic sources, such as plants, wood, or paper products, also helps to control the growth of mold. Less obvious sources of water include damage due to prior flooding or rainwater and condensation on pipes and ductwork within interior or exterior structure walls.

### Outdoor Air Pollution and Allergens
In communities with recognized periods of increased ozone, pediatricians should counsel their patients with asthma (and parents) about the health impacts of ozone. Parents and coaches should consider modifying sports practice schedules on days with high ozone (see Chapter 7).

Identification of seasonal allergens that trigger a patient's asthma is important. This will allow the practitioner to initiate prophylactic

antihistamine or anti-inflammatory therapies and/or to recommend
the use of air conditioning, if available. Staying indoors during the
afternoon hours may help symptoms. Outdoor molds, especially
*Alternaria,* may be present in moderate climates, but are greatly
reduced following the onset of frost or recurrent freezing temperatures.
Affected individuals should be instructed to follow pollution alerts for
high pollen counts, especially during summer months.

## Frequently Asked Questions

Q *Do you recommend any special air filtration system for patients*
*with asthma?*

A Avoid room humidifiers, and keep central furnace system humidifi-
cation below 45% to 50% during winter months. Filters on central
forced air systems and furnaces should be changed periodically,
according to manufacturers' recommendations. Upgrading to a
medium-efficiency filter (rated at 20% to 50% efficiency at removing particles between 0.3 and 10 μm) will improve air quality and
is economical. Electrostatic filters/precipitators in central furnace
and air-conditioning systems may be beneficial for airborne particles (eg, cat allergen) but only are effective when turned on.
Room HEPA filters also are beneficial. However, they only work
in a single room, and the noise generated may not be acceptable.
Preferably, they should be used in the child's bedroom, but are
of little benefit in reducing exposure to ETS. Avoid the use of
air cleaners that generate ozone.

Q *Do you recommend a special vacuum cleaner for patients*
*with asthma?*

A Other strategies to reduce allergen exposure are more beneficial.
However, an efficient vacuum cleaner that avoids resuspension of
allergen may be useful for removing allergen, especially from hard
surfaces. Leakage of allergen is minimized in vacuum cleaners that
incorporate a double-thickness bag and have tight-fitting junctions

within the cleaner; a HEPA filter is not always necessary, depending on vacuum design. Unfortunately, there is no certification process to guide consumers. Important features for an efficient vacuum cleaner have been reviewed.[41]

Q *How can we better prepare the house to prevent asthma attacks from occurring?*

A Quit smoking if you smoke and eliminate all sources of ETS. Reduce or eliminate dust mites, cockroaches, and home dampness or molds. Remove pets to which the child demonstrates specific allergy. If removal of the pet is not possible, routinely perform allergen reduction measures. Consider using a vacuum cleaner that is efficient at cleaning and avoids resuspension of allergens (such as one equipped with a HEPA filter).

Q *Can odors of cooking foods cause an allergic reaction (eg, asthma) in susceptible patients?*

A Although rare, odors from foods may cause reactions in some patients. For example, a patient with known anaphylactic/anaphylactoid response to peanuts may react to aerosolized peanut oil used for cooking. The presence of a positive skin-prick test or RAST or an elevated IgE level to a given food should not necessarily lead to an elimination diet, however, because only one third of individuals have an allergic response when challenged orally with the specific food.

Q *Should I use a humidifier?*

A Humidifiers should be avoided. A relative humidity of greater than 50% promotes the growth of dust mites and mold. If used, the humidifier must be cleaned frequently to prevent mold growth.

Q *Are foam pillows safe for children or can they also be allergenic?*

A Foam pillows generally are hypoallergenic, although occasionally they may produce allergic responses. Polyester pillows may be less allergenic. However, all pillows, regardless of content, may serve as reservoirs for dust mites. An allergen-impermeable pillow cover should be used as a physical barrier between dust mite reservoirs in pillows and the child.

Q *What can be done when a family lives in a multi-unit building where there are barriers to asthma control due to pest infestation and cigarette smoking in common areas?*

A If families share concerns about issues such as pest control, mold problems, and cigarette smoking, they may want to organize as a group to alert management to their concerns for their children's health.

## Resources

American Lung Association, phone: 800-LUNG-USA, Internet: http://www.lungusa.org

Asthma and Allergy Foundation of America, phone 202-466-7643, Internet: http://www.aafa.org

California Indoor Air Quality Program Infosheets, Internet: http://www.cal-iaq.org/iaqsheet.htm; Air cleaners, Internet: http://www.arb.ca.gov/research/indoor/acdsumm.htm

Mothers of Asthmatics, Inc, phone: 800-878-4403

National Institutes of Health (NIH), phone: 301-496-4000.

## References

1. Busse WW, Lemanske RF Jr. Asthma. *N Engl J Med.* 2001;344:350–362
2. Gern JE, Lemanske RF Jr, Busse WW. Early life origins of asthma. *J Clin Invest.* 1999;104:837–843
3. National Institutes of Health, National Asthma Education Program. *Expert Panel Report 2: Guidelines for the Diagnosis and Management of Asthma.* Bethesda, MD: National Institutes of Health, National Heart, Lung, and Blood Institute; 1997. Publication NIH 97-4051. Available at: http://www.nhlbi.nih.gov/guidelines/asthma/asthgdln.pdf
4. Strachan DP. Family size, infection and atopy: the first decade of the "hygiene hypothesis." *Thorax.* 2000;55(suppl 1):S2–S10

5. Platts-Mills TA, Blumenthal K, Perzanowski M, Woodfolk JA. Determinants of clinical allergic disease. The relevance of indoor allergens to the increase in asthma. *Am J Respir Crit Care Med.* 2000;162:S128–S133

6. Platts-Mills TA. Paradoxical effect of domestic animals on asthma and allergic sensitization. *JAMA.* 2002;288:1012–1014

7. Celedon JC, Litonjua AA, Ryan L, Platts-Mills T, Weiss ST, Gold DR. Exposure to cat allergen, maternal history of asthma, and wheezing in first 5 years of life. *Lancet.* 2002;360:781–782

8. Etzel RA. How environmental exposures influence the development and exacerbation of asthma. *Pediatrics.* 2003;112:233–239

9. Pirkle JL, Flegal KM, Bernert JT, Brody DJ, Etzel RA, Maurer KR. Exposure to the US population to environmental tobacco smoke: the Third National Health and Nutrition Examination Survey, 1988 to 1991. *JAMA.* 1996;275:1233–1240

10. Ehrlich RI, DuToit D, Jordaan E, et al. Risk factors for childhood asthma and wheezing. Importance of maternal and household smoking. *Am J Respir Crit Care Med.* 1996;154:681–688

11. Martinez FD, Cline M, Burrows B. Increased incidence of asthma in children of smoking mothers. *Pediatrics.* 1992;89:21–26

12. Weitzman M, Gortmaker S, Walker DK, Sobol A. Maternal smoking and childhood asthma. *Pediatrics.* 1990;85:505–511

13. Abulhosn RS, Morray BH, Llewellyn CE, Redding GJ. Passive smoke exposure impairs recovery after hospitalization for acute asthma. *Arch Pediatr Adolesc Med.* 1997;151:135–139

14. Menon P, Rando RJ, Stankus RP, Salvaggio JE, Lehrer SB. Passive cigarette-smoke-challenge studies: increase in bronchial hyperreactivity. *J Allergy Clin Immunol.* 1992;89:560–566

15. Committee of the Environmental and Occupational Health Assembly of the American Thoracic Society. Health effects of outdoor air pollution. *Am J Respir Crit Care Med.* 1996;153:3–50

16. Institute of Medicine. *Clearing the Air: Asthma and Indoor Air Exposures.* Washington, DC: National Academies Press; 2000

17. Delfino RJ. Epidemiologic evidence for asthma and exposure to air toxics: linkages between occupational, indoor, and community air pollution research. *Environ Health Perspect.* 2002;110(suppl 4):573–589

18. Shim C, Williams MH Jr. Effect of odors in asthma. *Am J Med.* 1986;80:18–22

19. Wood RA, Eggleston PA. Management of allergy to animal danders. *Pediatr Asthma Allergy Immunol.* 1993;7:13–22

20. Luczynska CM, Li Y, Chapman MD, Platts-Mills TA. Airborne concentrations and particle size distribution of allergen derived from domestic cats *(Felis domesticus)*. Measurements using cascade impactor, liquid impinger, and a two-site monoclonal antibody assay for *Fel d I. Am Rev Respir Dis.* 1990;141:361–367

21. Almquist C, Wickman M, Perfetti L, et al. Worsening of asthma in children allergic to cats, after indirect exposure to cat at school. *Am J Respir Crit Care Med.* 2001;163:694–698

22. de Groot H, Goei KG, van Swieten P, Aalberse RC. Affinity purification of a major and a minor allergen from dog extract: serologic activity of affinity-purified *Can f I* and of *Can f I*-depleted extract. *J Allergy Clin Immunol.* 1991;87:1056–1065

23. Lindgren S, Belin L, Dreborg S, Einarsson R, Pahlman I. Breed-specific dog-dandruff allergens. *J Allergy Clin Immunol.* 1988;82:196–204

24. Phipatanakul W, Eggleston PA, Wright EC, Wood RA. Mouse allergen. I. The prevalence of mouse allergen in inner-city homes. The National Cooperative Inner-City Asthma Study. *J Allergy Clin Immunol.* 2000;106:1070–1074

25. Phipatanakul W, Eggleston PA, Wright EC, Wood RA. Mouse allergen. II. The relationship of mouse allergen exposure to mouse sensitization and asthma morbidity in inner-city children with asthma. *J Allergy Clin Immunol.* 2000;106:1075–1080

26. Rosensteich DL, Eggleston P, Kattan M, et al. The role of cockroach allergy and exposure to cockroach allergen in causing morbidity among inner-city children with asthma. *N Engl J Med.* 1997;336:1356–1363

27. Peat JK, Dickerson J, Li J. Effects of damp and mould in the home on respiratory health: a review of the literature. *Allergy.* 1998;53:120–128

28. Bornehag CG, Blomquist G, Gyntelberg F, et al. Dampness in buildings and health. Nordic interdisciplinary review of the scientific evidence on associations between exposure to "dampness" in buildings and health effects (NORDDAMP). *Indoor Air.* 2001;11:72–86

29. Nafstad P, Oie L, Mehl R, et al. Residential dampness problems and symptoms and signs of bronchial obstruction in young Norwegian children. *Am J Respir Crit Care Med.* 1998;157:410–414

30. Dales RE, Miller D. Residential fungal contamination and health: micro bial cohabitants as covariates. *Environ Health Perspect.* 1999;107(suppl 3): 481–483

31. Landwehr LP, Boguniewicz M. Current perspectives on latex allergy. *J Pediatr.* 1996;128:305–312

32. White MC, Etzel RA, Wilcox WD, Lloyd C. Exacerbations of childhood asthma and ozone pollution in Atlanta. *Environ Res.* 1994;65:56–68

33. American Academy of Pediatrics Committee on Environmental Health. Ambient air pollution: respiratory hazards to children. *Pediatrics.* 1993;91:1210–1213

34. McConnell R, Berhane K, Gilliland F, et al. Asthma in exercising children exposed to ozone: a cohort study. *Lancet.* 2002;359:386–391

35. Licorish K, Novey HS, Kozak P, Fairshter RD, Wilson AF. Role of *Alternaria* and *Penicillium* spores in the pathogenesis of asthma. *J Allergy Clin Immunol.* 1985;76:819–825

36. O'Hollaren MT, Yunginger JW, Offord KP, et al. Exposure to an aeroallergen as a possible precipitating factor in respiratory arrest in young patients with asthma. *N Engl J Med.* 1991;324:359–363

37. Targonski PV, Persey VW, Ramekrishnan V. Effect of environmental molds on risk of death from asthma during the pollen season. *J Allergy Clin Immunol.* 1995;95:955–961

38. Dales RA, Cakmak S, Judek S, et al. The role of fungal spores in thunderstorm asthma. *Chest.* 2003;123:745–750

39. Etzel RA. Indoor air pollution and childhood asthma: effective environmental interventions. *Environ Health Perspect.* 1995;103(suppl 6):55–58

40. Tovey E, Marks G. Methods and effectiveness of environmental control. *J Allergy Clin Immunol.* 1999;103:179–191

41. Platts-Mills TA, Vaughan JW, Carter MC, Woodfolk JA. The role of intervention in established allergy: avoidance of indoor allergens in the treatment of chronic allergic disease. *J Allergy Clin Immunol.* 2000;106:787–804

42. Krieger JK, Takaro TK, Allen C, et al. The Seattle-King County healthy homes project: implementation of a comprehensive approach to improving indoor environmental quality for low-income children with asthma. *Environ Health Perspect.* 2002;110(suppl 2):311–322

43. de Blay F, Chapman MD, Platts-Mills TA. Airborne cat allergen (Fel d I). Environmental control with the cat in situ. *Am Rev Respir Dis.* 1991;143:1334–1339

44. von Mutius E. Towards prevention. *Lancet.* 1997;350(suppl 2):SII14–SII17

45. Tovey ER, Taylor DJ, Mitakakis TZ, De Lucca SD. Effectiveness of laundry washing agents and conditions in the removal of cat and dust mite allergen from bedding dust. *J Allergy Clin Immunol.* 2001;108:369–374

46. Call RS, Smith TF, Morris E, Chapman MD, Platts-Mills TA. Risk factors for asthma in inner city children. *J Pediatr.* 1992;121:862–866
47. O'Connor GT, Gold DR. Cockroach allergy and asthma in a 30-year-old man. *Environ Health Perspect.* 1999;107:243–247

# 35
# Cancer

## Occurrence and Characteristics of Childhood Cancers

Childhood malignancies are relatively rare, with only approximately 8700 cancers of all types diagnosed per year among US children younger than 15 years, and 12 400 among US children and adolescents younger than 20 years (corresponding to average annual incidence rates of 13.4 per 100 000 and 14.9 per 100 000 per year, respectively).[1] In contrast, 1.22 million cancers (excluding non-melanoma skin cancers) are diagnosed annually among adults in the United States, corresponding to an average annual incidence rate of 398 per 100 000 for all cancers. Despite the rarity of childhood cancers, this category of diseases is the fourth most common cause of death among children younger than 15 years. While carcinomas predominate among adults, the major pediatric cancers are non-epithelial, with the most common malignancies being the leukemias (representing 30.2% of all cancers diagnosed in children younger than 15 years), brain and central nervous system (CNS) cancers (21.7%), and lymphomas (10.9%); these 3 categories (together comprising 63% of all childhood malignancies) and the remaining 37% of pediatric neoplasms are characterized by substantial histological and biological diversity.[2,3] The classification system used for pediatric neoplasms, updated in 1996 and designated as the International Classification of Childhood Cancer, includes 12 major categories that use histologically based subtypes.[4] For adult malignancies, anatomic site-based categories are employed.

The major categories of childhood cancers and subtypes within each category often are distinguished by differing age, ethnic/racial, and gender-related characteristics.[1] For example, some unique features of childhood leukemia include a notable peak at ages 2 to 3 years of the common form of acute lymphoblastic leukemia; the substantially lower incidence and absence of a striking age peak at ages 2 to 3 years in black Americans compared with white Americans; the long-term, changing trends for common acute lymphoblastic leukemia in white Americans, with little evidence of a peak at very young ages until the 1920s in Britain and until the 1930s in the United States; and the relatively flat incidence of acute myeloid leukemia throughout childhood, with the only small peak apparent in infancy.[5] In addition to acute lymphoblastic leukemia, ethnic or racial differences are apparent for sympathetic nervous system tumors (low in black Americans), renal tumors (notably reduced in Asian Americans), and Ewing sarcoma (very low in black Americans). These ethnic or racial differences may be related to genetic factors or perhaps environmental exposures that differ by ethnic/racial group. It also is possible that ethnic/racial differences in genetic factors that affect carcinogen metabolism, immune function, or other functional processes could be important. Gender differences may distinguish certain types of childhood malignancies, such as the high male-female ratios for Hodgkin disease and for ependymomas and primitive neuroectodermal tumors in contrast to other forms of brain and CNS tumors.[1] In contrast to the higher male-female ratio for acute lymphoblastic leukemia, the ratio is lower for acute myeloid leukemia. A notable female predominance is apparent for thyroid carcinoma and for malignant melanoma in children and adolescents.

### Time Trends in Incidence and Mortality

Public concern about possible increases in childhood cancer incidence in the United States led to recent analyses of childhood cancer time trends in incidence and mortality.[1,6] In a detailed evaluation of the trend patterns for cancers diagnosed among 14 450 children younger than 15 years from 1975 through 1995 in 9 population-based registries, a modest rise in the incidence of leukemia was largely due to an abrupt increase from 1983 to 1984; rates declined from 1989 through 1995.[6] For brain and other CNS cancers, incidence rose modestly, although statistically significantly, from 1983 through 1986 but rates subsequently stabilized. A few rare childhood cancers demonstrated upward trends (eg, a 40% increase in skin cancers designated as dermatofibrosarcomas, adrenal neuroblastomas, and retinoblastomas, the latter 2 in infants only). Incidence of other cancers has decreased modestly but statistically significantly for Hodgkin disease. Overall, there was no substantial change in incidence for the major pediatric cancers, and rates remained relatively stable from the mid-1980s through 1995. The patterns of the modest increases observed in the mid-1980s (for brain/CNS cancers, leukemia, and infant neuroblastoma) suggest that the increases likely reflected diagnostic improvements or reporting changes. Dramatic steady declines in mortality have occurred for all major childhood cancer categories (albeit less dramatic for brain/CNS malignancies) for several decades. The dramatic declines in mortality represent treatment-related improvements in survival.

## Risk Factors

Some characteristic features of the major categories (and a limited number of subtypes) are shown in Tables 35.1 through 35.4. More detailed characterization of childhood cancers can be found in the recent National Cancer Institute monograph.[1] While epidemiologic studies of childhood cancers have evaluated a large number of postulated risk factors, the few known or suspected risk factor associations are summarized in Tables 35.1 through 35.4. Familial and genetic factors seem to occur in no more than 5% to 15% of different categories of childhood cancer.[7] Some risk factors, such as ionizing radiation (which in moderate to high doses has been linked with increased risks for acute lymphoblastic and acute myeloid leukemias, CNS tumors, malignant bone tumors, and thyroid carcinoma), have been established as causal for several types of pediatric cancers, while others, such as treatment with alkylating agents (which in some children has been linked with acute myeloid leukemia), have been linked with

**Table 35.1**

**Risk Factors (Known and Suggestive) Associated With Childhood Leukemias and Lymphomas**

| Exposure or Characteristic | Leukemia | | Lymphoma | |
|---|---|---|---|---|
| | Acute Lymphoblastic | Acute Myeloid | Hodgkin Lymphoma | Non-Hodgkin Lymphoma |
| **Known** | | | | |
| Male-to-female ratio | 1.3 | 1.1 | 1.3 | 3.0 |
| Age peak | 2–4 years | Infancy | Adolescence | Adolescence |
| Average annual age-adjusted incidence per million | 26.3 | 6.5 | 13.8 | 9.9 |
| White-to-black ratio | 2.0 | 1.0 | 1.3 | 1.4 |
| Other factors | Birth weight >4000 g <br>• Ionizing radiation <br>  - Diagnostic, in utero acute lymphoblastic leukemia and acute myeloid leukemia <br>• Down syndrome <br>  - ALL and AML M7 <br>• Congenital disorders, ataxia-telangiectasia, Fanconi syndrome, Bloom syndrome, neurofibromatosis | | Monozygotic twins of young adults <br><br>Affected siblings <br><br>Epstein-Barr virus linked with some forms <br><br>Infectious mononucleosis | Immuno-suppresive therapy <br><br>Congenital immuno-deficiency syndromes (eg, ataxia-telangiectasia) <br><br>AIDS |
| **Suggestive** | | | | |
| | Maternal fetal loss <br><br>Mother older than 35 years at pregnancy <br><br>First born | Maternal alcohol use during pregnancy <br><br>Parental occupational exposures <br>  – Benzene <br>  – Pesticides | | |

**Table 35.2**
**Risk Factors (Known and Suggestive) Associated With Childhood Brain Tumors and Sympathetic Nervous System Tumors**

| Exposure or Characteristic | Brain Tumors | | | Sympathetic Nervous System Tumors | |
|---|---|---|---|---|---|
| **Known** | | | | | |
| | Type | Male-to-Female Ratio | Average Annual Incidence per Million | Male-to-Female Ratio | Average Annual Incidence per Million |
| | All brain tumors | 1.2 | 25.9 | 1.1 | 7.9 |
| | Astrocytomas | 1.1 | 13.4 | | |
| | Primitive neuroectodermal tumors | 1.7 | 5.0 | | |
| | Other gliomas | 1.0 | 4.4 | | |
| | Ependymomas | 2.0 | 2.1 | | |
| Age peak | Infancy | | | Infancy | |
| White-to-black ratio | 1.2 | | | 1.8 | |
| Other factors | Ionizing radiation | | | | |
| | Genetic disorders<br>- Neurofibromatosis<br>- Tuberous sclerosis<br>- Nevoid basal cell syndrome<br>- Turcot syndrome<br>- Li-Fraumeni syndrome | | | | |
| **Suggestive** | | | | | |
| | Maternal diet during pregnancy<br>- Cured meats | | | | |
| | Sibling or parent with brain tumor increases risk | | | | |

**Table 35.3**
**Risk Factors (Known and Suggestive) Associated With Childhood Malignant Bone Tumors, Soft Tissue Sarcomas, Renal Tumors, and Hepatic Tumors**

| Exposure or Characteristic | Malignant Bone Tumors | | Soft Tissue Sarcomas | | Renal Tumors | | Hepatic Tumors | |
|---|---|---|---|---|---|---|---|---|
| | Type | Male-to-Female Ratio | Type | Male-to-Female Ratio | Type | Male-to-Female Ratio | Type | Male-to-Female Ratio |
| **Known** | | | | | | | | |
| | All bone | 1.2 | All soft tissue | 1.2 | All renal | 0.9 | All hepatic | 1.2 |
| | Osteosarcoma | 1.2 | | | | | Hepatoblastoma | 1.2 |
| | Ewing sarcoma | 1.3 | | | | | Hepatocellular carcinoma | 1.0 |
| | Chondrosarcoma | 1.5 | | | | | | |
| Age peak | 13–18 years | | Infancy for rhabdomyosarcoma; 15–19 years for others | | Infancy for Wilms tumor; 5–19 years for renal cell carcinomas | | Infancy for hepatoblastoma; 15–19 years for hepatocellular carcinoma | |
| Average annual age-adjusted incidence per million | 8.6 | | 10.8 | | 6.4 | | 1.5 | |
| White-to-black ratio | 1.3 | | 0.9 | | 0.9 | | 1.2 | |
| Anatomic site | Osteosarcoma: long bones; Ewing sarcoma: central axis | | | | 7% of Wilms tumors are bilateral | | | |

**Table 35.3**

**Risk Factors (Known and Suggestive) Associated With Childhood Malignant Bone Tumors, Soft Tissue Sarcomas, Renal Tumors, and Hepatic Tumors,** *continued*

| Exposure or Characteristic | Malignant Bone Tumors | Soft Tissue Sarcomas | Renal Tumors | Hepatic Tumors |
|---|---|---|---|---|
| **Known** | | | | |
| Other factors | Radiation therapy for childhood cancer<br><br>Treatment with alkylating agents<br><br>High doses of radium<br><br>Genetic disorders<br>- Hereditary retinoblastoma<br>- Li-Fraumeni syndrome<br>- Rothmund-Thomson syndrome | Some concordance between anatomic location of rhabdomyosarcoma and major birth defects<br><br>Up to one third of patients with rhabdomyosarcoma have at least 1 congenital anomaly<br><br>Genetic disorders<br>- Li-Fraumeni syndrome<br>- Neurofibromatosis | Notably decreased incidence in Asians, compared with whites and blacks<br><br>Genetic disorders<br>- WAGR (Wilms tumor, aniridia, genitourinary abnormalities, mental retardation)<br>- Beckwith-Wiedemann syndrome<br>- Perlman syndrome<br>- Denys-Drash syndrome | Genetic disorders<br>- Beckwith-Wiedemann syndrome<br>- Hemihypertrophy<br>- Familial adenomatous polyposis<br>- Gardner syndrome |
| **Suggestive** | | | | |
| | — | — | Father employed as welder or mechanic increases risk | — |

**Table 35.4**
**Risk Factors (Known and Suggestive) Associated With Childhood Germ Cell Tumors, Carcinomas and Other Malignant Epithelial Tumors, and Retinoblastoma**

| Exposure or Characteristic | Germ Cell Tumors | | | Carcinomas and Other Malignant Epithelial Tumors | | | Retinoblastoma | | |
|---|---|---|---|---|---|---|---|---|---|
| | Type | Male-to-Female Ratio | Average Annual Incidence per Million | Type | Male-to-Female Ratio | Average Annual Incidence per Million | Type | Male-to-Female Ratio | Average Annual Incidence per Million |
| **Known** | | | | | | | | | |
| | All germ cell | 1.1 | 10.1 | All carcinomas | 0.5 | 14.1 | All retino-blastoma | 1.0 | 2.8 |
| | Gonadal | 1.5 | 6.1 | Thyroid carcinoma | 0.2 | 5.0 | | | |
| | Testicular | | 8.1 | Malignant melanoma | 0.6 | 4.5 | | | |
| | Ovarian | | 5.3 | | | | | | |
| Age peak | 15–19 years | | | 15–19 years | | | Infancy | | |
| White-to-black ratio | 1.5 | | | 1.5 | | | 0.9 | | |

**Table 35.4**

**Risk Factors (Known and Suggestive) Associated With Childhood Germ Cell Tumors, Carcinomas and Other Malignant Epithelial Tumors, and Retinoblastoma,** *continued*

| Exposure or Characteristic | Germ Cell Tumors | Carcinomas and Other Malignant Epithelial Tumors | Retinoblastoma |
|---|---|---|---|
| **Known** | | | |
| Other | Cryptorchidism | Thyroid carcincma<br>- Ionizing radiation exposure during childhood from environmental and medical sources<br>- Inherited cancer susceptibility syndromes (familial polyposis multiple endocrine neoplasia types I, II-A, II-B)<br><br>Malignant melanoma<br>- Ultraviolet sunlight exposure<br>- Number of nevi and dysplastic nevi | Parent with a history of bilateral retinoblastoma |
| **Suggestive** | | | |
| | High maternal hormone levels during pregnancy<br><br>Family history of germ cell tumor<br><br>Hernia<br><br>Preterm birth | | 13q deletion syndrome |

specific forms of childhood cancer. Increased incidence of several types of childhood cancers is found in children with genetic syndromes or congenital disorders. Suggestive or limited data (the latter not shown in the tables) link certain maternal reproductive factors, parental occupational exposures, residential pesticides, cured meats, paternal smoking, and other exposures with increased risk of some types of childhood cancers. The remainder of this chapter will focus on the sources of etiological information; important aspects of the mechanisms of carcinogenesis; routes of exposure; key biological processes involved in carcinogenesis and some clinical effects; selected physical, chemical, and biological carcinogens; and practical considerations and what to do when a possible cancer cluster is identified.

## Sources of Etiologic Information

Human carcinogens usually have been first recognized by clinicians who observed increased occurrence or clusters of cases and traced them to their causes. To determine whether a clinically recognized, postulated carcinogen is etiologically linked with childhood malignancy and to quantify the strength of the relationship, case-control studies generally are undertaken because of the rarity of virtually all forms of childhood cancer. Because childhood cancers are uncommon, a prospective study would need to collect exposure information from hundreds of thousands, if not millions, of children over several years to identify adequate numbers of pediatric cancers for assessing statistical associations; such a study would be too expensive to be feasible. Exposure assessment methods used in epidemiologic investigations of childhood cancer have improved with time, but studies continue to require collection of substantial exposure information from interviews with parents. In the absence of environmental or biological measurements, or more ideally molecular genetic evidence of a specific exposure, it is difficult to interpret responses of a parent about a child's exposure to many agents or devices, particularly because exposure levels or use change over time with growth, development, and behavioral change. Efforts to develop new methods for assessing exposures are under way. If epidemiologists consistently find that the exposure or agent is linked with a specific childhood cancer, the association is then considered too likely to be due to chance.

## Key Features of Carcinogenesis in Childhood Cancers

The latent period between exposure and onset of cancer is not established for most childhood malignancies because the etiologies are largely unknown. For carcinogenic exposures occurring during the prenatal (such as diagnostic x-rays to the pregnant mother) or postnatal (such as chemotherapy with epipodophyllotoxin drugs) periods, the latency interval between exposure and onset of childhood cancer is relatively short. The latency period may be longer for preconception carcinogenic exposures (such as paternal cigarette smoking) that increase the risk of childhood cancer in offspring. While a few carcinogenic exposures occurring during childhood (such as certain chemotherapy agents linked with increased risk of acute myeloid leukemia, moderate doses of ionizing radiation to bone marrow linked with increased risk of chronic myeloid leukemia, and the combination of Epstein Barr virus and malaria linked with endemic Burkitt's lymphoma in Africa) have been associated with increased risk of childhood cancer, most carcinogenic exposures occurring during childhood or adolescence (including exposures to moderate to high doses of ionizing radiation, ultraviolet sunlight, cigarette smoking, alcohol consumption, asbestos, benzene, and many other chemical and physical agents) will more likely result in occurrence of cancer during adulthood because of the substantially higher incidence and longer latent periods associated with most carcinogens. Diethylsilbestrol, ionizing radiation, and chemotherapy, however, have short latent periods for exposures that enable cancer to develop in childhood. About 60 chemical or physical agents are known to cause cancer in humans.[8] The carcinogenicity of environmental agents may be enhanced or diminished by interaction with one another or by genetic influences.

## Routes of Exposure

Carcinogens such as radiation may be ingested ($^{131}$I from fallout or accidents, such as Chernobyl), injected (radioisotopes), or inhaled (radon decay products). Similarly, chemical and biological carcinogens may be inhaled, ingested, or absorbed through the skin. These carcinogens occur in pollutants, tobacco products, naturally in the diet, or in medications. Occasionally, what is considered a therapeutic advance has proved to have deleterious effects, including cancer, so practitioners must remain vigilant to all therapeutic innovations and their potential hazards. In addition to exogenous agents and their associated routes of exposure, cancers also may result in children and adults from endogenous reactions, such as oxidation or other types of metabolic change. Several forms of exogenous chemical agents do not cause cancer until undergoing one or more endogenous chemical reactions.

## Biological Processes and Clinical Effects

The effects of environmental carcinogens, whether chemical or physical, have been attributed to the damage they do to deoxyribonucleic acid (DNA), changing its coding specificity and acting as initiators of cancer. Types of DNA damage vary from specific point mutations to wider effects, such as the double strand breaks associated with radiation exposure. The repair of DNA damage can ameliorate most of the exogenous or endogenous damage caused by carcinogens. The key role of DNA repair in control of the induction of cancer in humans was based on findings that patients with xeroderma pigmentosum, a disorder linked with high risk of skin cancer, had defects in nucleotide excision repair. Other important mechanisms of carcinogenesis derived from recognition of 2 major categories of cancer genes. Oncogenes are one class of latent cancer genes. When activated, they transform normal cells to cancer cells. Tumor suppressor genes are the other main class of cancer genes. Normally they regulate development (eg, of the eye or kidney). When these genes are inactivated (mutated),

they no longer regulate growth of the organ, and cancer develops
(eg, retinoblastoma or Wilms tumor). Substances that are immuno-
suppressants of all types act by diminishing immunosurveillance and
destruction of the earliest neoplastic cells. These cells appear throughout life but usually are eliminated, a defense that lessens with age.

The carcinogenic effect of a chemical is detectable when the dose
is high or chronic, as in medicinal, occupational, or large accidental
exposures. Note that if an effect has been sought but not found after
high exposures, it is unlikely to be found at lower ones.

## Physical Agents

**Solar Radiation.** A substantial proportion of all cancers in humans
involve the skin. Skin cancers may be induced by ultraviolet (UV)
light.[9] Because of the long latent period, skin cancers rarely occur in
childhood, except when there is markedly heightened sensitivity, as in
xeroderma pigmentosum, which has an inherent DNA repair defect,
or in albinism due to lack of pigment in the skin that protects against
UV damage. In the general population, the darker the complexion, the
lower the frequency of skin cancer. Maps that show cancer mortality
disclose that mortality due to malignant melanoma is significantly
higher in the southern United States than in the northern United
States. The incidence of melanoma has increased more rapidly than
that of most cancers, and children who experience repeated sunburns
are at risk (see Chapter 26).[10]

**Ionizing Radiation.** Children are more susceptible than adults to
radiation-induced leukemia, especially of the acute lymphocytic type.
The peak incidence occurs 5 years after exposure, and some excess
persists for 25 years. The excess of radiogenic thyroid cancer begins at
11 years of age and persists for decades. Breast cancer was induced by
childhood exposure to the atomic bomb in Japan, with diagnosis at
about 30 years of age; the risk was greater when exposure occurred to
people younger than 20 years.[11] The lowest dose after which an excess

of solid tumors can be detected in atomic bomb survivors is 0.10 Sv (10 rem).[12]

The carcinogenic effects of intrauterine exposure to radiation also have been studied. Diagnostic in utero exposures have been associated with various cancers in children younger than 10 years, but recent case-control studies show a significant excess only of childhood leukemia.[13] Several cohort studies have shown no increase in cancer occurrence among those exposed while in utero to diagnostic x-rays, but most of these cohorts were relatively small in size and lacked adequate statistical power to demonstrate a clear increase in risk. Atomic bomb exposure of children younger than 15 years did not increase the frequency of lymphoma, brain cancer, or embryonal cancers (which are among the most common cancers of childhood). While the observation of no significant excess of cancer occurrence among those Japanese atomic bomb survivors exposed while in utero sheds some doubt that in utero exposures can induce cancer occurrence, it also must be recognized that the relatively small number of individuals exposed while in utero and the rarity of childhood cancer and young adult cancer occurrence would be unlikely to have resulted in elevated occurrence of cancer at these young ages. Experimental data show little evidence of cancer risk in animals exposed to low doses of radiation while in utero. Thus, overall, the evidence for elevated risk of childhood cancer following in utero exposure to diagnostic radiation is not overwhelmingly consistent, but the precautionary principle would suggest that such exposures should be avoided.

Radiotherapy is associated with an increased risk of second primary cancers; treatment for Hodgkin disease, for example, has been associated with an excess of osteosarcoma, soft-tissue sarcoma, leukemia, skin cancer, and breast cancer.[14] In some genetic disorders, such as hereditary retinoblastoma and the nevoid basal cell carcinoma syndrome, there is increased susceptibility to radiogenic cancers. Exposure to radon decay products (also known as radon daughters or radon progeny), which come from uranium—ubiquitous in rocks and soil—is associated with an increased risk of lung cancer in adults. Whether children are more susceptible than adults to the carcinogenic effects of radon exposure is unknown.

The threat of accidental release of radiation from nuclear reactors was largely theoretical until 1979. Then, in Pennsylvania at Three Mile Island, an equipment failure resulted in radiation exposure to neighboring communities. The doses of radiation received by the general population nearby were too small to produce increases in cancer rates, mutations, or teratogenic effects. To protect the thyroid, potassium iodide therapy was recommended, but was not available.

In 1986 a partial meltdown at a nuclear reactor in Chernobyl, Ukraine, occurred. Substantial amounts of radioactive isotopes were released into the atmosphere. Fallout occurred primarily in the Ukraine and Belarus, in neighboring countries, and, to a lesser extent, throughout the world. Twenty-nine heavily exposed workers at the reactor died. Near the plant 135 000 people were evacuated. Twenty-five thousand people who lived 3 to 15 km from the plant were estimated to have received 350 to 550 mSv (35 to 55 rem) from external irradiation. This amount is 7 to 11 times the annual dose limit for radiation workers. Additional exposures occurred from the ingestion of radioisotopes (fallout) that contaminated food and water. Thyroid cancer developed in hundreds of children after a latent period of only 4 years.[15] Other such nuclear accidents may be expected to occur as a result of natural catastrophes, human error, deterioration of nuclear facilities, or terrorist events.

**Asbestos.** Exposure to asbestos fibers increases the frequency of lung cancer, especially in smokers, and, after a latent period as long as 40 years, can cause mesothelioma. During the 1950s, schoolroom ceilings were routinely sprayed with asbestos, which deteriorated with time. As a result of recent public health initiatives, the asbestos has been removed or walled off, but it is conceivable that mesothelioma may develop in adults exposed as school children, and those who smoke will have an increased risk of lung cancer (see Chapter 9).

### Chemical Agents

**Tobacco.** Active smoking is a well-established cause of cancer. Studies on the health effects of passive smoking indicate an increase in the frequency of adult lung cancer among nonsmokers chronically exposed to the cigarette smoke of others. This effect is biologically plausible given the known carcinogens in tobacco smoke. The risk of lung cancer is increased after exposure in childhood to environmental tobacco smoke (ETS) from parents who smoke (see Chapter 13).[16]

Smokeless tobacco causes oral cancer in young adults.[17] The habit of chewing tobacco has grown among high school students who are using professional athletes as role models. In 1985 a Consensus Development Panel of the National Institutes of Health estimated that at least 10 million people in the United States used smokeless tobacco and concluded that strong evidence exists that it causes cancer of the mouth.[17] The Council on Scientific Affairs of the American Medical Association concurred and urged that restrictions applied to the advertising of cigarettes be applied to the advertising of snuff and chewing tobacco. Pediatricians have an opportunity and responsibility to prevent tobacco-related cancers by educating their patients.

**Diet.** A variety of natural chemicals in food may be carcinogenic in people. Among them are aflatoxins, sassafras, cycasin, and bracken (their natural constituents are carcinogens), which can be found in peanuts, peanut butter, and many other foods, as well as protein pyrolysates produced when certain foods are cooked. Some food constituents protect against cancer in experimental animals. Among these anticarcinogens are carotenoids and dietary fiber.[18]

It has been difficult to derive strong evidence that individual components of the diet are carcinogenic in humans because of the long latent periods, the role of metabolic conversion, and possibly interactions that may potentiate or inhibit carcinogenesis.

Laboratory experimentation and human correlational studies suggest that overeating contributes to cancer of the endometrium, and fats in particular contribute to cancer of the breast and colon.[19] The composition of the diet is believed to affect the bacterial flora of the intestines, which in turn produce carcinogenic metabolites through degradation of bile acids and cholesterol. In addition, high fiber content is believed to diminish the frequency of colon cancer by speeding transit time and thus diminishing contact between dietary carcinogens and intestinal mucosa.

Data from epidemiologic studies, clinical observations, and animal experimentation are insufficient for strong recommendations to be made about specific dietary factors, but no harm would be done and other health benefits might result from following the recommendations that several medical organizations have issued about diet and cancer: reduce fat consumption from 40% to 30% of calories; include whole-grain cereals, citrus fruits, and green or yellow vegetables in the daily diet; limit consumption of salt-cured and smoke-cured foods and alcoholic beverages; and maintain optimal body weight.[18,19]

**Parental Occupation.** Since the mid-1970s, an expanding body of literature has implicated the role of parents' preconception, prenatal, and postnatal occupational exposures to a growing list of potential carcinogens in the etiology of many types of childhood cancers.[20] Agents such as ionizing radiation, asbestos, benzene, pesticides, and many other types of exposures have been implicated in the etiology of childhood cancers, but the strategy used to assess such exposures in most studies has been limited to identification of job exposure from job titles on birth or death certificates, or a job history obtained from one, or to a lesser extent both, parents. While the relationship between specific jobs or occupational exposures and specific childhood cancers has often not been consistent, the application of newer and more accurate methods to ascertain exposure is likely to clarify the relationship of specific occupational exposures with specific forms of childhood cancer.

**Environmental Chemical Exposures.** Children are exposed to a wide range of chemical agents in residential, school, child care, and other environments. Environmental chemical exposures of particular concern include pesticides; contaminants of drinking water, such as nitrate; mycotoxins; and cleaning agents used in residential settings. Recently, case-control studies assessing the possible role of pesticide exposures in the etiology of childhood leukemia have incorporated new methods, such as use of high-suction vacuum cleaners to obtain dust from carpets for measuring pesticide levels in carpet dust.

## What to Do When Clusters Are Observed

Occasionally a cluster of cancers occurs within a neighborhood or school district, often by chance. Clusters of cancers occasionally may be environmentally induced (ie, the histories of the affected persons reveal a large exposure in common, usually a drug or occupational chemical).[21] In office practice, pediatricians can make novel observations about environmental or inherent causes of specific types of childhood cancers. A single case may draw attention to the suspected carcinogen, as in respiratory cancers induced by war-time exposure to mustard gas during its manufacture in Japan or liver neoplasia due to oral contraceptives that was noted in Michigan.[21]

When a cluster is observed, the pediatrician should determine whether the cancers are of the same or related types. Cancers of the same type are more likely than diverse types to be induced by an environmental carcinogen. Diagnosis by cell type and primary anatomic site should be verified. Cases should be excluded if the latent period is too short or if the neoplasm was present before the child resided, attended school, or was otherwise exposed in the area. If the exclusions do not dispel the clusters, an environmental epidemiologist from the state health department should be consulted.

An association between 2 events need not be causal. Establishing causality is enhanced by showing (1) a logical time sequence (ie, the presumed causal event preceded the effect), (2) specificity of the effect (ie, one type rather than multiple types of cancer caused by a given exposure), (3) a dose-response relationship, (4) biologic plausibility (ie, the new information is consistent with previous knowledge), (5) consistency with other observations about cause and effect (eg, determining whether the relationship of fat consumption to colon cancer rates is demonstrated in other countries), (6) the exclusion of concomitant variables (alternative explanations) in the analysis, and (7) disappearance of the effect when the cause is removed. Not all of these elements can be evaluated or will hold true for even the most fully studied effects of an environmental exposure.[22] It is not the pediatrician's job to establish causality but to work with the epidemiologist and health department to evaluate the situation.

## Searching for Clues to Cancer Causes

In searching for clues to cancer causes, a careful history can produce a wealth of new information. Family history ranks first. Ideally, the medical record for a child with cancer should include a recent pedigree showing illnesses in each first-degree relative (parents, siblings, and children of the index case), as well as information about other relatives with cancer or other potentially related diseases, such as immunologic disorders, blood dyscrasias, or congenital malformations. Second, the pediatrician should inquire about the parents' occupations and other exposures during pregnancy (including smoking) and about the child's exposures to ETS, chemicals, radiation, and unusual infections. Other findings that may be important to determining the cause are coexistent disease, such as multiple congenital malformations, multifocal or bilateral cancer in paired organs (a possible clue to hereditary transmission), cancer of an unusual histologic type, cancer at an unusual age (eg, adult-type cancers in childhood), cancer at an unusual site, or marked overreaction to conventional cancer therapy (eg, acute reaction to radiotherapy for lymphoma in ataxia-telangiectasia). From such occurrences, new understanding of the origins of childhood cancer may be derived in the future, as they have been in the past.

## Frequently Asked Questions

Q  *What steps can I take to prevent cancer in my child?*

A  The causes of most childhood cancers are unknown. Most cases of cancer occur in adulthood, and we still do not know the steps to decrease the chances of the development of certain types of cancer in adulthood. Children should be encouraged not to smoke or use smokeless tobacco products. Adults should not be allowed to smoke when children are present. Children should not sunburn and should be encouraged to wear clothing and hats and to use sunscreen when outdoors. Important preventive measures for parents include testing the home for radon and making sure no friable asbestos exists in the home.

Q  *Why did neuroblastoma develop in my 3-month-old child?*

A  Almost all childhood cancer in the United States occurs at random. In one study, 500 children were studied, and no cause of neuroblastoma could be found. We know that damage to DNA occurs at a specific location in chromosome 1 in neuroblastoma, but rarely do we know what causes the mutation in this or other childhood cancers. We know, for example, that Japanese atomic bomb survivors had an excess of leukemia, among other cancers. The mutation may occur during normal reshuffling of genetic material. Usually the damage is repaired, and cancer does not develop, but unfortunately this defense is sometimes breached.

Q *The cat's been sick. Could the cat have caused my child's leukemia?*

A Cats develop a similar disease due to a virus, which they can transmit to other cats but not to humans. The same is true of chickens and cattle, in which a leukemia-like disease is virally induced. There is no evidence that pets transmit cancer to humans.

Q *Several children in our neighborhood have cancer. Could it be due to the same cause?*

A Most causes of cancer in humans have been first recognized by the occurrence of a cluster of cases. Such discoveries are infrequent and generally involve rare cancers due to heavy exposures to a carcinogen. The many types of cancer (more than 80) give rise to thousands of random clusters each year in the United States in neighborhoods, schools, social clubs, sports teams, and other groups of people. By drawing boundaries on a scatter map near the cases, random clustering can seem to be unusual. In any event, more evidence than a cluster is needed, including a dose-response effect (the bigger the dose the more frequent the effect) and biologic plausibility considering other knowledge about cancer. In most clusters there are many different types of cancers and many different causes, rather than a single cause.

Q *Will my child with cancer give my other children cancer?*

A Cancer is not transmitted from one child to another. Occasionally, a predisposition to specific cancers is transmitted through the ova or sperm cells of the parent. For example, retinoblastoma runs in families. Usually signs of predisposition to hereditary cancer can be detected in the histories of families with genetic disorders. For children at risk, early detection and treatment can improve survival and well-being. Thus few children die of retinoblastoma today.

Q *A member of our household smokes. Could that be the cause of my child's cancer?*

A There is no evidence that childhood cancer has been induced by exposure to ETS. Cancers in children younger than 15 years generally are of a different microscopic category (non-epithelial) from cigarette-induced cancers (epithelial), and no evidence currently exists that the childhood types are inducible by ETS. On the other hand, adult cancers, such as lung cancer, leukemia, and lymphoma, have been associated with exposure to maternal smoking that occurs before the child reaches age 10 years.

Q *Is it possible that the drugs I took during pregnancy started my child's cancer?*

A Drugs commonly used during pregnancy have not been shown to be carcinogenic in the offspring.

Q *I have heard that peanut butter may cause cancer. Is this true?*

A It is true that peanuts may become contaminated with molds producing aflatoxin, a carcinogen. The US Food and Drug Administration regulates the amount of aflatoxin permitted in foods such as peanut butter.

Q *Is childhood cancer increasing?*

A Overall, there has been no substantial change in the incidence for the major pediatric cancers since the mid-1980s in the United States. There were modest increases in the mid-1980s for certain types of childhood cancer (including the leukemias, brain/CNS cancers, and neuroblastoma). The type and pattern of these increases over a short period suggest that the increases likely reflected diagnostic improvements or reporting changes.

## Resource

National Cancer Institute, phone: 800-4-CANCER

## References

1. Ries LAG, Smith MA, Gurney JG, et al. *Cancer Incidence and Survival Among Children and Adolescents: United States SEER Program 1975–1995.* Bethesda, MD: National Cancer Institute, SEER Program, 1999. NIH Publication 99-4649

2. Miller RW, Myers MH. Age distribution of epithelial and non-epithelial cancers. *Lancet.* 1983;2:1250

3. Chow WH, Linet MS, Liff JM, Greenberg RS. Cancers in children. In: Schottenfeld D, Fraumeni JF Jr, eds. *Cancer Epidemiology and Prevention.* 2nd ed. New York, NY: Oxford University Press–USA; 1996:1331–1369

4. Kramarova E, Stiller CA. The international classification of childhood cancer. *Int J Cancer.* 1996;68:759–765

5. Smith MA, Simon R, Strickler HD, McQuillan G, Ries LA, Linet MS. Evidence that childhood acute lymphoblastic leukemia is associated with an infectious agent linked to hygiene conditions. *Cancer Causes Control.* 1998;9:285–298

6. Linet MS, Ries LA, Smith MA, Tarone RE, Devesa SS. Cancer surveillance series: recent trends in childhood cancer incidence and mortality in the United States. *J Natl Cancer Inst.* 1999;19:1051–1058

7. Birch JM. Genes and cancer. *Arch Dis Child.* 1999;80:1–3

8. Tomatis L, Kaldor JM, Bartsch H. Experimental studies in the assessment of human risk. In: Schottenfeld D, Fraumeni JF Jr, eds. *Cancer Epidemiology and Prevention.* 2nd ed. New York, NY: Oxford University Press; 1996:11–27

9. Council on Scientific Affairs. Harmful effects of ultraviolet radiation. *JAMA.* 1989;262:380–384

10. American Academy of Pediatrics Committee on Environmental Health. Ultraviolet light: a hazard to children. *Pediatrics.* 1999;104:328–333

11. Miller RW. Delayed effects of external radiation exposure: a brief history. *Radiat Res.* 1995;144:160–169

12. Pierce DA, Preston DL. Radiation-related cancer risks at low doses among atomic bomb survivors. *Radiat Res.* 2000;154:178–186

13. Miller RW, Boice JD Jr. Cancer after intrauterine exposure to the atomic bomb. *Radiat Res.* 1997;147:396–397

14. Bhatia S, Robison LL, Oberlin O, et al. Breast cancer and other second neoplasms after childhood Hodgkin's disease. *N Engl J Med.* 1996;334:745–751

15. Tronko MD, Bogdanova TI, Komissarenko IV, et al. Thyroid carcinoma in children and adolescents in Ukraine after the Chernobyl nuclear accident: statistical data and clinic morphologic characteristics. *Cancer.* 1999;86:149–156

16. Committee on Passive Smoking, Board on Environmental Studies and Toxicology, National Research Council. *Environmental Tobacco Smoke. Measuring Exposures and Assessing Health Effects.* Washington, DC: National Academies Press; 1986

17. Consensus conference. Health applications of smokeless tobacco use. *JAMA.* 1986;255:1045–1058
18. Willett WC. Diet and health: what should we eat? *Science.* 1994;264:532–537
19. Key TJ, Allen NE, Spencer EA, Travis RC. The effect of diet on risk of cancer. *Lancet.* 2002;360:861–868
20. Savitz DA, Chen JH. Parental occupation and childhood cancer: a review of epidemiologic studies. *Environ Health Perspect.* 1990;88:325–337
21. Miller RW. The discovery of human teratogens, carcinogens and mutagens: lessons for the future. In: Hollaender A, de Serres FJ, eds. *Chemical Mutagens: Principles and Methods for Their Detection.* Vol 5. New York, NY: Plenum Publishing Corp; 1978:101–126
22. Hill AB. The environment and disease: association or causation? *Proc R Soc Med.* 1965;58:295–300

# 36
# Chemical-Biological Terrorism

## History

Terrorism of all forms has the goal of producing injury, fear, or chaos. In recent years terrorist acts that once were confined to wartime have been directed against civilians, including children. The distribution of anthrax-containing letters through the US Postal Service in October 2001 is a recent example of a domestic terrorist incident; children were among the victims.

The release of a chemical or biological (chem-bio) weapon would have a tremendous impact on the environments in which children live.[1] In addition to the clinical issues that would arise after exposure to these agents, additional issues arise including the safety of water and food supplies and potential soil and air pollution. The principles of consequence management, designed to minimize morbidity and mortality after a chem-bio release, must involve multiple pediatric disciplines including environmental health, emergency medicine, behavioral medicine, and infectious diseases. Treatment plans must address the issues of recognition, triage, diagnosis, and management. Moreover, an effective partnership between government agencies and pediatricians must be forged to minimize the effects of terrorism on children.

The most common terrorist act directed at civilians is the hoax (eg, bomb threat, suspicious letter or package). True acts of destruction are placed in 5 categories: biological, nuclear, incendiary, chemical, and explosive. The creation of a weapon of mass destruction typically involves extensive planning, large amounts of money, and technological equipment. This is particularly true for biological weapons. Explosive, incendiary, and chemical devices can be much easier to prepare. Chemical and explosive weapons may simply be "weapons of opportunity" (ie, devices created for another purpose).[2] An example is a railcar carrying hazardous chemicals; an explosion could release the car's contents on a nearby community.

The 2 types of terrorism for which management plans have been best developed are chemical and biological.[1]

## Agents of Concern

### Chemical

The list of chemicals that have been developed for use as terrorist weapons is extensive (see Table 36.1). Agents in this class include nerve gases, mustard gas, and phosgene. Chemical agents may be designed for incapacitation rather than death (eg, lacrimators such as Mace).

**Table 36.1**
**Potential Chemical Agents for Use in Terrorism***

| Class | Examples |
|---|---|
| Nerve agents | Tabun<br>Sarin<br>Soman<br>VX |
| Vesicants | Mustard gas<br>Nitrogen mustard |
| Irritants/corrosives | Chlorine<br>Bromine<br>Ammonia |
| Choking agents | Phosgene |
| Cyanogens | Hydrogen cyanide |
| Incapacitating agents<br>  Central nervous system<br>    depressants | Cannabinoids<br>Barbiturates |
| Anticholinergics | 3-Quinuclidinyl benzilate (BZ) |
| Lacrimators | Capsaicin |

*From American Academy of Pediatrics Committee on Environmental Health, Committee on Infectious Diseases.[1]

Hallucinogens and other central nervous system (CNS) agents are designed to produce debilitating alterations in consciousness.[3-7]

The 1995 release of the nerve gas sarin in Japan demonstrated the ease with which a chemical agent can be dispersed and the resulting effects.[7] Relatively easy to manufacture, sarin, like all nerve agents, acts like an organophosphate pesticide, inhibiting the enzyme acetylcholinesterase. Victims of sarin gas exposure therefore present with a picture of cholinergic excess. Most common symptoms are miosis, nausea, and vomiting. More significant exposures produce lacrimation, salivation, and diarrhea. Moderate exposures to nerve agents result in stimulation of nicotinic receptors with muscle fasciculation and generalized weakness. Finally, severe exposures produce CNS toxicity, manifested as seizures and coma. Death from sarin results from respiratory failure or complications of CNS toxicity. Sarin also has unique chemical properties that enhance its toxicity. For example, it is denser than air and settles close to the ground, in the breathing zone of children. It is viscous and oily, leading to its deposition on clothing and skin. It is readily absorbed through intact skin as well as through standard barriers used by health care personnel, such as surgical gloves. Finally, because it can remain on clothing or skin until it is removed, it can secondarily affect anyone who handles a contaminated victim without wearing personal protective equipment. Sarin vapors can enter a building (or hospital) ventilation system and affect individuals throughout the structure.[8-10] Management of exposure to chemical weapons is found in several reviews.[2,3]

### Biological

Many infectious agents or their toxins have been weaponized to produce mass casualties after their dispersal. Unlike chemical agents in which the release is usually obvious and casualties appear promptly, biological agents can be released covertly. Further complicating bioweapon releases, victims appear over a period of days, with a significant delay to diagnosis.[11–13] Finally, because victims typically become ill away from the site of exposure, the release site can be very difficult to identify.

According to the National Academy of Sciences, there are 34 biological agents or toxins sufficiently developed for use as bioweapons (see Table 36.2).[6] Included among these are Category A agents that

- Can be easily disseminated or transmitted person-to-person
- Cause high mortality, with potential for major public health impact
- Have the greatest potential for causing public panic and social disruption

**Table 36.2**
**Potential Candidates for Biological Weapons Development\***

| Viruses | Rickettsia |
|---|---|
| Congo hemorrhagic fever | *Coxiella burnetii* (Q fever) |
| Eastern equine encephalitis | *Rickettsia prowazekii* (epidemic typhus) |
| Ebola virus | *Rickettsia rickettsii* (Rocky Mountain |
| Equine morbilli virus | spotted fever) |
| Lassa fever virus | Yellow fever virus |
| Marburg virus | |
| Rift Valley fever virus | **Fungi** |
| South American hemorrhagic fever | *Coccidioides immitis* |
| Tickborne encephalitis complex | (coccidioidomycosis) |
| Variola (smallpox) | |
| Venezuelan equine encephalitis virus | **Toxins** |
| Hantavirus | Abrun |
| Conotoxin | Aflatoxin |
| | Botulinum toxins |
| **Bacteria** | *C. perfringes* epsilon toxin |
| *Bacillus anthracis* (anthrax) | Ricin |
| *Brucella abortus, melitensis, suis* | Saxitoxin |
| *Burkholderia mallei* (glanders) | Shiga toxin |
| *Clostridium botulinum* (botulism) | Staphylococcal enterotoxin |
| *Francisella tularensis* (tularemia) | Tetrodotoxin |
| *Yersinia pestis* (plague) | T-2 toxin |
| | Microcystins |

\* From American Academy of Pediatrics Committee on Environmental Health, Committee on Infectious Diseases.[1]

The 6 Category A bioweapons are anthrax, plague, smallpox, tularemia, botulinum toxin, and viral hemorrhagic fevers. With public health efforts focusing on the Category A agents, hospitals, pediatricians, and government agencies are being called on to improve preparedness (eg, by stockpiling antibiotics, vaccines, and antidotes).[2,14,15] Assessment and treatment guidelines for exposure to biological weapons have been described.[1]

## Pediatric Implications
Children may be especially susceptible to the effects of biological agents because of their anatomic and physiologic differences from adults and their unique behavioral characteristics (see Table 36.3).[16]

## Identification of Sentinel Events
The many forms of terrorism require different needs in planning rapid and effective responses. Nuclear, incendiary, chemical, and explosive disasters have in common their immediate recognition. These types of events should be managed by existing principles of disaster management, including out-of-hospital triage, patient segregation, and

**Table 36.3**
**Factors Enhancing Children's Vulnerability to Biological Agents***

| Factor | Relevant Agents† |
|---|---|
| **Anatomic and physiologic differences**<br>- Increased surface area/volume ratio<br>- Higher minute ventilation | T-2 mycotoxins<br>All aerosolized agents |
| **Unique Susceptibility/Severity** | Smallpox, T-2 mycotoxins, VEE |
| **Developmental Considerations**<br>- Inability to flee dangerous situations<br>- Inability to cooperate with officials<br>- Inability to separate reality and fantasy | All agents |

*Adapted from Cieslak TJ, Henretig FM.[16]
†VEE, Venezuelan equine encephalitis.

careful appropriation of resources to receiving medical facilities. There will be additional needs (eg, decontamination of casualties) requiring the development of new protocols. Also, disaster systems may fail if care capacity is exceeded by patient volume. Appropriate planning for biological terrorism stands in stark contrast. After the covert release of a bioweapon, victims will appear over a period of several days; children and adults will seek medical attention with nonspecific complaints. Easily misdiagnosed, these victims may then go on to infect others before their clinical manifestations become more characteristic. Clinician education about biological weapons is therefore the cornerstone of effective planning.[17,18]

Key in the principles of consequence management for biological terrorism is the recognition that pediatricians, in emergency department and primary care settings, may be the first to encounter victims. Because early diagnosis and treatment have been shown to substantially reduce the number of affected individuals, it is essential for pediatricians to develop sufficient knowledge to recognize the first signal of a bioterrorist event. For example, initial cases of cutaneous anthrax in October 2001, including the sole pediatric patient, were mistaken for spider bite. All physicians must acquaint themselves with the signs and symptoms resulting from exposure to the most common of the biological weapons, namely anthrax, plague, smallpox, and botulism.[2]

## Triage, Management of Mass Casualties
Terrorist attacks commonly produce large numbers of casualties but an even larger number of "walking wounded" and "worried well," with the latter groups exceeding the seriously injured or infected patients by ratios as high as 10:1. This ratio would likely be magnified in a pediatric population because young children are unable to communicate effectively, leading parents to bring them to a health care provider for a thorough assessment. Depending on the number of victims in each group (well, wounded, and severely injured), clinical

sites, including pediatric offices and emergency departments, may become overwhelmed. In the 1995 sarin attack, patients came to emergency departments at a rate as high as 500 per hour, rapidly overwhelming hospital resources.[9] Moreover, because most of the patients came by foot, car, or taxi, there was no opportunity to perform out-of-hospital ("field") triage and separate healthy from contaminated patients. The principal lesson from that event is that office and hospital-based emergency planning must include contingencies for managing large numbers of victims (surge-capacity planning). Additional challenges will come in creating algorithms for the assessment of young, preverbal children.

### Treatment and Prophylaxis

Protocols for treatment and postexposure prophylaxis of children exposed to chem-bio weapons remain poorly developed. For example, in the case of chemical agents, some decontamination protocols have called for a 10-minute shower with soap or diluted bleach.[5] In children such a regimen risks hypothermia and serious skin or eye irritation. Also, management of children while wearing personal protective gear can be difficult. In the case of biological weapons, recommendations for pediatric patients have been poorly developed, although recommendations specific to children and pregnant women have been released.[16] With the exception of the smallpox vaccine, no vaccinations against bioweapons have been used in children. Antibiotics, antidotes, and other medical supplies may be quickly depleted. The Centers for Disease Control and Prevention (CDC), under its National Pharmaceutical Stockpile program, is amassing necessary materials for rapid delivery to any city in the event they are needed. A request for deployment of National Pharmaceutical Stockpile equipment is made to the CDC by a state or local board of health.

Hospital administrators also must consider how to protect hospitalized patients from an airborne release of chem-bio weapons. The

National Institute for Occupational Safety and Health has prepared guidance for protecting building environments from airborne chemical, biological, or radiological attacks.[19]

## Behavioral Consequences

All forms of terrorism, including hoaxes, can produce significant psychological trauma. However, the greatest potential for long-term or permanent behavioral disturbances is found in mass casualty incidents resulting in injury or death. As the events of September 11, 2001, proved, children can develop acute anxiety reaction, posttraumatic stress disorder, or other mental health illness after witnessing large-scale violence. Manifestations of anxiety in children can include difficulty sleeping, loss of appetite, headache, malaise, emotional lability, and difficulty concentrating.[20–22] Therefore, after a terrorist event pediatricians must educate parents about how to communicate with their children, limit their exposure to media reports, and recognize anxiety reactions. Additionally, community-level disaster preparedness should include the development of a network of mental health services for psychological victims of terrorism.

## Planning by Government

Rapid, effective response to terrorist acts relies on a number of government agencies. The federal public health infrastructure includes the US Department of Homeland Security, the US Department of Health and Human Services, the Federal Emergency Management Agency, the US Environmental Protection Agency, the US Department of Agriculture, and others. State and local agencies are essential collaborators in the process of disaster planning.

Acts of terrorism require not only the involvement of public health systems but also, as criminal acts, all branches of law enforcement including the Central Intelligence Agency, the Federal Bureau of Investigation, and state and local police. Terrorism, unlike natural disasters such as earthquakes, will, in unprecedented fashion, require that these systems work together. By necessity law enforcement may need to influence the clinical care provided (eg, collection of clothing and specimens as evidence, embargo of sensitive or classified information, immediate interrogation of victims). This poses challenges for pediatricians, emergency physicians, nurses, and other health care providers.

## Community Planning

Disaster planning also takes place at the community level. Important community activities include the identification of auditoriums and facilities capable of caring for large numbers in the event that a local area becomes uninhabitable. Alternate sites should be able to provide a 2- to 3-day supply of food, water, toiletries, and other basic needs.

Schools and child care facilities also must be included in community-level planning because children spend much of their time in these settings.[1] Issues in school planning include protocols for rapid evacuation of children, the identification of safe sites should a facility require immediate evacuation, mechanisms for notifying parents and reuniting them with their children as quickly as possible, arrangement of care for children whose parents are incapacitated or unable to reach them, the provision of first aid, and arrangements for *in loco parentis* treatment of children when their parents cannot be reached.

## Pediatrician Planning for Bioterrorism

The possibility of children or adolescents appearing in pediatricians' offices or health centers after exposure to a bioweapon requires that pediatricians in these settings (1) become knowledgeable about bioweapons and their clinical manifestations, (2) become effective educators and communicators to parents with anxieties and questions about bioterrorism and how its threat will affect their children, (3) ensure that their offices have plans and protocols that permit the evaluation of victims while protecting unaffected patients, and (4) develop surge-capacity protocols. Appropriate education of physicians about bioterrorism has been facilitated by the recent publication of Web sites, articles, monographs, brochures, and continuing education series. Additionally, Web sites that provide brochures and other reading materials for patients are being developed. The education and training of pediatricians will, in the future, be improved by the inclusion of a curriculum in medical schools and pediatric residencies. Office protocols for patient management will be necessary. Such planning may include a review of the office ventilation system and the availability of personal protective equipment. For many of these preparedness details, pediatricians can adopt algorithms currently being developed by federal agencies, the American Academy of Pediatrics and its Children, Terrorism & Disasters Web site (http://www.aap.org/terrorism/index.htm), and other organizations.

## Resource

The complete text of the *US Army Medical Research Institute of Infectious Diseases' Defense Against Toxin Weapons* is posted at: http://www.nbc-med.org/SiteContent/MedRef/OnlineRef/FieldManuals/datw/index.htm

## References

1. American Academy of Pediatrics Committee on Environmental Health, Committee on Infectious Diseases. Chemical-biological terrorism and its impact on children: a subject review. *Pediatrics*. 2000;105:662–670
2. Macintyre AG, Christopher GW, Eitzen EM Jr, et al. Weapons of mass destruction events with contaminated casualties: effective planning for health care facilities. *JAMA*. 2000;283:242–249
3. US Army Medical Research of Institute of Chemical Defense Chemical Casualty Care Division. *Field Management of Chemical Casualties Handbook*. Aberdeen Proving Ground, MD: US Army Medical Research Institute of Chemical Defense; 1996
4. Dunn MA, Sidell FR. Progress in medical defense against nerve agents. *JAMA*. 1989;262:649–652
5. Holstege CP, Kirk M, Sidell FR. Chemical warfare. Nerve agent poisoning. *Crit Care Clin*. 1997;13:923–942

6. National Research Council. *Chemical and Biological Terrorism—Research and Development to Improve Civilian Medical Response.* Washington, DC: National Academies Press; 1999

7. Okumura T, Takasu N, Ishimatsu S, et al. Report on 640 victims of the Tokyo subway sarin attack. *Ann Emerg Med.* 1996;28:129–135

8. Okumura T, Suzuki K, Fukuda A, et al. The Tokyo subway sarin attack: disaster management, Part 3: national and international responses. *Acad Emerg Med.* 1998;5:625–628

9. Okumura T, Suzuki K, Fukuda A, et al. The Tokyo subway sarin attack: disaster management, Part 2: hospital response. *Acad Emerg Med.* 1998;5:618–624

10. Okumura T, Suzuki K, Fukuda A, et al. The Tokyo subway sarin attack: disaster management, Part 1: community emergency response. *Acad Emerg Med.* 1998;5:613–617

11. Christopher GW, Cieslak TJ, Pavlin JA, Eitzen EM Jr. Biological warfare. A historical perspective. *JAMA.* 1997;278:412–417

12. Danzig R, Berkowsky PB. Why should we be concerned about biological warfare? *JAMA.* 1997;278:431–432

13. Holloway HC, Norwood AE, Fullerton CS, Engel CC Jr, Ursano RJ. The threat of biological weapons. Prophylaxis and mitigation of psychologic and social consequences. *JAMA.* 1997;278:425–427

14. Terriff CM, Tee AM. Citywide pharmaceutical preparation for bioterrorism. *Am J Health Syst Pharm.* 2001;58:233–237

15. Centers for Disease Control and Prevention. Update: Interim recommendations for antimicrobial prophylaxis for children and breastfeeding mothers and treatment of children with anthrax. *MMWR Morb Mortal Wkly Rep.* 2001;50:1014–1016

16. Cieslak TJ, Henretig FM. Bioterrorism. *Pediatr Ann.* 2003;32:154–165

17. Henretig FM, Cieslak TJ, Eitzen EM Jr. Biological and chemical terrorism. *J Pediatr.* 2002;141:311–326

18. Henretig FM, Cieslak TJ, Kortepeter MG, Fleisher GR. Medical management of the suspected victim of bioterrorism: an algorithmic approach to the undifferentiated patient. *Emerg Med Clin North Am.* 2002;20:351–364

19. Centers for Disease Control and Prevention. *Guidance for Protecting Building Environments from Chemical, Biological, or Radiological Attacks.* Washington, DC: National Institute for Occupational Safety and Health; 2002

20. American Academy of Pediatrics Committee on Psychosocial Aspects of Child and Family Health. How pediatricians can respond to the psychosocial implications of disasters. *Pediatrics.* 1999;103:521–523

21. Burkle FM Jr. Acute-phase mental health consequences of disasters: implications for triage and emergency medical services. *Ann Emerg Med.* 1996;28:119–128

22. Pynoos RS, Goenjian AK, Steinberg AM. A public mental health approach to the postdisaster treatment of children and adolescents. *Child Adolesc Psychiatry Clin North Am.* 1998;6:195–210

# 37
# Environmental Disparities

Children in poor or ethnic minority communities frequently suffer disproportionately from the effects of environmental pollution. Poor urban children often are in neighborhoods with poor air quality, live next to bodies of water contaminated with organic and inorganic pollutants, and occupy homes that are substandard, placing them at risk from exposure to environmental hazards.[1] These risks are much greater than those experienced by their wealthier classmates. Additionally, poor communities are relatively powerless compared with their more affluent neighbors and have fewer resources to protect their children from the environmental risks present.[2,3]

Disparities in the burden of illness and death experienced by minority groups such as blacks and American Indians/Alaska Natives, compared with the US population as a whole, have existed since the government began tracking health outcomes. Eliminating these disparities is a major goal of Healthy People 2010, the nation's health agenda for this decade.[4]

## Disparities in Mortality and Morbidity
Racial and ethnic differences in infant mortality and the prevalence and severity of many childhood diseases are well recognized. The degree to which environmental factors account for some of the differences in morbidity and mortality among race/ethnic groups is unknown, and further investigation is needed. There is no doubt, however, that environmental factors play a role in these differences.

### Infant Mortality
Since the early 1900s, the infant mortality rate in the United States has always been higher for black and American Indian infants than

for white infants.[5,6] The reasons for the racial disparities are not fully understood. Sudden infant death syndrome (SIDS) is a major contributor to excess infant mortality in nonwhites. The rate of deaths from SIDS is higher among Alaska Natives, American Indians, and blacks.[7,8] In addition to race/ethnicity, important environmental risk factors for SIDS include prone sleep position, maternal smoking during pregnancy, postnatal exposure to environmental tobacco smoke, and (possibly) exposure to outdoor air pollution.[9–11] Recent dramatic decreases have occurred in the infant mortality rate and the rate of SIDS among Alaska Natives and American Indians living in the Pacific Northwest.[12] The reason or reasons for the decreases are not fully understood.[13]

## Asthma

Puerto Rican, black, and Cuban American children in the United States have a higher prevalence of asthma than white children.[14–21] Black children are nearly twice as likely to have asthma as white children are. Blacks younger than 24 years are 3 to 4 times more likely to be hospitalized for asthma. Much of this increase is thought to be due to poverty rather than race.[22,23] Children of Hispanic mothers have a rate of asthma 2.5 times higher than that of whites and a rate more than 1.5 times higher than that of blacks.[24] Within the Hispanic population, the highest prevalence of asthma among children occurred in Puerto Ricans (11.2%), followed by Cuban Americans (5.2%) and Mexican Americans (2.7%). These data are in contrast to the incidence of asthma in non-Hispanic blacks (5.9%) and non-Hispanic whites (3.3%).[24]

## Infant Pulmonary Hemorrhage

Clusters of cases of acute pulmonary hemorrhage have been reported among infants in Cleveland, Chicago, and Detroit.[25–28] Most infants in these clusters have been black. It is not known whether race is a risk factor for infant pulmonary hemorrhage, or whether race is associated with socioeconomic status or with the prevalence of other specific risk factors, for which race may be a marker.[26]

## Disparities in Exposure

### Air Pollution Exposure

Minority children may experience greater exposure to polluted indoor and outdoor air. Indoors, they may have greater exposures to dust mites, molds, and cockroaches.[29] They also may live in neighborhoods with substandard outdoor air quality. For instance, 52% of all whites in the United States live in counties with high ozone concentrations. For blacks the figure is 62% and for Hispanics 71%. Higher percentages of blacks and Hispanics than whites reside in counties with higher levels of carbon monoxide, sulfur dioxide, nitrogen dioxide, lead, and particulate matter (see Table 37.1).[30]

### Food Exposure

Ethnic minorities may be exposed to certain chemical contaminants in the food supply due to dietary habits. Native Americans and subsistence fishing communities may be at much greater health risk from contaminants in fish. For example, the Penobscot Indian Nation has a fish consumption rate nearly twice the national average (see Chapter 27).

**Table 37.1**
**Proportions of Black, Hispanic, and White Populations Living in Air Quality Non-attainment Areas, 1992\***

|  | Percentage Living in Air Quality Non-attainment Areas | | |
| --- | --- | --- | --- |
| **Pollutant** | **Blacks** | **Hispanics** | **Whites** |
| Particulates | 16.5 | 34.0 | 14.7 |
| Carbon monoxide | 46.0 | 57.1 | 33.6 |
| Ozone | 62.2 | 71.2 | 52.5 |
| Sulfur dioxide | 12.1 | 5.7 | 7.0 |
| Lead | 9.2 | 18.5 | 6.0 |

\*From Department of Health and Human Services.[2,3]

## *Lead Exposure*

Despite recent large declines in blood lead levels, young children of low-income, urban minority families have a higher prevalence of blood lead levels above 10 µg/dL. From 1991 to 1994, an estimated 11.2% of black, 4% of Hispanic American, and 2.3% of white non-Hispanic children younger than 6 years had blood lead levels above 10 µg/dL.[31] Eight percent of low-income children had blood lead levels above 10 µg/dL, compared with 1% of children from high-income families (see Table 37.2). Heavy metal poisoning in disadvantaged populations is thought to be related to substandard housing. Some Latin American families use traditional ceramic ware for cooking and food storage, which has lead in the glazing and can leach into the food.

**Table 37.2**
**Percentage of Children Aged 1–5 Years With Blood Lead Levels (BLLs) ≥10 µg/dL and Weighted Geometric Mean (GM) by Year Housing Built and Selected Characteristics***

| Characteristic | Year Housing Built | | | Total | |
|---|---|---|---|---|---|
| | Before 1946 % | 1946–1973 % | After 1973 % | % | GM BLL (µg/dL) |
| **Race/Ethnicity** | | | | | |
| Black/non-Hispanic | 21.9 | 13.7 | 3.4 | 11.2 | 4.3 |
| Mexican American | 13.0 | 2.3 | 1.6 | 4.0 | 3.1 |
| White, non-Hispanic | 5.6 | 1.4 | 1.5 | 2.3 | 2.3 |
| **Income** | | | | | |
| Low | 16.4 | 7.3 | 4.3 | 8.0 | 3.8 |
| Middle | 4.1 | 2.0 | 0.4 | 1.9 | 2.3 |
| High | 0.9 | 2.7 | 0.0 | 1.0 | 1.9 |
| **Urban status** | | | | | |
| Population ≥1 million | 11.5 | 5.8 | 0.8 | 5.4 | 2.8 |
| Population <1 million | 5.8 | 3.1 | 2.5 | 3.3 | 2.7 |
| **Total** | 8.6 | 4.6 | 1.6 | 4.4 | 2.7 |

*From Centers for Disease Control and Prevention.[31]

## Pesticide Exposure

More than 3 decades ago, several surveys reported that levels of dichlorodiphenyltrichloroethane (DDT) and its metabolites (in fat or blood) were higher in blacks than in whites.[32] In a community in Florida, DDT and dichlorodiphenyldichloroethene levels in blood were significantly lower in the affluent groups than in the low-income groups, in blacks and whites. However, in comparable income groups, blacks had higher DDT levels than whites.[32]

Children of farmworkers may accompany their parents to the fields, live in housing contaminated by direct pesticide spray or drift from nearby fields, and work in the fields themselves.[33] Farmworkers can bring home pesticides on their shoes, clothes, and skin, and then transfer them to their children, food, and home environment. A recent California Department of Health Services pilot project suggests a potential for higher residential exposure to some pesticides for children of farmworkers as opposed to children of non-farmworkers. Dust samples were obtained from homes within a quarter mile of agricultural fields where approximately 50 agricultural pesticides were used. A total of 10 different pesticides were detected.[34] Half of the homes had at least 1 resident who was a farmworker. The pesticides diazinon and chlorpyrifos were detected only in the homes of farmworkers. In the homes of 2 farmworkers, risk estimates for diazinon ingestion suggested that the toddlers' exposure to house dust may exceed the US Environmental Protection Agency's chronic oral reference dose.

## Rituals

In certain ethnic groups, rituals may be potential sources of exposure to environmental contaminants. For example, some Hispanic Americans who practice Santeria may sprinkle elemental mercury in the house, possibly resulting in elevated levels of mercury in the indoor air (see Chapter 20). Lead and other toxic metals are used in some Latin American and Asian traditional medicines that are given to children.

## Water Exposure

Many small, rural, or low-income neighborhoods do not have access to safe and affordable drinking water supplies. Some water contamination problems may affect certain populations disproportionately. There are situations where certain racial and socioeconomic populations are exposed to higher levels of contaminants in water than is the general population, such as deteriorating pipes/solder in old homes and fertilizer runoff into rural water supplies.[35]

## Waste Sites

The siting of hazardous waste sites may occur disproportionately in minority neighborhoods. A report by the United Church of Christ's Commission for Racial Justice revealed that 3 of the 5 largest hazardous waste landfills in the United States were in black or Hispanic neighborhoods and that the mean percentage of minority residents in areas with toxic waste sites was twice that of areas without toxic waste sites.[36] Table 37.3 shows that a higher proportion of blacks and Hispanics and people living below the poverty level live in or near census tracts with waste treatment, storage, and disposal facilities. In 1994, in recognition of the disproportionate impact of environ-

**Table 37.3**
**Proportions of Certain Racial/Ethnic and Lower Socioeconomic Populations in Census Tracts Surrounding Waste Treatment, Storage, and Disposal Facilities (TSDF) Compared to the Proportions of Those Groups in Other Census Tracts, 1994**

| Location of TSDFs | Blacks % | Hispanics % | Persons Living Below the Poverty Level % |
|---|---|---|---|
| Census tracts containing TSDFs or with at least 50% of their area within 2.5 miles of a tract with TSDF | 24.7 | 10.7 | 19.0 |
| Census tracts without TSDFs | 13.6 | 7.3 | 13.1 |

*From Department of Health and Human Services.[2,3]

mental hazards on low-income communities, President Clinton issued an Executive Order seeking to achieve environmental justice.[37]

Children in poverty face an array of formidable challenges in their lives. Environmental health sciences education is an essential tool for achieving environmental equity and protecting children.[38] Pediatricians must work together to protect children, especially those living in low-income or minority communities, from environmental threats to their health.

## Practical Recommendations for Clinicians

Health supervision of children from ethnic minority groups requires a knowledge of the unique environmental risks of the neighborhood or community, a high index of suspicion for environmental causes of disease, and a willingness to work with local health officials to sort out public health issues and make the appropriate referrals. The pediatrician should consider the following:

- Build a network to learn about environmental concerns within the community. Meet and establish relationships with the local, county, or state environmental health unit.
- Actively learn the history of environmental illness that has affected various ethnic and minority groups within your practice. The special problems may vary between urban and rural settings, and between racial and minority groups. Ask parents and community leaders when possible for their perceptions of environmental exposure and disease.
- Tailor the environmental history to local conditions, risks, and concerns.
- Consider local cultural practices that may lead to environmental exposures and risk for illness. These may range from subsistence fishing in waters contaminated with polychlorinated biphenyls to use of unusual substances in cooking, home building, and home remedies.

- Speak out on behalf of these children before local, state, and national groups.

## Resource

National Institute of Child Health and Human Development (NICHD), Internet: http://www.nichd.nih.gov. The NICHD, the National Black Child Development Institute, and the Health Resources and Services Administration have developed the Resource Kit for Reducing the Risk of Sudden Infant Death Syndrome in African American Communities. To receive the resource kit, call 800-505-CRIB or go to the NICHD Web site at http://www.nichd.nih.gov/sids/sidspubskey.cfm.

## References

1. Powell DL, Stewart V. Children. The unwitting target of environmental injustices. *Pediatr Clin North Am.* 2001;48:1291–1305
2. Department of Health and Human Services. Understanding and improving health. In: *Healthy People 2010.* 2nd ed. Washington, DC: US Government Printing Office; 2000
3. Department of Health and Human Services. Objectives for improving health. In: *Healthy People 2010.* 2nd ed. Washington, DC: US Government Printing Office; 2000
4. Institute of Medicine. *Toward Environmental Justice—Research, Education, and Health Policy Needs.* Washington, DC: National Academies Press; 1999
5. MacDorman MF, Atkinson JO. Infant mortality statistics from the linked birth/infant death data set—1995 period data. *Mon Vital Stat Rep.* 1998;46 (6 suppl 2):1–22
6. Grossman DC, Baldwin LM, Casey S, Nixon B, Hollow W, Hart LG. Disparities in infant health among American Indians and Alaska Natives in US metropolitan areas. *Pediatrics.* 2002;109:627–633
7. Irwin KL, Mannino S, Daling J. Sudden infant death syndrome in Washington State: why are Native American infants at greater risk than white infants? *J Pediatr.* 1992;121:242–247
8. Oyen N, Bulterys M, Welty TK, Kraus JF. Sudden unexplained infant deaths among American Indians and whites in North and South Dakota. *Paediatr Perinat Epidemiol.* 1990;4:175–183

9. American Academy of Pediatrics, AAP Task Force on Infant Positioning and SIDS. Positioning and SIDS. *Pediatrics.* 1992;89:1120–1126

10. MacDorman MF, Cnattingius S, Hoffman HJ, Kramer MS, Haglund B. Sudden infant death syndrome and smoking in the United States and Sweden. *Am J Epidemiol.* 1997;146:249–257

11. Woodruff TJ, Grillo J, Schoendorf KC. The relationship between selected causes of postneonatal infant mortality and particulate air pollution in the United States. *Environ Health Perspect.* 1997;105:608–612

12. Centers for Disease Control and Prevention. Decrease in infant mortality and sudden infant death syndrome among Northwest American Indians and Alaskan Natives—Pacific Northwest, 1985–1996. *MMWR Morb Mortal Wkly Rep.* 1999;48:181–184

13. Centers for Disease Control and Prevention. Guidelines for death scene investigation of sudden, unexplained infant deaths: recommendations of the Interagency Panel on Sudden Infant Death Syndrome. *MMWR Morb Mortal Wkly Rep.* 1996;45(No. RR-10):1–22

14. Gergen PJ, Mullally DI, Evans R III. National survey of prevalence of asthma among children in the United States, 1976 to 1980. *Pediatrics.* 1988;81:1–7

15. Schwartz J, Gold D, Dockery DW, Weiss ST, Speizer FE. Predictors of asthma and persistent wheeze in a national sample of children in the United States. Association with social class, perinatal events, and race. *Am Rev Respir Dis.* 1990;142:555–562

16. Weitzman M, Gortmaker S, Sobol A. Racial, social, and environmental risks for childhood asthma. *Am J Dis Child.* 1990;144:1189–1194

17. Weitzman M, Gortmaker SL, Sobol AM, Perrin JM. Recent trends in the prevalence and severity of childhood asthma. *JAMA.* 1992;268:2673–2677

18. Cunningham J, Dockery DW, Speizer FE. Race, asthma, and persistent wheeze in Philadelphia schoolchildren. *Am J Public Health.* 1996;86:1406–1409

19. Centers for Disease Control and Prevention. Asthma mortality and hospitalization among children and young adults—United States, 1980–1993. *MMWR Morb Mortal Wkly Rep.* 1996;45:350–353

20. Ray NF, Thamer M, Fadillioglu B, Gergen PJ. Race, income, urbanicity, and asthma hospitalization in California: a small area analysis. *Chest.* 1998;113:1277–1284

21. Gergen PJ, Weiss KB. Changing patterns of asthma hospitalization among children: 1979 to 1987. *JAMA.* 1990;264:1688–1692

22. Wissow LS, Gittelsohn AM, Szklo M, Starfield B, Mussman M. Poverty, race, and hospitalization for childhood asthma. *Am J Public Health.* 1988;78:777–782

23. Crain EF, Weiss KB, Bijur PE, Hersh M, Westbrook L, Stein RE. An estimate of the prevalence of asthma and wheezing among inner-city children. *Pediatrics.* 1994;94:356–362

24. Beckett WS, Belanger K, Gent JF, Holford TR, Leaderer BP. Asthma among Puerto Rican Hispanics: a multi-ethnic comparison study of risk factors. *Am J Respir Crit Care Med.* 1996;154:894–899

25. Centers for Disease Control and Prevention. Acute pulmonary hemorrhage/ hemosiderosis among infants—Cleveland, January 1993–November 1994. *MMWR Morb Mortal Wkly Rep.* 1994;43:881–883

26. Centers for Disease Control and Prevention. Acute pulmonary hemorr-hage among infants—Chicago, April 1992–November 1994. *MMWR Morb Mortal Wkly Rep.* 1995;44:67, 73–74

27. Pappas MD, Sarnaik AP, Meert KL, Hasan RA, Lieh-Lai MW. Idiopathic pulmonary hemorrhage in infancy. Clinical features and management with high frequency ventilation. *Chest.* 1996;110:553–555

28. Dearborn DG, Smith PG, Bahms BB, et al. Clinical profile of 30 infants with acute pulmonary hemorrhage in Cleveland. *Pediatrics.* 2002;110:627–637

29. Sarpong SB, Hamilton RG, Eggleston PA, Adkinson NF Jr. Socioeconomic status and race as risk factors for cockroach allergen exposure and sensiti-zation in children with asthma. *J Allergy Clin Immunol.* 1996;97:1393–1401

30. Wennette DR, Nieves LA. Breathing polluted air. *EPA J.* March/April 1992

31. Centers for Disease Control and Prevention. Update: blood lead levels— United States, 1991–1994. *MMWR Morb Mortal Wkly Rep.* 1997;46:141–146

32. Davies JE, Edmundson WF, Raffonelli A, Cassady JC, Morgade C. The role of social class in human pesticide pollution. *Am J Epidemiol.* 1972;96:334–341

33. Zahm SH, Devesa SS. Childhood cancer: overview of incidence trends and environmental carcinogens. *Environ Health Perspect.* 1995;103 (suppl 6):177–184

34. Bradman MA, Harnly ME, Draper W, et al. Pesticide exposures to children from California's Central Valley: results of a pilot study. *J Expo Anal Environ Epidemiol.* 1997;7:217–234

35. Calderon RL, Johnson CC Jr, Craun GF, et al. Health risks from contaminated water: do class and race matter? *Toxicol Ind Health.* 1993;9:879–900

36. Commission for Racial Justice, United Church of Christ. *Toxic Wastes and Race in the United States: A National Study of the Racial and Socioeconomic Characteristics of Communities with Hazardous Waste Sites;* 1987

37. Presidential executive order on environmental justice. *Fed Regist.* 1994;54. EO 12898

38. Claudio L, Torres T, Sanjurjo E, Sherman LR, Landrigan PJ. Environmental health sciences education—a tool for achieving environmental equity and protecting children [commentary]. *Environ Health Perspect.* 1998;106:849–855

# 38
# Multiple Chemical Sensitivities

## Definition

Multiple Chemical Sensitivity (MCS), also known as "Environmental Illness" or "Idiopathic Environmental Intolerance" is a highly controversial condition. There is overlap between the MCS syndrome and other ill-defined conditions such as fibromyalgia, chronic fatigue syndrome, and Gulf War syndrome. Although the complaint of MCS most commonly is seen in adults, conditions attributed to MCS are reported to occur in children.[1] To answer parental concerns, pediatricians should be familiar with the condition.

Multiple Chemical Sensitivity has been defined as an acquired, chronic disorder characterized by recurrent symptoms, referable to multiple organ systems, occurring reproducibly in response to exposure to many chemically unrelated compounds at doses far below those established in the general population to cause harmful effects.[2,3] No single test or physiologic function correlates with MCS; the symptoms improve when the incitants are removed. In contradistinction to the "sick building syndrome," symptoms are not associated with a single physical environment, but can occur anywhere.

## Clinical Symptoms

People with MCS complain of a myriad of symptoms when exposed to low levels of a wide variety of chemically unrelated substances. Adults with MCS often can recall an initial sensitizing exposure to an overpowering chemical, often occurring in the workplace. Their symptoms can involve any organ system and commonly include headache, fatigue, gastrointestinal problems, joint and muscle pains, skin problems, and upper respiratory tract problems. Most patients will have neurologic or neuropsychological symptoms (such as "mental fog" or impaired cognition, confusion, memory loss, paresthesias, irritability, and depression) as prominent features of the syndrome. Other symptoms often include malaise, headache, dizziness, burning sensations, and breathlessness. In children, hyperactivity and attention deficits have been cited by some as developmental consequences of MCS.[4]

Over time, a person's sensitivity increases and decreases; sensitivity also expands from a single "inciting" chemical to a wide variety of unrelated substances. Pesticides, perfumes, aftershaves, copy machine emissions, cigarette smoke, formaldehyde, nylon fabrics, rayon material, and gases released from new carpets are substances commonly implicated in MCS.[5] Some people with MCS complain of foul odors (cacosmia) from chemicals or perfumes as triggers for their symptoms. The olfactory nerve mediates odor perception, while branches of the trigeminal nerve perceive irritation and pungency for taste and smell. Odor seems to be a prominent factor in precipitating the symptoms of MCS and serves as an important warning for the presence of toxic exposures. Most investigators agree that an explanation of the role of odor is a necessary component of any model of the causes of MCS.

Reportedly, symptoms also can migrate from one target organ system to another over time (switching). The progressive nature of symptoms titered to smaller and smaller doses of precipitants, the olfactory warning of offending odors, and the progressive restrictions on the patient's activities and habitable environments all characterize this condition.

### Epidemiology

One major difficulty in studying the epidemiology of MCS is the lack of a case definition agreed on by the medical and scientific community. Many published reports of MCS consist of case series or the clinical experiences of referral practices; none describe affected children. Small surveys have estimated the prevalence rates of self-reported MCS syndrome among adults to be about 12%,[6,7] although one subspecialty-based study (allergy, otolaryngology, occupational medicine) found an overall prevalence rate of MCS ranging from 5% to 27% of referrals.[8] None of these studies included children.

## Historical Background

The late Theron Randolph, an allergist from Chicago, IL, first described MCS during the 1950s.[9] He believed that traditional allergists defined "sensitivity" too narrowly by limiting it exclusively to antibody-antigen reactions. In contrast, Dr Randolph hypothesized that foods and chemicals might cause other derangements of the immune system. He postulated that increasing exposure to petroleum products, pesticides, synthetic textiles, and food additives in modern life were responsible for his patients' health problems, which included mental and behavioral disturbances, as well as rhinitis, headache, and asthma. A group of physicians, often called clinical ecologists, who supported Dr Randolph's concept of environmental illness founded the American Academy of Environmental Medicine.

In several position papers, traditional medical organizations have questioned the scientific basis of MCS. The subspecialty of allergy, as represented by the American Academy of Allergy, Asthma & Immunology, asserted that there were no adequate studies to support the theories of the clinical ecologists and, in 1986, issued a position statement stating that the diagnostic and therapeutic principles of clinical ecology were based on unproven and experimental methods.[10] Similarly, the American College of Physicians in 1989 and the American Medical Association in 1992 criticized clinical ecology.[11,12] A position statement by the American College of Occupational and Environmental Medicine in 1999 called for more research into the "phenomenon" of MCS.[13]

## Proposed Causative Mechanisms

A number of different models have been proposed to explain MCS. A model of immunologic dysfunction postulates that chemicals may damage the immune system so that it no longer functions normally. However, no clinical laboratory, other than those associated with clinical ecologists, has found consistent immune abnormalities in patients with MCS.[14] Investigators also have proposed a classic conditioned response to odor as an explanation for MCS. After an initial traumatic exposure to a strong-smelling odor, subsequent exposure may cause a conditioned response to much lower concentrations of the chemical. This conditioned response may be accompanied by varying degrees of "stimulus generalization" to the development of symptoms in response to other strong odors. Some researchers have suggested that an extreme form of this response be called an "odor-triggered panic attack."[15] Affective disorders, somatoform disorders, and anxiety are the most frequent psychological conditions used to explain MCS.[16] Some studies have shown that people in whom MCS develops have a high degree of preexisting psychiatric morbidity and a tendency toward somatization.[17] These findings suggest that psychological factors, although not necessarily causative, seem to predispose some people to the development of a generalized chemical sensitivity. Comorbidities such as posttraumatic stress disorder or childhood physical or sexual abuse also may have roles as underlying determinants of vulnerability to the later development of MCS.[18]

The limbic-olfactory model of MCS provides a speculative biological explanation for the affective and cognitive symptoms. The model depends on the anatomic links between the olfactory nerve, the limbic system, and other regions of the brain. Subconvulsive kindling (the ability of a subthreshold electrical or chemical stimulus to cause a response) and time-dependent sensitization are central nervous system constructs that provide a mechanism by which low-level chemical exposures can be amplified and produce symptoms referable to multiple organ systems.[19] Other proposed causes of MCS, such as neuropathic porphyria[20] or hypersensitization to yeast, are unsubstantiated.

## Clinical Evaluation of a Child Believed to Have Chemical Sensitivity

The pediatrician should approach the evaluation of a child whose parents believe that MCS is the cause of the child's symptoms in the same manner as any other problem: with a history, a physical examination, and a methodical work-up. Table 38.1 offers some diagnostic criteria that, while not studied systematically, may be applicable to children. By using the patient history and selecting appropriate clinical tests, the pediatrician should rule out conditions that are part of

Table 38.1
Diagnostic Elements of MCS Syndrome in Children*

| |
|---|
| **Nature of Incitants Provoking a Response** |
| • Responses to offending environmental toxicants occur at levels of exposure below the 2.5 percentile for responses in the general population. |
| • Child responds to multiple substances that are unrelated chemically. The symptoms are not confined to one environment (eg, only "sick" buildings). |
| **Biological Plausibility, Identifiable Exposure** |
| • Symptoms are reproducible with exposure with reasonable consistency. |
| • Symptoms resolve after removal of incitant exposures. |
| • An identifiable exposure preceded the onset of the problem. |
| **Topology of Responses** |
| • Adverse responses affect more than one body system. |
| • Primary complaints include neuropsychological symptoms. |
| • The child exhibits altered sensitivity to odor. |
| • The disorder is chronic. |
| **Diagnosis** |
| • No single, accepted test of physiological function correlates with the symptoms. |
| **Subjective Responses and Ameliorative Actions of Affected Children** |
| • The caretakers and/or child perceive the child's response as unpleasant. |
| • The family has sought professional advice. |
| • The individual's caretakers believe he or she has a disorder. |
| • The family takes action to avoid exposures to symptom-inducing chemicals. |

*Modified from Nethercott JR, Davidoff LL, Curbow B, Abbey H.[21]

the differential diagnosis. Other diseases to consider are those with symptoms that are nonspecific and inconstant, including Lyme disease, Munchausen by proxy, or psychosocial problems such as school phobia. The assessment should be directed toward the exclusion of other diagnoses, such as asthma, migraine, allergies, or an autoimmune disease. Specific environmental causes of systemic illness should be considered. Carbon monoxide poisoning, for example, can produce generalized complaints such as headache, fatigue, dizziness, nausea, and aches and pains. Chronic poisoning with heavy metals such as arsenic or lead can sometimes be manifested by behavioral symptoms and appetite disturbances. Upper respiratory tract symptoms often are encountered, and the possibility that the child has allergies should be considered. Although rhinorrhea, nasal obstruction, and sneezing are the most obvious allergic symptoms, atopic children may present with fatigue and irritability due to chronic upper respiratory tract problems and lack of sleep. Allergic stigmata found on physical examination, supported with appropriate skin testing, will suggest a diagnosis of allergy. Headache and dizziness, common complaints in MCS, can be manifestations of sinus disease.

Psychiatric disorders of the parents and/or children, dysfunctional family dynamics, or even child abuse and neglect must be considered in the evaluation of children presenting for assessment of MCS syndrome. A positive family history for psychiatric diagnoses and treatment may be common in children presenting with a possible diagnosis of MCS. The evaluation of MCS in children should include a careful family history of psychiatric conditions. For some families, the illness may serve as a coping strategy or a more socially acceptable medical condition within which to express depressive symptoms. Children may be attracted to the attention they gain when they are in the dependency role of patient.

## Diagnostic Methods

No laboratory tests are diagnostic for MCS, and none are recommended for its evaluation. A number of unproven tests have been proposed for the diagnosis of MCS. For example, the use of positron emission tomography and single photon emission computed tomography scans has not been standardized or validated and is not recommended. Diagnostic provocation-neutralization tests with different chemicals ("desensitization" routines of frequent injections or sublingual or dermal application of incitants), advocated by clinical ecologists, have been repudiated as being without scientific basis or validity. The American College of Physicians reviewed 15 studies of provocation-neutralization testing performed by clinical ecologists and criticized the introduction of bias, lack of controls, and their uniformly poor methodological designs.[11]

Testing of hair, blood, urine, or other tissues to screen for environmental chemicals generally is not helpful. When appropriate, laboratory testing to rule out other diagnoses or underlying medical conditions should be performed. Testing should be done only at laboratories that adhere to the guidelines for quality control established through the Clinical Laboratory Improvement Act.

## Treatment

The demands of adult patients with MCS on health care professionals, their high use of health care resources, and their dissatisfaction with proffered advice, especially if that advice suggests psychological counseling as a management option, are frustrating for patient and practitioner. They are high-frequency users of medical facilities and suffer a considerable amount of functional disability because of their complaints and the strategies they must employ to get through the day. Parental overuse of care services can be frustrating to pediatric health care providers, who must nevertheless continue to offer their availability and support in the best interests of the child.

Proposed therapies for MCS syndrome include restricted, rotating diets, provocation-neutralization, and the use of saunas for chemical detoxification. Patients with MCS syndrome seek out a variety of treatments, not only from physicians but also clinical ecologists, naturopaths, and other practitioners. Clinical ecologists and other alternative practitioners may recommend herbs, oxygen, oral nystatin, and minerals to treat their patients by improving their "tolerance" of the environment. Some postulate that MCS sufferers have deficits of essential cofactors or enzymes necessary for chemical "detoxification"; they prescribe dietary supplements, herbs, antioxidants, and vitamins to repair such deficiencies. Some therapies used to treat MCS hold special risks for children; their use should be discouraged. Parents should be warned against potentially harmful and expensive remedies, such as chelation, gamma globulin injections, catharsis, or "sweat therapies" as advocated by some practitioners, when there is little scientific evidence that these are effective for the treatment of MCS. Desensitization, herbs, or vitamins may be especially harmful to children who are still developing. Children may have limited capacity to detoxify certain herbs, minerals, hormones, and dietary supplements through the liver and kidneys, with a consequent higher risk of toxic reactions. They may experience allergic reactions to such substances as well as those used in "desensitization" routines.

Many patients restrict their activities and reconstruct their habitats so that they can avoid those environmental agents causing symptoms, essentially living in a relatively chemical-free environment. Some adults use barrier clothing such as special masks, gloves, coveralls, and even self-contained breathing apparatus in the attempt to avoid chemical triggers. The disability in adults is such that they often isolate themselves from others socially and cannot hold a job. Children who cannot attend school or develop normal peer relationships because of MCS syndrome would be similarly disabled.

Newer inventories show promise for standardizing the diagnosis and measuring the impact and severity of MCS.[22] Biopsychological modalities of management, including biofeedback, electrophysiological monitoring, coping strategies, family-centered therapy, and behavioral modification (psychological deconditioning) techniques are worth investigating in children.[23] Breaking through any mistrust of families and their hostility to allopathic medicine is important. Offering to work with families should extend to collaboration with school systems, social services, and other community-based agencies in helping families cope with the illness.

## Conclusions

Examining a child purported to have MCS is a challenge for the pediatrician who is faced with treating the child's health as it fits into the family's belief system. Exploring the basis for the beliefs and keeping an open mind to the different values that underlie them will allow effective and compassionate use of the pediatrician's medical knowledge and skills.

## Frequently Asked Questions

Q  *I have been told that my child has a short attention span and that he frequently is inattentive in class. The teacher has suggested psychological testing. My child is fine at home. Could these problems be related to chemical exposure at school?*

A  A thorough evaluation of the child's difficulty and appropriate testing are initial steps in dealing with this problem. Sources of potential environmental contamination cited in schools include cleaning agents, art supplies (glues, markers, and aerosol sprays), pesticides, and diesel exhaust fumes from school buses. Dust and molds also are sources of pollution. Symptoms in one setting only (the school) may suggest an environmental etiology. While performing a thorough evaluation, pediatricians also should keep in mind, however, that parental anxieties about learning and behavior problems might focus on concern about chemical exposure in the schools.

Q *My child is being made sick by the chemicals that she is exposed to in school. Can you, as my pediatrician, intervene and help me decrease my child's exposure to chemicals in the school?*

A Parents often ask pediatricians to write a letter supporting the child's withdrawal from some activity or area in the school. In these instances, the pediatrician should be open-minded but careful about fostering negative associations between the child and the child's environment. Another issue raised by this question is less obvious but of crucial importance in considering the problem of chemical sensitivity: the patient's causal attribution of symptoms to MCS. At present, MCS is defined in terms of the patient's report of a temporal relationship between perceived exposures to chemicals and the appearance of symptoms. In the case of children, the situation is complicated because it usually is the parent who attributes the child's symptoms to chemical exposure. While there might be a temporal relationship between the exposure and symptoms, the association may not be causal.

Q *What do I need to do to my home to prevent my child from being exposed to chemicals that might be toxic?*

A It is important for parents to understand that their child's exposure to chemicals is cumulative: the sum of inhalation, ingestion, and dermal exposures. Parents should be encouraged to consider all activities and situations in which their child might be exposed. The home inventory is designed to alert parents to potentially toxic exposures in the home (see Chapter 5). The school environment may be a source of additional exposures to chemicals (see Chapter 30). One of the most common environmental exposures is to environmental tobacco smoke (ETS)—thus one of the most important things parents can do is to try to decrease their child's exposure to ETS.

# References

1. Woolf A. A 4-year-old girl with manifestations of multiple chemical sensitivities. *Environ Health Perspect.* 2000;108:1219–1223

2. Cullen MR. The worker with multiple chemical sensitivities: an overview. *Occup Med.* 1987;2:655–661

3. Multiple chemical sensitivity: a 1999 consensus. *Arch Environ Health.* 1999;54:147–149

4. Kidd PM. Attention deficit/hyperactivity disorder (ADHD) in children: rationale for its integrative management. *Altern Med Rev.* 2000;5:402–428

5. Hu H, Stern A, Rotnitzky A, Schlesinger L, Proctor S, Wolfe J. Development of a brief questionnaire for screening for multiple chemical sensitivity syndrome. *Toxicol Ind Health.* 1999;15:582–588

6. Kreutzer R, Neutra RR, Lashuay N. Prevalence of people reporting sensitivities to chemicals in a population-based survey. *Am J Epidemiol.* 1999;150:1–12

7. Meggs WJ, Dunn KA, Bloch RM, Goodman PE, Davidoff AL. Prevalence and nature of allergy and chemical sensitivity in a general population. *Arch Environ Health.* 1996;51:275–282

8. Kutsogiannis DJ, Davidoff AL. A multiple center study of multiple chemical sensitivity syndrome. *Arch Environ Health.* 2001;56:196–207

9. Randolph TG. Sensitivity to petroleum including its derivatives and antecedents. *J Lab Clin Med.* 1952;40:931–932

10. Executive Committee of the American Academy of Allergy and Immunology. Clinical ecology. *J Allergy Clin Immunol.* 1986;78:269–271

11. American College of Physicians. Clinical ecology. *Ann Intern Med.* 1989;111:168–178

12. Council on Scientific Affairs, American Medical Association. Clinical ecology. *JAMA.* 1992;268:3465–3467

13. College of Occupational and Environmental Medicine. ACOEM position statement. Multiple chemical sensitivities: idiopathic environmental intolerance. *J Occup Environ Med.* 1999;41:940–942

14. Simon GE, Daniell W, Stockbridge H, Claypoole K, Rosenstock L. Immunologic, psychological, and neuropsychological factors in multiple chemical sensitivity. A controlled study. *Ann Intern Med.* 1993;119:97–103

15. Staudenmayer H. Multiple chemical sensitivities or idiopathic environmental intolerances: psychophysiologic foundation of knowledge for a psychogenic explanation. *J Allergy Clin Immunol.* 1997;99:434–437

16. Terr AI. Environmental illness. A clinical review of 50 cases. *Arch Intern Med.* 1986;146:145–149

17. Black DW, Rathe A, Goldstein RB. Environmental illness. A controlled study of 26 subjects with "20th century disease." *JAMA*. 1990;264: 3166–3170

18. Black DW, Okiishi C, Gable J, Schlosser S. Psychiatric illness in the first-degree relatives of persons reporting multiple chemical sensitivities. *Toxicol Ind Health*. 1999;15:410–414

19. Ross PM, Whyser J, Covello VT, et al. Olfaction and symptoms in the multiple chemical sensitivities syndrome. *Prev Med*. 1999;28:467–480

20. Ellefson RD, Ford RE. The porphyrias: characteristics and laboratory tests. *Regul Toxicol Pharmacol*. 1996;24:S119–S125

21. Nethercott JR, Davidoff LL, Curbow B, Abbey H. Multiple chemical sensitivities syndrome: toward a working case definition. *Arch Environ Health*. 1993;48:19–26

22. Miller CS, Prihoda TJ. The Environmental Exposure and Sensitivity Inventory (EESI): a standardized approach for measuring chemical intolerances for research and clinical applications. *Toxicol Ind Health*. 1999;15:370–385

23. Spyker DA. Multiple chemical sensitivities—syndrome and solution. *J Toxicol Clin Toxicol*. 1995;33:95–99

# 39
# Nontherapeutic Use of Antibiotics in Animal Agriculture

Antibiotic resistance in many pediatric pathogens is widespread, including infectious agents encountered in community-acquired (eg, *Campylobacter* spp, *Salmonella* spp) and hospital-acquired (eg, *Enterococcus* spp, *Staphylococcus aureus*) infections. Overuse or misuse of antibiotics in veterinary and human medicine is responsible for much of the resistance. Between 40% and 80% of the antibiotics used in the United States each year are used in chickens, turkeys, beef cattle, pigs, sheep, and other animals raised for human consumption (see Table 39.1).[1,2] Most use involves addition of subtherapeutic doses of antibiotics to the feed of healthy animals over prolonged periods to promote growth, increase feed efficiency, and prevent disease. These nontherapeutic uses create environmental reservoirs where bacteria are exposed to antibiotics and contribute significantly to the development and dissemination of antibiotic resistance. Infants and children are at increased risk of morbidity and mortality from infection with antibiotic-resistant food-borne organisms or those that acquire resistance indirectly from environmental reservoirs related to food animal production.[3]

## Antibiotic Use in Food Animal Production
Antibiotics are used in a variety of settings, but neither antibiotic manufacturers nor agricultural producers are required to report antibiotic use for either human uses or food animal production. Thus precise data on the magnitude of each specific use of antibiotics are not available. While no one disputes the fact that the major nonhuman use of antibiotics is in food animal production, there is considerable debate about the magnitude of and indications for such use. It is certain, however,

**Table 39.1**
**Estimates of Annual Antimicrobial Use in United States***

| Institute of Medicine |
| --- |
| Total: 50 million pounds |
| • 60% in human medicine |
| • 40% in agriculture |
|    • 32% nontherapeutic use in agriculture |
|    • 8% therapeutic use in agriculture |
| **Union of Concerned Scientists** |
| Total: 35 million pounds |
| • 13% in human medicine |
| • 3% in pets |
| • 84% in animal agriculture |
|    • 78% nontherapeutic use in agriculture |
|    • 6% therapeutic use in agriculture |

*From Institute of Medicine[1] and Union of Concerned Scientists.[2]

that millions of pounds of antibiotics per year are used during the production of food animals.

As in human medicine, therapeutic use in clinically ill animals involves use of curative doses of antibiotics for relatively short periods. However, in contrast to human medicine, therapeutic agents may not be delivered to individual sick animals only, but to entire herds or flocks depending on the disease, type of food animal, and type of production facility. For example, more than 90% of poultry in the United States is grown in large barns containing up to 60 000 animals.[4] When a sick animal is discovered, the entire population is considered at risk and treated by placing antibiotics in the drinking water. Animals receive variable doses of antibiotic depending on water intake, and environmental contamination from spilled and discarded water is inevitable. A wide variety of antibiotics is approved for therapeutic use in animals, many of which are identical or similar to drugs used in human medicine.[5] Only some of these approved antibiotics require a veterinarian's prescription.

The other 2 categories of antibiotic use in animal production, disease prevention and growth promotion/feed efficiency, employ the addition of subtherapeutic doses of antibiotics to the feed of healthy animals over long portions of their life cycle. Because both practices generate similar selective pressure on microbial populations, these uses will be discussed under the common term "nontherapeutic use." Growth promotion/feed efficiency refers to the ability to grow animals larger and faster on less food by adding small amounts of antibiotics to feed. Since the early 1950s, this practice has been used to shorten time to slaughter, improve profits for producers, and lower costs to consumers.[6] The biological basis for this acceleration of growth is unknown, but one theory is that subclinical infections are treated before becoming overt illness, animal health is preserved, and growth is enhanced.

Of the 22 antibiotics approved as growth promoters in the United States, more than half are closely related or identical to important human-use compounds.[5,7] A number of antibiotics also are used routinely to prevent high prevalence diseases in food animals. Administration of most growth promoters is accomplished by adding the drug to the feed or water over much of the life cycle. Use of antibiotics for these nontherapeutic indications does not require a veterinarian's prescription. Table 39.2 gives a list by drug class of several of these nontherapeutic uses.

### Selection of Antibiotic Resistance Resulting From Agricultural Uses of Antibiotics

Bacteria exposed to various concentrations of antibiotics select for resistance genes. In agriculture, the nontherapeutic dosing of healthy animals with antibiotics is known to produce reservoirs of resistant organisms, which ultimately reach humans and can cause disease.[8,9]

When animals become colonized with resistant organisms, these organisms eventually can reach humans through the food chain, via direct contact, or through contamination of water or crops by animal

**Table 39.2**
**Major Antibiotic Classes Approved for Use in Animals***

| Antibiotic Class | Species | Prophylaxis | Growth Promotion |
|---|---|---|---|
| Aminoglycosides | Beef cattle, goats, poultry, sheep, swine | Yes | No |
| Beta-Lactams (penicillins) | Beef cattle, dairy cows, fowl, poultry, sheep, swine | Yes | Yes |
| Beta-Lactams (cephalosporins) | Beef cattle, dairy cows, poultry, sheep, swine | Yes | No |
| Ionophores | Beef cattle, fowl, goats, poultry, rabbits, sheep | Yes | Yes |
| Lincosamides | Poultry, swine | Yes | Yes |
| Macrolides | Beef cattle, poultry, swine | Yes | Yes |
| Polypeptides | Fowl, poultry, swine | Yes | Yes |
| Streptogramins | Beef cattle, poultry, swine | Yes | Yes |
| Sulfonamides | Beef cattle, poultry, swine | Yes | Yes |
| Tetracyclines | Beef cattle, dairy cows, fowl, honey bees, poultry, sheep, swine | Yes | Yes |
| **Other** | | | |
| Bambermycin | Beef cattle, poultry, swine | Yes | Yes |
| Carbadox | Swine | Yes | Yes |
| Novobiocin | Fowl, poultry | Yes | No |
| Spectinomycin | Poultry, swine | Yes | No |

*From US General Accounting Office.[7]

excreta.[10] Modern animal production technology, which includes the use of nontherapeutic antibiotics, enhances selection and dissemination of antibiotic-resistant organisms and increases the likelihood of spread to humans. Increasingly, food animals are raised in large numbers under close confinement, transported in large groups to slaughter, and processed very rapidly.[11] These stressful conditions cause increased bacterial shedding and inevitable contamination of hide, carcass,[12] and meat[13] with fecal bacteria. Dissemination of resistant pathogens via the food chain is further facilitated by centralized food processing and packaging, particularly of ground meat products, and broad distribution through food wholesalers and retail chains.[14] Farmers, farmworkers, and farm families,[9] as well as casual visitors,[15] are at documented increased risk for infection with resistant organisms.

Resistance can develop from a new mutation under optimal conditions within hours or days.[8,16] Most resistance genes, however, are acquired from other bacteria via horizontal gene transfer.[17] Resistance genes frequently are located on extra-chromosomal plasmids containing 10 or more different resistance genes and can be transmitted between bacteria of the same or different species. This permits the selection of multidrug resistance as a response to the presence of a single antimicrobial agent. The diverse and efficient mechanisms whereby bacteria share genetic material has caused experts to go beyond consideration of movement of resistant bacterial cells to studies of the ecology and movement of resistance genes in reservoirs where bacteria and antibiotics coexist.[18] Important reservoirs include the rumen and/ or gut of food animals eating feed containing antibiotics, and the gut of humans exposed to antibiotics.[19] Increasing numbers of studies document resistance gene movement between commensal bacteria and pathogens, and transfer of these genes among animal species including humans.[20] Environmental reservoirs also are important contributors to the movement of resistance genes. Active antibiotics have been measured in water near animal waste lagoons,[21] surface waters, and river sediments.[22] Investigators have found resistance genes identical to those found in swine waste lagoons in groundwater and soil microbes hundreds of meters downstream.[23] Multiple environmental and animal reservoirs may ultimately be found, which are involved in dissemination of resistance genes.

Relatively few studies have attempted to document the impact of agricultural use of antibiotics on human health. Advances in molecular epidemiology over the past 2 decades have enabled investigators to document direct links between antibiotic use in animals and resistant infection in humans. For example, the dissemination of antibiotic-resistant *Salmonella* infections through the food chain is well documented. A 6-state outbreak of plasmid-mediated, multidrug-resistant *Salmonella newport* infections was traced through the food chain via consumed beef to a feedlot using nontherapeutic doses of chlortetracycline as a growth promoter in feed.[24] This study also found an elevated risk of illness with resistant versus sensitive strains occurring among patients taking antibiotics for other infections (odds ratio = 51.3, $P = 0.001$), suggesting that asymptomatic carriage of the epidemic strain was converted to symptomatic infection by the use of antibiotics. Two of 3 children younger than 10 years in the outbreak had received antibiotics prior to symptom onset.

Infants and young children are vulnerable to infections with resistant food-borne pathogens by indirect exposures as well. Bezanson and coworkers[25] described a plasmid-mediated, 6-drug–resistant strain of *Salmonella typhimurium* infection acquired asymptomatically by a pregnant woman from raw milk and passed to her infant at birth and secondarily to several other babies in the newborn nursery.[25] In another newborn nursery outbreak, multidrug-resistant *Salmonella heidelberg* caused bloody diarrhea in 3 infants.[26] The index case was a baby born at term by cesarean section after 18 hours of ruptured membranes to a farmer's daughter; until delivery, the mother had been working with new calves from a herd containing several sick animals. Child care centers, because of high concentrations of young children not yet toilet trained and cared for by shared staff, provide another unique pediatric environment where food-borne pathogens may be easily transmitted.[27]

Antibiotic resistance is an increasing and serious problem. Consumers, pediatricians, and public health and federal agencies should take steps to institute universal judicious use of antibiotics, promote better infection control, improve animal husbandry, and eliminate all unnecessary use of antibiotics to preserve efficacy and delay antibiotic resistance, thus providing increased time for development of new preventive and therapeutic strategies.

## Frequently Asked Questions

Q *If the use of antibiotic growth promoters is eliminated, will meat and poultry become very expensive?*

A No. Best estimates are that the cost to the consumer would increase by no more than a few pennies per pound.

Q *Can animals be successfully raised and brought to slaughter without the use of antibiotics to prevent illness?*

A Yes. Several European countries that have banned nontherapeutic use of antibiotics in food animal production have found that by improving animal husbandry practices and hygiene, animals can be raised successfully without requiring prophylactic antibiotics.

Q *Do the antibiotics added to animal feed stay in the animals and eventually reach humans who consume meat and poultry?*

A There are regulations requiring specific "washout" periods. Antibiotics must be stopped for a prescribed number of days or weeks, depending on the drug, prior to slaughter or harvest of meat, dairy, and poultry products. These have been designed to prevent dangerous residual levels of antibiotics in animal proteins at the time of slaughter or harvest. The success of these regulations is dependent on compliance of food animal producers and the adequacy of enforcement and inspection programs.

Q *What can pediatricians do to discourage use of unnecessary antibiotics in animals?*

A Pediatricians should educate patients on appropriate use of antibiotics in the clinical setting and consistently practice the judicious use of antibiotics in their therapeutic interventions. Health care providers also are in a powerful position to advocate for antibiotic-free food options in local grocery stores and food services, such as in schools and hospitals. Further, those pediatricians in farm states can advocate for reducing or eliminating use of nontherapeutic antibiotics in local animal agriculture through letters to the editor, communication with state legislators and regulators, and discussions with the media.

Q *What can parents do to discourage use of unnecessary antibiotics in animals?*

A Where available, consumers can support individual producers who do not use nontherapeutic antibiotics in their animal husbandry practices. Animal-based foods labeled with the "USDA Organic" seal have been raised without antibiotics. Some fast food chains also have pledged to use only animal protein raised antibiotic-free and are reducing their use of animal proteins raised with certain antibiotics. These are listed online at http://www.keepantibioticsworking.com/pages/home.cfm.

## References

1. Harrison PF, Lederberg J, eds. *Antimicrobial Resistance: Issues and Options. Workshop Report.* Forum on Emerging Infections, Division of Health Sciences Policy, Institute of Medicine. Washington, DC: National Academies Press; 1998

2. Mellon M, Benbrook C, Benbrook KL. *Hogging it! Estimates of Antimicrobial Abuse in Livestock.* Washington, DC: Union of Concerned Scientists; 2001

3. Shea KM, Florini K, Barlam T. *When Wonder Drugs Don't Work: How Antibiotic Resistance Threatens Children, Seniors, and the Medically Vulnerable.* Washington, DC: Environmental Defense; 2001. Available at: http://www.environmentaldefense.org

4. Humane Society of the United States. *Broiler Chicken—Life on a Factory Farm.* Available at: http://www.hsus.org/programs/farm/factory/life_on_factory.html

5. US Department of Agriculture, Center for Veterinary Medicine. *The 2002 Green Book On-Line.* Available at: http://www.fda.gov/cvm/greenbook/elecgbook.html

6. Animal Health Institute. *Backgrounder: Antibiotic Use in Farm Animals.* Available at: http://www.ahi.org/antibioticsdebate

7. US General Accounting Office. *Report to the Honorable Tom Harkin, Ranking Minority Member, Committee on Agriculture, Nutrition, and Forestry, US Senate: Food Safety: The Agricultural Use of Antibiotics and Its Implications for Human Health.* Washington, DC: US General Accounting Office; 1999. Publication GAO/RCED-99-74

8. Khachatourians GG. Agricultural use of antibiotics and the evolution and transfer of antibiotic-resistant bacteria. *CMAJ.* 1998;159:1129–1136

9. Levy SB, FitzGerald GB, Macone AB. Changes in intestinal flora of farm personnel after introduction of a tetracycline-supplemented feed on the farm. *N Engl J Med.* 1976;295:583–588

10. Witte W. Medical consequences of antibiotic use in agriculture. *Science.* 1998;279:996–997

11. Center for Science in the Public Interest, Environmental Defense Fund, Food Animal Concerns Trust, Public Citizen's Health Research Group, Union of Concerned Citizens. *Petition to Rescind Approvals for the Subtherapeutic Use of Antibiotics in Livestock Used in (or Related to Those Used in) Human Medicine.* Available at: http://www.cspinet.org/ar/petition_3_99.html

12. Barkocy-Gallagher GA, Arthur TM, Siragusa GR, et al. Genotypic analyses of *Escherichia coli* O157:H7 and O157 nonmotile isolate recovered from beef cattle and carcasses at processing plants in the Midwestern states of the United States. *Appl Environ Microbiol.* 2001;67:3810–3818

13. Millemann Y, Gaubert S, Remy D, Colmin C. Evaluation of IS200-PCR and comparison with other molecular markers to trace Salmonella enterica subsp enterica serotype typhimurium bovine isolates from farm to meat. *J Clin Microbiol.* 2000;38:2204–2209

14. Tauxe RV, Holmberg SD, Cohen ML. The epidemiology of gene transfer in the environment. In: Levy SB, Miller RV, eds. *Gene Transfer in the Environment.* New York, NY: McGraw-Hill; 1989:377–403

15. Centers for Disease Control and Prevention. Outbreaks of *Escherichia coli* O157:H7 infections among children associated with farm visits—Pennsylvania and Washington, 2000. *MMWR Morb Mortal Wkly Rep.* 2001;50:293–297

16. American Society of Microbiology. *Antimicrobial Resistance: An Ecological Perspective.* Available at: http://www.asmusa.org/acasrc/aca1.htm

17. Levy SB, Marshal BM. Genetic transfer in the natural environment. In: Sussman M, Collins GH, Skinner FA, Stewart-Tall DE, eds. *Release of Genetically-engineered Micro-organisms.* London, England: Academic Press; 1988:61–76

18. Mazel D, Davies J. Antibiotic resistance in microbes. *Cell Mol Life Sci.* 1999;56:742–754

19. Shoemaker NB, Wang GR, Salyers AA. Evidence of natural transfer of a tetracycline resistance gene between bacteria from the human colon and bacteria from the bovine rumen. *Appl Environ Microbiol.* 1992;58:1313–1320

20. Hummel R, Tschape H, Witte W. Spread of plasmid-mediated nourseothricin resistance due to antibiotic use in animal husbandry. *J Basic Microbiol.* 1986;26:461–466

21. Meyer MT, Kolpin DW, Bumgarner JE, Varns JL, Daughtridge JV. Occurrence of antibiotics in surface and ground water near confined animal feeding operations and waste water treatment plants using radioimmunoassay and liquid chromatography/electrospray mass spectrometry. Programs with Extended Abstracts, presented at: 219th Meeting of the American Chemical Society; March 26–30, 2000; San Francisco, CA. No. 1, p. 106

22. Halling-Sorensen B, Nors Nielsen S, Lanzky PF, et al. Occurrence, fate and effects of pharmaceutical substances in the environment—a review. *Chemosphere.* 1998;36:357–393

23. Chee-Sanford JC, Aminov RI, Krapac IJ, Garrigues-Jeanjean N, Mackie RI. Occurrence and diversity of tetracycline resistance genes in lagoons and groundwater underlying two swine production facilities. *Appl Environ Microbiol.* 2001;67:1494–1502

24. Holmberg SD, Osterholm MT, Senger KA, Cohen ML. Drug-resistant *Salmonella* from animals fed antimicrobials. *N Engl J Med.* 1984;311:617–622

25. Bezanson GS, Khakhria R, Bollegraaf E. Nosocomial outbreak caused by antibiotic-resistant strain of *Salmonella typhimurium* acquired from dairy cattle. *Can Med Assoc J.* 1983;128:426–427

26. Lyons RW, Samples CL, DeSilvan HN, Ross KA, Julian EM, Checko PJ. An epidemic of resistant *Salmonella* in a nursery. Animal-to-human spread. *JAMA.* 1980;243:546–547

27. Holmes SJ, Morrow AL, Pickering LK. Child-care practices: effects of social change on the epidemiology of infectious diseases and antibiotic resistance. *Epidemiol Rev.* 1996;18:10–28

# 40
# Environmental Threats to Children's Health in Developing Countries

Pediatricians in the United States, particularly in urban areas and areas with large immigrant populations, may likely examine and care for patients who were not born in this country. When a child comes from a developing country, it is important to be aware of the lifestyle, cultural, and environmental differences that can greatly affect a child's health status. This chapter is intended to provide an overview of the problems and to increase awareness of the types of environmental exposures that exist in developing countries. Additionally, consciousness of the environmental health conditions in other parts of the world provides a needed perspective to help understand the importance of the roles that the United States and other governments, nonprofit institutions, and international organizations take in shaping international solutions.

## Defining the Problems

Although there is no single accepted definition of a "developing country," the *Cambridge International Dictionary of English* defines the developing world as: "the poorer countries of the world, which include many of the countries of Africa, Latin America and Asia, which have less advanced industries."[1] The World Bank defines developing countries as those with low to middle income economies (below $9,205 gross national income per capita).[2] InterConnection, a nonprofit agency that provides technology assistance to nongovernmental organizations in developing countries, uses the following definition: "Developing countries include the most impoverished and deprived nations in the world. They are characterized by environmental misuse and/or human resource exploitation due to indebtedness, lack of viable alternative economic resources, education and political control."[3]

In 2001 the Population Reference Bureau estimated the world's population to be slightly more than 6 billion people.[4] Almost 5 billion of the world's people live in less developed countries. Nearly all of the world's population growth occurs in less developed countries, with 99% of the yearly increase occurring in Africa, Asia, Latin America and the Caribbean, and Oceania.[4] Thirty percent of the world population is younger than 15 years. In the developed countries, only 18% of the population is younger than 15 years, but in less developed countries 33% of the population is younger than 15 years.[4]

In developing countries, children often are exposed to higher levels of environmental contaminants in the air, water, soil, and food than are children in the more developed nations.

The costs of economic and industrial development often include environmental degradation. This deterioration often is fueled by urbanization, unregulated industrialization, population growth and displacement, and increased pressure on limited natural resources. In addition to the dumping of industrial and chemical wastes, problems include overcrowding in cities, poor sanitation, limited access to safe drinking water, and poor air quality.

The environmental health risk differential exists not only between rich and poor countries, but also between population groups within a given country. Environmental risks to children tend to disfavor rural populations compared with urban populations, and an unequal disease burden on the poor may be further aggravated by differences in access to health care.

Obstacles to protecting pediatric environmental health in developing countries are far greater than the obstacles in the developed countries.[5] Environmental health specialists and medical professionals in the developed countries are often concerned about imperfect datasets and outdated monitoring data. In many developing countries, even simple monitoring data are not collected. Very little is known about the body burdens of lead, mercury, dioxins, pesticides, persistent organic pollutants (POPs), and other environmental contaminants in the children of developing countries. The nature and magnitude of environmental pollution and contamination often is unknown.[5] Inadequate infrastructure and financial resources, shortage of laboratory equipment and trained technical personnel, inadequate and unreliable data, and the distrust that often exists between the public and governmental agencies are significant impediments to addressing these issues.

In September 1990 the United Nations (UN) sponsored the 1990 World Summit for Children.[6] At this historic summit, 7 major goals, all related to enhancing children's health and nutrition, were outlined. The goals were (1) reducing mortality in infants and children younger than 5 years, (2) reducing mortality in mothers, (3) reducing severe and moderate malnutrition in children younger than 5 years, (4) universal access to safe drinking water, (5) universal access to sanitary means of excreta disposal, (6) universal access to basic education, and (7) improved protection of children.[6] More than 155 countries prepared programs of action, and through the involvement of many UN agencies, nongovernmental organizations, universities, and research institutions, more than 100 countries conducted monitoring surveys.[6] A mid-decade review was held in 1996, and UNICEF has prepared progress reports, the latest being a September 2001 statistical review[7] and the *We the Children* report.[6] Great progress has been made, but as will be described in this chapter, the threats to the environment and children's health are still considerable.

## Child Mortality in the Developing World

Globally, it is estimated that 1 in 5 children in the poorest regions of the world will not live to see his or her fifth birthday.[6] The World Health Organization (WHO) estimates that more than 50% of the deaths of children younger than 5 years are directly attributable to respiratory infections, diarrhea, measles, malaria, and malnutrition.[6] Of all deaths in chidren younger than 5 years, 40% occur in Sub-Saharan Africa, 34% in South Asia, 13% in East Asia and the Pacific, 6% in the Middle East and North Africa, 4% in Latin America and Caribbean countries, and only 1% in industrialized countries.[7] This mortality is, to a large extent, theoretically preventable through cost-effective and sustainable environmental interventions. Realistically, many developing countries lack the infrastructure and financial resources, as well as the capacity to work toward sustainable development. The greatest environmental problems that still exist are related to air pollution, safe drinking water, and sanitation.[6]

## Air Pollution—Indoors and Outdoors

Half of the world's population, including up to 90% of rural households in low-income countries and a total of two thirds of the households in developing countries, rely on unprocessed biomass fuels.[8] These fuels include wood, dung, and crop residues. They typically are burned indoors on open fires or in poorly ventilated stoves, creating high levels of indoor air pollution. For example, in India, biomass is used in more than 80% of households.[9] For children, exposures occur not only at home, but also at school, where biomass is commonly used. In some countries, kerosene is beginning to be used as a substitute because it seems to burn cleaner. Unfortunately, as with the use of biomass fuel, indoor kerosene burning leads to the accumulation of volatile organic compounds and polyaromatic hydrocarbons. Additionally, in developing countries, most cooking is performed by women of childbearing age. Often young children, particularly females, spend time indoors with their mothers, thus potentially increasing their exposure and risk of adverse health effects due to indoor air pollutants.

Rapid industrialization in many countries has meant that better regulations and concerns over the environment have been left behind. Coal burning fuel plants, steel factories, and mining operations have

created severe air, water, and soil contamination in much of Eastern
and Central Europe.[5] Pollutants from these operations include, but
are not limited to, mercury vapor, sulfur dioxide, nitrogen oxides, particulate matter, lead, chromium, arsenic, cadmium, zinc, copper, and
varied heavy metal contamination in mine tailings.[5] Outdoor air pollution is made worse in many developing countries because of the
types of vehicles driven. In Southeast Asia, most vehicles are 2 and 3
wheelers, including mopeds, motorcycles, scooters, and autorickshaws.
These types of vehicles use the more polluting 2-stroke engine technology, which contributes greatly to air pollution in urban areas of
Southeast Asia and many other developing countries. In the United
States, less polluting 4-stroke internal combustion engines are most
commonly used. Compared with 4-stroke engines, the 2-stroke
engines burn more gasoline and a lot of oil. Additionally, because
leaded gasoline is still commonly used, many vehicles in developing
countries do not have catalytic converters, which help to reduce
carbon monoxide and hydrocarbon emissions.

Decreasing indoor and outdoor air pollution, improving access to
health care providers, and making available affordable antibiotics are
all needed to significantly decrease air pollution–related illnesses in
developing countries.

## Lead Contamination

As of 1999, leaded gasoline had been completely phased out in only
58 countries throughout the world. Lead contamination has been a
significant problem in rapidly industrializing countries, yet the resources to monitor and evaluate the levels in the environment are not
in place in most developing countries.[10] Where leaded gasoline has not
been phased out, it is responsible for 90% of the airborne lead pollution in cities.[11] In Africa, only high lead content gasoline is used. The
concentration of lead in this gasoline is more than twice the level that
the United States allowed in the 1970s. In many parts of the Middle
East, Latin America, and Eastern Europe, high lead content gasoline

still is the standard choice. Figure 40.1, shows the sales of lead-free gasoline throughout the world.

In 1996 the World Bank estimated that most of the 1.7 billion urban dwellers in developing countries were at risk for lead poisoning. In fact, it was suspected that all urban children younger than 2 years and more than 80% of those between 3 to 5 years of age, had blood lead levels exceeding health standards set by the WHO.[11] It was estimated that 15 to 18 million children in developing countries may suffer permanent brain damage due to lead poisoning.[11]

In Bangkok, Thailand, lead exposure has been linked to 200 000 to 500 000 cases of hypertension, resulting in 400 deaths per year in the late 1980s. In 1995 Thailand banned leaded gasoline.[11] In Cairo, Egypt, it is estimated that more than 800 infants die annually due to their mothers' exposure to lead.[11] In the center of Budapest, Hungary, in the mid-1980s, children had blood lead levels of 24.8 µg/dL, levels 3 times higher than those measured for suburban children in Hungary.[11] In Jakarta, Indonesia, it is estimated that reducing ambient lead concentrations to WHO standards could prevent more than 60 000 cases of hypertension, 70 cases of heart attacks, and almost 60 cases of premature mortality.[12] In a convenience sample of children in 6 large cities in India, more than 50% of the nation's children younger than 12 years living in urban environments had blood lead levels of 10 µg/dL or greater.[10]

Progress is being made to phase out leaded gasoline in many developing countries. Table 40.1 lists the countries that have phased out and are planning to phase out leaded gasoline. It is anticipated that the next round of epidemiologic studies will show significantly lower blood lead levels in children living in countries where leaded gasoline is no longer used.

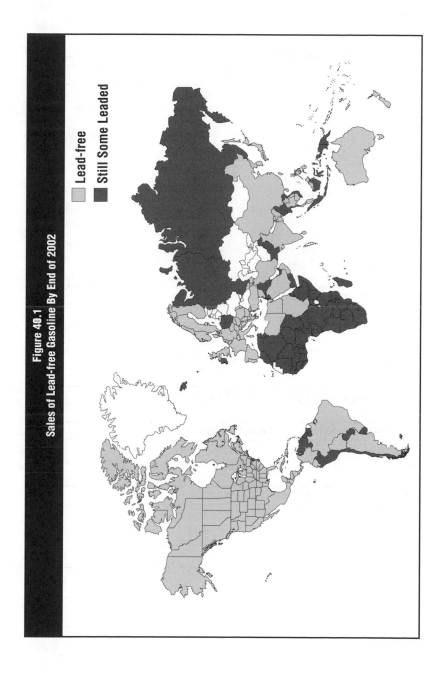

**Figure 40.1**

Sales of Lead-free Gasoline By End of 2002

Lead-free

Still Some Leaded

Table 40.1
Phase Out of Leaded Gasoline*

| Leaded Gasoline Phased Out by End of 2001 | | | |
|---|---|---|---|
| Argentina | Dominican Republic | India | Saudi Arabia |
| Austria | Ecuador | Jamaica | Singapore |
| Bahamas | Egypt | Japan | Slovakia |
| Belgium | El Salvador | Luxembourg | South Korea |
| Bangladesh | Finland | Malaysia | Sweden |
| Belize | France | Mexico | Switzerland |
| Bermuda | Germany | Monaco | Taiwan |
| Bolivia | Guam | Netherlands | Thailand |
| Brazil | Guatemala | New Zealand | United Kingdom |
| Canada | Haiti | Nicaragua | United States |
| Colombia | Honduras | Norway | Uruguay |
| Costa Rica | Hong Kong | Philippines | US Virgin Islands |
| Czech Republic | Hungary | Portugal | Vietnam |
| Denmark | Iceland | Puerto Rico | |
| **Countries Expected to Phase Out Leaded Gasoline in 2002** | | | |
| Australia | Ireland | Oman | Spain |
| Bahrain | Italy | Panama | United Arab |
| Greece | Kuwait | Qatar | Emirates |
| **Countries Expected to Phase Out Leaded Gasoline in 2003** | | | |
| Indonesia | | | |
| **Countries Expected to Phase Out Leaded Gasoline in 2005** | | | |
| Peru | | | |
| **Countries Likely to Phase Out Leaded Gasoline in 2005** | | | |
| Poland | | | |
| Chile | | | |
| Romania | | | |
| **Major Targets for Opportunity** | | | |
| Algeria | Iran | Libya | Syria |
| Confederation of | Iraq | Nigeria | Turkey |
| Independent | Israel | South Africa | Venezuela |
| States | | | |

*From MP Walsh, written communication, July 2002.

## Safe Drinking Water and Sanitation

Nearly 1.1 billion people in the world are still without access to safe drinking water.[13] Forty-two percent of these people are in East Asia and the Pacific, 25% are in Sub-Saharan Africa, and 19% are in South Asia.[7] Access is particularly low in the poor rural areas of developing countries. Nearly 2.4 billion people, including half of all Asians, lack access to sanitary means of excreta disposal.[13]

Although access to safe water has increased since 1990, during this period dangerous levels of arsenic in the groundwater have been identified in several Asian countries. In many rural areas, treatment of drinking water is poor or nonexistent. High levels of nitrates, arsenic, fluoride, and pesticides are common in the drinking water supply in many rural areas. In Eastern Europe nitrate levels have been found at concentrations high enough to cause methemoglobinemia.[14] Persistent organic pollutants also are being documented in water supplies throughout developing countries.[15] Pesticide and herbicide contamination from agricultural uses is common because approximately 80% of the rural populations in developing countries are engaged in agriculture.[6]

Rapid urbanization often is accompanied by rapid growth of cities. In developing countries, this represents a serious challenge to governments seeking to provide proper housing, drinking water, and sanitation for their people. With proper sanitation, proper hygiene, and safe drinking water, diarrhea can be decreased 22% and deaths resulting from diarrhea can be decreased 65%.[6] Because diarrhea accounts for 12% of the deaths of children younger than 5 years, improvements in water and sanitation are critical to improving the health of children. Additionally, improved sanitation and safe drinking water will help to eradicate guinea worm disease, hookworm, schistosomiasis, and other waterborne diseases that greatly influence the health and development of children in developing countries, especially in Sub-Saharan Africa.

## Arsenic Contamination

Natural contamination of groundwater by arsenic has become a critical water quality problem in many parts of the world. Arsenic toxicity in West Bengal, India; Bangladesh; Mongolia; China; and other countries is a major concern for public health. Globally, the number of children at risk who actually are suffering from arsenic toxicity is unknown. Tubewells, wells that tap directly into groundwater, have been established in many developing countries to prevent exposure to microbial contamination and other contamination that often is found in surface water.[16] Since establishing these wells, it has been determined that many of these natural aquifers are contaminated with high levels of naturally occurring arsenic. The world's 2 biggest cases of groundwater arsenic contamination, and those that affected the greatest number of people, are in Bangladesh and West Bengal, India.

Forty-two districts in Bangladesh and 9 districts in West Bengal, India, have arsenic levels in groundwater of about 50 μg/L. This amounts to 122.6 million people potentially being exposed to very high levels of arsenic through drinking water. Chowdhury et al[17] examined approximately 40 000 people from some of the affected districts and found that 15% to 25% of the people examined had arsenical skin lesions, a sign of arsenic toxicity. In Vietnam the average arsenic concentration measured in tubewells in rural districts surrounding Hanoi was 159 μg/L (WHO drinking water guideline is set at 10 μg/L).[16] Symptoms of chronic arsenic exposure have not yet been reported in Vietnam, despite the fact that several million people may be consuming drinking water with high levels of arsenic. The first private tubewells for drinking water were installed 7 years ago.[16] Severe symptoms often are not seen until 5 to 10 years of exposure, and early symptoms of exposure are difficult to diagnose, particularly in the absence of awareness.[16] In the Guizhou province of China alone, 200 000 people are at risk for overexposure to arsenic due to high levels of arsenic in the air, food, and water.[18] Arsenic in the air comes from the burning of coal that contains high levels of arsenic. This coal is used in households and is burned predominantly in unventilated stoves. Seventeen percent of the population examined has obvious skin lesions.[18] By physical examination in 1992, 37% of the population showed signs of hepatomegaly; by ultrasound examination in 1998, 21% of the population showed signs of hepatomegaly.[18]

These arsenic contamination examples may represent the tip of the iceberg. Potential contamination and subsequent health effects in many developing countries have not yet been examined.

## Fluoride Contamination and Skeletal Fluorosis

Fluorosis is a potentially crippling disease caused by the ingestion of too much fluoride in drinking water.[19] Fluorosis is endemic in at least 25 countries including, but not limited to, India, Mexico, China, and Bangladesh. High concentrations of fluoride occur naturally in groundwater and coal in many of these countries.[20] The upper recommended limit of fluoride in drinking water is about 1.0 mg/L.[20] Nutritional status plays a role in determining how much fluoride is maintained in the body, especially for children. Calcium and vitamins A and C can help prevent risks of skeletal fluorosis.[20] In India an estimated 6 million children younger than 14 years are victims of fluorosis.[20] Levels in groundwater used for drinking in India range from 0.2 mg/L to 48 mg/L.[21] Three types of fluorosis exist: dental, skeletal, and nonskeletal. The most debilitating is skeletal fluorosis, where skeletal abnormalities can include knock-knees, bowleg, and generalized skeletal deformities.[21]

UNICEF is working closely with the government of India on defluoridation programs and technologies, but there still is a great deal of work to be done in identifying and addressing the fluoride problem in other developing countries.

## Scavenging

Metal contamination, with mercury from gold mining and other heavy metals from uranium mines, is a serious problem because often these waste products are disposed of in open dumps. Scavenging in these open dumps, particularly by children, has become a cottage industry and a means of support for many young people (http://www.who.int/peh/ceh/Bangkok/Bangkokconfreport.pdf).

## Further Environmental Threats to Children

Air pollution, safe drinking water, and sanitation are at the top of the list of environmental concerns in developing countries. Malnutrition, vector-borne disease, food safety, lead poisoning, fluorosis, arsenic toxicity, pesticide exposures and poisonings, exposure to POPs and endocrine disrupting chemicals, ultraviolet radiation, proximity to industrial and municipal waste sites, and industrial dust are among emerging and reemerging environmental health threats. Children living in unsafe environments are more vulnerable to injuries resulting from traffic accidents, falls, drowning, burns, poisonings, and deliberate acts of violence, including child abuse. The spectrum of issues is as diverse and broad as the developing countries themselves.

## Resources

International Labour Organization, Internet: http://www.ilo.org/. This organization provides good information and links to other sites with information relating to child labor.

International Society of Doctors for the Environment, Internet: http://www.isde.org. The society has created a primer on international environmental and health politics. This primer, available online, provides an excellent resource for contacts in specific countries, international organizations, and nongovernmental organizations. The site also provides links to environmental topics and international programs within each topic area.

UNICEF, Internet: http://www.unicef.org

United Nations, Internet: http://www.un.org

World Health Organization, Internet: http://www.who.int/home-page
and http://www.euro.who.int/eprise/main/WHO/Progs/CHE/home

## References

1. *Cambridge International Dictionary of English.* Cambridge, UK: Cambridge University Press; 2001
2. World Bank. *Classification of Economies.* Washington, DC: World Bank; 2002. Available at: http://www.worldbank.org/data/countryclass/countryclass.html
3. Inter*Connection. What Is a Developing Country?* Seattle, WA: Inter*Connection;* 2002. Available at: http://www.info@interconnection.org/background/develop.htm
4. Population Reference Bureau. *2002 World Population Data Sheet.* Washington, DC: Population Reference Bureau; 2002. Available at: http://www.prb.org/pdf/WorldPopulationDS02_Eng.pdf
5. Fitzgerald EF, Schell LM, Marshall EG, Carpenter DO, Suk WA, Zejda JE. Environmental pollution and child health in central and Eastern Europe. *Environ Health Perspect.* 1998;106:307–311
6. UNICEF. *We the Children: Meeting the Promises of the World Summit for Children.* New York, NY: UNICEF; 2001. Available at: http://www.unicef.org/specialsession/about/sgreport-pdf/sgreport_adapted_eng.pdf
7. UNICEF. *Progress Since the World Summit for Children: A Statistical Review.* New York, NY: UNICEF; 2001. Available at: http://www.unicef.org/specialsession/about/sgreport-pdf/sgreport_adapted_stats_eng.pdf
8. World Health Organization. *Child Health Research: A Foundation for Improving Child Health.* Geneva, Switzerland: World Health Organization; 2002. Available at: http://www.who.int/child-adolescent-health/New_Publications/CHILD_HEALTH/GC/WHO_FCH_CAH_02.3.pdf
9. Shrestha B. Air pollution and children's health. In: Proceedings of the International Conference on Environmental Threats to the Health of Children; March 2002; Bangkok, Thailand. Geneva, Switzerland: World Health Organization; 2002

10. George AM, ed. *Lead Poisoning Prevention and Treatment: Implementing a National Program in Developing Countries.* Bangalore, India: The George Foundation; 1999. Available at: http://www.leadpoison.net/research.htm

11. World Bank. World Bank recommends global phase-out of leaded gasoline [press release #96/68S]. Washington, DC: World Bank; 1996. Available at: http://web.worldbank.org/WBSITE/EXTERNAL/NEWS/0,,contentMDK: 20014304~ menuPK:34465~pagePK:34370~piPK: 34424~theSitePK: 4607,00.html

12. Ostro B. *Estimating the Health Effects of Air Pollutants: A Method with an Application to Jakarta.* Washington, DC: World Bank; 1994. Policy Research Working Paper #1301. Available at: http://www-wds.worldbank.org/servlet/WDSContentServer/ WDSP/IB/1994/05/01/000009265_3970716141007/Rendered/PDF/ multi0page.pdf

13. World Health Organization. *Global Water Supply and Sanitation Assessment 2000 Report.* Geneva, Switzerland: World Health Organization; 2000. Available at: http://www.who.int/docstore/water_sanitation_health/ Globassessment/GlobalTOC.htm

14. Jedrychowski W, Maugeri U, Bianchi I. Environmental pollution in central and eastern European countries: a basis for cancer epidemiology. *Rev Environ Health.* 1997;12:1–23

15. European Environment Agency. Children's health and environment: a review of evidence. A joint report from the European Environment Agency and the WHO Regional Office for Europe. Environmental issue report No. 29. Luxembourg Office for Official Publications of the European Communities; 2002

16. Berg M, Tran HC, Guuyen TC, Pham HV, Schertenleib R, Giger W. Arsenic contamination of groundwater and drinking water in Vietnam: a human health threat. *Environ Sci Technol.* 2001;35:2621–2626

17. Chowdhury UK, Biswas BK, Chowdhury TR, et al. Groundwater arsenic contamination in Bangladesh and West Bengal, India. *Environ Health Perspect.* 2000;108:393–397

18. Liu J, Zheng B, Aposhian HV, et al. Chronic arsenic poisoning from burning high-arsenic-containing coal in Guizhou, China. *Environ Health Perspect.* 2002;110:119–122

19. UNICEF. *State of the Art Report on Fluoride and Resulting Endemicity for Fluorosis in India.* New York, NY: UNICEF; 1999

20. UNICEF. *Fluoride in Water: An Overview.* New York, NY: UNICEF; 2002. Available at: http/www.unicef.org/programme/wes/info/fluor.htm
21. Susheela AK, Bhatnagar M. Health benefits derived by children in endemic areas of fluorosis in India through early diagnosis of fluorosis and practice of interventions focusing on safe drinking water and nutritional supplementation. Presented at: International Conference on Environmental Threats to the Health of Children; Bangkok, Thailand. Geneva, Switzerland; World Health Organization; 2002

# 41
# Communicating About Risk

Risk communication can be defined as an exchange of information about the nature, magnitude, significance, and management of a risk. Physicians are among the most trusted sources of information on occupational and environmental health risks,[1] and health care professionals are increasingly being asked by parents to consider environmental toxicants among the possible causes of a child's ill health.[2] However, a 1995 survey found that although exposure to environmental poisons leads a list of parental health concerns, pediatricians rarely provide advice on this topic.[3] Several factors may help explain this disparity: time constraints, billing issues, lack of environmental health training, lack of toxicologic information specific to children, and lack of comfort in undertaking environmental health risk communication. This chapter will cover some of the basic information about environmental risk communication.

## Principles of Risk Communication
It is important to approach questions of risk with an understanding of the limitations of the current science and the importance of the role of individual and social perceptions.

For each health risk, there is an upper threshold risk level, above which a risk is perceived as completely unacceptable, and a lower threshold value, below which risks are considered negligible. Risk tolerance, like risk aversion, is affected by personal, social, and political factors.[4] Although each person perceives risk somewhat differently, researchers identify 3 factors that commonly influence risk perception: the nature of the hazard, the demographic background of the person perceiving the risk, and the social context of the risk.[5]

## Nature of the Hazard

A number of hazard characteristics influence the perception of risk (see Table 41.1).[6,7] Hazards that are unlikely but that have potentially catastrophic consequences generally are seen by the public as greater risks than hazards that are more likely but that would result in less serious outcomes. For example, the health risk from a nuclear power plant may be seen as far greater than the risk from a coal power plant, although the likelihood of emissions that are hazardous to health is higher from the coal power plant. Similarly, the risk of an exposure associated with a dreaded outcome, such as cancer or brain damage, is seen as worse than the risk of a disease that is less dreaded, such as a skin disease. Unfamiliar hazards generally are seen as riskier than familiar hazards, such as mine tailing piles that might have been in a community for generations. Manufactured hazards, such as high-voltage lines, are perceived as riskier than naturally occurring hazards such as radon.

**Table 41.1**
**Some Factors Related to Perception of Risk**

| Decrease Perceived Risk | Increase Perceived Risk |
|---|---|
| **Hazard Factors** | |
| Familiar<br>Natural, naturally occurring<br>Adults affected<br>Voluntary, under any individual's control | Unfamiliar or unusual<br>Man-made<br>Children or fetuses affected<br>Involuntary, imposed |
| **Demographic Factors** | |
| Male gender<br>White race | Female gender<br>Nonwhite race |
| **Social Context Factors** | |
| Trust in the risk communicator<br>Trust in the person or institution<br>  imposing the risk<br>Equal distribution of risk and benefits | Mistrust in the risk communicator<br>Mistrust in the risk imposer<br><br>Unequal or unfair distribution of risk<br>  and benefits |

A hazard to children often is judged as worse than a hazard to adults. Hazards that are perceived as involuntary almost always are judged as more serious and risky than hazards that are faced by choice.

This last characteristic is especially important in relation to risk communication because of the issue of risk comparisons. Comparisons of a voluntary risk (such as smoking or driving) with an involuntary risk (such as a local hazardous waste incinerator) usually are not seen by the public as equivalent risks or valid comparisons because of the issue of control. Parents might find such risk comparisons irrelevant or offensive. Risk comparisons should be used carefully because comparisons that are seen as inappropriate or misleading may hurt the credibility of the pediatrician.

### Demographic Characteristics

Not surprisingly, different groups of people tend to perceive risk differently. In particular, experts and scientists tend to view many risks as less significant than nontechnically trained individuals do.[7,8] Research has shown that white women perceive risks to be much higher than do white men. However, this gender difference is not true of nonwhite women and men, whose perceptions of risk are quite similar. Most striking was the finding that white males tend to differ from everyone else in their attitudes and perceptions. On average, they perceive risks as much smaller and much more acceptable than do other people. These results suggest that sociopolitical factors such as power, status, alienation, and trust are strong determinants of people's perception and acceptance of risk.[9]

### Social Context of the Risk

If the individual, business, or agency imposing a risk is known and trusted by the community, the risk often is perceived as less than if the risk is imposed by an outsider. Risks seen as unfair often are viewed as more serious than those seen as fairly distributed.[7] Similarly, if an individual or community perceives significant benefits from submitting to a risk, that risk seems smaller than if the benefits will only accrue to other communities or to a faceless corporation. Such context and history are particularly important when risk communication involves low-income communities or communities of color. In these communities, even a relatively small additional risk might be seen against a background of racial and socioeconomic discrimination in the distribution of risks and benefits, and could be perceived as adding to an already unacceptable background of risk and environmental health burden (see Table 41.2).[6]

## Seven Cardinal Rules of Risk Communication

The Seven Cardinal Rules of Risk Communication were initially written in 1988 for representatives of government as a communication framework for effective interactions with concerned communities about issues of technological risk.[7] Miller and Solomon[8] believe that it is helpful for pediatricians to be aware of these rules because the rules are pertinent to the process of communication in the pediatric professional arena and because the rules set standards for communi-

**Table 41.2**
**Perception of Risk Dichotomies***

| Acceptable or Reduces Apparent Riskiness | Unacceptable or Increases Apparent Riskiness |
|---|---|
| Risk assumed voluntarily or self-imposed | Risk borne involuntarily or imposed by others |
| Adverse effect immediate | Outcome delayed |
| Alternatives not available, a necessity | Alternatives available |
| Risk certain | Risk uncertain |
| Occupational exposure | Community exposure |
| Familiar hazard | Feared or "dreaded" hazard |
| Consequences reversible | Consequences irreversible |
| Some benefit gained from assuming risk | No apparent benefit to those at risk |
| Hazard associated with perceived good | Someone else profits at "my expense" |

*From Gochfeld M.[6]

cation that should be expected whenever a forum concerning an environmental hazard is held.

## Seven Cardinal Rules of Risk Communication (adapted)

- Involve the patient and parent in identifying and solving the problem.
- Have a communication plan and a clear message.
- Listen to the patient and parent's story.
- Be honest, open, and frank.
- Work with credible sources.
- Provide access to information.
- Speak clearly and with compassion.

## Planning for Risk Communication and Risk Management

1. If necessary, research the topic of concern. Consider the cultural background, employment, language barriers, education, and possible concerns about environmental disparaties of the patient and parents, as well as other factors that might influence their risk perceptions.
2. Determine the messages to be communicated. Remember that communication is a 2-way street and the other person(s) will have goals and messages too. What do the patient and parents need and want to know? Is there an action or change or new behavior that might need to be adopted? If possible, focus on no more than 3 key pieces of information.
3. It is usually a good idea to practice communication messages. Prepare for tough questions that can be anticipated. Emphasize any action-oriented message; what can and should be done to protect or promote the patient's health? Who should do it?
4. Implement the risk communication effort. Listen carefully to the questions and to the responses of the person you are communicating with. Answer questions as specifically as possible. If the question cannot be answered, explain why and discuss the type

of information that would be needed to provide an answer. Use simple, clear language. Reinforce the messages over time if necessary. Try to ensure that office staff and other health care providers present a consistent message. It may be helpful to provide printed materials that the patient and parent can take home and refer to. The American Academy of Pediatrics and other professional organizations have some patient education booklets available.

5. Honestly evaluate the effectiveness of the communication. In some instances, one of the other health care team members may be the more appropriate communicator.

6. Know how to contact other local physicians, local public health officials, local elected officials, and the media if they need to be alerted to identify or prevent exposure.

## References

1. Covello VT. Risk communication and occupational medicine. *J Occup Med.* 1993;35:18–19
2. Woolf A, Cimino S. Environmental illness: educational needs of pediatric care providers. *Ambul Child Health.* 2001;7:43–51
3. Stickler GB, Simmons PS. Pediatricians' preferences for anticipatory guidance topics compared with parental anxieties. *Clin Pediatr.* 1995;34:384–387
4. Norland O. A discussion of risk tolerance principals. *The Hazards Forum Newsletter.* Summer 1999; Issue 27
5. Hage ML, Frazier LM. Reproductive risk communication: a clinical view. In: *Reproductive Hazards of the Workplace.* New York, NY: John Wiley & Sons, Inc; 1998
6. Gochfeld M. Environmental risk assessment. In: Last JM, Wallace RB, eds. *Maxcy-Rosenau-Last Public Health and Preventive Medicine.* 13th ed. Norwalk, CT: Appleton & Lange; 1992:336
7. Covello VT, Allen FW. *Seven Cardinal Rules of Risk Communication.* Washington, DC; Environmental Protection Agency, Office of Policy Analysis; 1992
8. Miller M, Solomon G. Environmental risk communication for the clinician. *Pediatrics.* 2003;112:211–217
9. Flynn J, Slovic P, Mertz CK. Gender, race, and perception of environmental health risks. *Risk Anal.* 1994;14:1101–1108

# 42
# Environmental Health Advocacy

*"It should be our aim to discover neglected problems and, so far as in our power, to correct evils and introduce reform."*—Isaac Abt, MD, first president of the American Academy of Pediatrics

When it comes to political advocacy, pediatricians are powerful friends of children. This is especially true in the area of environmental health, where a pediatrician's education, training, and professional experience can help transform an environmental debate into a debate about public health. Simply put, by advocating for the health component of environmental health, pediatricians have the opportunity to significantly improve the lives of children and their families by improving the environment in which they live.[1]

Pediatricians have a long history of effectively advocating for children's environmental health at the federal and state level. These efforts have yielded the enactment of numerous state and federal laws, addressing such issues as air quality, lead poisoning prevention, pesticide safety, and environmental research. This chapter outlines several key tools and opportunities for pediatric environmental health advocacy. Additional advocacy resources also are provided.

## Know the Audience
Although pediatricians can act as advocates for individual patients in the office and at the bedside, major accomplishments for children can be realized at all levels of government—local, state, or federal. Each of these levels is composed of different audiences, including state representatives, members of Congress, and other public officials and the news media. Therefore, it is important for pediatricians to be familiar with the different audiences they may face while advocating for children's environmental health and safety.

## US Congress

The US Congress has 2 distinct chambers—the US Senate and the US House of Representatives. Each chamber has its own leadership, its own committee structure, and its own set of rules. Each chamber also has its own election cycle.

| US Senate | US House of Representatives |
| --- | --- |
| 100 senators, 2 from each state | 435 representatives; state populations determine distribution |
| Each senator represents entire state | Each representative represents one district within state |
| 6-year terms | 2-year terms |
| 1/3 of Senate up for re-election every 2 years | All representatives up for re-election every 2 years |

Laws are made in Congress by consideration and debate of legislation. There are 8 basic steps that govern the legislative process.

1. *Bill introduction.* To be considered by either the Senate or the House, a bill must first be introduced. Legislation can originate from concerns of a senator, a representative, or congressional staff. Legislation also can originate from concerns of a constituent. As such, pediatricians have a unique opportunity at this stage of the legislative process to suggest new proposals to improve children's environmental health and safety.

2. *Committee consideration.* After introduction, a bill is assigned a number and referred to an authorizing committee for study. While a bill is under committee consideration, it is scrutinized, analyzed, and modified by congressional members and staff. Hearings are held to review as much information as possible relevant to the bill under consideration. Hearings also allow committee members and staff to negotiate various legislative provisions. As committees complete their work, pediatricians have the opportunity to weigh

in with recommendations about the proposed legislative language. Such committee-level advocacy is often critical to the final outcome of a bill.

3. *Committee markup and vote.* This is the formal procedure by which all prior committee negotiations are approved. The result is a revised bill that is cleared for the next step in the process. In reality, this is usually a 2-step process because most bills are considered by a subcommittee, marked up and cleared by the subcommittee, and then sent to a full committee for a final markup and vote. The markup process therefore represents another opportunity for pediatricians to positively affect legislation because congressional members and staff determine which suggested revisions to include in the final bill.

4. *Floor consideration.* Once a bill has been passed by a committee, it is scheduled for floor debate and a vote. Before going to the floor, a committee chairperson usually knows how most members of that chamber will vote, regardless of their party affiliation. The floor manager of the bill also usually knows about all amendments to be offered in advance.

5. *Second chamber.* A bill passed by one chamber has completed only half of the legislative process. To advance further, the second chamber also must pass it. The legislation process outlined in the preceding 4 steps is repeated as the bill moves through the second chamber. As with the first chamber, pediatricians have several opportunities in the early stages of the legislative process to advocate for specific provisions affecting children's environmental health and safety.

6. *Conference committee.* A conference must be held to reconcile the differences between Senate and House versions of the same or similar bills. If an identical bill is passed by both chambers, a conference committee may not be held. If, however, different versions are passed by each chamber, effective advocacy by pediatricians can help to ensure that the best alternative is included in the final bill.

7. *Final vote.* Votes by both chambers are needed to approve the compromise agreed to by the conference committee.

8. *Presidential action.* Through party leadership in Congress, the president can attempt to influence a piece of legislation at any point during its course through the legislative process. However, when a bill reaches the president's desk, he or she has the ultimate authority to sign or veto it. The president has 10 days from the time the bill arrives on his or her desk to sign or veto it. If the bill is vetoed, it goes back to Congress for reconsideration. Overturning a veto requires a two-thirds vote of both the Senate and the House.

Once legislation is passed by Congress and is signed into law by the president, attention shifts to the relevant federal agency, or agencies, responsible for implementing the law.

### Federal Agencies

Once a bill is passed by Congress and approved by the president, it has little practical effect until it is implemented by the relevant federal agency or agencies. Currently there are 14 cabinet-level agencies, including the US Department of Health and Human Services and the Environmental Protection Agency, which are responsible for developing federal regulations to implement federal law. These regulations guide the activities of those industries, professions, and programs overseen by the agency. They also direct the work of the agency's employees.

Because federal regulations dictate how, and when, a new law will be enforced, participation in the regulatory process is just as important as participation in the legislative process. A legislative victory can be lost if the regulatory agency charged with implementing a new law issues a regulation with the adverse interpretation of a bill.[2] Similarly, a new law can be devastated by an agency that stalls its writing or implementation of a regulation.

Regular communication between pediatricians and the federal agencies can increase the opportunity for early and ongoing involvement in the promulgation of regulations. One key communication tool used to affect the development and implementation of federal regulations is the submission of public comments. Agencies are required to solicit public comment before finalizing most new regulations. This public comment period provides a critical time for pediatricians to review, analyze, and make recommendations about proposed regulations. Because so much rests on an agency's interpretation of the law, pediatric involvement at this level can dramatically affect the practical effect a new law will have on children's environmental health.

### State Legislatures

While national attention often focuses on Congress, much of the nation's legislative work is accomplished at the state level. In fact, state legislatures have been called "the guts of democracy" by political scientists such as Alan Rosenthal.[3] In 1997, for example, approximately 130 000 bills were introduced in state legislatures, nearly 30 000 of which became laws. That number translates into a nationwide passage rate of 80 state bills for every federal bill that Congress enacted in the same period.

Currently 49 states have bicameral, or 2-chamber, legislatures. The "upper" chamber is commonly known as the Senate and contains fewer members than the other chamber, known as the House of Representatives or the Assembly. Nebraska is the exception; its legislature is unicameral, or 1 chamber, and its nonpartisan members are referred to as senators.

There is less consistency among the states on the frequency and duration of legislative sessions. Some state legislative sessions are as short as 30 days, others last for 2 years; still others meet only during even- or odd-numbered years. No matter the structure or schedule of the legislature, however, an invaluable resource published in every state is the state "blue book." The "blue book" contains the names, addresses, and telephone numbers of state legislators and other public officials. It also contains the state departments, commissions, and agencies charged with implementing legislation once it is passed, as well as the state's judicial system.

The same 8-step legislative process seen in the US Congress governs the work of the state legislatures. Understanding this process, as well as the slight variations from state to state and chamber to chamber, is critical to effective advocacy on any issue, including children's health.

## Advocacy Tools

Many people experience some uneasiness when they hear the word "lobbying." In fact, some people still envision lobbying as a less than desirable activity conducted in smoke-filled rooms by shady characters. Although there may be some historical truth to that characterization, lobbying today is quite different. Today lobbying is the process of informing, educating, negotiating, and influencing policy makers. It is advocacy in the simplest form, and it is a powerful opportunity to use knowledge and expertise to contribute to the development of sound public policy.

There are many ways that pediatricians can advocate for children at the local, state, and national levels. The following are just a few of the advocacy tools pediatricians can use to advocate for children in the political arena:

- Meeting with public officials
- Writing to public officials
- Providing testimony
- Working with the media

### Meeting With Public Officials

Meeting with public officials enables pediatricians to become more acquainted with their appointed and elected representatives. Pediatricians can schedule appointments to discuss specific issues or to follow up on letters. Pediatricians also can invite public officials to their clinics or offices to learn more about pediatric practice.

Generally, state legislators and public officials are more personally accessible than members of Congress or federal executives. However, federal and state legislators typically return home on weekends and during legislative breaks. Federal officials often request that constituents meet with their staff rather than with them personally; in Congress it is the staff who are largely responsible for initially developing policy positions on specific issues.

When meeting with a public official, it is important to

1. *Be prepared.* Before meeting with a public official, prepare for the visit by reading available background material on the issue to be discussed. Try to discuss the issue or problem in a manner that is relevant to the lawmaker, drawing examples from personal experience to demonstrate how an issue affects children in his or her hometown. Prepare a brief fact sheet or backgrounder to serve as a "leave-behind" that can remind the public official of the key points that were discussed.
2. *Present the most important points first.* Because a public official's time may be limited, convey the strongest arguments first. Time permitting, elaborate with more details. Include additional information, as appropriate, on any leave-behind.
3. *Demonstrate expertise.* Public officials recognize pediatricians as children's health experts and welcome the information they can provide on issues related to children's health.
4. *Be honest.* Never make up an answer to a question. Instead, offer to provide any requested information at a later time.
5. *Follow up on your visit.* Send a follow-up letter thanking the public official and staff for taking the time to meet. In the letter, review the issues discussed and any actions agreed on during the visit.

### *Writing to Public Officials*
The constituent letter is one of the most effective ways to gain the attention of a public official. These personalized letters typically

receive more attention than form letters, preprinted postcards, or petitions combined. When writing a public official—and this applies to electronic mail communications too—it is important to

1. *Be brief.* A single page clearly presenting the opinions, facts, and reasons for supporting or opposing an issue is ideal.
2. *Include names, addresses, and telephone numbers.* By providing this identifying information, public officials can more easily distinguish constituents from non-constituents and respond accordingly.
3. *Identify bill number and author.* When writing a public official to urge support or opposition to a specific bill, be sure to reference the bill number and author in the first paragraph of the letter. If the bill number is unknown, use the popular name of the bill if it has one, such as the "Children's Health Plan."
4. *Discuss one issue per letter.* Presenting several issues in one letter can be confusing and may dilute the effectiveness of a request for action.
5. *Offer expertise.* Public officials and their staff appreciate information from constituents who have special expertise on issues under consideration. Pediatricians, by their education and training, are experts in children's health and therefore can help guide public officials on issues affecting children and their families.
6. *Time the arrival of all correspondence.* A convincing message that provides insight on a children's health matter will do little to change the outcome if it arrives too soon or too late in the public policy process.
7. *Be courteous and express gratitude.* Use reason and never threaten or make demands. Consider writing letters of appreciation when you feel a public official has done a commendable job. Lawmakers value thank-you letters and appreciate encouragement from constituents.

### Providing Testimony

Another effective means of advocating to state and federal officials is to testify at a hearing. Providing testimony is an opportunity to publicly endorse, oppose, or express concerns about a specific piece of legislation. Pediatricians can testify in person or in writing. At the congressional level, only invited witnesses are permitted to provide oral testimony.

As with any presentation, testifying effectively depends on thorough preparation. If specific legislation is to be discussed, be sure to read the bill and any available analyses of the legislation carefully. If the hearing is on an issue only, research the topic and collect facts that support the points that need to be made. Either way, secure the most current data available, and be sure to check that all facts and background materials are accurate.

Whether the testimony is written or oral, there are a few key points that should be included in all remarks.

1. *Identify the speaker and the speaker's credentials.* Begin by giving the speaker's name, title, residence, and any other relevant credentials.
2. *Speak from personal experience.* Anecdotes and specific examples pertaining to individual children are more likely than generalities to sway legislators.
3. *Be positive and constructive.* Offer solutions to problems whenever possible.

It is important to be skilled in all the available ways of communicating with public officials. Whether by telephone, letter, electronic mail, personal visit, or formal testimony, the effectiveness and persuasiveness of the message in content and presentation can be vital to success.

### Working With the Media

Another audience for effective advocacy is the media. Using the news media to increase public awareness of an issue can help to produce positive change in public policy. Radio, television, and print media also are excellent channels through which pediatricians can disseminate their knowledge and expertise while undertaking a public policy initiative. When working with the media, there are a few specific tools that should be kept in mind.

1. *The pitch letter.* These personalized letters to editors, reporters, or producers can help generate interest in an issue that is important to the pediatric community. Because curiosity is the heart of news gathering, it is best to start letters with a probing question— followed by a startling answer. Providing current and accurate statistics also can serve as a hook to grab the reporter's attention.

2. *Letters to the editor.* Letters to the editor are exactly that—letters written to the editor of a newspaper with the objective of being published on the editorial page. These letters generally respond to specific articles or editorials that already have been published. A letter to the editor may clarify a point, refute a charge, or simply react to a recent situation or occurrence that received media coverage. Brief letters that offer important information for readers are more likely to be published. Letters to the editor are often the simplest and most commonly used advocacy tool.

3. *Op/Ed pieces.* These are so-named because the opinion page generally appears opposite the editorial page in a newspaper. The letters or articles that appear on this page are submitted by the general public. Effective op/eds define an issue or state a current problem, and they provide background and historical information to support the claims that have been made. Op/ed pieces should always include suggestions that can change or improve the situation.

4. *Feature stories.* Because many feature stories are based on human interest topics, this arena is excellent for stories on pediatric issues. Write a pitch letter to the feature writers or the editor of a feature section suggesting a story about children's environmental health and safety. If government action is needed to help remedy the situation, suggest that during an interview.

5. *Television.* Although the reach of television is vast, it is an intimate medium. News reporters can spend anywhere from 20 minutes to

several weeks investigating and developing a story for the television news. Pediatricians can provide reporters with an expert's opinion on a children's health issue through interviews. Pediatricians also can serve as expert panelists on community talk shows.

6. *Radio.* Radio reporters and interviewers often work on much more restricted timelines than do television or even print reporters. As such, it is crucial to present the main message and catchphrase up front. As with television, radio talk shows or call-in shows provide another media outlet for advocacy.

No matter which communications medium is used, it is important to present advocacy views accurately, professionally, and personally. The more sincere and understandable the message, the more widely it will be considered.

## Conclusion

The very nature of pediatric practice extends beyond the office and the bedside to involve advocacy at the community and governmental level on behalf of children. This is especially true in the area of environmental health because children are so clearly affected by the air, water, food, and general environment around them. Whether serving on a governor's advisory committee, providing public comments on a proposed regulation, visiting or writing a public official, or leading the support of a legislative proposal, pediatricians can make a difference in the lives of children through effective public advocacy.

The American Academy of Pediatrics (AAP) has numerous resources to assist these advocacy efforts. The AAP Committee on Federal Government Affairs and Committee on State Government Affairs can assist members with legislative and regulatory activities at the federal and state levels. Similarly, the staff of the AAP Department of Federal Affairs and the Division of State Government Affairs are available to answer member questions and provide support.

Please also see the *AAP Government Affairs Handbook,* from which much of this material was drawn.

## Resources

*American Academy of Pediatrics*
Department of Federal Affairs, Internet:
http://www.aap.org/advocacy/washing/mainpage.htm
Division of State Government Affairs, Internet:
http://www.aap.org/advocacy/stgov.htm
Members Only Channel, Internet: http://www.aap.org/moc

*Federal*
White House, Internet: http://www.whitehouse.gov

*Congressional*
Thomas: Legislative Information on the Internet: http://thomas.loc.gov
US House of Representatives, Internet: http://www.house.gov
US Senate, Internet: http://www.senate.gov

*State*
National Association of Counties, Internet: http://www.naco.org
National Conference of State Legislatures, Internet: http://www.ncsl.org
National Governors Association, Internet: http://www.nga.org
US Conference of Mayors, Internet: http://www.usmayors.org

## References

1. Paulson JA. Pediatric advocacy. *Pediatr Clin North Am.* 2001;48:1307–1318
2. Blum JO, Bowers HH, eds. *Beyond Washington: An Association Guide to Shaping a State Government Affairs Program.* Washington, DC: American Society of Association Executives; 1990:45
3. Rosenthal A. The legislative institution: transformed and at risk. In: Van Horn CE, ed. *The State of the States.* Washington, DC: CQ Press; 1989:69

# 43
# Risk Assessment and Risk Management

Environmental health risk assessment in the broadest terms is any method of systematic collection and interpretation of scientific information relating environmental hazard(s) to adverse human health outcome(s). While it has many forms (from expert judgment as exercised by individual clinicians during clinical practice to highly proscribed mathematical determinations of probability statements of risk from experimental data), the term risk assessment has come to be synonymous with the standard practices of the federal regulatory agencies used to set regulations. Risk management is the sociopolitical process that results in policy. This chapter gives a brief history of the evolution of federal regulatory assessment and reviews the key concepts of environmental risk assessment and risk management. (Risk perception and risk communication are discussed separately in Chapter 41.)

## Risk Assessment

Risk assessment has its roots in 19th century industrial toxicology and public health, but has gained its current form during the past 3 decades of rapid expansion of US federal environmental laws and regulatory agencies.[1] Beginning in the 1950s, the US Food and Drug Administration (FDA) began to establish acceptable daily intake levels for noncarcinogenic food additives or contaminants using animal toxicology studies and the application of safety factors.[2] This regulatory approach assumes that for a given substance there exists an exposure level below which no harm to human health will occur, such an exposure level is measurable, and it can be inferred from experimental data from animal studies. During this same period, the Atomic Energy and Nuclear Regulatory Commissions developed "probabilistic risk analysis" in their attempts to develop regulatory standards for the use of nuclear technology.[2] This approach, developed to address the carcinogenic capacity of ionizing radiation, assumes that any exposure level can cause harm to susceptible individuals and sets regulatory limits anticipated to cause tolerably low, but non-zero, elevations of the incidence of cancers. These 2 approaches have been developed in parallel by the federal regulatory agencies with input from academicians, industry representatives, and the federal courts. Numerous models for evaluation of laboratory data, extrapolation from animal toxicity to human risk, approaches for incorporating issues of incomplete data, and scientific uncertainty in toxicity and exposure data evolved over the next decades. Scholarly debate is ongoing about the relative merits of standardized assumptions and general approaches to risk assessment, but decisions by the federal courts require that quantitative risk assessment be used by federal agencies in rule setting.[2]

In 1983, in an attempt to standardize environmental health risk assessment, the National Research Council proposed a 4-step risk assessment model that has been widely adopted and applied[3] (see Table 43.1). The 4 steps are (1) hazard identification, (2) dose-response assessment, (3) exposure assessment, and (4) risk characterization. In this schema, risk assessment is considered separately from risk management. The former is performed using predetermined criteria by scientists. The latter is performed by policy makers in the

**Table 43.1**
**Steps of Risk Assessment***

| Hazard identification | characterization of innate adverse toxic effects of agents |
|---|---|
| Dose-response assessment | charcterization of the relation between doses and incidences of adverse effects in exposed populations |
| Exposure assessment | measurement or estimation of the intensity, frequency, and duration of human exposure to agents |
| Risk characterization | estimation of the incidence of health effects under the various conditions of human exposure |

*From National Library of Medicine.[4]

political/policy sector. A brief overview of each step is discussed here and illustrated by US Environmental Protection Agency (EPA) and FDA standard approaches. Other agencies may apply quite different techniques.

## Hazard Identification

Hazard identification is a qualitative step that seeks to identify and review health effects data associated with exposure and determine whether a particular substance or chemical is causally linked to particular health effects. The EPA has developed a "weight of evidence classification scheme," which gives guidelines to risk assessors for interpretation of the data reviewed.[5] The standard scheme assigns highest confidence to direct human exposure studies followed (in descending order) by laboratory animal studies, in vitro studies, and structure-activity relationships (predicting a chemical's possible activity based on knowledge of its chemical structure). The scope of hazards identified usually is limited to direct adverse health effects on individual humans. In general, if a toxicant is judged to be carcinogenic, this is the endpoint targeted for risk assessment (as opposed to other possible endpoints such as neurotoxicity or reproductive toxicity). With noncarcinogens, a variety of other approaches may be taken depending on what human toxicities are anticipated.[6]

## Dose-Response Assessment

Hazard identification is followed by dose-response assessment. This step seeks to determine the relationship between the administered dose and the occurrence of health effects. Dose-response almost always is based on animal toxicity data. To generate a useful dose-response curve, sophisticated toxicology studies, extrapolation schemes, and pharmacokinetic modeling are all used with the goal of finding the maximal safe exposure of an individual to a specific chemical. Depending on the primary toxic effect, different experimental designs are employed to generate data. Carcinogens are considered to be "non-threshold" hazards. That is, there is no exposure level below which a carcinogen is considered "safe." Groups of animals are exposed to several high doses of the toxicant, and the data are fitted to a simple linear model extrapolated to zero. The assumption of a linear relationship is believed to be conservative and protective of human health. The slope of the dose-response line is used to calculate increased risk of cancer at various exposure levels.

Most noncarcinogens such as neurotoxicants or developmental toxicants (teratogens) are considered to exhibit a threshold of toxicity, and groups of animals are tested at lower doses to find the lowest dose where toxicity begins to appear (Figure 43.1). The highest dose tested without any measurable effect is called the NOEL (no observable effect level). The highest dose tested without a clear adverse health effect is called the NOAEL (no observable adverse effect level).

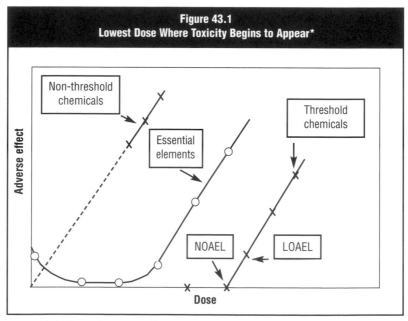

**Figure 43.1**
**Lowest Dose Where Toxicity Begins to Appear\***

*From World Health Organization.[7]

Correspondingly, LOEL (lowest observable effect level) and LOAEL (lowest observable adverse effect level) are the first doses in the experimental exposures that cause discernible effects and adverse health effects respectively. The shape of the dose-response curve for noncarcinogens often is found to approximate a sigmoid curve, with the true threshold of toxicity somewhere between the NOEL and LOAEL (see Risk Characterization).

## Exposure Assessment

Exposure assessment is the step used to determine the likely human exposures to a hazard or chemical. To be useful, it must accurately characterize all important sources of a particular toxicant in the environment (eg, point or non-point source, mixture, chemical form), identify sources of exposure (eg, groundwater, surface water, air, soil, food, breast milk), and quantify exposures (eg, microgram per liter in drinking water, microgram per gram in soil). Realistic exposure scenarios must be considered that identify at-risk populations or subpopulations, duration of exposure, routes of exposure, types of substances, etc. The chemical characteristics of the environmental toxicant must be evaluated in the context of entry point into the environment (eg, point source into air), climate and weather, topography and geology, level of urban/rural development, etc. Because of the complexity of this task, exposure assessment frequently is the most incomplete portion of the risk assessment, particularly with respect to pediatric exposures that are less well studied and poorly characterized. Increasingly in recent years, biomarkers for various envionmental toxicants have been developed that can be measured directly in representative exposed populations to eliminate some of the uncertainties in modeled exposures.[8]

## Risk Characterization

Risk characterization is the final step of risk assessment and involves the synthesis of the dose-response and exposure assessments. The result is expressed as the maximum acceptable exposure that is protective of health in an exposed population. Assumptions made in the first 3 steps of risk assessment generate significant uncertainties in the risk characterization step (ie, non-threshold toxicants, such as carcinogens, are handled differently from threshold-exhibiting toxicants).

For a carcinogen, risk traditionally has been characterized as the proportion of excess cancers following continuous, low-dose exposure at a specific average level over a 70-year lifetime. Risk is generally considered acceptable if the exposure results in an increase of less than 1 in 1 million ($10^{-6}$) cancers over a lifetime. This approach does not distinguish exposures to fully mature humans from exposures in utero, during infancy, childhood, or adolescence.

Noncarcinogens, thought to have thresholds for adverse health effects, are evaluated by comparing the projected exposure from the exposure assessment to the acceptable exposure level generated from the dose-response curve. Here extrapolation from animal toxicity testing is required to determine a reference dose (RfD, used by EPA) or an acceptable daily intake (ADI, used by FDA), that if not exceeded over a lifetime should not result in any unacceptable effects in exposed humans. Extrapolation from experimentally determined toxic levels of exposure in animals to likely safe levels of exposure in humans frequently is accomplished by taking the most reliable animal NOAEL and dividing it by some number of uncertainty or safety factors. The rationale for this practice is that humans may be more susceptible than laboratory animals to toxicity, so permissible levels of exposure could be well below those found to be nontoxic in animals. Safety or uncertainty factors usually are multiples of 10, an arbitrary multiplier. The FDA, which pioneered this approach, usually applies a safety factor of 100 (1 factor of 10 to account for the potential differences between animal and human susceptibility and an additional factor of 10 to account for differences in human susceptibility). These factors are applied to the NOAEL from the most reliable study(ies) to determine the acceptable daily intake. The EPA uses a similar approach to calculate RfDs (see Table 43.2). Additional safety factors may be added if the quality of the toxicity data is inadequate, if there is no determined NOAEL, or to account for increased risk to certain groups such as children. It is important to realize that the selection of a specific body of experimental data for use in the calculation, choice of NOAEL versus NOEL, and decisions about the number and magnitude of safety factors to be used are all based on expert judgment, standards of practice, and various protocols. Each of these individual decisions can affect the magnitude of the risk prediction by orders of magnitude. It is unclear how well these practices protect children whose exposure and vulnerabilities often are quite different from those of adults (see Chapter 2).

The output of this 4-step risk assessment process is an expression of risk, most commonly quantified as the proportion (or probability) of a specific population(s) exposed to a toxicant(s) at a particular level(s) that will express a particular toxic effect(s). For carcinogens this risk characterization attempts to identify regulatory levels below

**Table 43.2**
**Extrapolation From Animal Toxicity Data to Reference Dose (RfD)\*†**

$$RfD = \frac{NOAEL \text{ or } LOAEL}{UF_1 \times UF_2 \ldots}$$

| Examples of Uncertainty Factors | |
| --- | --- |
| 10X | human variability |
| 10X | extrapolation from animals to humans |
| 10X | use of LOAEL instead of NOAEL |
| 0.1–10X | modifying factor |

\* Adapted from National Library of Medicine.[4]
† RfDs are calculated by the US Environmental Protection Agency. Similar measures include acceptable daily intake (same calculation except modifying factors not used) and minimal risk levels (calculated by the Agency for Toxic Substances and Disease Registry for noncancer endpoints). UF, uncertainty factor

which expected exposure to populations would result in a "negligible" increased risk of cancer rate. For non-threshold toxicities, this process seeks to determine acceptable levels of toxicant in a particular medium (eg, water, food) that is anticipated to cause no adverse effects to humans assuming normal exposure scenarios. For single chemical exposures expected via a single route of exposure that cause a single adverse effect, the process of risk assessment can be quite straightforward. For mixed exposures, encountered by multiple routes from multiple sources that can cause multiple toxic effects, the process becomes extremely complex. Because virtually all real world environmental exposures are to complex mixtures of chemicals in air, water, soil, and food, which vary geographically and in time, the precision of standard risk assessments applied to non-theoretical populations may be quite limited.

Despite its limitations, risk assessment can provide useful information to policy makers when inherent scientific uncertainties and default assumptions (standard assumptions regarding exposures, mechanism of action, applicability of animal data to humans, etc) are fully understood and transparent. Historically, risk assessment and research on environmental hazards have considered mainly the outcomes of adult exposures and most default assumptions and safety factor calculations were geared to address lifetime exposures in an adult male. Most commonly, single toxicants (eg, benzene) and single outcomes (eg, leukemia) have been analyzed. Exposures to complex mixtures (such as environmental tobacco smoke) are increasingly studied, but present enormous methodological challenges.

In the early 1990s the special vulnerabilities of children emerged in the scientific, political, and policy debate over environmental risks.[9] As a result, there has been a substantial increase in research directed toward evaluating the toxicities of and exposures to environmental toxicants in children, which can be applied to risk assessment and risk management strategies.[10]

## Risk Management

Risk management is that process by which risks are compared, data gaps and uncertainties are judged, and risk/benefit–cost/benefit considerations are combined to produce specific policies that seek to minimize risk to individuals and groups. It is an iterative process that should remain flexible and be reviewed periodically (see Figure 43.2). While risk management may be informed by science, the process essentially is political because it involves weighing of societal values and perceptions of risks.[11] For environmental health risks, risk management is the work of policy makers in federal regulatory agencies such as the EPA, the US Department of Agriculture, the Nuclear Regulatory Commission, and state and local authorities. Despite the improved understanding of the special vulnerabilities of children to

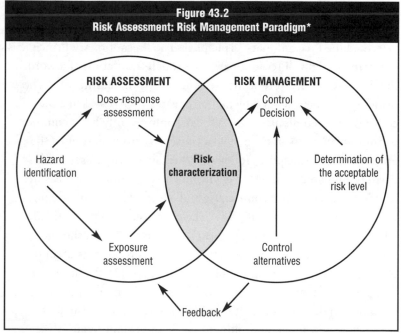

**Figure 43.2**
**Risk Assessment: Risk Management Paradigm\***

*From National Library of Medicine.[4]

environmental exposures, increasingly experts debate the feasibility of relying solely on the traditional risk assessment model to inform risk management when designing policy. Chemical-by-chemical risk assessment is a time-consuming and data-intensive process requiring generalizations and assumptions that are difficult to validate, particularly in children. While risk assessment can work well for simple environmental exposures with one adverse health outcome (eg, to determine the acceptable level of radon in indoor air to minimize excess lung cancer or the acceptable level of fluoride in drinking water to prevent skeletal fluorosis), most environmental exposures are much more complex and adverse outcomes much more varied and numerous. Generating adequate data for all the adverse health outcomes for children and exposure estimates at all developmental stages is a costly resource- and time-intensive task.

Because of the well-recognized limitations of risk assessment, other tools for risk management are being developed. One prominent model is termed the Precautionary Principle.[11] The Precautionary Principle is of German origin. "Precautionary" is a rough translation of a word that literally means "forecaring" (caring for a difficult future).[12] The principle is widely applied by the European Union.[13,14] While the concept has been discussed for 30 years, only recently has a common definition begun to arise. In 1998 a consensus group described the Precautionary Principle as follows: "When an activity raises threats of harm to human health or the environment, precautionary measures should be taken even if some cause and effect relationships are not fully established scientifically."[12,15] The consensus group identified 4 key components of the principle: (1) preventive action should be taken when uncertainty about safety exits, (2) proponents of a proposed activity bear the burden of proof of safety, (3) all alternatives to a possibly harmful action should be explored, and (4) public participation in decision making should be increased. In the area of children's environmental health, it may be important to apply the

Precautionary Principle as the default rather than await the data required for a full risk assessment.[15]

The task of protecting children from environmental hazards is a difficult one. Established approaches to chemical-by-chemical risk assessment are useful, but may not be adequate. Involvement of pediatric health care professionals in the regulatory process is critical as the vulnerabilities of children to environmental hazards are deliberated by regulatory agencies.

### Online Glossary

US Environmental Protection Agency:
http://www.epa.gov/ocepa111/OCEPAterms/ and
http://www.epa.gov/iris/gloss8.htm

### Resources

Association of Occupational and Environmental Clinics (AOEC), phone: 202-347-4976, fax: 202-347-4950, e-mail: aoec@aoec.org, Internet: http://www.aoec.org. *An Introduction to Basic Risk Assessment* is available on CD-ROM by contacting the AOEC.

The Precautionary Principle, Internet: http://www.biotech-info.net/precautionary.html

National Center for Environmental Risk Assessment, Internet: http://cfpub.epa.gov/ncea/cfm/nceahome.cfm

### References

1. Covello VT, Mumpower J. Risk analysis and risk management: an historical perspective. *Risk Anal.* 1985;5:103–120
2. Centers for Risk Analysis. *A Historical Perspective on Risk Assessment in the Federal Government.* Boston, MA: Harvard School of Public Health; 1994
3. Committee on the Institutional Means for Assessment of Risks to Public Health, Commission on Life Sciences, National Research Council. *Risk Assessment in the Federal Government: Managing the Process.* Washington, DC: National Academies Press; 1983

4. National Library of Medicine. Risk assessment. In: *Toxicology Tutor I. Basic Principles*. Washington, DC: US Department of Health and Human Services. Available at: http://sis.nlm.nih.gov/ToxTutor/Tox1/a61.htm

5. US Environmental Protection Agency. *Guidelines for Carcinogen Risk Assessment*. Washington, DC: US Environmental Protection Agency; 1999:A1–A11. Available at: http://www.epa.gov/ncea/raf/pdfs/cancer_gls.pdf Appendix A

6. *EPA Risk Assessment Guidelines*. Available at: http://www.epa.gov/ncea/raf/rafguid.htm

7. World Health Organization. *Programme on Chemical Safety. Hazardous Chemicals in Human and Environmental Health. A Resource Book for School, College and University Students*. Geneva, Switzerland: World Health Organization; 2001. WHO/PCS/00

8. Centers for Disease Control and Prevention. *Second National Report on Human Exposure to Environmental Chemicals*. Available at: http://www.cdc.gov/exposurereport/pdf/SecondNER.pdf

9. Guzelian PS, Henry CJ, Olin SS. *Similarities & Differences Between Children & Adults: Implications of Risk Management*. Washington DC: ILSI Press; 1992

10. Miller MD, Marty MA, Arcus A, Brown J, Morry D, Sandy M. Differences between children and adults: implications for risk assessment at California EPA. *Int J Toxicol*. 2002;21:403–418

11. Raffensperger C, Tickner J, Jackson W. *Protecting Public Health and the Environment: Implementing the Precautionary Principle*. Washington, DC: Island Press; 1999

12. Raffensperger C. The precautionary principle: bearing witness to and alleviating suffering. *Altern Ther Health Med*. 2002;8:111–115

13. Foster KR, Vecchia P, Repacholi MH. Risk management. Science and the precautionary principle. *Science*. 2000;288:979–981

14. Kriebel D, Tichner J, Epstein P, et al. The precautionary principle in environmental science. *Environ Health Perspect*. 2001;109:871–876

15. Tichner JA, Hoppin P. Children's environmental health: a case study in implementing the precautionary principle. *Int J Occup Environ Health*. 2000;6:270–280

# Appendix A
# AAP Policy Statements and Technical Reports
# From the Committee on Environmental Health

Please visit the American Academy of Pediatrics (AAP) public online policy site for updated information on AAP Policy Statements and to access current policies: http://www.aappolicy.org/.

## Current Statements
**Radiation Disasters and Children**
PEDIATRICS, Vol 111, No 6, 1455–1466, June 2003

**Pediatric Exposure and Potential Toxicity of Phthalate Plasticizers**
PEDIATRICS, Vol 111, No 6, 1467–1474, June 2003

**Mercury in the Environment: Implications for Pediatricians**
PEDIATRICS, Vol 108, No 1, 197–205, July 2001

**Irradiation of Food**
PEDIATRICS, Vol 106, No 6, 1505–1510, December 2000

**Chemical-Biological Terrorism and Its Impact on Children: A Subject Review**
PEDIATRICS, Vol 105, No 3, 662–670, March 2000

**Ultraviolet Light: A Hazard to Children**
PEDIATRICS, Vol 104, No 2, 328–333, August 1999

**Screening for Elevated Blood Lead Levels**
PEDIATRICS, Vol 101, No 6, 1072–1078, June 1998

**Toxic Effects of Indoor Molds**
PEDIATRICS, Vol 101, No 4, 712–714, April 1998

**Noise: A Hazard to the Fetus and Newborn**
PEDIATRICS, Vol 100, No 4, 724–727, October 1997

**Environmental Tobacco Smoke: A Hazard to Children**
PEDIATRICS, Vol 99, No 4, 639–642, April 1997

**Hazards of Child Labor**
PEDIATRICS, Vol 95, No 2, 311–313, February 1995

**Ambient Air Pollution: Respiratory Hazards to Children**
PEDIATRICS, Vol 91, No 6, 1210–1213, June 1993

## Retired Statements

**Thimerosal in Vaccines—An Interim Report to Clinicians**
PEDIATRICS, Vol 104, No 3, 570–574, September 1999
Retired 11/02

**Risk of Ionizing Radiation Exposure to Children: A Subject Review**
PEDIATRICS, Vol 101, No 4, 717–719, April 1998
Retired 4/02

**PCBs in Breast Milk**
PEDIATRICS, Vol 94, No 1, 122–123, July 1994
Retired 2/01

**Use of Chloral Hydrate for Sedation in Children**
PEDIATRICS, Vol 92, No 3, 471–473, September 1993
Retired 2/00

**Lead Poisoning: From Screening to Primary Prevention**
PEDIATRICS, Vol 92, No 1, 176–183, July 1993
Retired 6/98

**Radon Exposure: A Hazard to Children**
PEDIATRICS, Vol 83, No 5, 799–802, May 1989
Retired 2/01

**Childhood Lead Poisoning**
PEDIATRICS, Vol 79, No 3, 457–465, March 1987
Retired 10/93

**Asbestos Exposure in Schools**
PEDIATRICS, Vol 79, No 2, 301–305, February 1987
Retired 2/01

**Involuntary Smoking: A Hazard to Children**
PEDIATRICS, Vol 77, No 5, 755–757, May 1986
Retired 4/97

**Smokeless Tobacco — A Carcinogenic Hazard to Children**
PEDIATRICS, Vol 76, No 6, 1009–1011, December 1985
Retired 2/01

**Special Susceptibility of Children to Radiation Effects**
PEDIATRICS, Vol 72, No 6, 809, December 1983
Retired 4/98

**Environmental Consequences of Tobacco Smoking: Implications for Public Policies that Affect the Health of Children**
PEDIATRICS, Vol 70, No 2, 314–315, August 1982
Retired 2/87

**National Standard for Airborne Lead**
PEDIATRICS, Vol 62, No 6, 1070–1071, December 1978
Retired 2/87

**PCBs in Breast Milk**
PEDIATRICS, Vol 62, No 3, 407, September 1978
Retired 9/94

**Infant Radiant Warmers**
PEDIATRICS, Vol 61, No 1, 113–114, January 1978
Retired 6/95

**Hyperthermia from Malfunctioning Radiant Heaters**
PEDIATRICS, Vol 59, No 6, 1041–1042, June 1977
Retired 2/87

## Carcinogens in Drinking Water
PEDIATRICS, Vol 57, No 4, 462–464, April 1976
Retired 2/87

## Effects of Cigarette Smoking on the Fetus and Child
PEDIATRICS, Vol 57, No 3, 411–413, March 1976
Retired 9/94

## Noise Pollution: Neonatal Aspects
PEDIATRICS, Vol 54, No 4, 476–478, October 1974
Retired 10/97

## Animal Feedlots
PEDIATRICS, Vol 51, No 3, 582–592, March 1973
Retired 9/94

## Lead Content of Paint Applied to Surfaces Accessible to Young Children
PEDIATRICS, Vol 49, No 6, 918–921, June 1972
Retired 2/87

## Pediatric Problems Related to Deteriorated Housing
PEDIATRICS, Vol 49, No 4, 627, April 1972
Retired 2/87

## Earthenware Containers: A Potential Source of Acute Lead Poisoning
Newsletter, Vol 22, No 13, 4, August 15, 1971
Retired 2/87

## Neurotoxicity from Hexachlorophene
Newsletter, Vol 22, No 7, 4, May 1971
Retired 2/87

## Acute and Chronic Childhood Lead Poisoning
PEDIATRICS, Vol 47, No 5, 950–951, May 1971
Retired 11/86

**Pediatric Aspects of Air Pollution**
PEDIATRICS, Vol 46, No 4, 637–639, October 1970
Retired 2/87

**More on Radioactive Fallout**
Newsletter Supplement, Vol 21, No 8, April 15, 1970
Retired 2/87

**Smoking and Children: A Pediatric Viewpoint**
PEDIATRICS, Vol 44, No 5, Part 1, 757–759, November 1969
Retired 2/87

**Present Status of Water Pollution Control**
PEDIATRICS, Vol 34, No 3, 431–440, September 1964
Retired 2/87

**Hazards of Radioactive Fallout**
PEDIATRICS, Vol 29, No 5, 845–847, May 1962
Retired 2/95

**Statement on the Use of Diagnostic X-Ray**
PEDIATRICS, Vol 28, No 4, 676–677, October 1961
Retired 2/87

## Pediatrics Supplements
**A Partnership to Establish an Environmental Safety Net
for Children**
Supplement to PEDIATRICS, Vol 112, No 1, Part II, July 2003

**The Susceptibility of the Fetus and Child to Chemical Pollutants**
Supplement to PEDIATRICS, Vol 53, No 5, Part II, May 1974

**Conference on the Pediatric Significance of Peacetime
Radioactive Fallout**
Supplement to PEDIATRICS, Vol 41, No 1, Part II, January 1968

# Appendix B
# Resources for Environmental Health

The American Academy of Pediatrics has not reviewed the material on these Web sites. Inclusion in this list does not imply endorsement.

| Organization | Contact Information |
|---|---|
| **Governmental** | |
| Agency for Toxic Substances and Disease Registry (ATSDR) US Department of Health & Human Services (DHHS) 1600 Clifton Rd NE; Mail Stop E-28 Atlanta, GA 30333 | Web: http://www.atsdr.cdc.gov/ Information Center Clearinghouse: Phone: 404-639-6360 Fax: 404-639-0744 Emergency Response Branch Phone: 404-639-0615 |
| ATSDR Child Health Initiative | Web: http://www.atsdr.cdc.gov/child/ |
| ATSDR GATHER (Geographic Analysis Tool for Health and Environmental Research) | Web: http://gis.cdc.gov/atsdr |
| ATSDR Toxicological Profiles | Web: http://www.atsdr.cdc.gov/toxpro2.html |
| ATSDR Regional Offices | Web: http://www.atsdr.cdc.gov/oro_contact.html |
| California Electric and Magnetic Fields (EMF) Program 1515 Clay St, Suite 1700 Oakland, CA 94612 | Web: http://www.dhs.ca.gov/ehib/emf |
| National Center for Environmental Health (NCEH) 4770 Buford Hwy, NE Mail Stop F-28 Atlanta, GA 30341-3724 | Web: http://www.cdc.gov/nceh/ E-mail: ncehinfo@cdc.gov NCEH Health Line: 888-232-6789 |
| NCEH Asthma Program | Web: http://www.cdc.gov/nceh/airpollution/asthma |
| NCEH Lead Poisoning Prevention Program | Web: http://www.cdc.gov/nceh/lead/lead.htm |
| NCEH Human Exposure Report | Web: http://www.cdc.gov/nceh/dls/report/ |

| Organization | Contact Information |
|---|---|
| **Governmental** | |
| State Health Department Search (CDC) | Web: http://www.cdc.gov/search2.htm |
| CDC Bioterrorism Information | Web: http://www.bt.cdc.gov<br>Emergency Number: 770-488-7100<br>Emergency Chemical & Biological<br>  Hotline: 888-422-8737<br>Public Inquiry Number: 404-639-3534 or<br>  800-311-3435 |
| National Institute for Occupational Safety and Health (NIOSH) | Web: http://www.cdc.gov/niosh/homepage.html<br>E-mail: eidtechinfo@cdc.gov<br>Phone: 800-35-NIOSH<br>(800-356-4674) |
| Consumer Product Safety Commission (CPSC)<br>4340 East West Hwy<br>Bethesda, MD 20814 | Web: http://www.cpsc.gov<br>Phone: 800-638-2772<br>Fax: 301-504-0124 |
| US Environmental Protection Agency (EPA)<br>1200 Pennsylvania Ave NW<br>Washington, DC 20460 | Web: http://www.epa.gov<br>Administrative Phone: 202-272-0167 |
| EPA Office of Children's Health Protection | Web: http://yosemite.epa.gov/ochp/<br>  ochpweb.nsf/homepage<br>Office of Child Health Protection Phone:<br>  202-564-2188 |
| EPA Office of Pesticide Programs | Web: http://www.epa.gov/pesticides<br>Office of Pesticide Programs Phone:<br>  703-305-5017<br>National Pesticides Hotline: 800-222-1222 |
| EPA Office of Air and Radiation | Office main Web : http://www.epa.gov/oar<br>Indoor air Web : http://www.epa.gov/iaq<br>Indoor Air Quality Information Clearinghouse<br>  Phone: 800-438-4318<br>Tools for Schools Program Web:<br>  http://www.epa.gov/iaq/schools/index.html<br>Air Now–ground-level ozone Web:<br>  http://www.epa.gov/airnow |
| EPA Endocrine Disruptor Screening Program | Web: http://www.epa.gov/scipoly/oscpendo |

| Organization | Contact Information |
|---|---|
| **Governmental** | |
| EPA Children's Environmental Health Research Initiative | Web: http://es.epa.gov/ncer/centers |
| EPA Chemical Emergency Preparedness and Prevention | Web: http://yosemite.epa.gov/oswer/cep poweb.nsf/content/index.html <br> Chemical Spills Emergency Hotline: 800-424-8802 <br> Hazardous Waste/Community Right to Know Hotline: 800-424-9346 |
| EPA Office of Water | Web: http://www.epa.gov/water/index.html <br> Safe Drinking Water Hotline: 800-426-4791 <br> Drinking Water Advisories Web: http://www.epa.gov/waterscience/drinking <br> Fish Consumption Advisories Web: http://www.epa.gov/ost/fish/ |
| EPA Office of Pollution Prevention & Toxics | Web: http://www.epa.gov/opptintr/index.html <br> Toxic Substances Control Act (TSCA) Information Line: 202-554-1404 |
| EPA Toxics Release Inventory Program | Web: http://www.epa.gov/tri |
| Center for Food Safety and Applied Nutrition (CFSAN) <br> Food and Drug Administration (FDA) <br> 5100 Paint Branch Parkway <br> College Park, MD 20740-3835 | Web: http://www.cfsan.fda.gov <br> Phone: 888-SAFEFOOD |
| Food Safety: Gateway to Government Food Safety Information | Web: http://www.FoodSafety.gov |
| Food Safety and Inspection Service <br> Food Safety Education Office <br> 1400 Independence Ave, SW <br> Washington, DC 20250 | Web: http://www.fsis.usda.gov <br> E-mail: fsis.webmaster@usda.gov <br> Phone: 301-504-9605 <br> Fax: 301-504-0203 |
| National Institute of Environmental Health Sciences (NIEHS) <br> US DHHS <br> PO Box 12233 <br> Research Triangle Park, NC 27709 | Web: http://www.niehs.nih.gov <br> Phone: 919-541-1919 <br> Fax: 919-541-3592 |
| The Environmental Genome Project | Web: http://www.niehs.nih.gov/envgenom/home.htm |

| Organization | Contact Information |
|---|---|
| **Governmental** | |
| NIEHS Children's Environmental Health Research Initiative | Web: http://www.niehs.nih.gov/external/ resinits/ri-28.htm http://www.niehs.nih.gov/dert/programs/ translat/children/children.htm |
| The National Toxicology Program (NTP) | Web: http://ntp-server.niehs.nih.gov/ |
| Center for the Evaluation of Risks to Human Reproduction | Web: http://cerhr.niehs.nih.gov |
| National Cancer Institute (NCI) US DHHS National Institutes of Health (NIH) 9000 Rockville Pike Bethesda, MD 20892 | Web: http://www.nci.nih.gov SEER Web: http://seer.cancer.gov/Publications/ raterisk/riskstoc.html Phone: 800-4-CANCER |
| National Library of Medicine | Web: http://www.nlm.nih.gov |
| TOXNET | Web: http://toxnet.nlm.nih.gov |
| Office of Healthy Homes and Lead Hazard Control US Department of Housing & Urban Development 451 7th St SW Washington, DC 20410 | Web: http://www.hud.gov/offices/lead |
| National Institute for Occupational Safety and Health 200 Independence Ave, SW Washington, DC 20201 | Phone: 800-356-4674 |
| **Nongovernmental** | |
| Alliance to End Childhood Lead Poisoning 227 Massachusetts Ave NE, Suite 200 Washington, DC 20002 | Web: http://www.aeclp.org E-mail: aeclp@aeclp.org Phone: 202-543-1147 Fax: 202-543-4466 |
| Ambulatory Pediatric Association 6728 Old McLean Village Dr McLean, VA 22101 | Web: http://www.ambpeds.org E-mail: info@ambpeds.org Phone: 703-556-9222 Fax: 703-556-8729 |

| Organization | Contact Information |
|---|---|
| **Governmental** | |
| American Association of Poison Control Centers 3201 New Mexico Ave NW, Suite 310 Washington, DC 20016 | Web: http://www.aapcc.org Phone: 202-362-7217 |
| American Cancer Society 1599 Clifton Rd NE Atlanta, GA 30329 | Web: http://www.cancer.org Phone: 404-320-3333 or 800-ACS-2345 Fax: 404-329-7530 |
| American Lung Association 61 Broadway 6th Floor New York, NY 10016 | Web: http://www.lungusa.org Phone: 800-LUNG-USA |
| American Public Health Association 800 I St NW Washington, DC 20001 | Web: www.apha.org Phone: 202-777-2742 |
| **Association of Occupational and Environmental Clinics (AOEC)** | **Web: http://www.aoec.org** |
| Association of State and Territorial Health Officials (ASTHO) | Web: http://www.astho.org/?template= environment.html |
| Asthma and Allergy Foundation of America 1233 20th St NW Suite 402 Washington, DC 20005 | Web: http://www.aafa.org Phone: 202-466-7643 Fax: 202-466-8940 |
| Beyond Pesticides 701 E St SE, #200 Washington DC 20003 | Web: http://www.beyondpesticides.org/main.html E-mail: info@beyondpesticides.org Phone: 202-543-5450 Fax: 202-543-4791 |
| Canadian Association of Physicians for the Environment 208-145 Spruce St Ottawa, ON K1R 6P1 Canada | Web: www.cape.ca/children.html E-mail: info@cape.ca Phone: 613-235-2273 Fax: 613-233-9028 |
| Canadian Institute of Child Health 384 Bank St, Suite 300 Ottawa, ON K2P 1Y4 Canada | Web: http://www.cich.ca E-mail: cich@cich.ca Phone: 613-230-8838 Fax: 613-230-6654 |

| Organization | Contact Information |
|---|---|
| **Nongovernmental** | |
| Center for Health, Environment and Justice (CHEJ) PO Box 6806 Falls Church, VA 22040 | Web: http://www.chej.org E-mail: chej@chej.org Phone: 703-237-2249 |
| Child Proofing Our Communities Campaign | Web: www.childproofing.org E-mail: childproofing@chej.org Phone: 703-237-2249, ext 21 Fax: 703-237-8389 |
| Children's Environmental Health Network 110 Maryland Ave NE, Suite 511 Washington, DC 20002 | Web: http://www.cehn.org E-mail: cehn@cehn.org Phone: 202-543-4033 Fax: 202-543-8797 |
| Children's Health Environmental Coalition PO Box 1540 Princeton, NJ 08542 | Web: http://www.checnet.org |
| Columbia University Mailman School of Public Health Center for Children's Environmental Health | Web: http://www.niehs.nih.gov/centers/ center/col-ctr.htm |
| North American Commission for Environmental Cooperation (CEC) 393, rue St-Jacques Ouest Bureau 200 Montréal, QC H2Y 1N9 Canada | Web: http://www.cec.org/programs_projects/ pollutants_health/342/index.cfm? varlan=english E-mail: info@ccemtl.org Phone: 514-350-4300 Fax: 514-350-4314 |
| EMR Network PO Box 5 Charlotte, VT 05445 | Web: http://www.emrnetwork.org/index.htm E-mail: info@emrnetwork.org Phone: 978-371-3035 |
| Environmental Defense 257 Park Ave S New York, NY 10010 | Web: http://www.environmentaldefense.org Phone: 212-505-2100 Fax: 212-505-2375 |
| Scorecard | Web: http://scorecard.org |
| Environmental Justice Resource Center at Clark Atlanta University 223 James P Brawley Dr SW Atlanta, GA 30314 | Web: http://www.ejrc.cau.edu Phone: 404-880-6911 Fax: 404-880-6909 |

| Organization | Contact Information |
|---|---|
| **Nongovernmental** | |
| Environmental Working Group (EWG) 1436 U St NW Suite 100 Washington, DC 20009 | Web: http://www.ewg.org |
| FoodNews | Web: http://www.foodnews.org |
| EXTOXNET InfoBase | Web: http://ace.ace.orst.edu/info/extoxnet |
| Farm*A*Syst 303 Hiram Smith Hall 1545 Observatory Dr Madison, WI 53706-1289 | Web: http://www.uwex.edu/farmasyst Phone: 608-262-0024 E-mail: farmasys@uwex.edu |
| Generations at Risk Greater Boston Physicians for Social Responsibility 11 Garden St Cambridge, MA 02138 | Web: http://www.igc.org/psr/gar-proj.htm E-mail: psrmabo@igc.org Phone: 617-497-7440 Fax: 617-876-4277 |
| Health Care Without Harm 1755 S St, NW, Suite 6B Washington DC 20009 | Web: http://www.noharm.org E-mail: info@hcwh.org Phone: 202-234-0091 |
| Healthy Schools Network, Inc. 773 Madison Ave Albany, NY 12208 | Web: http://www.healthyschools.org E-mail: info@healthyschools.org Phone: 518-462-0632 Fax: 518-462-0433 |
| Home*A*Syst Program 303 Hiram Smith Hall 1545 Observatory Dr Madison, WI 53706 | Web: http://www.uwex.edu/homeasyst E-mail: homeasys@uwex.edu Phone: 608-262-0024 Fax: 608-265-2775 |
| In Harm's Way Greater Boston Physicians for Social Responsibility 11 Garden St Cambridge, MA 02138 | Web: http://www.igc.org/psr/ihw.htm E-mail: psrmabo@igc.org Phone: 617-497-7440 Fax: 617-876-4277 |
| Institute for Agriculture and Trade Policy 2105 1st Ave S Minneapolis, MN 55404 | Web: http://www.iatp.org Phone: 612-870-0453 Fax: 612-870-4846 |

| Organization | Contact Information |
|---|---|
| **Nongovernmental** | |
| Institute for Children's Environmental Health 1646 Dow Rd Freeland, WA 98249 | Web: www.iceh.org and www.partnersforchildren.org Phone: 360-331-7904 E-mail: emiller@iceh.org Fax: 360-331-7908 |
| International Research and Information Network for Children's Health, Environment and Safety (INCHES) | Web: http://www.inchesnetwork.org/index.html |
| Johns Hopkins University Center for Civilian Biodefense Strategies | Web: http://www.hopkins-biodefense.org/ index.html Phone: 410-223-1667 |
| Learning Disabilities Association of America 4156 Library Rd Pittsburgh, PA 15234-1349 | Web: http://www.ldanatl.org E-mail: info@ldaamerica.org Phone: 412-341-1515; 412-341-8077 Fax: 412-344-0224 |
| March of Dimes Birth Defects Foundation 1275 Mamaroneck Ave White Plains, NY 10605 | Web: http://www.modimes.org Phone: 914-428-7100 Fax: 914-428-8203 |
| Allergy & Asthma Network Mothers of Asthmatics 2751 Prosperity Ave, Suite 150 Fairfax, VA 22031 | Web: http://www.aanma.org Phone: 800-878-4403 Fax: 703-573-7794 |
| National Association of County and City Health Officials (NACCHO) 1100 17th St, 2nd Floor Washington, DC 20036 | Web: http://www.naccho.org Phone: 202-783-5550 Fax: 202-783-1583 |
| National Center for Healthy Housing 10227 Wincopin Circle, Suite 100 Columbia, MD 21044 | Web: http://www.centerforhealthyhousing.org/ index.htm Phone: 410-992-0712 Fax: 410-715-2310 |
| National Environmental Education & Training Foundation 1707 H St NW, Suite 900 Washington, DC 20006-3915 | Web: http://www.neetf.org Phone: 202-833-2933 Fax: 202-261-6464 |

| Organization | Contact Information |
|---|---|
| **Nongovernmental** | |
| National Lead Information Center<br>422 S Clinton Ave<br>Rochester, NY 14620 | Web: http://www.epa.gov/lead/nlic.htm<br>Phone: 800-424-LEAD (5323) |
| National Pesticide Information<br>Center (NPIC) | Web: http://npic.orst.edu |
| National Safety Council,<br>Environmental Health Center<br>1025 Connecticut Ave NW;<br>Suite 1200<br>Washington, DC 20036 | Web: http://www.nsc.org/ehc.htm |
| National Safety Council (NSC),<br>Environmental Health Center,<br>Indoor Air | Web: http://www.nsc.org/ehc/indoor/wctoc.htm |
| Natural Resources Defense Council<br>40 West 20th St<br>New York, NY 10011 | Web: http://www.nrdc.org<br>E-mail: nrdcinfo@nrdc.org<br>Phone: 212-727-2700<br>Fax: 212-727-1773 |
| Pediatric Environmental Health<br>Specialty Units (PEHSUs) | Web: http://www.aoec.org/pesu.htm<br>(includes links to all PEHSUs) |
| Pediatric Environmental Health<br>Center at Children's Hospital/<br>Occupational &Environmental<br>Health Center at Cambridge<br>Hospital | Web: http://www.childrenshospital.org<br>(enter keywords "pediatric environmental"<br>for link)<br>Phone: 888-CHILD 14 (888-244-5314)<br>or 617-355-8177 |
| Pediatric Environmental Health<br>Specialty Unit<br>Mount Sinai School of Medicine | Web: http://www.mssm.edu/cpm/<br>peds_environ.shtml<br>Phone: 866-265-6201 (toll-free) or<br>212-241-0938 |
| Mid-Atlantic Center for Children's<br>Health and the Environment<br>(MACCHE) | Web: http://www.health-e-kids.org<br>Phone: 866-MACCHE1 (866-622-2431) or<br>202-994-1166<br>Fax: 202-994-4861 |
| Pediatric Environmental Health<br>Specialty Unit, Southeast Region | Web: http://www.sph.emory.edu/PEHSU<br>Phone: 877-33PEHSU (877-337-3478)<br>(toll-free) or 770-956-9636 |

| Organization | Contact Information |
|---|---|
| **Nongovernmental** | |
| Great Lakes Center for Children's Environmental Health | Web: http://www.uic.edu/sph/glakes/kids<br>Phone: 800-672-3113 (toll-free) or 312-633-5310 |
| Southwest Center for Pediatric Environmental Health | Web: http://research.uthct.edu/swcpeh<br>E-mail: swcpeh@uthct.edu<br>Phone: 888-901-5665 (toll-free) or 903-531-0830 (local)<br>Fax: 903-877-7982 |
| Midwest Regional Pediatric Environmental Health Center | Web: http://www.uihealthcare.com/depts/ pediatricenvironmentalhealth<br>E-mail: MWRPEHC@uiowa.edu<br>Phone: 866-MWR-PEHC (697-7342) or 319-384-8311 (local)<br>Fax: 319-384-5518 |
| Rocky Mountain Regional Pediatric Environmental Health Specialty Unit | Web: www.rmrpehsu.org<br>Phone: 877-800-5554 (toll-free) |
| Pediatric Environmental Health Specialty Unit University of California San Francisco & University of California Irvine | Web: www.ucsf.edu/ucpehsu<br>Phone: 866-UC-PEHSU (866-827-3478) (same toll-free phone for both sites— San Francisco and Irvine), 415-206-4320 (local San Francisco), or 949-824-8961 (local Irvine) |
| Northwest Pediatric Environmental Health Specialty Unit 325 9th Ave Mail Stop 359739 Seattle, WA 98104-2499 | Web: http://depts.washington.edu/oemp/ grants/PEHSU.html<br>Phone: 877-KID-CHEM (877-543-2436) (restricted to west of the Mississippi River) |
| Pediatric Environmental Health Clinic Misericordia Child Health Centre Edmonton, AB Canada | E-mail occdoc@connect.ab.ca<br>Phone: 780-930-5731 |
| Unidad Pediatrica Ambiental–Mexico Pediatric Environmental Health Specialty Unit (UPA-PEHSU) Cuernavaca, Morelos Mexico | Web: www.upa-pehsu.com<br>Phone: 800-001-7777, 52-777-102-1259 (outside of Mexico) |

| Organization | Contact Information |
|---|---|
| **Nongovernmental** | |
| Organization of Teratology Information Services | Web: http://www.otispregnancy.org/index.html |
| Our Stolen Future | Web: http://www.ourstolenfuture.org/index.htm |
| Pew Environmental Health Commission | Web: http://pewenvironhealth.jhsph.edu |
| Physicians for Social Responsibility 1875 Connecticut Ave NW, Suite 1012 Washington, DC, 20009 | Web: http://www.psr.org E-mail: psrnatl@psr.org Phone: 202-667-4260 Fax: 202-667-4201 |
| School Integrated Pest Management | Web: http://schoolipm.ifas.ufl.edu |
| Teratology Society 1821 Michael Faraday Dr Suite 300 Reston, VA 20190 | Web: http://www.teratology.org E-mail: tshq@teratology.org Phone: 703-438-3104 |
| Tulane/Xavier Center for Bioenvironmental Research 1430 Tulane Ave, SL-3 New Orleans, LA 70112 | Web: http://www.cbr.tulane.edu E-mail: cbr@tulane.edu Phone: 504-585-6910 Fax: 504-585-6428 |
| University of Minnesota Environmental Health & Safety Program W-140 Bayton Health Service 410 Church St SE Minneapolis, MN 55455 | Web: http://www.dehs.umn.edu E-mail: dehs@tc.umn.edu |
| World Health Organization (WHO) Task Force for the Protection of Children's Environmental Health | Web: http://www.who.int/peh/ceh |

# Appendix C
# Curricula for Environmental Education in Schools

Environmental education is defined as "an active process that increases awareness, knowledge, and skills that result in understanding, commitment, informed decisions, and constructive action that ensure stewardship of all interdependent parts of the earth's environment" (North Carolina Environmental Education Plan, April 1995). Environmental education should begin early and continue through high school. Children who receive environmental education may be able to prevent environmental exposures through personal health choices and through community involvement. As adults, these children should be well prepared to participate in the political process as informed and environmentally literate citizens.

A number of excellent environmental education curricula have been developed. Environmental health education curricula also are emerging. The most successful environmental education programs result from combining excellent curricula with the efforts of enthusiastic individuals at the local level.

Health professionals can stimulate environmental health education efforts in the schools through volunteerism in the classroom, school health programs, and technical partnerships with local school boards and state departments of education. Direct classroom volunteerism can take the form of assisting teachers in designing and executing hands-on environmental science and environmental health activities that actively link human health to the state of the physical environment. Within the tradition of school health is the concept of the "healthy school environment." Enthusiastic clinicians can help local schools identify ways in which the school environment can be made healthier. A specific agent or toxicant should be selected for such work.

Examples could be developing a plan for the school to reduce pesticide use or working with students and faculty to ensure that the school is in compliance with state and federal health and safety regulations. They can participate in Parent-Teacher Association activities and teacher training on environmental health issues pertinent to their community, drawing examples from their practices. Finally, they can work at the district or state department of education level to introduce environmental health education systemically. Increasingly, states are creating offices of environmental education within departments of education to stimulate preservice and in-service teacher training as well as inclusion of environmental sciences in K–12 curricula. Health professionals can add valuable insight and expertise to this process by stimulating discussion of the links between the environment and human health.

## Environmental Education Curricula

### *General Environmental Education*

1. Project Learning Tree, 1111 19th St NW, Suite 780, Washington, DC 20036, phone: 202-463-2462, Internet: http://www.plt.org/. Project Learning Tree uses the forest and trees as a "window on the world" to increase students' understanding of our complex environment, stimulate critical and creative thinking, develop the ability to make informed decisions on environmental issues, and instill the confidence and commitment to take responsible action on behalf of the environment (K–12).

2. Project WILD, 5555 Morningside Dr, Suite 212, Houston, TX 77005, phone: 713-520-1936, Internet: http://www.projectwild.org. The *Project WILD K–12 Activity Guide* focuses on wildlife and habitat, while the *Project WILD Aquatic Education Activity Guide* emphasizes aquatic wildlife and aquatic ecosystems. The guides are organized thematically and are designed for integration into existing courses of study.

3. Project WET, 201 Culbertson Hall, Montana State University, Bozeman, MT 59717-0057, phone: 406-994-0211, Internet: http://www.projectwet.org. The goal of Project WET is to promote awareness, appreciation, knowledge, and stewardship of water resources through the development and dissemination of classroom-ready teaching aids and the establishment of state and internationally sponsored programs (K–12).

4. Environmental Education Link: Environmental Education on the Internet: http://eelink.net. Environmental Education Link is a project of the National Consortium for Environmental Education and Training, a major environmental education professional group, with support from the US Environmental Protection Agency.

5. California Department of Education, Office of Environmental Education, 1430 North St, Sacramento, CA 95814, Internet: http://www.cde.ca.gov/cilbranch/oee. This office has reviewed and rated hundreds of environmental education curricula (K–12) and published them in a compendium.

### *Environmental Health Education*

1. National Institute of Environmental Health Sciences (NIEHS), Marian Johnson-Thomason, Director of NIEHS Office of Institutional Development, PO Box 12233, Research Triangle Park, NC 27709, phone: 919-541-1919, Internet: http://www.niehs.nih.gov/od/k-12/best.htm. The NIEHS sponsors demonstration projects around the country for the purpose of developing environmental health curricula for K–12.

2. Environmental and Occupational Health Sciences Institute (EOHSI), Brenda Steinberg, Director of Resource Program, 170 Frelinghuysen Rd, Piscataway, NJ 08854, phone: 732-445-0200, Internet: http://eohsi.rutgers.edu/rc. The institute is jointly sponsored by the University of Medicine and Dentistry of New Jersey; Robert Wood Johnson Medical School; and Rutgers, the State

University of New Jersey. They have developed and widely disseminated environmental health curricula for K–12 throughout New Jersey and other states. The Toxicology, Risk Assessment and Pollution (ToxRAP™) curriculum series includes 3 modules: Early Elementary (K–3), Intermediate Elementary (4–6), and Middle School (6–9). The Early Elementary Module *(The Case of the Green Feathers)* focuses on pollen and other air pollutants that can cause allergic reactions in children. The Intermediate Elementary Module *(What is Wrong with the Johnson Family?)* discusses indoor air pollution, with special attention to carbon monoxide. The Middle School Module *(Mystery Illness Strikes the Sanchez Household)* investigates air contaminants that include dust from lead-based paint. Additional information is available at http://www.eohsi.rutgers.edu/rc/toxrap.html.

3. Baylor College of Medicine Division of School-Based Programs, Nancy Moreno, PhD, *My Health, My World* Project Director, 1709 Dryden, Suite 545, Houston, TX 77030, phone: 800-798-8244, Internet: http://www.bayloreducationaloutreach.org. The *My Health, My World* project has developed teaching units on current environmental issues for students in grades K–4. Each unit weaves physical, earth, and life sciences together to promote understanding of environmental processes and how they affect health and well-being. Three units are available. *My World Indoors* creatively explores air quality in the home, school, and work. *Water and My World* provides a perspective on water and why it is important to health and well-being. *My Home, My Planet* looks at changes in the upper atmosphere, such as global warming, and how the changes may affect human health.

# Appendix D
## Common Abbreviations

| | |
|---|---|
| ADI | acceptable daily intake |
| AChE | acetylcholinesterase |
| ACMI | Art & Craft Materials Institute |
| ACS | American Cancer Society |
| AHERA | Asbestos Hazard Emergency Response Act |
| AQI | Air Quality Index |
| ASTM D4236 | American Society for Testing and Materials Standard (art materials) |
| AT | ataxia-telangiectasia |
| ATSDR | Agency for Toxic Substances and Disease Registry |
| BAL | dimercaprol |
| BLL | blood lead level |
| BRI | building-related illness |
| CAM | complementary and alternative medicine |
| CCA | copper chromium arsenate |
| CDC | Centers for Disease Control and Prevention |
| CERCLA | Comprehensive Environmental Response, Compensation, and Liability Act |
| CFC | chlorofluorocarbon |
| CFU | colony forming unit |
| CPSC | Consumer Product Safety Commission |
| dB | decibel |
| dBA | decibels weighted by the A scale |
| DDE | dichlorodiphenyldichloroethene |
| DDT | dichlorodiphenyltrichloroethane |
| DEET | N-N diethyl-m-toluamide also known as N,N-diethyl-3-methyl-benzamide |
| DHEA | dehydroepiandrosterone |

| | |
|---|---|
| DMSA | dimercaptosuccinic acid (succimer) |
| DSHEA | Dietary Supplement Health and Education Act |
| EMF | electromagnetic fields |
| EPA | Environmental Protection Agency |
| ETS | environmental tobacco smoke |
| eV | electron volts |
| FLSA | Fair Labor Standards Act |
| FDA | Food and Drug Administration |
| FQPA | Food Quality Protection Act |
| FSIS | Food Safety and Inspection System |
| GIS | geographic information systems |
| Gy | gray |
| HEPA | high-efficiency particulate air |
| HBO | hyberbaric oxygen |
| HHS | Department of Health and Human Services |
| HUD | Department of Housing and Urban Development |
| HVAC | heating, ventilation, and air conditioning |
| HVOD | hepatic veno-occlusive disease |
| Hz | hertz |
| IAQ | indoor air quality |
| IPM | integrated pest management |
| kGy | kilogray |
| KI | potassium iodide |
| kV | kilovolt |
| LOAEL | lowest observable adverse effect level |
| LOEL | lowest observable effect level |
| MCL | maximum contaminant level |
| MCS | multiple chemical sensitivities |
| MHz | megahertz |
| MMT | methylcyclopentadienyl manganese tricarbonyl |
| mrem | millirem |
| MSDS | Material Safety Data Sheet |

| MTBE | methyl tertiary butyl ether |
|------|------|
| NAAQS | National Ambient Air Quality Standards |
| NAS | National Academy of Sciences |
| NCI | National Cancer Institute |
| NHANES | National Health and Nutrition Examination Survey |
| NIEHS | National Institute for Environmental Health Sciences |
| NIHL | noise-induced hearing loss |
| NIOSH | National Institute for Occupational Safety and Health |
| NITS | noise-induced threshold shift |
| NMSC | nonmelanoma skin cancer |
| NOAEL | no observable adverse effect level |
| NOEL | no observable effect level |
| NPL | National Priorities List |
| NRC | National Research Council |
| OP | organophosphate |
| OSHA | Occupational Safety and Health Administration |
| Pa | pascal |
| PAH | polycyclic aromatic hydrocarbon |
| PBB | polybrominated biphenyl |
| PCB | polychlorinated biphenyl |
| PCDD | polychlorinated dibenzodioxin |
| PCDF | polychlorinated dibenzofuran |
| pCi | picocurie |
| PCP | pentachlorophenol |
| PDCB | p-dichlorobenzene |
| PEHSU | Pediatric Environmental Health Specialty Unit |
| $PM_{10}$ | particles smaller than 10 μm |
| $PM_{2.5}$ | particles smaller than 2.5 μm |
| ppb | parts per billion |
| ppm | parts per million |
| ppt | parts per trillion |

| | |
|---|---|
| PSI | Pollutant Standards Index |
| R | roentgen |
| Rad | radiation absorbed dose |
| RBE | relative biological effectiveness |
| RCRA | Resource Conservation and Recovery Act |
| rem | roentgen equivalent man |
| RfD | reference dose |
| SARA | Superfund Amendments and Reauthorization Act |
| SBS | sick building syndrome |
| SPF | sun protection factor |
| Sv | sievert |
| T-2 | trichothecene mycotoxin |
| TCDD | 2,3,7,8 tetrachlorodibenzo-p-dioxin |
| THM | trihalomethane |
| TEQ | toxic equivalent |
| TSCA | Toxic Substances Control Act |
| TSDF | waste treatment, storage, and disposal facilities |
| UL | Underwriters Laboratories |
| UPF | UV protection factor |
| USDA | US Department of Agriculture |
| UV-A | ultraviolet A |
| UV-B | ultraviolet B |
| UVR | ultraviolet radiation |
| VEE | Venezuelan equine encephalitis |
| VOC | volatile organic compound |
| WHO | World Health Organization |
| XP | xeroderma pigmentosum |

# Appendix E
# Chairs of the AAP Committee
# on Environmental Health

**Committee on Radiation Hazards and Epidemiology of Malformations**

Robert A. Aldrich, MD, 1957–1961

In 1961 the committee was split in 2: a short-lived Committee on Malformations and the Committee on Environmental Hazards

**Committee on Environmental Hazards**

Lee E. Farr, MD, 1961–1967

Paul F. Wehrle, MD, 1967–1973

Robert W. Miller, MD, DrPH, 1973–1979

Laurence Finberg, MD, 1979–1980

In 1979 the AAP established the Committee on Genetics with Charles Scriver, MD, as chair. In 1980 the AAP combined this committee with the Committee on Environmental Hazards to form the:

**Committee on Genetics & Environmental Hazards**

Laurence Finberg, MD, Cochair, 1980–1983

Charles Scriver, MD, Cochair, 1980–1983

In 1983 the 2 committees were separated again.

**Committee on Environmental Hazards**

Philip J. Landrigan, MD, MSc, 1983–1987

Richard J. Jackson, MD, MPH, 1987–1991

In 1991 the committee was renamed the Committee on Environmental Health.

**Committee on Environmental Health**
J. Routt Reigart, MD, 1991–1995
Ruth A. Etzel, MD, PhD, 1995–1999
Sophie J. Balk, MD, 1999–2003
Michael W. Shannon, MD, MPH, 2003–

# Appendix F
# AAP Patient Education Materials Related to Environmental Health Issues

Following is a list of patient education materials from the American Academy of Pediatrics (AAP) relating to environmental health issues. To obtain pricing information or to order the materials, contact the AAP bookstore at 888/227-1770 or visit the bookstore online at http://www.aap.org/bookstore.

HE0106  Allergies in Children
HE0236  Anemia and Your Young Child
HE0193  Ear Infections and Children
HE0168  Environmental Tobacco Smoke: A Danger to Children
HE0181  Fun in the Sun: Keep Your Baby Safe
HE0177  How to Help Your Child With Asthma
HE0251  Lead Poisoning: Prevention and Screening
HE0180  Middle Ear Fluid in Young Children
HE0065  The Risks of Tobacco Use: A Message to Parents and Teens
HE0189  Smokeless Tobacco
HE0088  Smoking: Straight Talk for Teens
HE0218  Your Child and the Environment

# Index

## F

# X

X-rays, 215, 229–230
m-Xylene, *56*
o-Xylene, *56*
p-Xylene, *56*
Xylenes (total), *406*

# Y

Youth employment, 41–42, 493–497
    hours and hazards in, regulation of,
        495–497

# Z

Zearalenone, 171
Zinc supplementation, 208